Burnside's
Working with Older Adults

Group Process and Techniques

FOURTH EDITION

Edited by,

Barbara Haight, PhD, RN, FAAN
Professor Emeritus
College of Nursing
Medical University of South Carolina
Charleston, South Carolina

Faith Gibson
Emeritus Professor of Social Work
University of Ulster
Northern Ireland

JONES AND BARTLETT PUBLISHERS
Sudbury, Massachusetts
BOSTON   TORONTO   LONDON   SINGAPORE

World Headquarters
Jones and Bartlett Publishers
40 Tall Pine Drive
Sudbury, MA 01776
978-443-5000
info@jbpub.com
www.jbpub.com

Jones and Bartlett Publishers Canada
2406 Nikanna Road
Mississauga, ON L5C 2W6
CANADA

Jones and Bartlett Publishers International
Barb House, Barb Mews
London W6 7PA
UK

Jones and Bartlett's books and products are available through most bookstores and online booksellers. To contact Jones and Bartlett Publishers directly, call 800-832-0034, fax 978-443-8000, or visit our website www.jbpub.com.

Substantial discounts on bulk quantities of Jones and Bartlett's publications are available to corporations, professional associations, and other qualified organizations. For details and specific discount information, contact the special sales department at Jones and Bartlett via the above contact information or send an email to specialsales@jbpub.com.

Library of Congress Cataloging-in-Publication Data
Burnside's working with older adults : group process and techniques
  / [edited by] Barbara Haight and Faith Gibson. -- 4th ed.
     p. ; cm.
  Rev. ed. of: Working with older adults. 3rd ed. c1994.
  Includes bibliographical references and index.
  ISBN 0-7637-4770-X (pbk.)
   1. Social work with older people. 2. Social group work. 3. Group
psychoanalysis.   I. Haight, Barbara K. II. Gibson, Faith.
  III. Working with older adults. IV. Title: Working with older
adults.
   [DNLM: 1. Aged. 2. Group Processes. 3. Psychotherapy, Group.
  4. Social Work.   WT 30 B967 2005]
  HV1451.B88 2005
  362.6--dc22

    2004020288

Production Credits
Acquisitions Editor: Kevin Sullivan
Production Director: Amy Rose
Associate Production Editor: Tracey Chapman
Associate Editor: Amy Sibley
Associate Marketing Manager: Emily Ekle
Manufacturing and Inventory Coordinator: Amy Bacus
Composition: AnnMarie Lemoine
Cover Design: Timothy Dziewit
Photo Research: Kimberly Potvin
Cover Image: © Keith Brofsky/Photodisc/Getty Images
Printing and Binding: Malloy, Inc.
Cover Printing: Malloy, Inc.

Printed in the United States of America
09 08 07 06 05   10 9 8 7 6 5 4 3 2 1

To our families,

My children, Heidi, Tim, Dan, Kelly, and Mike; and their partners, Robin, Trixie, Matt, and Joelle; and my spouse, Barrett; and our grandchildren, Sam, Meaghan, Brian, Carey, Mackenzie, Alex, Abby, and Ben, for being such a loving, supportive, and challenging group.

—BH

For Norman, Michael, Kathryn, Patrick, and Janice with love.

—FG

Contributors

Elaine J. Amella, PhD, APRN, BC, GNP
Associate Professor
Associate Dean for Research
College of Nursing
Medical University of South Carolina
Charleston, SC

E. Frederick Anderson, PhD, LCSW
Professor and Founding Director
School of Social Work and Master of Social
Work Program
California State University, Los Angeles
Los Angeles, CA

James Birren, PhD
Professor Emeritus and Associate Director
Andrus Gerontology Center
University of California, Los Angeles
Pacific Palisades, CA

John A. Blando, PhD
Assistant Professor, Coordinator
Gerontological Counseling,
Department of Counseling
San Francisco State University
San Francisco, CA

Jan Black, MSW, LCSW
Professor Emeritus
Department of Social Work
California State University, Long Beach
Long Beach, CA

Barry Bortnick, PhD
Program Director, Humanities and
Behavioral Sciences
Artistic Director, Senior Musicals
University of California (UCLA) Extension
Los Angeles, CA

Sandra S. Brotherton, PT, PhD
Assistant Professor
Department of Rehabilitation Sciences
College of Health Professions
Medical University of South Carolina
Charleston, SC

Jerry K. Burik, MHS, OTR/L
Assistant Professor, College of Health Professions
Medical University of South Carolina
Charleston, SC

Roger Delgado, MSW, LCSW, PhD
Professor and former Bachelor's Program Director
School of Social Work
California State University
Los Angeles, CA

Donna E. Deutchman
President/CEO
ONEgeneration
Van Nuys, CA

Brian de Vries, PhD, FGSA
Professor and Director
Gerontology Programs
San Francisco State University
San Francisco, CA

Barbara J. Edlund RN, PhD, ANP-BC
Gerontological Coordinator and Associate Professor
College of Nursing
Medical University of South Carolina
Charleston, SC

Nancy J. Finch RN, PhD
Assistant Professor, College of Nursing
Medical University of South Carolina
Charleston, SC

Sally Friedlob, LCSW, OTR/L
Private practice
Los Angeles, CA

Faith Gibson, MA, BEd, Dip. Soc.St, Dip. Ed.
Emeritus Professor of Social Work
University of Ulster
Northern Ireland

Barbara K. Haight, RNC, DRPH, FAAN
Professor Emeritus
College of Nursing
Medical University of South Carolina
Charleston, South Carolina

Robin Stull Haight, PsyD
Clinical Psychologist
Private practice
Vienna, VA

James J. Kelly, MSSW, PhD
Associate Vice President
Continuing and International Education
Hayworth, CA

John Kunz, MSW
Director, Continuing Education
University of Wisconsin, Superior
Superior, WI

Maralynne D. Mitcham, PhD, OTR/L, FAOTA
Director, Occupational Therapy and Professor
College of Health Professions
Medical University of South Carolina
Charleston, South Carolina

Jane B. Neese, PhD, APRN, BC
Associate Dean for Academic Affairs and Associate
Professor, College of Health and Human Services
University of North Carolina at Charlotte
Charlotte, NC

Thomas W. Pierce, PhD
Professor of Psychology
Radford University
Radford, VA

Molly J. Ranney, PhD, LCSW
Assistant Professor, Department of Social Work
California State University, Long Beach
Long Beach, CA

Susan Rice, DSW
Professor
Department of Social Work
California State University, Long Beach
Long Beach, CA

Patricia Shafer, MA, MBA
Consultant and President
Compel, Ltd.
Organizational Excellence Alliance
Charlotte, NC

Marv Westwood, PhD
Professor and Associate Member Faculty of Medicine
Counseling and Psychology Program
University of British Columbia
Vancouver, Canada

Alison Wicks, PhD, MHSc OT,
BAppSc OT, AccOT
Consultant
Occupational Perspectives
Nowra, NSW, Australia

Elizabeth M. Williams, RN, MSN, C
Case Manager/Fall Program Coordinator
Eastern Colorado Health Care System
Denver Veterans Administration Hospital
Denver, CO

Carole A. Winston, PhD, ACSW, LCSW
Assistant Professor, Department of Social Work
College of Health and Human Services
University of North Carolina at Charlotte
Charlotte, NC

Holly Wise, PT, PhD
Assistant Professor
College of Health Professions
Medical University of South Carolina
Charleston, SC

Contents

Part Five   A Multidisciplinary Perspective 353

About the Authors

Dr. Barbara Haight is a Professor Emeritus at the College of Nursing, Medical University of South Carolina. Recently retired, Dr. Haight served the University for over 20 years in various roles including Associate Dean of Research and Practice, Department Chairperson, and Senior Scholar. She was the first nurse faculty member to be awarded the Distinguished Service Award by the Medical University.

Dr. Haight received funding to start three separate graduate programs in gerontological nursing and eight research projects on the structured role of life review. She opened a primary care clinic in a subsidized housing high-rise where nurses and social workers were reimbursed for conducting life reviews. She was the first president of the Life Review and Reminiscing Society, now the International Institute of Reminiscence and Life Review, and has conducted life review projects in the United States, England, Japan, and most recently Northern Ireland, where she worked with coauthor Faith Gibson.

Dr. Haight is coeditor of two books on reminiscing and life review and is widely published in the field of life review and gerontology. She is a fellow in the Gerontological Society of America, and the American Academy of Nursing. She is married to Col. Barrett Haight, an attorney, retired from the US Army and from the Citadel. They have five children and eight grandchildren.

Faith Gibson OBE, is an Emeritus Professor of Social Work in the University of Ulster, Northern Ireland. She is a graduate of the Universities of Sydney, Queensland, and the University of Chicago and holds degrees in psychology, social work, and education.

Although her earlier social work career was in childcare and psychiatric social work, she has been involved in social work practice, policy development, research, and teaching concerned with aging and dementia for more than thirty years. She has published widely on social work education, social gerontology, dementia care, and reminiscence theory and practice. She has authored or coauthored six books concerned with reminiscence work with individuals and small groups.

She is a member of the British Association of Social Workers, the British Society of Gerontology, and the Northern Ireland, UK, and European Reminiscence Networks. She is married to Norman Gibson, an Emeritus Professor of Economics, and they have three children and four grandchildren.

Acknowledgments

First, we must acknowledge two scholars, now deceased, Irene Burnside and Mary Gwynne Schmidt, who envisioned the idea for this book and produced its third edition. We also acknowledge those authors from the previous edition whom we could not locate and whose contributions we used in this fourth edition.

We gratefully acknowledge the current contributors who worked with us in a timely and professional manner to produce an interesting and updated manuscript.

We thank Barrett Haight who generously gave his time to review and critique multiple chapters, making this text decidedly more understandable, and we thank Norman Gibson for all his assistance and encouragement.

Our gratitude to Peggy Mauldin, librarian at the Medical University of South Carolina, who was always available to search for references and citations.

Thanks to Kevin Sullivan, Amy Sibley, Mark Goodin, and others from Jones and Bartlett for providing immediate guidance and assistance when asked.

Preface

Dr. Irene Burnside first published this book in 1978 when she was already well known to nursing and gerontology students as the author of one of the earliest texts on gerontological nursing. When Irene was 60 years old, after many years of teaching about aging, she earned her doctoral degree. A role model for what she taught, she continued to influence the world's attitudes toward aging and older people until the end of her life. She had a poignant way with words that caused us to grasp, remember, and apply what she so eloquently taught. When she talked of an old lady who hadn't been hugged or touched with love in over twenty years, we could feel the loneliness. When today we hear of new developments and innovations, we find that so many were tried long ago and reported by Irene Burnside. She was first to try Snoezelen, known then as multisensory stimulation, and she advocated many of the new techniques used by Edenizing. Irene was a pioneer, a woman before her time, a woman who will long be remembered in history by nurses and others studying gerontology.

—Barbara K. Haight, friend and colleague.

Dr. Mary Gwynne Schmidt was an indefatigable scholar who taught in the Aging Concentration of the School of Social Work at California State University, San Diego. Her commitment to the development of new knowledge in aging and in gerontology was focused, as was her commitment to probity and accuracy in the depiction of older people. She was a warm, caring individual who encouraged others and was always excited about her research and her teaching. She was an inspiration and a welcome addition to the faculty.

—E. Frederick Anderson, friend and colleague

Two giants have gone before us. We hope we represent their expertise and understanding of older people in this fourth edition of *Working with Older Adults*.

Irene Burnside was notable in gerontological nursing and group work for a significant number of years. Having produced two earlier editions of this book, Irene found she needed a social worker as a coeditor to include the social worker viewpoint. Irene was fortunate to find Mary Gwynne Schmidt; together they produced a memorable third edition.

Since the third edition, they've both departed this world, thus we have created this fourth edition in their memory. We hope to carry on their rich generative tradition and continue to influence students and care workers in their work with older people. It is our intent to enlarge on their wisdom while retaining their humor, and update their knowledge to apply to the issues of the 21st century. Thus, we have added several new chapters by new authors and revised existing ones.

Following the same format as Burnside and Schmidt, we as present editors who are also a nurse and a social worker, provide a background for group work with older people in Part 1 which provides an overview of the changing world of aging. In this section we review the history and theory of group work and examine present day demographics.

Part 2 provides the practical principles of group work. The information will supply the service worker with guidelines and cautions for running groups. With this knowledge base, new group leaders will have more confidence and direction when designing and running a group.

Armed with the basics, we approach Part 3 with excitement as we review the possibilities for innovative group work. Capable practitioners have written about their own group experiences and provided the reader with ideas and direction. Students of group work can formulate their own ideas for therapeutic groups after enjoying these examples, or they may wish to replicate a group as it is represented in a chapter in this section. Part 3 presents many possibilities for the beginner or for experienced practitioners looking for fresh ideas.

Many group workers get most of their experience and ideas from their own workplaces. Students spend most of their time in a university and have only a vague idea of the assorted venues and opportunities available for group work in various types of residential facilities and community settings. The possibilities for multidisciplinary team work in board and care homes, for example, are endless. The acute care setting requires the involvement of other types of groups, but all with a psychoeducational purpose nonetheless. Many long established staff members in health and social care facilities find that the immediate demands of their job often leave little time or energy for thinking about new ways of reaching out to older people. We hope that this book will encourage them, and students too who may so far have had little experience of group work to try out some of the approaches suggested in this book. Many examples of groups used as a means of responding to diverse needs are included.

In Part 5, we look at multidisciplinary perspectives. Of course, the nurse and the social worker are represented, but we have added the perspectives of the occupational therapist and the physical therapist. In other sections we have included the work of a psychotherapist, a psychologist, and an artist. Each of these professionals has written chapters that contribute to the overall multidisciplinary perspective. To see a multidisciplinary team operate, read Chapter 23 on board and care homes.

Finally in Part 6 we examine issues in group work: from the ethics involved in group work, to the need for evaluation of our group work. Chapter 33 on research issues is also an informative chapter on designing a research project. Chapter 33 fits well with Chapter 34, the final evaluation chapter. As the world becomes more multicultural, it is imperative that we address multicultural differences that become more profound as people age or develop dementia. The ethics of group work must always be at the forefront of our thinking and inform all our practice because we are dealing with frail elderly people, a group at risk.

To The Student

After acquiring the basics of group work, this book will act as a reference for various types of groups. As a student, you can also pick chapters that interest you and are applicable to your specific studies. This book is not necessarily meant to be read from cover to cover but primarily to serve as a ready reference when needed, or as a guidebook when preparing to organize a group. Some teachers, however, may require the book to be read cover to cover as a comprehensive guide to group work practice.

To The Instructor

We recommend that you select the chapters most germane to your discipline and to your educational objectives if there is limited time for teaching the content. However, the book is easy reading, and some instructors like to assign the entire book for a quarter or semester class.

To facilitate teaching, each chapter includes a list of key words, learning objectives, and student exercises. Some teaching resources relevant to a specific chapter have been included at the end of chapters but resources of general interest, particularly national organizations, have been consolidated in a new comprehensive resources section in order to avoid repetition.

To The Clinician

There is nothing as rewarding as gathering together six strangers in a nursing home and six months later finding a strong and cohesive group of friends, or watching a group of women with breast cancer build confidence as they learn to cope with their illness, or seeing a group of regressed people with dementia eagerly respond to group activities. We hope that this book will excite, encourage, and assist clinicians so that they experience the joys and satisfactions inherent in working with groups of older people.

Part One

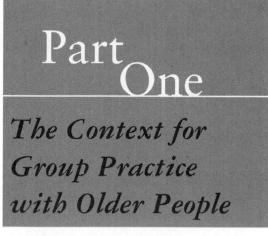

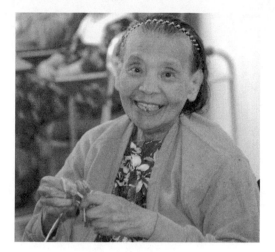

The Context for Group Practice with Older People

Part 1 is the foundation upon which the rest of the book is built. Part 1 provides background and context to better understand the state of the older person today. Part 1 is also devoted to explaining the theoretical underpinnings of group work. In Chapter 1, there is an introduction to and overview of group work practice. Chapter 2, written by Barbara Haight, a gerontologist of long standing, describes the demographics of the 21st century and discusses issues and problems for this aging population—from the baby boomers to the centenarians. In Chapter 3, Haight goes on to give a history of group work from a psychotherapeutic viewpoint, leading to the present day state of the art and science of group work. Chapters 4 and 5, written by Molly Ranney, a social worker and professor who teaches group work to students, clarify the linchpins of all group work in a discussion of the principles of Linden and Yalom so readying us for the guidelines and directions given in Part 2.

Introduction

Faith Gibson
Barbara Haight

Key Words

- Group work
- Multidisciplinary teams
- Innovations
- Multisite interventions

Learning Objectives

- Review the state of aging today
- Analyze the basics of group work
- Explore the existence of therapeutic groups
- Describe the multidisciplinary approach to group work
- Evaluate the settings used for group work
- Synthesize present day issues in group work

For age is opportunity no less than youth itself, though in another dress.

—*H. W. Longfellow*

Aging Today

In the ten years since the last edition of this book, there have been many changes concerning the lives and livelihoods of older people. The changing demography, long anticipated by gerontologists, is now becoming a reality of everyday life,

affecting individuals, families, policy makers, and politicians (Estes, 2001). The practice environment in which health and social care professionals are required to deliver services is becoming increasingly home and community based, whereas previously it was largely located in institutions. The inexorable rise in the costs of health provision, a tide of rising expectations, and the rapid march of technological advances have contributed to the pressure to find better and more cost-effective ways of supporting people in their own homes. Innovative developments in service provision increasingly seek to postpone for as long as possible—or for many aging people, avoid altogether—admission to health and social care facilities that cater to various levels of frailty, dependency, and income. Recognizing the multicultural nature of society and responding to the multiplicity of health and social care needs of diverse groups within an aging population demand imaginative, courageous responses from all members of the human service professions.

Basics of Group Work

Many different interlocking factors influence the provision of group work services for older people. These factors include cultural characteristics of potential participants, assessment of the health and social needs of individuals and groups, the objectives and ideologies of health and social service agencies, the theoretical orientation and professional socialization of workers, the financial resources available for programs, broader national, regional, and local public policy issues, and the ethics and values of the staff involved. The overarching intention of all group work undertaken by human service professionals should be to foster resiliency, to identify and build on people's strengths and remaining abilities, to foster mutual aid, to stress the local public empowerment of participants, and to promote well-being, stability, or change (Gitterman & Shulman, 1994; Kelly, Berman-Rossi, & Palombo, 2001).

Therapeutic Groups

Groups provide a positive context for changing beliefs and influencing behavior. The aims may be either to produce stability or to effect changes that are openly agreed as desirable by the people who participate. There are several good reasons for involving older people in group work. In a group, people who face similar difficulties, problems, or challenges can be brought together to pool their experience and support one another. In so doing they experience companionship; they have opportunities to give as well as to receive, to contribute and to benefit as equals—not always a common experience in later life, as common misperceptions abound and older people are frequently expected to assume the passive roles of recipient and beneficiary.

Multidisciplinary Approach

Some of the objectives and outcomes sought by group workers vary according to their different professional backgrounds, while other objectives are common to all professions. Although some objectives may differ, the background knowledge needed to facilitate successful groups is similar and the need to understand structural, develop-

mental, and process aspects of leading groups is identical. Most groups led by nurses emphasize treatment or therapeutic goals, although increasingly many nurses are leading psychoeducational and support groups. Many groups led by social workers seek similar therapeutic goals, but others aim to promote social and economic justice for the most vulnerable members of society. This is not a clear cut dichotomy because groups led by public health nurses may also seek change in communities or neighborhoods and seek to influence the physical and social environments in which people live as well as being interested in interpersonal relationships.

The therapy of group work is supported by the multiple disciplines using group work as a tool. Not only do nurses and social workers run groups but, as expected, psychologists and psychotherapists run them as well. And less expected are the groups described in this book that are run by occupational therapists, movement therapists, physical therapists, music specialists, professors, and business consultants. Group work is international and ubiquitous.

A veteran social worker, Rose Dobrof, wrote eloquently of the need for her profession to expand its vision and equip its members to meet the demanding challenges that lie ahead. Her words could readily be matched with a similar appeal for nurses, physical therapists, and occupational and recreation therapists to do likewise. Dobrof (2002) drew attention to one condition only, but the challenge is more general than this. She noted that there are now 4 million Americans with Alzheimer's disease but by 2010 there will be 5.8 million. By 2050, when the youngest of the baby boom generation will be in their mid eighties, 14.3 million of them are likely to have dementia. Given these forecasts, it is not surprising that she wrote:

The need for professionally qualified, trained social workers, knowledgeable about older people and their families, skilled in meeting the needs of these people, and committed to careers

{ in aging, is a need which will become even more urgent in the coming decades of the 21st century (p. 18). }

Irene Burnside (1984) almost twenty years earlier wrote about the power of group involvement for people who have dementia: they feel they belong and can communicate again, even if considerable effort is required to read and respond to their nonverbal language and unravel their perplexing speech.

Settings

Managed care and the emergence of geriatric case managers are changing institutional-based care and the delivery of community and home-based services for older people. These developments are linked with increasing recognition of the needs of family caregivers, who are most frequently aged spouses. Their need for information, support, respite, and domestic assistance is being increasingly recognized. A growing willingness to hear the voices of older people—including those with dementia—and to build on their existing strengths is also emerging. These changes have led to the increasing provision of day care services, assisted living facilities, dementia-specific day and residential services, and an upsurge in interdisciplinary and multiprofessional domicillary responses.

Synthesis

This book seeks to provide theoretical understanding about the nature of groups and processes of interaction between members of groups and between members and leaders throughout the stages of any group's development. In this sense the book takes a generic approach, although it recognizes many different types of groups and many variations within these broad categories, which include:

- Psychotherapeutic groups—Focus on changing relationships, feelings, perceptions, and behavior—managing life stresses and new or unresolved problems.
- Mutual aid groups—Focus on common experience, needs, and interests.
- Problem solving groups—Seek solutions to inter- and intrapersonal or practical problems.
- Brief solution focused groups—Focus on finding solutions within one to six sessions.
- Task-centered groups—Focus on achieving defined tasks external to the group, such as fund raising or social action.
- Action-oriented groups—Focus on social action, campaigning, and empowerment.
- Psychoeducational groups—Focus on information, attitude change, emotional support, and practical problem solving.
- Activity groups—Focus on creativity through artistic modalities for facilitating expressiveness, resolution, occupation, recreation, and diversion.
- Work groups—Focus on staff groups or teams, and committees.

Within each of the above categories there are many variations and different approaches. This is particularly pronounced within psychotherapy, where psychoanalytic, humanistic, cognitive/behavioral, brief solution, and creative artistic approaches, among others, all flourish. These categories do not always refer to pure types because intentions and approaches may overlap or mix and merge as an inevitable consequence of the dynamism which groups release. A support group for spouse caregivers of people with dementia, for example, may embrace elements of therapeutic support, mutual aid, problem solving, and social action.

Summary

Participation in groups is relevant to all age groups, including older people. Throughout this book contributors have sought to identify modifications which may be required to accommodate age-related differences and special needs. Because the book seeks to contribute to the development of knowledge, understanding, and practice skills of the various helping professions, it rightly includes many examples of practice with physically and cognitively frail older people. The book assumes that effective group leaders must exercise both creative and technical skills, and that successful group work reflects a dynamic mix of art and science. Students, experienced practitioners, the student's teachers, supervisors, and mentors are encouraged to plan carefully, reach out to others empathetically, and work creatively so that older people enjoy and benefit from meeting together in groups. Shura Saul, a pioneer educational coordinator working in a nursing home in the 1980s, emphasized the potential contribution groups can make to the lives of older people. Her convictions are equally relevant today:

> Creative approaches leap beyond the double stigma of aging and frailty. They are geared to meet the dependencies, to support the frailties; and, thereby, to free each person to function at the highest point of individual capability . . . Groups, in all their diversity, are viewed as creative approaches through which frail elderly persons may be reached for a variety of purposes; whose common denominators are affirmation of human identity, identification with others within a constructive social atmosphere, and enhancement of the life experience (Saul, 1983, p. 5).

All students who expect to work in professions concerned with human relationships, in caring, health, and helping services need to learn to view aging and old age within an interdisciplinary framework. They need to appreciate that "aging is not an illness but a phase of life; and that each of us expects someday to grow old." (Saul, 1974, p. 7). It is within this developmental lifelong framework that teaching and learning concerned with single-profession and multiprofession group work practice with older people should be located.

References

Burnside, I. (1994). Group work with the cognitively impaired. In I. Burnside & M. Schmidt (Eds.), *Working with older adults: Group processes and techniques.* Boston: Jones and Bartlett Publishers.

Dobrof, R. (Ed.). (2002). Editorial. *Advancing gerontological social work education.* Binghamton, NY: Haworth Press.

Estes, C. L. (Ed.). (2001). *Social policy and aging.* Thousand Oaks, CA: Sage.

Gitterman, A., & Shulman, L. (2004). *Mutual aid groups, vulnerable populations and the life cycle.* New York: Columbia University Press.

Kelly, T. B., Berman-Rossi, T., & Palombo, S. (Eds.). (2001). *Group work: Strategies for strengthening resiliency.* Binghamton, NY: Haworth Press.

Saul, S. (1974). *Aging: An album of people growing old.* New York: John Wiley & Sons.

Saul, S. (1983). Group work with the elderly. *Social Work with Groups, 5*(2). New York: Haworth.

Chapter 2

Demographic and Psychosocial Aspects of Aging

Barbara Haight

Mary Gwynne Schmidt

Irene Burnside

Key Words

- Age cohort
- Baby boomers
- Centenarians
- Continuity theory
- Dementia, Alzheimer's type
- Developmental tasks
- Disengagement theory
- Young-old
- Old
- Oldest-old
- Successful ager

Learning Objectives

- Apply a theory of aging to group goals and objectives
- Tell three ways the oldest-old as a group differ from people in their sixties and seventies
- Describe three characteristics of today's nursing home residents that may influence group choice
- List 10 normal age changes a group leader needs to consider in planning a group

This chapter provides a background for group work with older people by introducing who they are and describing how their aging changes them. You will also learn how both the demographic and the psychosocial differences affect the process of conducting groups. The chapter describes selected theories of aging and the wide distribution of cohorts of people within the older ages. Additionally, this chapter highlights normal aging changes and other aging issues that may affect a group process. This information will help you better understand the group of elderly people with whom you work. The chapter examines the impact that aging has on such group work. To not impede readers already familiar with the terms of gerontology, some terms, such as median age and ageism, are defined in the glossary in Appendix A of this chapter.

Theories of Aging

When studying gerontology, one must remember that the original gerontologists came from three separate disciplines—sociology, biology, and psychology. The field of gerontology is growing, due in no small part to the significant number of theories about aging being formulated in all three domains that continually contribute to the study of gerontology. Gerontology has presently broadened to include nurses, social workers, doctors, counselors, and other disciplines. Thus, the theories reflect these particular disciplines and address problems related to those disciplines. Because both past and present theories try to serve specific disciplines and practices, they are not full theories but rather models that guide study. For a theory to be comprehensive for gerontology, a theory must be holistic, multidisciplinary, and consider the life span from birth to the present. (Haight, Barba, Tesh, & Courts, 2002.) A theory is the construction of explicit explanations to account for empirical findings. Few gerontological theories meet these requirements. A selected few are offered here in a historical account as helpful background knowledge for the student of gerontology; however, they do not meet the test of an encompassing theory.

Disengagement Theory

One of the first, best-known, and most controversial theories in gerontology is the disengagement theory, which states that society and the older person withdraw from one another simultaneously and satisfactorily as the older person ages. This theory emerged in 1960 in a study commonly referred to as the Kansas City Study of Adult Life. For a more complete bibliography on disengagement theory, the reader should consult Hochschild (1975). The four premises of the theory are:

- Disengagement is a gradual process.
- Disengagement is inevitable.
- Disengagement is a mutually satisfying process for both the society and the individual.
- Disengagement is the norm.

The research into this theory has stimulated a great deal of discussion, including differing positions by theorists who do not see disengagement as an intrinsic or inevitable part of the aging process.

Activity Theory

Some theorists who do not agree with the disengagement theory use the activity theory to describe normal aging. This theory advances the idea that the individual needs to develop a high level of physical, mental, and social activities. Thus, if younger roles in society are given up by older adults, for example, working, then new roles must be found to take their place. The major criticism of this activity theory is that activities may not ensure high morale. Not all older people want high activity; they are happy to reduce their activity and enjoy a more relaxed schedule. There have been relatively few empirical attempts to test activity theory (Marshall, 1999).

Continuity Theory

Dissatisfaction with the first two theories led to continuity theory. This theory proposes that people became more of themselves as they age. Consequently, activities in late life should fit with lifelong personalities for people to age successfully. Therefore, a bank president wishing to remain active and content in later life might volunteer as the leader for a community project. Supposedly, raising money for this project and accomplishing a goal would lead to his particular happiness. Whereas a man who labored physically all his life because he had to, might find great joy in doing nothing but rocking in his chair and enjoying the present (Neugarten, 1968).

Developmental Theories

Also popular in the past and often used today are developmental theories of aging. The best-known developmental theorist is Erikson. He was one of the first to believe people changed and continued to grow after childhood. Erikson (1950) believed that an individual must successfully complete each stage of life and each task related to it before passing to the next stage. Erickson's eighth and last stage, which he calls "ego integrity versus despair," states that those people who can accept their lives as they were lived with no substitutions reach a state of wisdom and happiness and achieve ego integrity. Conversely he states that if in fact they cannot accept the past, they fall into despair, a combination of hopelessness and depression. This eighth and last stage is the least developed in his writings and covers the span of life ranging from age 50 to death. Some authors who criticize the Eriksonian model assert that it is "idealistic and not culturally nor gender sensitive" (Gatz & Zarit, 1999). In fairness to Erikson, however, one must admit that beginning students take to this model, and it seems to give them an understanding of the "life span approach" and the concept of developmental tasks across the life span. Erikson also spawned a group of developmental theorists who created tasks for people to accomplish as they aged through life. These included Peck and Havinghurst, whose theories are included in gerontology textbooks.

Of late, theory has become more creative and useful, and, though not encompassing, shows promise in dealing with the important questions of the day. For example, there are theories of cognition that promise to contribute to the study of the aging mind. Other theories look at anthropology and the elements of a narrative gerontology. Gerontology itself is developing, and yet because it still includes many basic disciplines, theories abound and one can and should find a specific theory to explain the phenomena with which one is working (Bengston & Schaie, 1999).

Older Adults: Distribution and Demography

Normal life expectancy in the United States is approximately 79.5 years. The United States ranks 21st in the world in life expectancy. The country with the longest living population is Japan with a life expectancy of 84 years (Centers for Disease Control and Prevention: National Center for Health Statistics, 2003). In the United States, there is still a difference of 5 years between men and women in the expected life span, with men purported to live until age 74.1. A disparity has always existed in the life expectancy among people of color. For the whole population, both men and women, the black population typically lives to age 71.7, while the white population life expectancy is 79.4 (Arias, 2002) In the year 2000, those over 65 accounted for 13% of the population in the United States, and by the year 2030 that percentage will double (Federal Interagency Forum on Aging-Related Statistics, 2000). Over the next 30 years, the population aged 85 and older is expected to grow faster than any other age group. This growth is especially important to our health care system as this age group uses the largest number of health care services.

In Western industrialized society today, old age is defined principally by sanctioned withdrawal from the workforce. Historically, people have been described as "old" when they have reached pensionable age, usually 65. However, now that the life span has become more extended, the older-aged group is enormous indeed, with a wide range of ages with differing needs for differing cohorts. Thus the following descriptions and grading of age will be divided into groups known as the young-old (55–75), the old (75–85), and the oldest-old (85–100). Each of these groups faces different developmental issues and thus needs to be treated differently.

Young-Old (55–75)

Many persons leave the workforce before age 65 and as a result face many of the same issues as older people considering retirement. Neugarten (1968) set 55 as a "meaningful lower limit" and spoke of persons between the ages of 55 to 74 as the young-old. Because of advances in health practice, today's 70 year old is like the previous generation's 60 year old (Trafford, 2000). Not only does the general public see older people as *appearing* younger, older people today perceive *themselves* as younger than past generations perceived themselves. The young-old today are among the most educated and the wealthiest of any preceding generation.

One issue for the young-old in America today involves the lack of good faith treatment by corporations toward their employees. Many young-old are laid off without pensions that they believed they would have as they neared retirement age, thus creating critical problems for this aging group. This unpensioned, retired group must not only learn to deal with increased longevity, they must learn to do it with fewer and smaller resources. Many are baby boomers who changed the face of the workplace as they progressed through their work life. Because of their impact on the workplace, we also expect them to influence and change the demands of the aging as they become part of this group. One can already see the affects of their influence as older retirement centers hastily add wellness centers and gyms to their list of existing facilities.

The growth rate for numbers of older people will accelerate again as the baby boomer cohort reaches old age. One of the most important future issues is the effect of this large and aging baby boomer population on the country and the economy. By 2011 the boomers will begin to turn 65 and by 2030 they will compose 20% of the total population. Because boomers have not continued to have children at the same high rate as their parents, there will be a shortage of workers in the future to fill available vacant jobs. The direct consequence of fewer available workers on the baby boomers will be the minimal number of workers available to serve as their caregivers.

Notably, the baby boomers have been interested in politics and public policy and probably will remain so (Hodge, Gordon, & Lambert, 2004). In considering their likes and dislikes, therefore, we find a group who has grown up with technology and frequently uses the Internet. They also use e-mail for communication, differing from the older cohort who have not so widely adopted computer technology. Thus, we will have to think about how to serve each diverse group. This dilemma of vastly different interests creates a conundrum for the person in the nursing home who is trying to create groups with like interests (Lazer and Mayer-Schonberger, 2004).

Old (75–85)

Those in the old age group begin to experience functional decline and chronic illness. The most common chronic illnesses in the United States for this group are heart disease, arthritis, hypertension, obesity, diabetes, and Alzheimer's disease. Each of these diseases brings some functional decline causing difficulty with activities of daily living (ADLs). By age 80 the percentage of people having difficulty with ADLs is 28%, nearly double that of the young-old (Haber, 2003). Additionally, by age 85 nearly 42% of older people experience some cognitive decline and have Alzheimer's disease (Alzheimer's Association, 2000). As people in this age group decline, they begin to lose the ability to function independently, they require more health care services, and they place more demands on societal resources and the health care system (Haber, 2003).

Another source of functional decline in this age group is falling, causing hip fracture and other injuries. Falls are the leading cause of injury-related deaths in older people with the incidence rising with age. Persons age 75 and older account for 82% of fall-related deaths among older adults (National Center for Injury Prevention and Control, 2000). Age alone does not cause functional limitations, but the impact of age-related health problems causes a loss of ADLs (Fukukawa et al., 2004), and health problems increase with age (Wang, van Belle, Kukall, & Larson, 2002). Stress levels and psychosocial issues also affect ADLs. Depression is a major cause of illness and lost function (Lyness, King, Cox, Yoediono, & Caine, 1999).

Oldest-Old (86 and older)

The oldest-old require the most health care services. As people age they develop more comorbidities with 70% having more than one chronic illness. Their illnesses and needs are varied and include both mental and physical illness as well as normal sensorial losses occurring with aging. Among those 85 and older, sensory impairments, particularly vision, cause as much disability as chronic disease (Robert Wood Johnson Foundation, 1996). Older adults also commit the greatest number of suicides; they have had the highest suicide rate since 1933 (20% of all deaths by suicide). Rates tend to rise with age and are highest among white men (Koplan & Thacker, 2000). Thus work groups could serve many needs for this cohort, from social support to an ongoing system of monitoring.

The oldest-old are also becoming the largest category of the nation's nursing home population, though only 5% of the total population lives in a nursing home at one time. Because women live longer than men, the majority of the residents in nursing homes are white, widowed, and functionally dependent females (Gabrel, 2000a). The leading diagnosis upon admission is disease of the circulatory system with the average number of days in the home at 870 days. Three fourths of the residents require assistance with more than three ADLs. The most common reason for discharge is death.

A part of the oldest-old group that is growing rapidly and of interest to researchers are those who are over 100 years old, the centenarians. Centenarians seem to be an elite group of people with better genes and better health habits that allow them to survive (Martin, Long & Poon, 2002). Centenarians are being studied in several countries in a coordinated way. Some of the findings show that centenarians have many individual differences, but as a group they practiced health habits now known to prolong life (Nickols-Richardson, Johnson, Poon, & Martin, 1996.) Their patterns of nutrition are especially interesting. Nutritionally, centenarians consumed 20–30% more carotenoids and vitamin A foods than younger-aged cohorts, ate breakfast more regularly, and avoided great weight fluctuations. They drank more whole milk and did not avoid dietary cholesterol (Williams, Johnson, Poon, & Martin, 1995). In terms of personality, centenarians were more dominant, suspicious, practical, and relaxed than younger cohorts. Their children act as their support system and they report fewer emotional symptoms than younger cohorts (Maddox et al., 2001)

The Impact of Cohorts

In the year 2000, there were 26 times as many Americans over the age of 85 as there were in 1900. It is popular to attribute population graying to greater survival, but this is only part of the story. As important as greater survival is, the effect of cohort size has a greater influence on the population as a whole. All age cohorts have not been advancing at the same rate. The number of persons in any cohort reaching old age depends in part on the number at the start. Today's oldest-old were born before the United States entered World War I when immigration and large families were the rule. Therefore, more of the very old in groups are likely to have been foreign born or to have had parents who were. After World War I, immigration decreased. More importantly, the oldest-old are a "fat" cohort, meaning the cohort had a large beginning, because theirs was a generation that grew up in large families. The size of succeeding cohorts was limited by the Great Depression and World War II, and many socioeconomic factors such as the birth control pill that reduced the birth rate. The rate of growth of the oldest-old will slow during the next two decades when the "skinny" cohort of Depression and wartime babies moves up.

When we speak about the percentage of older adults, more than the size of a particular cohort is involved. The percentage reflects the proportion of the elderly in a total population that includes the young and middle aged. In 1900, there were fewer old people in relation to a very large number of infants and children—older people were just 4% of the population. In 1990, the 31 million Americans over age 65 constituted 12.56% of the population. The size of the younger cohort groups had gotten smaller: there were fewer babies and children to rebalance the proportion. Middle-range projections predict 52 million older Americans, about 17.7% of the whole, by 2020, compared with the 4% reported above. Remember the limitations of projections. These projections assume that current conditions will continue. They cannot fully take into account the effect on specific cohorts of epidemics such as acquired immune deficiency syndrome (AIDS) or socioeconomic factors that may alter the birthrate, such as economic depressions.

Selected Aging Issues

Dementia

Nearly 18 million people have dementia in the world today. By the year 2025, that number will rise to over 34 million (National Institute on Aging, 2003) The most prevalent dementia, Alzheimer's disease, is the eighth leading cause of death in the United States. More importantly, the disease consumes the lives of two people, the Alzheimer caregiver and the Alzheimer-affected individual. Viewed in this way, approximately 30 years of productive life are lost when one person develops Alzheimer's disease. Even more devastating are the statistics showing that 49% of those over 85 will get Alzheimer's disease (National Institute on Aging, 2003). With the largest population increase expected in the over 85 age group (38% by 2020 in South Carolina), there is a press-

ing need to help families manage Alzheimer's disease at home, particularly those who are poor or not eligible for available resources (Alzheimer's Disease Registry, 1998).

CARE GIVING

Some of your participants will have problems with dementia, either their own or that of a parent or a spouse, and some will be caregivers. Caregivers of people with dementia often seek out support groups to assist them with social support as well as to learn more about the disease (Buckwalter, Maas, & Reed, 1997). All aspects of the disease are highly stressful for both patient and caregiver, and this additional stress can impair health (Perry & Olshansky, 1996). Functional impairment may arise from physical or cognitive causes or a combination of both. These impairments and the ability of the caregiver to leave the demented person alone must be taken into account when planning groups for this population in the community. Some successful groups have met with both caregiver and the afflicted person in the same group, while others have arranged to run two separate groups, one for caregivers and one for the people with Alzheimer's disease. Each type of group has its strengths, and consideration of the facilities as well as the group members should enter into your decision making regarding how to run your group (Schultz et al., 2002).

Adult children will be dealing with their own children, retirement, aging, and with concerns about their parents. Close to three quarters of disabled older adults have either a spouse or an adult child as the primary caregiver. Seventy-two percent of the caregivers are wives or daughters. The role of care giving is not static, and often the burden becomes heavier over time. The trajectory of health outcomes associated with care giving is generally downward, with those carrying the heaviest burdens having the poorest health or experiencing the greatest declines in health (Burton, Zdaniuk, Schulz, Jackson, & Hirsch,

2003). Chappel and Reid (2002) suggest that we should consider well-being, rather than burden, when looking at the effect of that role on the care-giver because well-being is affected by four variables, burden being only one of them. They see the other three variables of social support, self-esteem, and hours of care making a difference, with burden being directly related to the present behavior of the person who is ill. Burdened care-givers can benefit from group work such as psychoeducational skills training to manage their own anger and depression (Coon, Thompson, Steffan, Sorocco, & Gallagher-Thompson, 2003). Thus, when working with care-giving groups the effect of their burden should be considered when choosing an activity for the group.

The Disabled

A vulnerable cluster within the aging population are those people with lifelong disabilities. People with disabilities face difficult employment conditions that affect their health and well-being throughout their lives, resulting in poverty, lower levels of emotional well-being, and increased stress in old age. In the Healthy People 2010 report, it was shown that disability in older adults is more prevalent in the southern United States, requiring increased community support and skilled personal assistants (Department of Health and Human Services, 2003). Healthy People 2010 created a focus area on disability noting that disabled people face unique risks and require unique services. Often they are able to live independently while they are young, but as they grow older they become more dependent and require increased care-giving services. Working with each type of disability requires a different tailored approach. For example, those who are mentally retarded will respond to interventions differently from those who are paralyzed.

Individuals with mental retardation are living longer than they did in the past but aging faster than the general population. Often, they outlive their parents and this lengthened life span creates additional care-giving issues. Persons with Downs syndrome, epilepsy, and cerebral palsy have slightly shorter life expectancies than many other categories of developmentally disabled persons, but they, too, are living longer than they did before. As a group worker, you may be planning groups for the retarded when they have "retired" from sheltered workshops, are confronted with the death of a parent, or have moved into a group home. You may also be running a group for victims of stroke. One exciting group conducted by students was a group for aphasic elders who liked to sing. Though stroke victims often have difficulty communicating verbally, they thoroughly enjoyed singing old hymns together and were often surprised at the music coming out of their mouths because they could not speak. The lesson learned is that it is important for the group leader to be well informed about the disability with which he or she is working and to be able to help people with such disabilities reach their potential.

Nursing Homes

Many of the oldest-old will be in nursing homes at some time during their life or at least in need of home health services (Gianopoulos, Bolda, Baldwin, & Olsen, 2001). The baby boomer cohort in the United States will strain the current system which had an 88% occupancy rate in 1997 and has not grown considerably since then due to the push for home health care. Currently there are 17,000 nursing homes nationwide (Gabrel, 2000b), housing two basic and different types of patients: short stay and long term. Those who are there for rehabilitation after being discharged from the hospital are usually the short-stay Medicare patients. They are often recovering physically and not interested in being a member of a group because they are still ill. Then when they are better, they are close to being discharged and still not interested. Many of these short-stay patients are relatively younger and more alert than long-term residents.

On the other hand, the long-term patient is sicker and frailer when entering a nursing home. The average length of stay for such a patient is only three years before death occurs. Rising costs and more careful screening by many states of their Medicaid clients lead to later entry by older persons chiefly in need of personal care (Branch, 2001). Also, in many places there are more community resources to help frail older persons stay at home thus delaying entry into a nursing home. Between 1973 and 1985, the rate of nursing home entry for persons 65 to 84 dropped, and the rate of entry for those 85 and older remained steady. In response, nursing homes are evolving into two types of facilities: traditional homes offering personal care and Medicare facilities that are becoming more like minihospitals (Kliempt, Ruta, & McMurdo, 2000).

People entering a Medicare-funded nursing home since the prospective payment system came into effect are more likely to have orthopedic problems, stroke, and generally poorer health (Yip, Wilber, & Myrtle, 2002). Presently, nursing home patients fall under two different Medicare payment systems, managed care systems and fee-for-service. Researchers found that those using fee-for-service received significantly more therapy units and had significantly longer lengths of stay in rehab units than those in managed care (Angelelli, Wilber, & Myrtle, 2000).

In the past, older persons with schizophrenia and other mental illnesses were formally "deinstitutionalized" from mental hospitals to nursing homes. In the same period, nursing homes were viewed as suitable settings for older individuals with mental retardation. However the mandated preadmission screening and annual resident review (PASAR) provisions of the Nursing Home Reform Amendments to the Omnibus Reconciliation Act of 1987 (OBRA '87) changed the mix of residents by precluding both groups (mentally ill and men-

tally retarded) unless they truly needed skilled nursing care (Department of Health and Human Services, 1992). Individuals who have been previously diagnosed with a mental illness now need to be screened before they can enter a nursing home, and the only nursing homes that can accept mentally ill elders are those with the proper care providers to care for them. This change results in quieter nursing homes for older people but leaves older mentally ill people with no place to go other than the street if there are no vacancies in homes with the proper care available.

This list of aging issues only highlights some of the most common present day problems of older people, but should serve to give the reader a sense of some of the limitations that they will face as they begin group work. In addition to these dilemmas, as people age, they experience numerous physical and mental changes that are considered normal but noteworthy because of the accommodations that must be made by the older persons themselves and by the group leader when selecting and running a group.

Normal Aging Changes

Knowledge of some of the variables in the patterns of normal and abnormal aging is useful to the group leader (Reuben, 2000). The important variables fall into the triad used by most gerontologists: social, psychological, and physical/physiological. These variables ultimately have a great influence on the type of group chosen, the knowledge needed by the leader, and the adaptations that have to be made.

Normal aging, according to Atchley and Barusch (2004), refers to usual, commonly encountered problems of aging. Normal aging is different from culture to culture because of the sociocultural overlay. Pathological aging means there is physical or mental disease. A successful ager can meet needs—for example, income, housing, health care, nutrition, clothing, and recreation. Atchley and Barusch contend these positive outcomes occur because older people use "continuity strategies" to help them adapt to the changes that occur with normal aging.

Aging and Physical Changes

The physical changes that occur during aging require that a group leader maintains a constant health orientation. The leader needs to be aware of physical changes (or mental changes that may indicate a physical problem) because such changes may require adaptations in the group structure and format. Illness that precludes a member's attendance at a meeting may be a reason for the leader to see or call the individual outside of the group. Group leaders must be aware of the common disorders that occur in later life, both because they may cause absenteeism or loss of members through death, and also so that the leader can encourage prevention or early detection of diseases.

Table 2–1 contains a detailed list of aging changes. Remember that oldness is not to be equated with illness. Chapter 12 presents common diseases that occur in later life and suggests how the disease process can affect a group member's participation. Regarding normal aging, changes in vision and hearing will have a great impact on the group communication. Leaders should be prepared to work with these impairments. Leaders should also encourage healthy aging at every opportunity. Table 2–2 may be helpful when teaching healthier habits to older members of a group.

Table 2–1 Normal Age-Related Changes

Understanding normal age-related changes is the foundation to understanding health and disease in older people. The following section highlights changes within each organ system that are known to decline with age.

Skin and connective tissue

- Loss of dermal thickness produces transparent, thin skin appearance.
- In the epidermis, number and activity of melanocytes (pigment-producing cells) decrease, making skin more sensitive to ultraviolet sunlight.
- Loss of subcutaneous fat makes the person more sensitive to heat and cold.
- Progressive loss of melanocytes in hair bulbs and decreased number of hair follicles result in graying and thinning of hair.
- Decrease in epidermis turnover contributes to slower wound healing.
- Sebaceous and sweat glands decrease in number, size, and function, therefore producing less oil and sweat.
- Decreased vascular bed and responsiveness (and sweating) predispose older people to hypothermia and hyperthermia.
- Decreased vitamin D production and decreased exposure to sunlight may contribute to osteoporosis and osteomalacia.

Nervous system

- Moderate cortical atrophy.
- Loss of neurons in the neocortex, substantia nigra, and limbic system.
- Lipofuscin pigment accumulates primarily in glial tissues.
- Certain neurotransmitters decline.
- Binding sites for dopamine and serotonin decrease.
- Peripheral nerve fibers decrease in number and size.

(continued)

Table 2–1   NORMAL AGE-RELATED CHANGES (CONTINUED)

Motor and sensory nerve conduction decreases
- A decrease in vibratory sensation in feet and ankles may occur.
- Longer transmission time between neurons makes information flow and response slower.

Senses

Vision
- Atrophy of periorbital tissue may cause upper and lower lids to droop.
- Visual acuity may decrease due to changes in the retina or neural components.
- Loss of accommodation causes hyperopia.
- Nuclear sclerosis causes myopia.
- Decreased tear secretion may cause dryness of eyes.
- Less able to perceive colors in the cool range; blues and purples all appear grey.
- Glare sensitive, should not face windows or sunlight or walk in rooms with shiny floors.
- Less able to perceive change from floor to wall, therefore incorporate borders such as base boards in different colors to provide contrast.

Hearing
- Pure tone loss is greater at high frequencies than at low frequencies.
- Pitch discrimination declines primarily at very high and low frequencies.
- Speech discrimination declines and is worsened with background noise.
- Unable to hear high-pitched female voices.
- Unable to hear vowels clearly, therefore speech is garbled.

Smell
- Poor detection and discrimination by the eighth decade.

Oral
- A reduction in the integrity of epithelial and connective tissue causes a thinning of the oral mucosa and affects bone pulpal tissues.
  Blood supply is decreased.
  - Nerve innervation is compromised.
  - Tissue quality is modified.
  - Calcifitic tissue changes occur.
- A compositional change occurs in the nature of saliva.
  - Altered sodium levels.
  - Increase in potassium.
  - Decrease in secretory proteins.
- A reduction in taste perception.
  - Increase in threshold potentials for salt and bitter tastes.
- Structural changes to the teeth occur.
  - Erosion.
  - Abrasion.
  - Attrition.
- Gingival recession.
  - Alveolar dehiscence.
  - Compromised spatial position of teeth.

Table 2–1   NORMAL AGE-RELATED CHANGES (CONTINUED)

Cardiovascular
- Conducting system loses cells and fibers and becomes infiltrated with fat.
- Heart rate at rest and achievable maximum declines [maximum HR = (220 − age)].
- Increase in stroke volume (S.V.) compensates for lower heart rate (H.R.) and maintaining cardiac output (C.O.) [C.O. = H.R. × S.V.].
- Intrinsic contractile function declines.
- Vascular compliance decreases due to changes in the vessel walls with intima cellular proliferation, fibrosis, media elastin fragmentation, and calcification.
- In Western and developed countries, systolic blood pressure increases with lower rate of increase in diastolic pressure.

Respiratory
- Lung elastic recoil decreases as a result of collagen and elastin changes.
- Chest wall compliance decreases due to stiffening of the chest wall.
- Respiratory muscle strength decreases.
- Lung volumes change as a consequence of the above changes.
  - Increase in residual volume and functional residual capacity.
  - Decrease in vital capacity and expiratory flow rates.
- Gas exchange
  - Decrease in arterial PO_2, due to ventilation-perfusion mismatch.

Gastrointestinal
- Esophageal motility decreases due to lower amplitude contractions after swallowing (presbyesophagus).
- Gastric mucosa thins, acid-producing parietal cells atrophy, and gastric acid secretion decreases.
- Small and large intestinal mucosa atrophies, reducing absorptive surface area and decreasing the ability to absorb sugars, calcium, vitamin B_{12}, and iron.
- Liver decreases in size but maintains function; however, the microsomal enzyme function declines.

Renal
- Renal mass decreases with primarily cortical losses of nephrons, glomeruli, and capillaries.
- Renal plasma flow decreases.
- Glomerular filtration rate (GFR) falls.
- Creatinine clearance progressively declines 1% per year after age 40 with no change in serum creatinine level, because creatinine generation also decreases.
- Ability to retain sodium (Na) declines.
- Ability to concentrate urine declines.

Musculoskeletal
- Decrease in muscle weight compared to total body weight occurs.
- Decreased muscular strength and endurance associated with decrease in number of muscle fibers
  - Thigh muscle strength decreases first, making it difficult to get out of a chair without arms.
- Hyaline cartilage water content declines.
- Bone loss is universal, but rate is highly variable; loss is more rapid in women after menopause than in men.

Hematopoietic
- Overall red cells, hemoglobin, hematocrit, white cells, and platelets maintain normal values and functions.
- Active bone marrow decreases and marrow fat increases but remains adequate for hematopoiesis.

(continued)

ble 2–1 NORMAL AGE-RELATED CHANGES (CONTINUED)

Immune system
- Thymic involution begins about age of puberty.
- Number of T- and B-lymphocytes does not change.
- T-lymphocyte function declines.
    - Decreased response to skin tests.
    - Production of interleukin-2 is reduced.
- B-lymphocyte function is not as clear.
    - Immunoglobulins IgM and possibly IgG levels decline.
    - Immunoglobulin production to a challenge (vaccine or antigen) is lower response and shortened duration.

Endocrine
- Progressive decline in carbohydrate tolerance.
    - Primary defect in insulin resistance as post-receptor defect.
- Metabolic clearance rate of thyroid hormone decreases, but thyroxine (T4) levels are normal.

Genital/Sexual Function
Women
- With menopause, rapid decline of estrogen and progesterone.
- Hormonal changes cause atrophic changes of uterus, vagina, external genitalia, and breasts.
- Sexual activity decreases, but exact roles of biological changes and sociocultural factors are unknown.

Men
- Testosterone levels decrease with age.
- Prostate gland increases in size due to hyperplasia.
- Erectile and ejaculatory function declines; postejaculatory refractory period increases.
- Sexual response is delayed due to reduced penile sensitivity and increased threshold for tactile stimulation.

Table 2–2 TEN TIPS FOR HEALTHY AGING

1. Eat a balanced diet.
2. Exercise regularly and wisely.
3. Get regular medical check-ups.
4. Don't smoke. It's never too late to quit.
5. Practice safety habits at home to prevent falls and fractures. Always wear your seatbelt when traveling by car.
6. Maintain contacts with family and friends, and stay active through work, recreation, and community activities.
7. Avoid overexposure to the sun and the cold.
8. If you drink, moderation is the key. When you drink, let someone else drive.
9. Keep personal and financial records in order to simplify budgeting and investing. Plan long-term housing and financial needs.
10. Keep a positive attitude toward life. Do things that make you happy.

Source: National Institute on Aging, 2003

Exercises

EXERCISE 1

You have been engaged to organize three groups at Sunnyvale Nursing Facility. In view of today's demographic trends, what sex and age distributions would you expect to find among residents? What age groups would you be likely to find attending meetings of the family council?

EXERCISE 2

On the blackboard, draw four horizontal parallel lines. Write 1900 above one end and the current year above the other, marking the intervening years at 10-year intervals in between the two. Indicate major events that would have affected ordinary people's lives, such as World War I, autos becoming common, the Great Depression, World War II, television becoming common, the baby boom beginning and ending, and the like. On the four lines indicate the birth and overlapping life spans of four generations: mother, daughter, granddaughter, and great-granddaughter, or father, son, grandson, and great-grandson. Discuss how their lives and outlooks might differ because of the years in which they were born.

EXERCISE 3

Take the quiz in Appendix B, "What's Your Aging IQ?" Study the questions you missed by reading the explanation for the answers. Then select three of the quiz questions and explain how they might be relevant to a group you plan to lead.

References

Angelelli, J., Wilber, K., & Myrtle, R. (2000). A comparison of skilled nursing facility rehabilitation treatment and outcomes under Medicare managed care and Medicare fee-for-service reimbursement. *The Gerontologist, 40*(6), 646–653.

Arias, E. (2002). United States life tables, 2000. *National Vital Statistics Reports, 51*(3), 3–4.

Atchley, R., & Barusch, A. (2004). *Social forces and aging* (10th ed.). Montery: Wadsworth.

Alzheimer's Disease Registry. (1998). *Statewide Alzheimer's disease and related disorders registry*. Columbia, SC: Author.

Bengston, V., & Schaie, K. (Eds.). (1999). *Handbook of theories of aging*. New York: Springer.

Branch, L. (2001). Community long-term care services: What works and what doesn't. *The Gerontologist, 41*(3), 305–307.

Buckwalter, K. C., Maas, M., & Reed, D. (1997). Assessing family and staff caregiver outcomes in Alzheimer's disease research. *Alzheimer's Disease and Associated Disorders, 11*(Suppl. 6), 105–116.

Burton, L., Zdaniuk, B., Schulz, R., Jackson, S., & Hirsch, C. (2003). Transitions in spousal caregiving. *The Gerontologist, 43*(2), 230–241.

Chappel, N., & Reid, R. (2002). Burden and well-being among caregivers: Examining the distinction. *The Gerontologist, 42*(6), 772–780.

Coon, D., Thompson, L., Steffan, A., Sorocco, K., & Gallagher-Thompson, D. (2003). Anger and depression management: Psychoeducational skill training interventions for women caregivers of a relative with dementia. *The Gerontologist, 43*(5), 678–689.

Department of Health and Human Services. (2000). *Healthy people 2010* (Conference Edition). Washington, DC: Author.

Department of Health and Human Services. (2003). *Healthy people 2010: Progress review, disability and secondary conditions*. Washington, DC: Author.

Erikson, E. (1950). *Childhood and society*. New York: W. W. Norton.

Federal Interagency Forum on Aging-Related Statistics. (2000). *Older Americans 2000: Key indicators of well-being*. Washington, DC: U.S. Government Printing Office.

Fukukawa, Y., Nakashima, C., Tsubou, S., Niino, N., Ando, F., Kosugi, S., & Shimokata, H. (2004). The impact of health problems on depression and activities in middle aged and older adults: Age and social interactions. *Journal of Gerontology, 59*(B1), 19–26.

Gabrel, C. (2000a). *Characteristics of elderly nursing home current residents and discharges: Data from the 1997 National Nursing Home Survey*. Hyattsville, MD: National Center for Health Statistics.

Gabrel C. (2000b). *An overview of nursing home facilities: Data from the 1997 National Nursing Home Survey*. Hyattsville, MD: National Center for Health Statistics.

Gatz, M., & Zarit, S. (1999). A good old age: Paradox or possibility. In V. Bengston & K. Schaie (Eds.). *Handbook of theories of aging*. New York: Springer.

Gianopoulos, C., Bolda, E., Baldwin, M., & Olsen, L. (2001). What works? Maine's statewide uniform assessments and home care planning system tells all. *The Gerontologist, 41*(3), 309–311.

Haber, D. (2003). *Health promotion and aging: Practical applications for health professionals* (3rd ed.). New York: Springer.

Haight, B., Barba, B., Tesh, A., & Courts, N. (2002). Thriving: A life span theory. *Journal of Gerontological Nursing, 28*(3), 14–22.

Hochschild, A. (1975). Disengagement theory: A critique and proposal. *American Social Review, 40*(5), 553–569.

Centers for Disease Control and Prevention: National Center for Health Statistics. (2003). *Special excerpt: Health, United States Trend tables on 65 and older population.* Atlanta, GA: Author.

Hodge, P., Gordon, L., & Lambert, J. (2004). The age explosion: Baby boomers and beyond. *Harvard Generations Policy Journal, 1*, 67–77.

Kliempt, P., Ruta, D., & McMurdo, M. (2000). Measuring the outcomes of care in older people: A non-critical review of patient-based measures: III, Pain, physical disability and handicap, and social health instruments. *Reviews in Clinical Gerontology, 10*(3), 235–244.

Koplan, J., & Thacker, S. (2000). *Working to prevent and control injury in the United States: Fact book for the year 2000.* Atlanta, GA: Centers for Disease Control and Prevention, National Center for Injury Prevention and Control.

Lachs, M., Williams, C., O'Brien, S., & Pillemer, K. (2003). Adult protective service use and nursing home placement. *The Gerontologist, 42*(6), 734–739.

Lazer, D. Mayer-Schonberger, V. (2004). Staying connected: Baby boomers and the Internet. *Harvard Generations Policy Journal, 1*, 67–76.

Lyness, J. M., King, D. A., Cox, C., Yoediono, Z., Caine, E. D. (1999). The importance of subsyndromal depression in older primary care patients: Prevalence and associated functional disability. *Journal of the American Geriatric Society, 47*, 647–652.

Maddox, G., Atchley, R., Evans, J., Hudson, R., Kane, R., Masoro, E., Mezey, M., Poon, L., & Siegler, I. (Eds.). (2001). *The encyclopedia of aging* (3rd ed., Vols. 1, 2). New York: Springer.

Marshall, V. (1999). Analyzing social theories of aging. In V. Bengston & K. Schaie (Eds.), *Handbook of theories of aging.* New York: Springer.

Martin, P., Long, M. V., & Poon, L. W. (2002). Age changes in personality traits and states of the old and very old. *The Journal of Gerontology Series B, 57*(2), 144–152.

National Institute on Aging. (2003). *Progress report on Alzheimer's disease.* Washington, DC: Author.

Neugarten, B. (Ed.). (1968). *Middle age and aging: A reader in social psychology.* Chicago: University of Chicago Press.

Nickols-Richardson, S., Johnson, M., Poon, L., & Martin, P. (1996). Mental health and number of illnesses are predictors of nutritional risk factors in elderly persons. *Experimental Aging Research, 22*, 141–154.

Perry, J., & Olshansky, E. F. (1996). A family's coming to terms with Alzheimer's disease. *Western Journal of Nursing Research, 18*(1), 12–28.

Reuben, D. (2000). Multidimensional assessment in the community. In D. Osterweil, K. Brummel-Smith, & J. Beck (Eds.), *Comprehensive geriatric assessment.* New York: McGraw-Hill.

Robert Wood Johnson Foundation. (1996). *Chronic care in America: A 21st century challenge.* Princeton, NJ: Author.

Schultz, R., O'Brien, A., Czaja, S., Ory, M., Norris, R., Martire, L., Belle, S., Gallagher-Thompson, D., & Stevens, A. (2002). Dementia caregiver intervention research: In search of clinical significance. *The Gerontologist, 42*(5), 589–602.

Schulz, R., Burgio, L., Burns, R., Eisdorfer, C., Gallagher-Thompson, D., Gitlin, L., & Mahoney, F. (2003). Resources for enhancing Alzheimer's caregiver health (REACH): Overview, site-specific outcomes, and future directions. *The Gerontologist, 43*(4), 514–520.

Trafford, A. (2000, July3). What will people do with the extra decade? *Houston Chronicle*, p. 3C.

Wang, L., van Belle, G., Kukall, W. B., & Larson, E. B. (2002). Predictors of functional change: A longitudinal study of nondemented people aged 65 and older. *Journal of the American Geriatric Society, 50*(9), 1525–1534.

Williams, L., Johnson, M., Poon, L., & Martin, P. (1995). Oral health and demographic risk factors for poor nutrient intake in the elderly. *Age and Nutrition, 6*(1), 4–9.

World's Alzheimer Conference, Washington, DC, July 6–9, 2000.

Yip, J., Wilber, K., & Myrtle, R. (2002). The impact of the 1997 balanced budget amendment's prospective payment system on patient case mix and rehabilitation utilization in skilled nursing. *The Gerontologist, 42*(5), 653–660.

Appendix A

Glossary

activities of daily living (ADLs)—Skills necessary for self-care, usually listed as bathing, dressing, feeding oneself, toileting, and transferring oneself between bed and chair.

age cohort—A group of people born about the same time and therefore likely to share some experiences and values because they have passed through the same period of history.

ageism—Generalizing about persons on the basis of a single common characteristic, their age; a form of negative stereotyping. Rarely acknowledged but expressed through various subtle—and not so subtle—forms of discrimination, such as planning *for* rather than *with* older persons.

average age—All the ages added together and divided by the number of persons. The average can be skewed by extremes: the average age of Latinos is low, for example, because the high birthrate means there are many children.

centenarians—Individuals 100 years of age or older.

developmental tasks—These are responses to normal life stressors that occur throughout life, including the aging process.

disengagement theory—A debatable theory that contends that there is a mutual withdrawal of the elderly and society from one another.

instrumental activities of daily living (IADLs)—Include meal preparation, house-cleaning, handling money, shopping, and getting around in the community.

median age—The point in the age distribution at which there are an equal number of persons above and below.

modal age—The mode, the most common age, may fail to express the range.

Omnibus Budget Reconciliation Act of 1987 (OBRA '87)—This is also referred to as the Nursing Home Reform Amendments. These are amendments to Title XIX of the Social Security Act. They spell out the rights of residents and their families, require multidisciplinary assessments and individually tailored care plans, limit the use of physical and chemical restraints, and require that psychosocial approaches to problem behavior be tried before recourse to either. They emphasize activities programs, which includes group work.

personhood—Is characterized by the qualities that confer distinct individuality to each person. Personhood is the self that individuals strive to keep through the vicissitudes of loss and institutionalization in old age.

prospective payment—Medicare payments to hospitals predicated on the average cost of caring for patients in each diagnosis-related group (DRG). Although it was intended that length of stay average out among patients who recuperated quickly and those needing extra hospital days, hospitals tend to use this mean as the ceiling.

self-concept—A person's total sense of self; how the older individual feels about himself or herself and the person's attitudes, values, and all of life's experiences.

self-perception—The process of questioning the image that one has of oneself. This questioning may present conflict, which might include dependency on others, devaluation of one's contributions, and a multitude of losses. Such factors can create fear, a sense of powerlessness, and an overall diminished quality of life.

Appendix B

What's Your Aging I.Q.?

Answer the following true or false questions.

1. Baby boomers are the fastest growing segment of the population.
2. Families don't bother with their older relatives.
3. Everyone becomes confused or forgetful if they live long enough.
4. You can be too old to exercise.
5. Heart disease is a much bigger problem for older men than for older women.
6. The older you get, the less you sleep.
7. People should watch their weight as they age.
8. Most older people are depressed. Why shouldn't they be?
9. There's no point in screening older people for cancer because they can't be treated.
10. Older people take more medications than younger people.
11. People begin to lose interest in sex around age 55.
12. If your parents had Alzheimer's disease, you will inevitably get it.
13. Diet and exercise reduce the risk of osteoporosis.
14. As your body changes with age, so does your personality.
15. Older people might as well accept urinary accidents as a fact of life.
16. Suicide is mainly a problem for teenagers.
17. Falls and injuries "just happen" to older people.
18. Everybody gets cataracts.
19. Extremes of heat and cold can be especially dangerous for older people.
20. "You can't teach an old dog new tricks."

Answers

1. **False**—There are more than 3 million Americans over the age of 85. That number is expected to quadruple by the year 2040, when there will be more than 12 million people in that age group. The population age 85 and older is the fastest growing age group in the United States.
2. **False**—Most older people live close to their children and see them often. Many live with their spouses. An estimated 80% of men and 60% of women live in family settings. Only 5% of the older population lives in nursing homes.
3. **False**—Confusion and serious forgetfulness in old age can be caused by Alzheimer's disease or other conditions that result in irreversible damage to the brain. But at least 100 other problems can bring on the same symptoms. A minor head injury, high fever, poor nutrition, adverse drug reactions, and depression also can lead to confusion. These conditions are treatable, however, and the confusion they cause can be eliminated.
4. **False**—Exercise at any age can help strengthen the heart and lungs and lower blood pressure. It also can improve muscle strength and, if carefully chosen, lessen bone loss with age. See a physician before beginning a new exercise program.
5. **False**—The rise of heart disease increases dramatically for women after menopause. By age 65, both men and women have a one in three chance of showing symptoms. But risks can be significantly reduced by following a healthy diet and exercising.
6. **False**—In later life, it's the quality of sleep that declines, not total sleep time. Researchers have found that sleep tends to become more fragmented as people age. A number of reports suggest that

older people are less likely than younger people to stay awake throughout the day and that older people tend to take more naps than younger people.

7. **True**—Most people gain weight as they age. Because of changes in the body and decreasing physical activity, older people usually need fewer calories. Still, a balanced diet is important. Older people require essential nutrients just like younger adults. You should be concerned about your weight if there has been an involuntary gain or loss of 10 pounds in the past six months.

8. **False**—Most older people are not depressed. When it does occur, depression is treatable throughout the life cycle using a variety of approaches, such as family support, psychotherapy, or antidepressant medications. A physician can determine whether the depression is caused by medication an older person might be taking, by physical illness, stress, or other factors.

9. **False**—Many older people can beat cancer, especially if it's found early. Over half of all cancers occur in people 65 and older, which means that screening for cancer in this age group is especially important.

10. **True**—Older people often have a combination of conditions that require drugs. They consume 25% of all medications and can have many more problems with adverse reactions. Check with your doctor to make sure all drugs and dosages are appropriate.

11. **False**—Most older people can lead an active, satisfying sex life.

12. **False**—The overwhelming number of people with Alzheimer's disease have not inherited the disorder. In a few families,

scientists have seen an extremely high incidence of the disease and have identified genes in these families which they think may be responsible.

13. **True**—Women are at particular risk for osteoporosis. They can help prevent bone loss by eating foods rich in calcium and exercising regularly throughout life. Foods such as milk and other dairy products, dark green leafy vegetables, salmon, sardines, and tofu promote new bone growth. Activities such as walking, biking, and simple exercises to strengthen the upper body also can be effective.

14. **False**—Research has found that, except for the changes that can result from Alzheimer's disease and other forms of dementia, personality is one of the few constants of life. That is, you are likely to age much as you've lived.

15. **False**—Urinary incontinence is a symptom, not a disease. Usually, it is caused by specific changes in body function that can result from infection, diseases, pregnancy, or the use of certain medications. A variety of treatment options are available for people who seek medical attention.

16. **False**—Suicide is most prevalent among people age 65 and older. An older person's concern with suicide should be taken very seriously and professional help should be sought quickly.

17. **False**—Falls are the most common cause of injuries among people over age 65. But many of these falls, which result in broken bones, can be avoided. Regular vision and hearing tests and good safety habits can help prevent accidents. Knowing whether your medications affect balance and coordination also is a good idea.

18. **False**—Not everyone gets cataracts, although a great many older people do. Some 18% of people between the ages of 65 and 74 have cataracts, while more than 40% of those between 75 and 85 have the problem. Cataracts can be treated successfully with surgery; more than 90% of people say they can see better after the procedure.

19. **True**—The body's thermostat tends to function less efficiently with age, making the older person's body less able to adapt to heat or cold.

20. **False**—People at any age can learn new information and skills. Research indicates that older people can obtain new skills and improve old ones, including how to use a computer.

Source: National Institute on Aging, Bethesda, MD.

Chapter 3

History and Overview of Group Work

Barbara Haight
Irene Burnside

Key Words

- Age-specific groups
- Member-specific groups
- Psychotherapy
- Social-emotional area
- Topic-specific groups

Learning Objectives

- Describe the origin of group work in the United States
- Discuss the work of the pioneers in group work with older adults
- Discuss three principles of group work with older people
- Describe four levels of group work with older adults
- Describe two member-specific groups
- Discuss age-specific groups

Understanding is obtained by explaining what we know.

—*Robert L. Causey (1969, p. 24)*

This chapter provides a brief history of group work with older adults and an overview of current group work procedures. The following sections introduce some principles of group work, the most common types of groups, and the group methods used with older clients. Since World War II, therapists have used groups as a cost-effective method of delivering care. Groups are especially helpful to older people because of the social support that comes from the other group members. Group work is effective and should be used more widely for the prevention of disease and maintenance of psychosocial health in older people. In this book, group work covers a wide range of groups for older people that may be conducted by professionals and nonprofessionals. Group psychotherapy, as used in this book, designates only groups that are led by professionals with a background in mental health.

Historical Background of Group Work

The accepted originator of group psychotherapy was Joseph Henry Pratt, MD. In 1905, Dr. Pratt developed a plan for using groups for the treatment of tuberculosis in poor patients. Dr. Elwood Worchester, director of the Emmanuel Church in Boston, funded him. At that time, the disease was often called "consumption"; however, Pratt called the group meetings "tuberculosis classes." The group consisted of 15 to 20 patients who met with him once a week. Although aimed at fostering an understanding of tuberculosis, the group members also improved their psychosocial status. Unfortunately, other physicians who tried to emulate his classes were not nearly as successful. Some writers conclude that Pratt's outgoing personality had a great deal to do with the success of his group and that he tended to conduct the group work successfully by intuition (Burnside, 1994).

The improvement of the emotional status of the tuberculosis patients in these groups led to the use of group treatments for patients who suffered from mental illness. At a later date, Dr. Worchester, assisted by one of the first members of the American Psychoanalytic Association, began seeing patients in group meetings to assist them with health problems; these groups were not restricted to tuberculosis patients. Pratt continued to work in the group modality but switched his attention to patients who had emotional problems. At that time, no theoretical basis for group psychoanalytic therapy existed for teaching the method. Also, no worthwhile research had yet appeared. Pratt applied the ideas of Joseph Deperine who emphasized persuasion and reeducation. Pratt continued his work as a group psychotherapist into the 1950s (Burnside, 1994).

Psychiatric patients were treated by group psychotherapy as early as 1921. L. C. Marsh worked with psychotics in lectures and classes. Although Marsh's groups probably would not be recognized as psychotherapy today, he did realize the therapeutic value of group treatment for psychotics. He also used formal lectures, art classes, and dance classes in his group work (Ruitenbeck, 1970).

In the 1920s and 1930s, Louis Wender, a psychiatrist, worked with institutionalized borderline cases of mentally ill people. He thought of his groups as psychoanalytic rather than educational

or orientational, compared to similar groups at that time. Wender's method was to see groups of six to eight patients two or three times a week. Group members were of the same sex and each group meeting lasted for one hour. He also combined individual therapy with group psychotherapy and suggested that the group might represent a "family" to its members (Burnside, 1994). In 1934, Paul Schilder, at Bellevue, worked with groups using a psychoanalytic framework (Pinney, 1970). J. L. Moreno, who came to the United States from Germany in 1930, later introduced the concept of sociometry and diagramming the interactions that occur in groups (Hardy & Conway, 1978). In fact, the term "group psychotherapy" originated with Moreno (Ruitenbeck, 1970). He was the leading exponent of a treatment technique called "psychodrama" and his widow carried on the teaching of psychodrama.

Also in the 1930s, Samuel Slavson, a civil engineer, practiced group psychotherapy with children for the Jewish Board of Guardians. In 1943, he published *An Introduction to Group Therapy*. Later he was instrumental in the formation and development of the American Group Psychotherapy Association. He became the first editor of the *International Journal of Group Psychotherapy* in 1951 and was an active force in the advancement of group psychotherapy for both social work and psychiatry (Burnside, 1994). Finally, during World War II, group psychotherapy began to be used extensively as a treatment modality in military hospitals. The army psychiatrists then returned to civilian practice and applied group therapy in their own settings.

Review of the Literature

According to Toseland and Rivas (2002), group work with older persons in the United States developed in three distinct settings and occurred in settlement houses and community centers, homes for the aged, and state mental hospitals.

Since World War II, group work has become an increasingly popular form of treatment in the care of the aged—partly because it is economical. The efficacy of group treatments can be noted in the savings of the therapist's time. Therapists report savings of between 15 and 40% using groups. In any time of economic straits, with cutting back noted across the health care system, these figures become important. Moreover, according to Gotestman, Quarterman, and Cohn (1973, p. 422), "Small-group treatment can be used in both contrived settings like psychotherapy and naturalistic ones like families or communities of aged persons. This technique is valuable because it can be more naturalistic and more long lasting than individual therapy."

The literature is beginning to include more about both the benefits and the limitations of such work, but book chapters and journal articles on the topic are still widely scattered. For instance, Yalom's (1975) excellent book on group psychotherapy does not discuss psychotherapy with the aged at all, while Gwen Marram's (1973) book on the group approach in nursing only briefly describes some of the aspects of working with older people. Although there is more literature on group work itself, there is still a deficit in the literature regarding group work for and with older people. Nevertheless, the available literature does indicate that such work with older adults is conducted by a diverse occupational group, including psychiatrists, recreational, occupational, and physical therapists, social workers, psychologists, nurses, and administrators of skilled nursing facilities (Burnside, 1970). Thus, Linden (1953), a psychiatrist, pioneered group work with the aged when he co-led a group of 40 to 51 regressed women in a state hospital. In the same year, Kubie and Landau (1953) published a book about their nine years of group work in a recreation center for older people. Kaplan (1953) was one of the first social workers to write about group work with older adults, and Shere (1964), a psychologist, wrote a classic article on group work with the very old.

The trend for nurses to publish reports about their group work with the aged occurred later. The first collection of papers appeared in *Psychosocial Nursing Care of the Aged* (Burnside, 1973). During the 1970s and 1980s, types of groups for older persons included: short-term educational groups; skills-building groups; reminiscence and life-review groups; and self-help, support, and advocacy groups (Toseland, 1990). Publications on group work from the 1990s to the present are still scarce when it comes to looking at group work with older people, unless one looks to the specialty journals in gerontology. For example, in the *Journal of Gerontological Nursing*, there is a description of a psychosocial group nursing intervention for the purpose of overcoming the fear of falling (Gentleman & Malozemoff, 2001). Because older people have this fear, they restrict their own activities, leading to both social and functional decline. Although the outcomes were mixed, these authors highly recommend group work for solving some of the institutional problems of elderly people. Others report the use of groups in the community to deliver education on diabetes to older patients (Wendel, Durso, Zable, Loman, & Remsburg, 2003). Another community group was used to educate older women at a senior center about drug and alcohol use (Eliason & Skinstad, 2001). Groups provide an economical way to reach large numbers of people for educational purposes and that seems to be the most common use in this new century.

General Group Processes

Space limitations here preclude all but a few comments on interaction in groups. Kurt Lewin (1948) organized and developed field theory, which offered "a method of analyzing causal relations and building scientific constructs." His work at the University of Iowa in the 1930s and later at the Massachusetts Institute of Technology established the field of group dynamics. Group dynamics refers to the study of individuals who are interacting in small groups. Dynamics means "the motive and controlling forces, also the study of such forces" (Webster, 1976). Other terms used are "group processes," "group interaction," "group psychology," and "human relations."

Basic group process theory is explained in:

- *Groups: Facilitating Individual Growth and Societal Change*, by Walter Lifton (1972)
- *Group Processes: An Introduction to Group Dynamics*, by Joseph Luft (1963)
- *The Small Group*, by Michael Olmsted (1959)
- *The Process of Group Communication*, by Ronald Applbaum et al. (1974)
- *Groups in Social Work*, by Margaret Hartford (1972)

These works deal generally with groups, but do not include specific group work with older adults. Those interested or engaged in group psychotherapy, should consult Yalom's *The Theory and Practice of Group Psychotherapy* (1975) and Chapter 5 of this book.

Selected Principles of Group Work

The differences between group work with older adults and work with other age groups must be mentioned. In general, group work with older people involves a more direct approach (Corey & Corey, 1992). Leaders must take a more active role in giving information, answering questions, and sharing themselves with the group members. Group leaders need to provide support, encouragement, and empathy because older people often have unique problems that must be recognized and dealt with. On an emotional level, older people may be preoccupied with loss of loved ones and their own death and may refer to these topics again and again. A major objective in group work is to alleviate such anxiety by helping group members solve immediate problems. Thus, psy-

chotherapy groups for older people emphasize problem solving more than gaining insight or changing personality traits (Burnside, 1994).

Group leaders also must contend with the physical conditions of older people. The presence of people with sensory defects, for example, requires special techniques. Speaking slowly and clearly, sitting close to the members, and keeping the groups and circles small are all helpful. Assessing the energy level of each member is another important aspect of group work with older adults who often experience fatigue.

Psychological support from the leader increases group members' confidence and promotes cohesiveness. For example, group members may use their advancing age and/or illness as defenses against attending group sessions. Making meticulous contracts between leaders and members (see Chapter 7), attending to physical complaints, and personally visiting or telephoning members outside the group may help reduce the perceived need for such defensive behavior. Of course, leaders must feel comfortable with the dependency that may develop among their group members.

Group leadership can be much easier if a member-leader emerges from the group itself. Even mentally impaired older people diagnosed as having an organic brain syndrome can become helpers and try to assist the leader. The common frailty of most members in institutions has an impact on their leadership potential, and their own dependency needs preclude leadership roles for them. Nonetheless, leaders need to praise and encourage a member who demonstrates an inclination toward group leadership. This reward, in itself, can help raise the low self-esteem that so many aged people experience.

All the above principles of group work with older adults presuppose thoughtful communication among leaders and members, leaders and staffs, and leaders and families. Poor communication creates confusion, ill feelings, and lack of interest. With forgetful, confused, or disoriented older adults especially, it is crucial to communicate clearly and consistently.

Toseland (1990, p. 9) makes the important point that "groups will take on quite different dynamics if members are energetic and healthy, or if they are cognitively or physically impaired." Appropriate group membership is one of the basic reasons for carefully screening all potential group members. When screening, the leader must have the group purpose and objectives clearly in mind before selecting a group.

Common Groups and Group Methods

The varied possibilities for group work with aged persons makes it a challenging and exciting form of treatment. This introduction briefly describes current groups and group methods that are described in detail in subsequent chapters.

The following list illustrates possible types of group work. Variables affecting the types include the cognitive condition of the members, and the leaders knowledge base, skill, and profession. Examples are:

- Reality orientation
- Remotivation
- Reminiscing
  - Music (creative movement), art, and poetry
  - Bibliotherapy
  - Scribotherapy
  - Current events Family therapy
- Health teaching/educational/psychoeducational
- Group psychotherapy
- Validation therapy
- Snoezelen

These types of group work and some general information about each can be seen in **Table 3–1**.

Reality Orientation

Reality orientation (RO) groups have been very popular in the past, especially for regressed older

persons affected with dementia. A nurse and a psychologist at The Veterans Administration Hospital in Tuscaloosa, Alabama, first started these groups (Taulbee & Folsom, 1966).

Reality orientation groups were originally designed for confused, disoriented older adults but now may be more appropriate for forgetful adults to help them remain oriented. Meetings are half an hour, held daily, Monday through Friday, and led by a nursing assistant, a volunteer, or an activities coordinator. (Although regular meetings are scheduled, the reality-orienting process should be continued around the clock.) A group should not have more than four members because of the tremendous demands such a group places on the leader. A large reality orientation board is kept in the meeting room. Common information such as the weather, the date, and the next meal is posted daily. Correct information must be constantly given to the confused, disoriented older person. One way to keep the board current is to assign the upkeep to a more alert patient who would like to keep busy. It is sometimes important to reduce disorientation in the three spheres of time, place, and person. Also, proper names should be used to remind the confused members who the leader is and to confirm the member's own identity. Note that reality orientation groups are often mistakenly called reality therapy groups, but reality therapy is a specific type of psychotherapy begun by William Glasser (1965) for delinquent adolescents. (See also Chapter 13.) Because RO has been immensely popular and has garnered its share of published articles in the past, the concept is presented in detail in Chapter 13 where it is contrasted to validation therapy, a newer modality that is attracting many followers especially in Europe.

Validation Therapy

Naomi Feil (2002) pioneered validation therapy between 1963 and 1980. It can be administered individually or in groups. Based on Erikson's theory of the ages of man, validation teaches those

Table 3–1 Levels of Group Work with Older Adults

Group modality	Number of members	Type of leader	Length of meeting	Props useful	Refreshments
Reality orientation	4	Nurses' aide with special training	As tolerated: 15 or 30 minutes to 1 hour	Yes	Yes
Remotivation	12–14	Student, nurses' aide, or psychiatric technician with special training	1 hour	Yes	No (according to founder of remotivation therapy)
Validation therapy	6–8	Worker with training	30 minutes to 1 hour	No	Optional
Snoezzelen	2	Worker with training	1 hour	Yes	Yes
Reminiscence	6–8	Activity director, psychologist, nurses' aide, bibliotherapist, nurse, occupational therapist, social worker, or student volunteer	1–1 ½ hours	Yes	Yes
Art	4–6	Artist or art major	1 hour	Yes	Optional
Music	6–8 (or a very large group)	Musician or a person who is musically talented	1 hour	Yes	Optional
Poetry	6–8	Poet or teacher of poetry	1 hour	Yes	Optional
Bibliotherapy	6–8 (if frail aged); otherwise, 10–12	Librarian, volunteer	1 hour	Yes	Optional
Health teaching	Variable	Health-related professional, nurse, health educator	1 hour	Optional	Optional
Psychotherapy	6–8	Psychiatric nurse, psychiatric social worker, psychologist, psychiatrist, certified counselor	1 hour or 2 times weekly	No	Usually no

who care for disoriented old people to understand their behaviors. Feil categorizes these behaviors in successive stages. Stage one, malorientation, is characterized by confabulation and defensive behavior. Stage two is time confusion, which presents as a lack of awareness of the time, the day, or even the month. Stage 3 is known as repetitive motion where the victim is inner focused and totally unaware of others. Finally, stage 4 is the vegetative stage when motion is essentially stopped, eyes are closed, and the end is near. Feil

offers interventions and communication skills for each of these stages. First and foremost the caregiver must accept the beliefs, values, and reality of the person with dementia while gently redirecting their behavior. Many nursing home workers see this validation intervention as more appropriate for advanced dementia patients than reality orientation (Feil & deKlerk-Rubin, 2003).

For many years validation therapy has been criticized because the theory and interventions are not research based but are observational and adopted without proof of effectiveness. Recently there have been studies examining the impact of validation therapy (Toseland, Diehl, Freeman, Naleppa, & McCallion, 1997) that improve its credibility. Others are writing of its positive impact in nursing homes (Touzinsky, 1998; Woodrow, 1998).

Snoezelen

Snoezelen is a multisensory intervention, started in the Netherlands, which is presently capturing the imagination of caregivers working with folks who manifest advanced dementia. Originally, Snoezelen was used to provide a relaxing experience to profoundly disadvantaged children. The term Snoezelen is based on two Dutch words meaning "to sniff" and "to doze" and has recently been trademarked by Rompa, a company selling high-tech equipment. The purpose of Snoezelen in dementia settings is to entertain the bored dementia patient and to provide a relaxing experience. Snoezelen is designed to stimulate the primary senses of sight, hearing, touch, taste, and smell, using high-tech equipment in a white room known as a Snoezelen room.

Hulsegge and Verheul (1986) developed Snoezelen in 1975. Snoezelen rooms for older people were initiated in the Netherlands in the early 1980s. Researchers began to test it as a group intervention in the 1990s for older adults with dementia. Bryant (1991) compared four different activity groups with a Snoezelen group. All groups, including the Snoezelen group, decreased wandering and anxiety and improved mood and behavior. Additional research shows great promise for this group intervention. The Snoezelen process reduces agitation (Pinkney, 1997), increases psychological well-being (Witucki & Twibell, 1997), and encourages better relationships between staff and patients while preventing burnout in staff (Morrissey, 1997). Additionally, those patients participating in Snoezelen groups did not deteriorate as quickly as their peers

(Baker, Dowling, Wareing, Dawson, & Assey, 1997). The Snoezelen group intervention is widespread in Europe with more than 2000 Snoezelen rooms in use, even though it is just becoming recognized and implemented in the United States.

Remotivation Therapy

Another used group modality is remotivation. The focus of remotivation therapy is on simple, objective aspects of day-to-day living for older people who have been isolated and dependent. The leader arranges a very structured classroom setting with props and tries to get the patients to discuss their experiences in regard to a specific topic. As patients in remotivation groups are helped toward resocialization, they begin to converse and ask questions after not having spoken for several years. They also begin to ambulate and feed themselves, and to ask for bathroom assistance after long periods of incontinence. The model of the remotivation technique and its application to the mentally ill originated with Dorothy Hoskins Smith, an English literature teacher from Claremont College, in California. She trained a large group of personnel at the Philadelphia State Hospital in 1956. Because this treatment method was developed in a state hospital for use with mental patients, adaptations are necessary if it is to be used with older persons in other settings (Burnside, 1994).

Although many remotivation groups seem to have been successful, such groups do have drawbacks. There are several reasons that remotivation groups may lack appeal and challenge for the leader: They do not (1) explore feelings; (2) permit the leader to touch the members; (3) focus on leisure, but rather are based on the "work world" (which is fine for young institutionalized persons but is unrealistic for very old persons who are in extended care or intermediate care facilities or even boarding homes); (4) do not allow for much spontaneity or originality in leadership; and (5) they do not permit refreshments to be served. All these characteristics violate the generally accepted principles and philosophy so vital to group work with the aged. It seems especially inappropriate for an older group to have the work world as part of its focus—that implies being a producer. To old people who no longer work, it is a reminder that they not only cannot produce but may also be in a quite dependent role. That remotivation groups were launched in a state hospital has influenced the model. We need new and different models for individuals in extended care facilities and perhaps for community residents as well.

Reminiscence Groups

The power and the typology of the past and present are emerging as reminiscence therapy enters its fourth decade as a treatment modality. The reminiscence therapy group is one of the most widely used therapeutic modalities for older persons, and the literature is on the increase. One of the differences between reminiscence groups and traditional group therapy models is that reminiscence groups are more theme-oriented in the past than traditional models. Reminiscence groups are designed to explore memories with a group of six or eight older persons, meeting in either an institutional or a noninstitutional setting. Meetings are held once or twice weekly, according to the leader's and the group's wishes, for approximately one hour. The leader encourages the sharing of memories that run the gamut from happy to sad, carefree to somber, including all stages of life. Many subjects can be discussed in a reminiscence group—holidays, birthdays, major events, families, geographical places, travel, and modes of transportation, and so on. Reminiscence groups are enjoyable for both leader and patients and many authors report therapeutic results (Haight & Webster, 1995; Webster & Haight, 2002). Because reminiscence therapy (RT) is so important as a treatment modality with the aged population, a chapter in this text is devoted to RT (see Chapter 14).

Topic-specific Groups

MUSIC GROUPS

Music groups can accommodate a large number of members and can be led by a registered music therapist or a musically talented person with leadership skills. A solid base in gerontology is needed. Some leaders also incorporate creative movement into their music groups. Many types of groups incorporate appropriate music into their meetings. The type of music group—whether sing-along, listening group, instrumental group, or any other—depends on several factors: available space for meetings; available musical instruments; talent of the leader, members, staff personnel, and family members; and budget for sheet music, rental or purchase of instruments, and so on.

It is not the primary goal of music groups to teach music per se. The goals can vary; common ones are to improve the quality and enjoyment of daily living, to increase body movement, to reach withdrawn members, to provide props in group work, to increase or enhance reminiscing within the group through music, and to increase feelings of relatedness to cohorts through familiar music.

ART THERAPY AND POETRY GROUPS

Art therapy and poetry groups are highly recommended and are increasingly popular with older people. Chapter 16 describes similarly creative groups, which might be used with older people.

BIBLIOTHERAPY

Bibliotherapy is a special form of therapy that can be done individually or in a group. It uses reading aloud as a therapeutic approach to problems and problem solving.

SCRIBOTHERAPY

Scribotherapy, derived from the Latin *scribo*, which means to write, is "writing therapy." The benefits of scribotherapy include:
- A chance for self-expression
- The enhancement of self-esteem

- The encouragement of reminiscence
- An increase in social interaction

Autobiographical writing groups are one type of scribotherapy, and their process is fully described in Chapter 15.

Health-related Groups

Health-related groups are often conducted at nutrition centers, retirement homes, aging centers, and assisted-living communities. Trained persons from a variety of disciplines lead them. A podiatrist might teach foot care, a dentist might teach dental care, a cardiologist might teach about heart problems, and a nurse or health educator may coordinate the group. Older people do need more information about such things as glaucoma, cataracts, hearing problems, diabetes, arthritis, strokes, organic brain syndrome, and sexuality and aging. These groups can be organized as large, formal classes with a lecture approach, or they can be small and informal discussion groups. Although few kinds of groups for older people lend themselves to being large, health-related groups can be larger than most other groups because of their educational nature. Regardless of size or subject matter, prevention should be a recurring theme in any health-related group.

Member-specific Groups

GRIEVING

Some groups use grief as the common denominator for membership. Such groups can be especially beneficial for the older but recently widowed, many of whom may have little or no preparation for the widow role. These groups are often conducted in high-cost or low-cost housing units, senior citizen centers, extended care facilities, day care centers, and in the community. Many funeral homes offer grieving groups and advice for widows, and their connection with the grieving family makes this venue ideal.

The leader who chooses to conduct a group of recently widowed older women must have much patience and empathy. The leader must be able to listen openly and not judgmentally and should discourage verbalizations of "I can top that" (that is, descriptions of the most tragic suffering or demise). The leader must also be aware of the pacing necessary for widow groups and not attempt to accelerate the process of grief work. Important decision making should be held to a minimum, and here other members as well as the leader can be helpful. Chapter 19 offers greater insight into the process of death, dying, and grieving.

Groups for Family Members

Group work with family members may be initiated for a variety of reasons. Family group work:

- Reduces hostility, anxiety, and guilt feelings of the family
- Orients the family to nursing home life
- Educates the family about the aging process or about the pathological processes occurring
- Encourages family interest in the progress of the relative
- Reduces family conflicts detrimental to the aged person
- Provides care givers of dementia patients with insight and support.

Administrators of nursing homes, chaplains, nurses, social workers, or psychologists often conduct such family groups.

Establishing a group experience for family members can provide an opportunity for catharsis and can help them: identify incongruencies, realign their expectations with the aged member's present level of functioning, and focus on the potential for future rehabilitation and change. Also, group work with families of newly institutionalized older people can be therapeutic for the expression of guilt feelings and anticipatory grief. Such groups can be particularly helpful when those family members also are elderly. Parent and child may both be aged, but we are not accustomed to thinking of old children. An incident that occurred in a state hospital illustrates this. A very confused old man kept saying that he was going on pass for the weekend with his mother. As he was so old, the staff did not believe him until Friday afternoon, when a spry old lady in her nineties drove up to take her son home (Stange, 1973).

Age-specific Groups

There are four cohorts between 60 and 100 and each cohort group has had a different existence with different experiences, thus similar age specific groups will guarantee groups with like experiences to share.

As life experiences are shared, empathic listening increases both the cohesion and the desirability of the group. Burnside (1994) once grouped six nonagenarians for an evening meal each week. The frailties of the group made it a difficult one to lead. However, one day a woman wheeled herself into the office and stated, "Today I'm 90! Where is that group that I'm now eligible to join?" The elite character of the aged group had not dawned on the leaders until she asked to join it.

Conversely, leaders who choose to work with intergenerational groups will need to have a solid knowledge base in developmental tasks across the life span as well as a familiarity with the history each person has witnessed. Leaders of such groups must understand changes in puberty, young adulthood, midlife, and later years. Always when there are older persons in a group, the leader must be sensitive to the developmental tasks of later life. Handling sensory loss, sad themes of personal loss, and increasing illness or frailty are a few of the responsibilities inherent in the leadership role. Leaders of intergenerational groups might be from the disciplines of nursing, psychiatry, psychology, social work, or theology. Group methodology might depend on: the leader's style, philosophy, training, and experience; the ages of the group members; and the size and disabilities of the group.

Psychotherapy Groups

Group psychotherapy is often the preferred treatment for older psychotic patients because it is the more effective and economic use of the therapist's time. There are benefits for the aged person too. Supportive psychotherapy with aged patients is best carried out in a group context. The group experience enhances a sense of belonging, an appreciation for the value of external sources of satisfaction, and the effectiveness of reality testing. Reality testing in a group context is an important component in therapy, as was mentioned earlier in this chapter regarding reality orientation groups. Rationales for group therapy with older adults can be found in **Table 3–2**.

Group therapy is also the treatment of choice for the nonpsychotic elderly who are experiencing difficulty adjusting to loss. Groups offer a number of advantages for the older person: they decrease the sense of isolation, facilitate the development of new roles or the reestablishment of familiar roles, provide information on a variety of topics from other group members, and afford group support for effecting change or enhancing self-esteem.

Table 3–2 RATIONALES FOR GROUP THERAPY FOR OLDER ADULTS

1. Frequent later-life presenting problems
2. Reduce social isolation, depression, loneliness
3. Reduce feelings of inadequacy
4. Change sense of anonymity
5. Opportunity for camaraderie
6. Opportunity for social exercise
7. Opportunity for meaningful interpersonal interactions
8. Forum for personal feedback
9. Work through unresolved conflicts
10. Transference is "divided"; not as intense as in standard psychotherapy
11. Offer cognitive stimulation
12. Offer emotional responsiveness
13. Reduce feeling of being rejected by family
14. Offer almost immediate relief

There are two major obstacles to outpatient group therapy: transportation (particularly during the winter), and economics. Paradoxically, though group therapy is less costly than individual psychotherapy, its longer-term nature means additional cost as well as additional benefit. Medicare limitations particularly deter those of modest means. Clergy, nurses, psychiatrists, psychologists, and social workers all conduct therapy groups. Because there are so few geropsychiatric nurses, the leaders are usually psychiatric nurses. Chapter 18 describes in detail various methods of group psychotherapy.

Contraindications for Group Work

Although group work may be therapeutic for many older clients, remember that it is not appropriate for everyone, and it also involves some possibility of risk. It is especially inappropriate for persons who are so preoccupied and overwhelmed by their own problems that they are unable to listen or respond to other people. Some people are so concerned about their privacy that they will not be able to discuss personal matters in a group meeting. Extremely disoriented people may be detrimental in the functioning of a group. It is important to consider the mix of the group members as well as the goal of the group.

A very skillful leader will be able to handle some categories of participants that might overwhelm a neophyte group leader. Some of the categories are: disturbed or very active wandering persons, incontinent adults, those with psychotic depression, members recommended solely by the staff, bipolar individuals, very deaf persons, and hypochondriacal persons. Pronounced hostility due to paranoia or schizophrenia can be detrimental to a group. Also consider again the practical and economic limitations previously discussed.

Older people who are inappropriate for groups do know that about themselves. If older persons adamantly refuse to join a group, it is better not to coax them to join. If there is severe pathology and a low frustration level, it may create too much stress for the older person to be in a group. This is especially true if there is an expectation regarding responses, interactions, relationships, or competition for the time of the leader.

Summary

This chapter presents a brief history of group work with the aged and an overview of current group work. Since World War II, group work with older adults has become increasingly popular—partly because it is economical. Group work with the aged is more directive than group work with other age groups. Because older adults often have special emotional and physical problems, leaders need to provide much encouragement and empathy. Groups provide psychological support for their members and focus on ego enhancement rather than confrontation. A cardinal principle of such group work is careful and effective communication between leaders and members, leaders and staffs, and leaders and families.

There are a variety of types and levels of group work: reality orientation, remotivation, Snoezelen, reminiscence (which may include art, poetry, creative and autobiographical writing, and music), and group psychotherapy. These levels also indicate the knowledge, skill, and experience needed by the leader. See Table 3–1 for a more detailed explanation of the levels of groups.

The research to date indicates that a variety of disciplines conduct groups. The techniques and approaches are of a wide range—from very basic reality orientation group work to sophisticated psychotherapy. However, gaps in knowledge do remain regarding groups and their effectiveness.

Exercises

EXERCISE 1

Prepare a list of types of group work with the aged, indicating the important publications pertaining to each type. List chronologically the important articles about group work you have read. Study the list, and write one thoughtful page on each of the following:

1. A classic book or article that influenced subsequent group work with older clients. Your answer should include:
   a. Complete documentation of the book or article
   b. Whether it was a pioneering effort
   c. How you think it influenced subsequent group work
   d. A description of the leadership style
2. A discipline that has influenced group work (selected from your readings of the literature). Give reasons why.
3. The aspects of group work that are not covered in the literature. Select one or two readings and state the missing aspect in each. This missing aspect can be based upon your own group work with older adults, or it can be an omission you have discerned in your reading of the literature.

EXERCISE 2

To test your understanding of the cognitive ability and the physical and emotional requirements necessary for group participation, write a one-paragraph description of a person you would place in each of the following groups. For each individual, state cognitive level, physical abilities, and emotional requirements.

- Reality orientation group
- Remotivation group
- Reminiscence group
- Music group
- Art therapy or poetry group
- Health-related group
- Member-specific group
- Psychotherapy group

EXERCISE 3

You are about to implement an age-specific group for centenarians. Write your goals and objectives for the group.

References

Applbaum, R., Bodaken, E., Sereno, K., & Anatol, K. (1974). *The process of group communication*. Chicago: Science Research Associates.

Baker, R., Dowling, Z., Wareing, L., Dawson, J., & Assey, J. (1997). Snoezelen: Its long term and short term effects on older people with dementia. *British Journal of Occupational Therapy*, 60(5) 213–218.

Bryant, W. (1991). Creative group work with confused older people: A development of sensory integration therapy. *British Journal of Occupational Therapy*, 54(5), 187–192.

Burnside, I.M. (1970). Group work with the aged: Selected literature. Part 1. *The Gerontologist,* 10(3), 141–246.

Burnside, I. M. (1973). Long-term group work with hospitalized aged. In I. M. Burnside (Ed.), *Psychosocial nursing care of the aged* (1st ed. pp. 202–214). New York: McGraw-Hill.

Burnside, I. M. (1975, June). *Overview of group work with the elderly.* Paper presented at Nursing Symposium, Tenth International Congress of Gerontology, Jerusalem, Israel.

Burnside, I. M. (1994). *Working with older adults: Group processes and techniques*. Boston: Jones & Bartlett.

Corey, G., & Corey, M. (1992). Groups for the elderly. In G. Corey, & M. Corey (Eds.), *Groups: Process and practice* (pp. 399–430). Monterey, CA: Brooks/Cole.

Eliason, M., & Skinstad, A. (2001). Drug and alcohol intervention for older women: A pilot study. *Journal of Gerontological Nursing*, 27(12), 18–24.

Feil, N. (2002). *The validation breakthrough: Simple techniques for communicating with people with Alzheimer's-type dementia*. Baltimore: Health Professions Press.

Feil, N., & deKlerk-Rubin, V. (2003). *V/F Validation: The Feil method*. Cleveland, OH: Edward Feil Productions.

Gentleman, B., & Malozemoff, W. (2001). Falls and feelings: Description of a psychosocial group nursing intervention. *Journal of Gerontological Nursing*, 27(10), 35–39.

Glasser, W. (1965). *Reality therapy: A new approach to psychiatry*. New York: Harper & Row.

Gottestam, K., Quarterman, C., Cohn, G. (1973). Psychosocial treatment of the aged. In M. Lawton & C. Eisdorfer (Eds.), *The psychology of adult development and Aging*. Washington, DC: American Psychological Association.

Haight, B., & Webster, J. D. (Eds.). (1995). *The art and science of reminiscing: Theory, research, methods and applications*. Washington, DC: Taylor & Francis.

Hardy, M., & Conway, M. (1978). *Role theory*. New York: Appleton-Century-Crofts.

Hartford, M. (1972). *Groups in social work*. New York: Columbia University Press.

Hulsegge, J. & Verheul, A. (1987). *Snoezelen: Another world*. Chesterfield, UK: Rompa.

Kaplan, J. (1953). *A social program for older people*. Minneapolis: University of Minnesota Press.

Kubie, S., & Landau, G. (1953). *Group work with the aged*. New York: International Universities Press.

Lewin, K. (1948). *Resolving social conflicts: Selected papers on group dynamics*. New York: Harper & Row.

Lifton, W. (1972). *Groups: Facilitating individual growth and societal change*. Nework: Wiley.

Linden, M. (1953). Group psychotherapy with institutionalized senile women: Study in gerontological human relations. *International Journal of Group Psychotherapy*, 3, 150–170.

Luft, J. (1963). *Group process: An introduction to group dynamics*. Palo Alto, CA: National Press.

Marram, G. (1973). *The group approach in nursing practice*. St. Louis: Mosby.

Morrissey, M. (1997). Snoezelen: Benefits for nursing older clients. *Nursing Standard*, 12(3), 38–40.

Olmstead, M. (1959). *The small group*. New York: Random House.

Pinckney, L. (1997). A comparison of the Snoezelen environment and a music relaxation group on the mood and behavior of patients with senile dementia. *British Journal of Occupational Therapy*, 60(5), 209–212.

Pinney, E. (1970). *A first group psychotherapy book*. Springfield, IL: Thomas.

Ruitenbeck, H. (1970). *The new group therapies*. New York: Avon.

Shere, E. (1964). Group therapy with the very old. In R. Kastenbaum (Ed.), *New thoughts on old age*. New York: Springer, 140–160.

Stange, A. (1973). Around the kitchen table: Group work on a back ward. In I. M .Burnside (Ed.), *Psychosocial nursing care of the aged* (1st ed. pp. 174–186). New York: McGraw-Hill.

Taulbee, L., & Folsom, J. (1966). Reality orientation for geriatric patients. *Hospital Community Psychotherapy*, 17(5) 133–135.

Toseland, R. (1990). *Group work with older adults*. New York: New York University Press.

Toseland, R., & Rivas, R. (2002). *An introduction to group work practice* (4th ed.). Boston: Allyn & Bacon.

Toseland, R., Diehl, M., Freeman, K., Naleppa, M., & McCallion, P. (1997). The impact of validation group therapy on nursing home residents with dementia. *Journal of Applied Gerontology*, 16(1), 31–50.

Touzinsky, L. (1998). Validation method: Restoring communication between persons with Alzheimer's disease and their families. *American Journal of Alzheimer's Disease*, 13(2), 96–102.

Webster's new twentieth century dictionary. (1976). New York: Collins & World.

Webster, J., & Haight, B. (Eds.). (2000). *Critical advances in reminiscence work: From theory to application*. New York: Springer.

Wendel, I., Durso, S., Zable, B., Loman, K., & Remsburg, R. (2003). Group diabetes patient education: A model for use in a continuing care retirement community. *Journal of Gerontological Nursing*, 29(2), 37–45.

Witucki, J., & Twibell, R. (1997). The effect of sensory stimulation activities on the psychological well being of patients with advanced Alzheimer's disease. *American Journal of Alzheimer's Disease*, 12(1), 10–15.

Woodrow, P, (1998). Interventions for confusion and dementia, part 4: Alternative approaches (validation method, resolution therapy, and multisensory environments). *British Journal of Nursing*, 12(20), 1247–50.

Yalom, I. D. (1975). *The theory and practice of group psychotherapy* (2d ed.). New York: Basic Books.

BIBLIOGRAPHY

Burnside, I. M. (1969a). Group work among the aged. *Nursing Outlook*, 17(6), 68–72.

Burnside, I. M. (1969b). Sensory stimulation: An adjunct to group works with the disabled aged. *Mental Hygiene*, 33(3), 331–388.

Burnside, I. M. (1971). Long-term group work with the hospitalized aged. Part 1. *The Gerontologist*, 11(3), 213–218.

Burnside, I. M. (1976). Overview of group work with the aged. *Journal of Gerontological Nursing*, 2(6), 14–17.

Rose, S. R. (1991). Small group processes and interventions with the elderly. In P. K. H. Kim (Ed.), *Serving the elderly: Skills for practice* (pp. 167–186). New York: Aldine de Gruyter.

Chapter 4

Principles of Linden

Molly Ranney
Irene Burnside

Key Words

- A good reality
- Catalytic
- Contract
- Cotherapist
- Cotherapy
- Dual leadership
- Group psychotherapy
- Psychotic
- Regressed

Learning Objectives

- Discuss Maurice Linden's pioneer research in group psychotherapy
- List five outcomes of therapeutic intervention in groups
- Compare and contrast the group led by Burnside with the one led by Linden
- Define *dual leadership*
- Discuss five considerations in the development of a contract between cotherapists
- List four indicators that a group leader may need supervision
- Write six questions coleaders might ask one another before beginning cotherapy

The therapist's mode of managing . . . is to create out of himself, out of the treatment situation, and out of the group a "good" reality

—*Maurice Linden (1955, p. 64)*

Maurice Linden was one of the early presidents of the American Group Psychotherapy Association and pioneered the use of group therapy with older mentally ill patients (Burnside, 1994). Linden died in 1984, but he left a rich legacy to group leaders who work with older clients.

Beginning leaders of groups of older adults often think that they have discovered new principles of group work. However, a thorough search of the literature in different disciplines would reveal that many of the dynamics of group work have already been discovered, refined, and published. Linden's (1953, 1954, 1955) articles on his group psychotherapy with older women in a state hospital are classic examples of this early work. Also, Toseland (1995) cited Kaplan (1953), Konopka (1954), Kubie and Landau (1953), Shore (1952), and Vickery (1952) as being other classic examples that may help the reader.

Although Linden's articles were written many years ago, his techniques are relevant. All that dates the articles is his frequent use of the term *senile*, which gerontologists no longer use. In fact,

Linden (1955) in a paper cautioned against promiscuous use of the term. The articles are still recommended reading for group leaders working with older adults with mental illness (especially those who have psychoses or neuroses). This chapter discusses a number of principles derived from Linden's articles that are applicable to group work with older adults in geropsychiatric units, partial hospitalization programs, and or adult day care centers. Besides Linden, Toseland's (1995) book, *Group Work with the Elderly*, provides an overview of the theoretical issues that are unique to older adults, and it is also recommended to the reader.

Principles of Group Psychotherapy

Linden's (1953) first article, *"Group psychotherapy with institutionalized senile women: Study in gerontologic human relations,"* contained several statements that are relevant to group work with older adults.

1. "Modification of behavior does occur in group work with older adults" (p. 152). Because the modification in the behavior of older adults may be slow in appearing, leaders may fail to realize the impact of their leadership and the catalytic quality of the group. It is important that leaders are patient and realize that evidence of therapeutic change takes time in group work.

2. "Hospital discharges alone do not reflect the actual degree of response to therapy" (p. 153). This point is especially important to remember in group work with regressed older adults. This is because the leader may become discouraged by the seemingly insignificant changes. Also, clients often perceive behavior changes that seem small to the leader as life changing. For example, Linden discusses the fact that most of the women paid more attention to their hygiene once they began attending the group. While this may seem minor, it can be life changing for the client. With so much stigma shown towards people with a mental illness in our society, helping those affected with their appearance typically results in them being treated better by others.

3. Four important areas to evaluate in group work with older adults are mood, alertness, memory, and orientation (p. 154). For example, members with memory impairment can become very agitated with slight changes in their routine. If mood is routinely assessed, the leader should be prepared to handle the agitation in the group.

4. Therapeutic intervention assists in the "resolution of depressive affects, increases alertness, diminishes confusion, improves orientation, and replenishes memory hiati, all this being reflected in bettering of the many minute factors inherent in ward socialization" (p. 154). Life in an inpatient unit can be very depressing for patients. While there have been many reforms made to improve the quality of care for mentally ill people, being hospitalized is still by and large an unpleasant experience. Linden's quote is an important reminder that providing group work is one way to improve the quality of care for older adults in an inpatient unit.

5. Senility "is the logical culmination of the combined social rejection of the late mature person and the senescent person's self-rejection" (p. 154). Unfortunately, we have done little to banish the pejorative word *senility* and to raise the self-esteem of older adults. Ageism is still very prevalent in our society. More work needs to be done to reach out to isolated and disaffected older adults in our society.

All of these statements are as relevant for group work today in geropsychiatric units, partial hospitalization programs, and adult day care centers as they were for Linden's state hospital residents. Burnside (1994) compared and contrasted Linden's group of aged women and a group she led alone for 14 months in a mental facility. The group consisted of six persons, three men and three women, all of whom were diagnosed as having chronic brain syndrome. **Tables** 4–1 through 4–4 show the results of the analysis. Although Linden's group was much larger, the similarities are obvious.

We have certainly benefited, as have many others, from Linden's writings and philosophy about older adults. His courage in leading groups of women with dementia in a state hospital has inspired others to work with such individuals. For the fact that Linden successfully led a group of 40 women, one must admire him. As with all group work models, leaders have to adapt the techniques so that they are congruent with their style. For

Table 4–1 POSITIVE AND NEGATIVE CRITERIA USED BY LINDEN AND BURNSIDE FOR ADMITTANCE TO GROUPS

Positive criteria used by Linden (after Slavson)	Positive criteria used by Burnside (compared with Linden's)
Expressed desire to join the group	Given choice; could attend and leave later if wanted to
Appearance of relative alertness	No
A fair degree of good personal hygiene	Not considered
Ability to understand English	Same
Ability to walk or to be wheeled to the meeting	Same
At least a minimal range of emotions	No
Evidence of some degree of adult adjustment prior to entrance into senile state	Unable to secure data to assess
Capacity for evoking interest and affection from nursing and attendant personnel	Not considered
Sardonic hostility	Not considered
Negative criteria used by Linden	**Negative criteria used by Burnside**
Dementia	All diagnosed chronic brain syndrome or "senile"
Advanced physical debility	Accepted many
Systematized and chronic paranoia throughout life	Did not apply
Manic behavior	Did not apply
Intense chronic hostility with assaultiveness	Same
Unremitting bowel and bladder incontinence	Same
Advanced deafness	Accepted one very deaf woman
Monothematic hypochondriasis	Did not apply
Undirected restlessness with inability to sit still	Same
Unwillingness to participate	Same
Inability to understand English	Same

Source: Burnside, 1994, p. 43.

Table 4-2   Characteristics of Linden's and Burnside's Group Members

Linden	Burnside
Mean = 70 (mode = 69). Three persons < 60; one member aged 89 at group's beginning	Mean = 79 (mode = 79), age range 64–82 years. No member < 60; one man aged 90 at group's end
All were women	Both men and women
All were institutionalized	All confined to nursing homes or light mental facilities from 2 weeks to 10 years
All had needs inherent in pathological later maturity	Severe physical disabilities plus mental problems, mostly depression
All had same kind of care and daily experiences, as environmental factors could be fairly well controlled	Same
Diagnoses	**Diagnoses**
Psychosis with cerebral arteriosclerosis: alcoholism with	Male, 68: postfracture, right hip; ASCVD[1];
12 Involutional psychosis: 8 Schizophrenia: 6	secondary OBS[2]
Senile psychosis: 5 Paranoid condition: 4	Female, 82: ASCVD with CBS[3]; postfracture, right hip
Senile dementia: 3 Character neurosis: 2	with prosthesis; neurofibroma of scalp
Psychosis with intracranial neoplasm: 2 (operated) secondary	Male, 64: CBS associated with arteriosclerosis; polyneuritis
Psychoneurosis: 1 Huntington's chorea: 1	Female, 79: ASCVD with associated CBS
	Female, 81: ASCVD with associated CBS
	Male, 80: CBS due to arteriosclerosis; CNS[4] lues; blindness; anemia

[1]*arteriosclerotic cardiovascular disease;* [2]*organic brain syndrome;* [3]*chronic brain syndrome;* [4]*central nervous system disorder (syphilis).*
Source: Burnside, 1994.

example, many leaders would not feel comfortable using the sarcasm that Linden (1953) described, but may be comfortable using some humor.

Dual Leadership

Linden's (1954) second article was titled "The significance of dual leadership in gerontologic group psychotherapy: Studies in gerontologic human relations III." In this article, he used the term *dual leadership* to describe what is currently called *coleadership*, although his definition refers to male and female leaders. The female leader in this instance was a registered nurse, and one can only wish that she too had written about her coleadership experience. About the first six months of the group work, before the nurse became his coleader, he wrote, "The temptation to give up the group as an unsuccessful experiment was very strong" (p. 265). The true challenge of being a group leader is conveyed in Linden's statement. New leaders are often impatient and may be tempted to give up their group as an unsuccessful venture. They, and even experienced group leaders, can learn from Linden's perseverance and leadership skills.

Table 4–3   Types of Groups Led by Linden and Burnside

Group characteristics	Linden	Burnside
Physical setting	Day hall	Half of dining room (folding door shut)
Number asked to join	25	6
Number later attending	40	6
Type of group	Open	Closed
Time of meetings	Twice weekly (1 hour)	Once weekly (45 minutes to 1 hour)
Duration of group	2 years	14 months
Group arrangement	Semicircles before table in tastefully decorated room	Close circle; round table
Visitors welcomed (catalytic effect on group)	Yes	Yes
Staff in other disciplines visited	Yes	Never, although invited; used as a teaching group for students from many disciplines represented among students
Group leader	Male ward psychiatrist	Psychiatric nurse (a volunteer)
Coleader	In 6 months, ward nurse	None
Auxiliary leaders emerged	Yes	No
Formal approach	Yes	No
Rules	No violence or physical acting out; confidentiality	Basically none

Source: Burnside, 1994.

Seating of Coleaders

Another point of interest in Linden's (1954) article is the seating of the coleaders during the meetings. They sat side by side at a central table (see Chapter 9, Figure 9–2a, for an example of this type of seating). Although the older women in the group certainly must have been impressed with the importance of the nurse because she sat so close to the authority figure on that ward, the arrangement leaves one wondering about communication between the leaders.

Most group leaders find that sitting across from each other is most effective for continual group assessment, eye contact, and nonverbal messages (Burnside, 1994; Toseland, 1995). The patient sitting next to the therapists can also be more easily and quickly assessed for mood, group participation, anxiety, and nonverbal cues than those seated further away. This arrangement is also helpful when there are several members with hearing impairments in the group (Toseland, 1995). It is also helpful when there are monopolizers because it better enables the leaders to use nonverbal gestures to redirect the group (Toseland, 1995).

One of the main advantages of coleadership in groups of older adults is that there is someone to take over during the times when one feels bogged down, bored, or unable to fulfill the commitments of the original contract with the group. Linden (1954) stated:

It is a common experience among organizers of gerontologic groups, formed for whatever

Table 4–4   PROGRESS IN LINDEN'S AND BURNSIDE'S GROUPS

Areas of progress	Linden	Burnside
In the beginning, group quiet	Yes	Yes
Gripe sessions	Yes	No
Deft, good-humored sarcasm	Yes	Never used; leader's role supportive; always took ego-enhancing stance (staff provided sarcasm)
Leaders patient and persevering	Yes	Yes
Welcomed any amount of complaining	Yes	Members rarely complained; often denied problems
Change in morale throughout building	Yes	Did not occur; interest in classes, groups began; reminiscence groups started later by licensed vocational nurse and activity directors
Strong affectional ties between group members	Yes	Yes
Group identity evolved	Yes	Yes
Cliques of patients formed	Yes	No
Saving things to tell the leader	Yes	Rarely
Improved personal appearances	Yes	Yes (perhaps partly due to the fierce pride the aides had in their assigned residents)
Both leaders complimented	Yes	Leader always responded
Method of group approach at one time or another "opportunistic group therapy"	Yes	Yes
Every opportunity for fun and laughter exploited to the fullest	Yes	Yes
Mutual support and protectiveness	Yes	Yes
Benefits through group dynamics other than verbal participation	Yes	Yes

Source: Burnside, 1994.

purpose, that it is difficult to obtain a group *esprit* with aged people.... The elements characteristic of senility of vacillating amnesia, capricious disorientation, and variable confusion which may have presented an insurmountable obstacle to therapy were partially overcome by two factors: the spacing and frequency of the sessions and dual leadership. The first gave the group a predictable, routinized, serial continuity generating a rhythmic expectation in the participants. This allowed them to bind other realities as well to space-time guideposts (pp. 266–267).

Linden's second factor, dual leadership, reinforces the first factor. The primary (i.e., Linden) therapist frequently had to miss meetings; then the nurse led the group. She was a benevolent authority on the ward, so she was a supportive and therapeutic factor in the interim between meetings. However, Linden's dual leadership evolved out of necessity rather than preplanning. See Chapter 9 for more on coleadership.

Summary

This chapter discusses salient points made by Maurice Linden, one of the pioneers in group psychotherapy with older adults. His writings are now classic and should be read by all those who intend to work with older adults with mental health diagnoses. According to Linden, the emphasis in gerontological group psychotherapy should be on resocializing the individual and should promote tranquility, a chance for happiness, and a return to some self-sufficiency. An intelligent system of care and group management can help to decrease defenses and stimulate the return of object interest.

Coleadership is termed *dual leadership* by Linden (1954). The coleader played an important role in Linden's work. The reader is referred to Figures 9–1 and 9–2 to contrast usual seating arrangements with that of Linden and his coleader.

Linden "introduced directive techniques into analytic practice, an innovation necessitated by the functional capacity of patients" (Tross & Blum, 1983, p. 5). It seems appropriate to end a chapter about Linden's (1995) work with a repetition of his excellent admonition for all group leaders working with older adults: The leader's focus should be to "create a 'good' reality" for and from the group (p. 64).

Exercises

EXERCISE 1

Describe how you think Linden or the nurse coleader went about accomplishing "a good reality" out of themselves and the treatment situation in the groups they led.

EXERCISE 2

List "directive techniques" Linden introduced into his group work with members in a state hospital.

EXERCISE 3

Linden's own therapeutic style was to use sarcasm as a way to introduce humor into the group. Describe your own therapeutic style and relate it to Linden's.

EXERCISE 4

Describe what your future goals for group work are and relate them to Linden's work.

References

Burnside, I. (1994). Principles of Linden. In I. Burnside, & M. Schmidt (Eds.), *Working with older adults: Group process and techniques* (3rd ed. pp. 41–46). Boston: Jones & Bartlett.

Kaplan, J. (1953). *A social program for older people.* Minneapolis: University of Minnesota Press.

Konopka, G. (1954). Social group work in institutions for the aged. In G. Konopka (Ed.), *Group work in the institution: A modern challenge* (pp. 276–285). New York: Whiteside & Morrow.

Kubie, S., & Landau, G. (1953). *Group work with the aged.* New York: International Universities Press.

Linden, M.E. (1953). Group psychotherapy with institutionalized senile women: Study in gerontologic human relations. *International Journal of Group Psychotherapy, 3,* 150–170.

Linden, M. E. (1954). The significance of dual leadership in gerontologic group psychotherapy: Studies in gerontologic human relations III. *International Journal of Group Psychotherapy, 4,* 262–273.

Linden, M. E. (1955). Transference in gerontologic group psychotherapy: Studies in gerontologic human relations IV. *International Journal of Group Psychotherapy, 5,* 61–79.

Shore, H. (1952). Group work program development in homes for the aged. *Social Service Review, 26*(2), 181–194.

Toseland, R. (1995/1999). *Group work with the elderly and family caregivers.* New York: Springer.

Tross, S., & Blum, J. (1983). Review of group therapy with the older adult: Practice and research. In B. Maclennan, S. Saul, & M. Weiner (Eds.), *Group psychotherapies for the elderly* (pp. 3–29). Madison, CT: International Universities Press.

Vickery, F. (1952). A place in the sun for the aged: Group work activities for older people with an emphasis on club programs. *Group*, 14(2), 3–8; 23–24.

BIBLIOGRAPHY

Burlingame, V. S. (1999). *Ethnogerocounseling: Counseling ethnic elders and their families*. New York: Springer.

Dick, B., Lesser, K., & Whiteside, J. (1980). A developmental framework in co-therapy. *International Journal of Group Psychotherapy*, 30(3), 273–285.

Duffy, M. (Ed.). (1999). *Handbook of counseling and psychotherapy with older adults*. New York: Wiley.

Linden, M. (1976). Medicare and care of the aged. *Journal of the National Association of Private Psychiatric Hospitals*, 8(3), 7–9.

Linden, M. (1974). The challenge of aging: It means growing up...not down. *Mental Health*, 58(3), 34–38.

Linden, M. 1963. The aging and the community. *Geriatrics*, 18, 404–410.

Linden, M., & Courtney, D. (1953). The human life cycle and its interruptions: Studies in gerontologic human relations 1. *American Journal of Psychiatry*, 109(12), 906–915.

McInnis-Dittrich, K. (2002). *Social work with elders: A biopsychosocial approach to assessment and intervention*. Boston: Allyn & Bacon.

Sheikh, J. I. (Ed.). (1996). *Treating the elderly*. San Francisco: Jossey-Bass.

Whitbourne-Krauss, S. (Ed.). (2000). *Psychopathology in later adulthood*. New York: John Wiley & Sons.

Chapter 5

Principles of Yalom

Molly Ranney
Irene Burnside

Key Words

- Subgrouping
- Fractionalization
- Culture building
- Here-and-now
- Social reinforcement
- Curative factors

Learning Objectives

- Discuss subgrouping
- Describe crises in older adult group members
- State an important area of expertise of the group therapist
- Discuss culture building of a group
- Explain the use of the "here-and-now"
- Describe two roles of the group leader
- Discuss the eleven curative factors developed by Yalom

In the fourth edition of Yalom's (1995) seminal book, *The Theory and Practice of Group Psychotherapy*, he does not specifically discuss group psychotherapy with older adults. While Yalom, a psychiatrist, does not focus on group therapy with older adults, his text offers core principles and techniques that are applicable to all age groups. As such, students, health care workers, administrators, and instructors can benefit from adapting his ideas for group work with older people. It is important to note that Yalom's text is most applicable to psychotherapy groups.

This chapter discusses a number of Yalom's principles in relation to group work with older adults, including the maintenance of stable groups, culture building, the use of the here-and-now, subgrouping, crises in group life, the group leader as a transitional object, roles of the group leader, social reinforcement, and curative factors in group work. Yalom's book is extremely comprehensive and very technical. For example, Yalom uses a lot of psychiatric jargon that can be somewhat intimidating if you have not been schooled in that field. Nevertheless, Yalom's (1995) book is widely viewed as the lead text on group therapy, and it is important that group leaders are exposed to its content. In addition to this book chapter, several authors (e.g., Corey & Corey, 2002; Erwin, 1996; Sprenkle, 1999; Toseland, 1995) have applied Yalom's principles to group work with older adults and their books will also assist the reader.

The Maintenance of Stable Groups

According to Yalom (1995), an important task of leaders is the maintenance of stable groups. He states, "Stability of membership seems to be a sine qua non of successful therapy" (p. 107). This is most certainly true in group work with older adults. If members do leave the group, they should be replaced. Yalom suggested that the optimal size of an interactional group "is seven or eight, with an acceptable range of five to ten members" (p. 276). However, the optimal size of the older adult group is also dependent on the type of group, whether or not there is a coleader, and the functional impairment of the older adult members (e.g., if all or most members are in wheelchairs, the size of the group needs to be smaller so that the leader is able to offer assistance).

For new group leaders, it is common to make inappropriate choices for group membership. From Burnside's (1994) experience, usually the persons who demonstrated a lack of toleration or disrupted the meetings were those who dropped out. Such dropouts do provide valuable lessons for the leader, which prepares them to be more skilled in selecting future group members. In other cases, older adults may be required by staff to attend, and, as a result, are passive in the beginning stages of the group. Later, as these members gain self-confidence, they may choose to assert more control over their own lives by dropping out of the group. One way to minimize the likelihood of premature dropouts is to make sure that the group leader screens each member for the group (Yalom, 1995). While it may be challenging to convince facility staff of this need, there is general consensus among theorists and researchers that being prepared (i.e., through screening and/or pregroup meetings) for groups is predictive of a more positive outcome for members (Anderson, 1997; Bednar & Kaul, 1994; Corey & Corey, 2002; Toseland, 1995; Yalom, 1995).

Death is, of course, a much more common cause of attrition among older adult groups than younger age groups (Burnside, 1994; Toseland, 1995). After a death occurs, leaders are immediately faced with three tasks: (1) dealing with their personal feelings of loss for that member, (2) helping the group deal with the death of a peer, and (3) finding a replacement to join the group. In institutions, there is often a waiting list for entry into the group, so someone is ready to move into the group immediately (Burnside, 1994). Well-established groups soon become a topic of interest and concern to nongroup patients, and if these patients do not request to be in the group, very often their relatives will request participation for them.

Such interest in a group may not occur as readily with psychotherapy groups. For one thing, the present generation of older people, especially the 85+ age cohort group, are not particularly impressed by psychiatric interventions, and many of them still prefer pastoral counseling (Burnside, 1994). It may also be difficult to replace a member in a noninstitutional group because of transportation problems and other environmental challenges (Burnside, 1994; Toseland, 1995).

In spite of all these problems, stable groups do frequently occur among older adults, especially if the leader is conscientious about dealing with tardy and absent members. The effect of day-to-day crises on attendance can be minimized if the leader is alert for them (Burnside, 1970a). Another reason for tardiness and absenteeism in groups of elderly people in institutions is staff apathy, neglect, or lack of information about group schedules (Burnside, 1994; Toseland, 1995). If the patients need staff help to manage the activities of daily living, they may be having their hair done at meeting time, be in the process of being dressed, or lack the necessary help to get to the meeting.

Subgrouping

Yalom (1995) states that subgrouping, or "fractionalization—the splitting off of subunits—

occurs in every social organization" (p. 326). Further, Yalom contends that "the process may be transient or enduring, helpful or harmful" but it is inevitable (pp. 326–327). Yalom finds that subgrouping is usually disruptive. The authors of this chapter have found subgrouping quite the opposite in group work with older adults. Perhaps the need for friendship, mutual support, and a confidant makes subgrouping less threatening than in other groups.

Subgrouping does not seem to be as common among institutionalized older people as it is in other groups. These persons tend to avoid one another in a search for privacy. One member of a group that Burnside led always sat in a corner of the patio when the weather permitted. His reasons were "to get away from the old folks," "to read in peace and quiet," and "to be outdoors." Yet, group meetings had great meaning for him, and eventually he made friends with another man in the group and asked to be transferred to his room.

Leaders may choose to encourage subgrouping outside the meetings because they realize that it is unrealistic to expect older adults, who are often socially isolated, to refrain from it. Meetings outside the group need not be detrimental to the group process. To date, research has not been conducted on the impact of subgrouping on the outcomes of group work with older people. It is safe to say, however, that many friendships begin and increased socialization occurs when group members gather outside regular meetings. Thus, leaders of older adult groups must expect subgrouping and have a plan for how they intend to handle it.

Crises in Group Life

Many large and small crises plague old people and can be the reasons for absenteeism. We should redefine the term crisis in group work with older adults. Group crises can include fires, employee strikes, serious illnesses, losses of pets, high staff turnovers, and rejections by family (Burnside, 1970b). The cumulative effect of small crises also

needs to be considered. What seems to be a simple, easily solved problem may not be one in the eyes of the older person experiencing the problem. Small crises can include losing one's glasses, teeth, or hearing aid, or being constipated. One seemingly small crisis could represent the last element of control an older adult had over his or her life, or represent the loss of the last remembrance of preinstitutional life. Even slight falls can distress older adults considerably and markedly reduce their level of functioning. For example, a small fraternity pin was stolen from a member of a group Burnside led in a nursing home. He had had the pin for more than 50 years, and his wife had worn it for much of that time. I thought it was the value of the small diamond in the pin that concerned him, but it was the sentimental value of the pin. As he said, "I can always buy another diamond." He never got the pin back even though he offered a $50 reward for it, and he mentioned the loss to me frequently both in and outside the group. Another man's watch was stolen while he was in the same group. These were both sharp, alert men who might misplace their canes occasionally but who always managed to find them. This man said bitterly in a group meeting, "They'd steal the eye out of a snake here!" (Burnside, 1970b).

Much group time can be spent discussing the losses members have experienced (Burnside, 1970b; Burnside, 1994; Corey & Corey, 2004; Toseland, 1995). It is very important to allow these expressions of grief and to create a supportive atmosphere that encourages the older person to interpret the meaning for his or her own self. Additionally, Toseland cautioned group leaders to not assume "that all losses are devastating to older persons" (p. 14).

> For example, the husband of a member of a group that Ranney led at an adult day health care center died. Both the husband and wife had been blind since birth and worked very hard to live independently in the community.

They raised a child together, bought a home, and were very proud of their accomplishments. During the last few years of his life, the husband became very angry over his increased debility and growing dependence on others. According to his wife, "he was very difficult to live with because he shut out all of our friends and family members." At the time of his death, the wife expressed some sadness but mostly relief to the other group members that she was finally free to live her own life as she would like.

A nonjudgmental stance by the group leader is important because it permits the expression of feelings that may not be perceived as socially acceptable.

Tasks of the Group Leader

The three basic tasks of the group leader are the creation and maintenance of the group, culture building, and activation and illumination of the here-and-now (Yalom, 1995, p. 107). The leader has the sole responsibility for creating and carrying the group. According to Yalom, a considerable part of the maintenance task is performed before the first meeting: "The leader's expertise in the selection and the preparation of members will greatly influence the group's fate" (p. 107). Group maintenance also includes gatekeeping functions to prevent absenteeism and member attrition. Continued tardiness, absences, disruptive socializing, and scapegoating are all factors that can be harmful to a group; the leader must constantly watch for them and intervene when they occur.

Culture building is assisting the group to develop therapeutic norms. The group will turn to the leader for direction, and the leader must help the group establish norms consistent with the goals of therapy. The members are strangers as the group begins, so the therapist serves as a "transitional object" and is the group's primary unifying force. This is especially true in working

with older adults. The members may ignore one another and relate to, and sometimes speak only to, the group leader in meetings (Burnside, 1994; Toseland, 1995). This sort of behavior seems to be particularly characteristic of depressed, socially isolated, and regressed individuals. Thus, the group leader must focus his or her facilitation on encouraging member-to-member interactions. The leader must, however, remember that norms "are created relatively early in the life of a group and once established are difficult to change" (Yalom, 1995, p. 112). The following anecdote from Burnside's group experience is an illustration of a norm set by a member of a group of 80-year-olds who met weekly in a nursing home.

A group member, a man of 85, attended the meetings regularly each week. He admitted that the intellectual stimulation and the camaraderie meant a great deal to him, and even when he did not feel up to par he came to the meetings. On several occasions when he was not feeling well, he arrived at the meeting in his bathrobe and pajamas. The leader hesitated to comment on his attire, since the man's energy level was low and he was making the effort to attend. After he had come to his second or third meeting in his nightclothes, one of the women in the group eyed him and said tartly that she thought he could dress up a little bit for the meetings and have enough respect not to come in a robe and pajamas. Her statement had a marked effect; thereafter the man's grooming improved, and he never again came to the meetings in his robe and pajamas (Burnside, 1994).

Yalom (1995) devotes a great deal of time to the task of activating the "here-and-now." This task requires the leader to focus his or her facilitation efforts on the immediate events in the meeting. The emphasis on the present encourages members to engage in more authentic communication and involves them in the therapeutic process. At first glance, the emphasis on the present may seem at odds with the need for older adults to review their past. Yalom does, however, also encourage leaders to use the past. Specifically, Yalom states that the group should use the past "for the help it offers in understanding (and changing) the individual's mode of relating in the present" (p. 142).

In our work, we have observed that older adults are both present and past oriented in their group interactions. This view is congruent with Toseland's (1995) assertion that older adults make less distinction between the past and present than do younger groups. The ability to move freely between the past and present should be viewed as a strength of the older adult generation and group leaders must be prepared to view it as such. Further, older adults tend to be very direct with their communications with each other so it is not difficult to operate in the "here-and-now."

Two Roles of the Group Leader

According to Yalom (1995), group leaders use two roles to accomplish their basic tasks and to influence the group: the technical expert and model-setting participant (p. 112). The technical expert role involves using all the leader's technical knowledge and skill. One important task is to develop a pattern of communication that helps the group move toward a "social microcosm." The group becomes a "social microcosm" when members become comfortable enough with each other that they begin to behave like they do in their relationships outside of the group therapy" (p. 28).

The role of a model-setting participant is congruent with the role of technical expert. The leader role models behavior to help the group members develop therapeutic norms. The safety of the group can be enhanced as the members see the leader engaging in authentic communication, or interacting freely, without adverse effects. According to Yalom (1995), the leader who models "nonjudgmental acceptance and appreciates

the strengths of others as well as their problem areas, helps to shape a group that is health oriented" (p. 115). In agreement with Yalom, Toseland (1995) suggested that employing a strengths perspective in group work with older adults builds trust because it "helps members to be more understanding and empathetic" (p. 63).

Patience is an important attribute in a leader. Apathy in institutionalized aged people may be overpowering at times. Group leaders must always keep in mind that such apathy may be a mask for depression (Burnside, 1994; Levin, 1967) and social isolation. Group members who are depressed can benefit from attending groups, but may need the assistance of antidepressant medication to fully participate in the group.

Social reinforcement in group psychotherapy may be subtle or nondeliberate. More often, in group therapy with older adults, it is very deliberate, as in the use of touch in group meetings. Touch is important in working with older adults (Burnside, 1975; Corey & Corey, 2004; Toseland, 1995). Its use—a quick hug, a pat on the hand or shoulder—can be a simple, positive reinforcement. Sheer enjoyment of older adults is another positive and powerful kind of reinforcing—a hearty laugh by the leader may go a long way to convince old people that they still have a sense of humor and that they are appreciated. The use of empathy, versus sympathy or pity, communicates to older adults that the leader perceives them to be capable and of value to the group. Corey & Corey (2004) defined empathy as "the ability to tune in to what others are subjectively experiencing and to see their world through their eyes" (p. 135).

Active listening is important in all therapy situations with older adults. Again, the leader must role model for active listening, because many older people are often impatient with one another. In the effort to make someone listen to them, they may not be able to listen to others effectively. Such behavior is often due to high anxiety and diminishes after a few meetings.

Curative Factors in Group Work

Yalom developed 11 general categories of curative factors from the data he received from patients in group therapy:

1. Instillation of hope
2. Universality
3. Imparting information
4. Altruism
5. The corrective recapitulation of the family group (i.e., family reenactment)
6. Development of socializing techniques
7. Imitative behavior
8. Interpersonal learning
9. Group cohesiveness
10. Catharsis
11. Existential factors

Yalom does not state the ages of the patients who reported the curative factors, but seven of the categories seem especially important in older adult groups: instillation of hope, universality, altruism, interpersonal learning, group cohesiveness, catharsis, and existential factors.

Instillation of Hope

Many institutionalized older people have little hope left in their lives. The weekly group meeting offers something to look forward to, instilling hope. Older members can inspire each other in the group. The leader can also inspire them by helping them discover that they still have power over their own lives. By being empowered in the group meetings, members can also learn that autonomy exists outside group meetings. Instilling hope and working on establishing future goals are important for members. Further, if the group atmosphere encourages honest and authentic communications, members have a way of encouraging each other that is far more profound than what could ever be accomplished in individual therapy.

Universality

Late life can be a very lonely and isolating experience (Sprenkle, 1999). Isolated older adults can believe that the problems they experience are unique to them. Learning that others have had many of the same feelings and experiences can be very reassuring. Groups also give older people the chance to discuss the problems of aging, so that the members begin to feel that they are not so different after all. Sometimes listening to how others have coped with their losses, illnesses, and tragedies can inspire a group member toward better adjustment. Skillful leaders can maximize the universality aspect of groups.

A health background is a special advantage in work with disabled older adults. This is because the leader can do some health teaching during group work. If a group leader does not have a health background, inviting guest speakers to educate members on common health problems can be beneficial.

Altruism

Feeling useful to others is a developmental need for all age groups. For older adults, the ability to give to and feel needed by others often diminishes with increased debility. From our experience, feeling useless is one of the major sources of depression for institutionalized older adults. Membership in a support group can offer older adults the chance to feel useful again. According to Sprenkle (1999), groups "not only offer the elderly patient opportunities to assist others but actually also places a certain responsibility on him to do so" (p. 221). Being able to give to others has a strong therapeutic value for older adults.

Interpersonal Learning

Many older people suffer from conversation deprivation. The need to talk and share is very important for these people, and finding persons who will listen and take them seriously is a problem.

This need for human interaction occurs not only in institutions, but also in private homes. Older people, as a rule, get very little feedback. They need to know what relatives, peers, and staff members think about them and also how they are coming across. Without this interaction and feedback, older adults can become self-absorbed which can further isolate them (Toseland, 1995).

Group membership gives such people a chance to learn about their own habits and their ability to communicate with others. For example, members can get feedback from each other on their relationships with their children and grandchildren. This type of feedback, from others who are in the same or similar situations, represents the true value of group work. Although membership can be one means of working out difficulties with peers—or of communicating dislike—the personal closeness generated by group meetings may be one of their most important contributions. In our own work, both of us have observed that interpersonal learning is where real growth tends to occur for members.

Group Cohesiveness

One way of defining group cohesiveness is the togetherness feeling that a group develops over time. The relationships among members become very meaningful as Coyle (1930), a pioneer of social group work also stressed. Building on Yalom (1995), Toseland defines it "as the force which binds members together, attracting individuals to each other and the group as a whole" (p. 39). This is extremely important for older adults, who are slowly losing their relationships with others. In cohesive groups, the members remember the basic acceptance they had in the group and again feel that they belong even after the group disbands.

Numerous theorists and researchers have argued that for a group to be truly effective it must be cohesive (Anderson, 1997; Burnside, 1994; Corey & Corey, 2004; Evans & Dion, 1991; Hartford, 1972; Reid, 1997; Yalom, 1995). Groups tend to reach this stage in the middle phase of group work (Anderson, 1997; Corey & Corey, 2004; Reid, 1997). Evidence of cohesion appears when the members refer to the group as *we* and when they begin to take hold of an idea or a problem and go to work on it as a group. In work with older adults, Toseland (1995) stated that dependence and conformity are two potential negative aspects of group cohesiveness. In our experience, these can be avoided if group leaders continue to encourage authentic communication, including differences of opinion.

Catharsis

The importance of catharsis in groups becomes apparent early in the meetings. Once older adults find that the leader is not going to write down their every word, they feel free to express many feelings, especially harsh ones. According to Yalom (1995), members are likely to experience catharsis when they are able to freely share their thoughts and feelings in a group, and feel universal acceptance for who they really are by other members. With no fear of retribution, older people are quick to use the group as a sounding board.

Catharsis is especially important for groups in institutional settings, such as assisted living facilities and nursing homes. Group meetings give members a place to complain about the coffee, the food, the bathing procedures, the pills, the night nurse, and so forth—usually in that order. The book *As We Are Now* (1973), by May Sarton, is recommended for group leaders to understand the tremendous need for institutionalized people who feel powerless to have a place to air their feelings. For older adults in community settings, day-to-day living problems, discouragement about living conditions, and problems with agencies are fertile ground for the content of group discussions.

Summary

This chapter describes various extrapolations from Irvin Yalom's *The Theory and Practice of Group Psychotherapy* (1995) and their application to group psychotherapy with older adults. The chapter's focus is on how the leader can maintain stable groups and underlines the importance of that aspect of leadership. Subgrouping, or fractionalization of groups, is usually considered deleterious, but it may have benefits for older adults.

Crises both large and small can occur during a group's life. Large crises include loss of loved ones (including pets), suicide, employee strikes, staff turnover, and rejections by family. Little crises are day-to-day problems that may decrease the functional ability of the older adult.

Three tasks of group therapists are group maintenance, culture building, and activation of the here-and-now. The leader must use considerable technical expertise to prevent absenteeism, tardiness, and attrition. Culture building is accomplished through development of therapeutic group norms.

The group leader must fulfill the two roles of a technical expert and a model-setting participant. The group has to be helped to move toward a social microcosm, but growth and learning also need to occur in the group. Social reinforcement is a powerful shaper of behavior and may be used knowingly or unknowingly by a leader. A wise leader is generous with the use of touch as a social reinforcer with older adult group members.

Curative factors selected for discussion from Yalom's book are instillation of hope, universality, altruism, interpersonal learning, group cohesiveness, and catharsis. Each curative factor has an application and ramifications in groups of older people.

The depth and breadth of Yalom's book cannot easily be covered in one chapter. The group leader who is facilitating groups with older adults with mental health diagnoses (especially psychotic or neurotic persons) should read the entire book.

Exercises

EXERCISE 1

Write a biographical sketch of yourself as an older adult. Select an age you think is really old. Describe your living arrangements and family situation. Also, as a majority of older adults have at least one chronic health condition, discuss which one you think that you will have and how it will affect your life.

EXERCISE 2

Take one of the seven curative factors described in this chapter and write an in-depth analysis of what that term means to you related to the biographical sketch you wrote for Exercise 1. Also, discuss instances in your life when you felt that a particular curative factor was operating.

EXERCISE 3

Make a list of behaviors occurring in a group that would indicate group cohesiveness.

EXERCISE 4

Norms are created early in a group. What would be some of the norms that you might help establish in a group of older people?

References

Anderson, J. (1997). *Social work with groups: A process model.* New York: Longman Press.

Bednar, K., & Kaul, T. (1978). Experimental group research: Current perspectives. In A. Garfield & A. Bergin (Eds.), *Handbook of psychotherapy and behavior change* (2nd ed. pp. 769–816). New York: John Wiley & Sons.

Burnside, I. (1970a). Crisis intervention with geriatric hospitalized patients. *Journal of Psychiatric Nursing*, 8(2), 17–20.

Burnside, I. (1970b). Loss: A constant theme in group work with older adults. *Hospital & Community Psychiatry*, 21(6), 173–177.

Burnside, I. (1975, December). *The therapeutic use of touch.* Paper presented at conference entitled Sensory Processes and Aging, Dallas, TX.

Burnside, I. (1994). Principles of Yalom. In I. Burnside & M. Schmidt's (Eds.), *Working with older adults: Group process and techniques* (3rd ed. pp. 48-56). Boston: Jones and Bartlett.

Corey, M., & G. Corey. (2002). *Theory and practice of group counseling* (6th ed.). Belmont, CA: Brooks/Cole.

Coyle, G. (1930). *Social process in organized groups*. New York: Smith.

Evans, C., & Dion, K. (1991). Group cohesion and performance. *Small Group Research*, 22(2), 175–186.

Erwin, K.T. (1996). *Group techniques for aging adults: Putting geriatric skills enhancement into practice*. Washington, DC: Taylor & Francis.

Hartford, M. (1972). *Groups in social work*. New York: Columbia University Press.

Levin, S. (1967). Depression in older adults. In M. Berezin & S. Cath (Eds.), *Geriatric psychiatry: Grief, loss and emotional disorders in the aging process* (pp. 203–225). New York: International Universities Press.

Reid, K. (1997). *Social work practice with groups: A clinical perspective*. Pacific Grove, CA: Brooks/Cole.

Sarton, M. (1973). *As we are now*. New York: Norton.

Sprenkle, D. (1999). Therapeutic issues and strategies in group therapy with older men. In M. Duffy (Ed.), *Handbook of counseling and psychotherapy with older adults* (pp. 214–227). New York: John Wiley & Sons.

Toseland, R. (1995). *Group work with the elderly and family caregivers*. New York: Springer.

Yalom, I. (1995). *The theory and practice of group psychotherapy* (4th ed.). New York: Basic Books.

BIBLIOGRAPHY

Burnside, I., Preski, S., & Hertz, J. (1998). Research instrumentation and elderly subjects. *Journal of Nursing Scholarship*, 30(2), 185–190.

Burnside, I., & Schmidt, M. (1994). *Working with older adults: Group process and techniques* (3rd ed.). Boston: Jones and Bartlett.

Vinogradov, S., & Yalom, I. (1996). Group therapy. In R. Hales & S. Yudosky (Eds.), *American psychiatric press synopsis of psychiatry* (pp. 1063–1095). Washington, DC: American Psychiatric Association.

Yalom, I. (2002). *The gift of therapy: An open letter to a new generation of therapists and their patients*. New York: HarperCollins Publishers.

Yalom, I. (1999). *Memories and the meaning of life: Tales of psychotherapy*. New York: Basic Books.

Yalom, I. (1966). Problems of neophyte group therapists. *International Journal of Social Psychiatry*, 12(1), 52–59.

Yalom, I., Houts, P., Newell, G., & Rand, K. (1967). Preparation of patients for group therapy: A controlled study. *Archives of General Psychiatry*, 17(4), 416–427.

Yalom, I., Houts, P., & Zimberg, S. (1967). Prediction of improvement in group therapy: An exploratory study. *Archives of General Psychiatry*, 17(2), 159–168.

Yalom, I., & Terrazas, F. (1968). Group therapy for psychotic elderly patients. *American Journal of Nursing*, 68(8), 1690–1694.

Resources

- Videotape by Irvin Yalom, Volume 1. Outpatients consists of two 50-minute tapes that are part of the series *Understanding Group Psychotherapy*. Contact: Brooks/Cole Publishing, Pacific Grove, CA 93950-5098.
- Videotape by Irvin Yalom, Volume 2. Inpatients consists of two 50-minute tapes that are part of the series *Understanding Group Psychotherapy*. Contact: Brooks/Cole Publishing, Pacific Grove, CA 93950-5098.

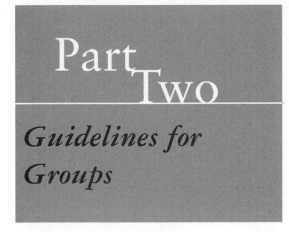

Part Two

Guidelines for Groups

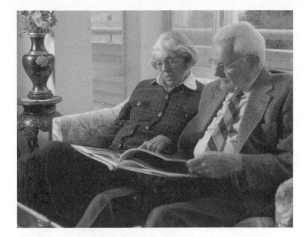

Part 2 is concerned with introducing beginning group leaders to basic general or generic characteristics of small groups. It identifies issues and important practice principles to guide their introduction to working with groups of older people. There is increasing interest in identifying different types of group work with older people as well as considering how group work practice with older people resembles and differs from group work with younger people. The increasing number of older people is encouraging professionals of many kinds to develop new ways of serving this disparate population. Chapter 6 discusses current needs, contexts for practice, and the necessary training for health and social care workers who wish to undertake group work with older people. Chapter 7 considers the central idea of basing group work with elders on explicitly agreed goals set out in a contract. It explores the ethical and procedural advantages of doing so and highlights some inherent obstacles. Chapter 8 focuses on criteria for group membership, group settings, and group goals. Chapter 9 examines a number of issues that leaders and coleaders commonly encounter when working together with groups of older adults. Common group concerns and steps that can be taken to improve the chances of effective leadership are discussed.

Chapter 6

Education and Preparation for Group Work

Faith Gibson
Irene Burnside

Key Words

- Affection
- Control
- Inclusion
- Power
- Primary aging
- Primary prevention
- Secondary aging
- Secondary prevention
- Sense of coherence or meaning
- Tertiary prevention

Learning Objectives

- List three needs of older people in groups
- Identify how a leader might seek to meet these needs
- Discuss the basic values and objectives of the education of health and social workers concerned with the care of older people
- Describe four power resources of an older person
- Differentiate between primary and secondary aging
- Define primary prevention
- Define secondary prevention
- Define tertiary prevention
- List one example of group work for each of the three stages of prevention

The question today is not whether "older people are no longer educable" but whether we, the mental health professionals, are.

—*J. L. Ronch & J. S. Maizler*
(1977, p. 283)

The first part of this chapter discusses the education, preparation, and support of beginning group leaders in order for them to develop style and confidence. The need for them to be supported as they seek to meet the needs of older group members for inclusion, control, and affection is emphasized. Because group leaders intervene across all three levels of prevention in their efforts to work through groups to maintain the health and well-being of older members, all three levels—primary, secondary, and tertiary—are discussed in the second part of the chapter.

Education Philosophy and Practice

The basic philosophy underpinning the education of health and social work professionals serving

Cautions for Beginning Leaders

Some of the secrets of successful group leadership are meticulous preparation, empathic communication, careful scheduling, and attention to detail. Students often create problems through inadequate preparation, lack of communication, and consideration for the families of group members and the staff in facilities in which the group is meeting. For instance, they might come to an agency without clear goals and specific objectives. Poor scheduling and general disorganization lead to unnecessary demands on the staff and increase everyone's anxiety level and/or frustration.

One potentially serious problem is that it is not always possible for the group leader to limit or control what occurs in a group meeting. Difficult situations that new leaders need to be cautioned about include agitated members; hostile, belligerent members attacking other group members physically or verbally; sad sessions where crying may prevail; and discussion of suicide by a member. Nonprofessionals should be cautioned not to probe or encourage expression of strong feelings and emotions and should be reminded that they are doing group work, not group psychotherapy. If at any time a student leader encounters a group member becoming exceedingly distressed beyond what can be handled in the group or in a subsequent one-to-one meeting, she or he should seek further assistance from a more experienced practitioner.

Some psychiatrists, psychologists, and social workers challenge instructors who place students in a facility to do group work because they fear just that—they may be doing psychotherapy. Protection of territorial turf may account for this reaction, but sometimes they seem to think that a student will unearth strong emotions and that the old people will go flying out of control. Although this may happen, and new leaders need to be prepared for the possibility, the expression of emotion is not to be feared. Old people are far less emotionally frail than is suggested by many professionals.

A more common problem is both subtle and not-so subtle sabotage by staff members in institutions or agencies. On the day of group meetings, the members may be out, or they may be having an X-ray, or they may still be in bed. The cook may not know that coffee is needed. It may take time to break through the wall of resistance. However, resistance is not always the reason for the problem: Sometimes it is simply a brouhaha in the facility or the lack of organization and efficiency, or perhaps a lack of preparation, communication, and organization on the part of the group leader (Rice, 2004). (See Chapter 23 for an example of how coleaders handled such problems in a board and care home.)

A well-run facility can take group work in its stride and encourage both the older members and the group leaders in the endeavor. Such cooperation and support have to come from the top. A supportive administrator and director will pass support down to other staff. But students usually have to prove themselves before much support from the staff in agencies is forthcoming. Students doing group work—or any new group leader, for that matter—should have strong preceptor support. Without this support, students may get discouraged with the group process and staff interpersonal relationships. (See Chapter 30 for more on consultation and supervision.)

It is hoped that group leaders will have been taught about the special biopsychosocial needs of older people. Normal aging is succinctly covered in Chapter 2, Table 2–3, and the physical limitations of older people are discussed in Chapter 12.

Background Knowledge

Leaders need to understand about the basic needs of people of all ages in groups, and they should appreciate the fundamentals of group dynamics as well as the special skills needed for leading groups of older people. It is important to be able to place older people within a life span framework and to understand the developmental tasks associated with each stage of the life cycle (Erikson, 1950, 1982). Everyone, especially older people experiences the need for inclusion, control, and affection (Schutz, 1966). Membership in a small group can assist with meeting these needs.

The Need for Inclusion

The need for all members to experience inclusion in each meeting is vital. Some people are very gregarious, while others want much less interpersonal contact and may not wish to participate in groups. If they do join a group, they may be content with much less attention directed to themselves in the presence of others. This is why it is important to know each member as an individual and to respond accordingly. A personal hello and goodbye to each member is a basic way to make each person feel included. In the early meetings a handshake is appropriate; in later meetings when everyone is better acquainted, both the leader and members often display more affection. Verbal inclusion is achieved by addressing each person by name and by creating opportunities to ensure that silent members are drawn into the discussion.

Sometimes, inviting each person in the group, in turn, to contribute can be a useful technique for achieving involvement, providing that no one feels overwhelmed by this degree of attention. Eye contact can provide nonverbal inclusion. Because some members may have serious vision problems or may not be wearing their glasses, they should be seated where they can best see the leader. Vision difficulties are increased if the leader sits in front of a window or bright lights. Group meetings should not be held in dimly lit rooms for the same reason. Sitting close to a person or holding their hand may satisfy the need for inclusion and can be used to support shy, withdrawn, or anxious individuals.

Nonverbal communication is particularly helpful for people who have dementia, as their verbal skills are frequently impaired. Burnside, for example, was leading such a group in which a 90-year-old man was very anxious and noisily stamping his feet on the wheelchair footrest. As she was talking to another member, she reached over and placed her hand on his knee. His agitation decreased. Try to touch two members simultaneously; frequently the two members will interact with each other, suggesting that the leader has bridged the gulf between them. A Spanish proverb says, "Habits are first cobwebs, then cables." As leadership skills are refined and developed, it is hoped that the cobwebs may develop into cables.

The Need for Control

The issue of control is particularly relevant to working with groups of older people who frequently in contemporary society have lost control over many aspects of their lives. It is of particular concern with older institutionalized people where increasing feelings of satisfaction and well-being are frequently defined as central objectives for group work. Young students may be reluctant to reflect upon the relevance of control within their own lives while fearing they may "lose control" within a group.

We all need to maintain a satisfactory balance of power and influence in our relationships with other people. One reason is that we need to make our environment predictable to some degree. Keeping it predictable often amounts to controlling other people, because they are the main agents creating unpredictable and uncontrollable situations. The degree of predictability each of us needs varies widely. Some individuals want to control their whole environment, while others do not want to control anyone in any situation, no matter how appropriate controlling them would be.

Older people who have lived alone and made their own decisions for many years are accustomed to feeling in control. Institutionalized older people, however, lose so much control over their lives that a group meeting provides one area where the individual can say adamantly "no" or vie for control. New group leaders need to be helped with feelings of rejection when such challenging occasions arise in group meetings. Students often do not realize the great need of older adults to maintain an inner locus of control as a positive defense against the loss of authority in so many aspects of their lives (Gitterman, 2002).

Despite this need, lack of exertion to secure control is also common in groups of apathetic institutionalized people. Some of the reasons may be lack of energy, inertia, depression, boredom, or lack of finesse in groups. It may be necessary for the leader to encourage older persons to exert more control in group meetings as well as over other aspects of their own lives.

Student leaders need to be guided into encouraging aged members in institutions to take more initiative and control. **Table 6–1** gives examples of these coping strategies in action. The over-

controlling group member is usually less of a leadership problem than the passive, submissive member. The dependency and helplessness exhibited by many groups can often frustrate or depress a new group leader.

New leaders often feel a loss of control of the group when a member leaves abruptly during a session, although older members generally do not leave their groups as abruptly as some younger persons do because they are physically slowed down for one reason or another. Older persons, however, may leave the group before it is dismissed if their anxiety is high. Anxiety in both new group members and the leader may result in especially tight control of the group by the leader. Overcontrol may be demonstrated by the leader making all the decisions alone, not giving proper attention to contracting, by showing impatience or irritation with tardiness or absenteeism, or by ignoring the needs of the members.

Table 6–1　MILLER'S POWER RESOURCES

Physical strength and reserve
A 96-year-old woman residing in a nursing home began the group in a wheelchair, but began walking to group with help, and now comes on her own.

Psychologic stamina and support network
A reminiscence group is begun with isolated women in low-cost housing, many of whom are coping with chronic illness. They receive much support from one another and begin to call other members their "neighbors."

Positive self-concept (self-esteem)
A group of residents, all in wheelchairs, begin to meet in a resident council's group. As they are empowered, their self-esteem rises.

Energy
A group of six nonagenarians residing in a nursing home meet weekly. Low energy was observed initially. But as the group progressed, they became more animated and saved their energy to attend group meetings.

Knowledge
A discussion group in a senior center forms to discuss special problems affecting older people with chronic illness (e.g., heart problems, strokes).

Motivation
A group of poorly motivated older veterans in a Veterans Hospital joins a small bingo group. The motivation to win becomes an important factor in getting them out of their rooms.

Belief system (hope)
A group meets weekly in an adult day care center. One member, who is losing her sight, receives great courage from talking to a blind member and feels more hopeful that she too can cope.

Source: Based on Miller, J. F. (1992). Used with permission.

Older people who are not accustomed to groups may take some time to warm to the group experience, or they may try the forms of control they used in their own families. Many of the present generation of older persons came from large families, and the place they had in the family constellation may influence how they behave in a group; thus, you find the mother (she was the oldest girl in the family) or the father (he was the oldest boy) or the baby of the family, the clown, the teaser, and so forth.

In general, the style of leadership in group work with older people is somewhat different from that required for leading groups of younger people. In groups of older people, while being enablers, the leaders are more often required to be more active, cautiously to be *completers*, the ones who enable the group and its individual members to accomplish any task the group is unable to do for itself.

The Need for Affection

We all need to maintain a balance between ourselves and others regarding love and affection. At one extreme, some people like very close, very personal relationships with each individual they meet. At the other extreme are those who like their relationships to be quite impersonal and distant, friendly perhaps, but not close and intimate.

The affectional (or intimacy) needs of the members are an important component of group work with older people. **Table 6–2** identifies sources of affection open to older members of groups. Older people may need much more affection than younger ones because they have lost so many peers and significant others. How the leader demonstrates and uses affection may also be different. The easy flow of affection between the leader and a group of older people would probably not be appropriate, for example, if the same leader were working with schizophrenic young people.

Lack of affection and warmth in a group is to be expected in the beginning meetings if all the members are strangers, and the leader needs to be very conscious of reaching out at this stage of a group's development. Affection grows as the group engages in shared work of mutual significance. Expression of affection may occur sooner if the group members have known one another before meeting as a group. The responses of aged persons in group meetings mirror the way they are treated in the facility or in their homes. If they receive affection, they tend to give affection in the group. If they live in a hostile or punitive environment, they are likely to be guarded, shy, or they may draw away from affectionate gestures offered them.

The importance of body image, self-esteem, and sexual drives may all appear to some degree in group work with older adults. As leaders display interest and affection (both verbally and nonverbally), they model behavior that can be emulated by the group. The leader's touching the very obese person, the jaundiced patient, or the unattractive aged person, for example, may make a great impression on all involved in the care of and interaction with that person.

Basic Understanding About Groups

Tolson, Reid, and Garvin (2003, p. 251) provide the following definitions of basic terms:

- **Group structure**—The pattern of relationships between members
- **Group cohesiveness**—How attractive the group is to its members
- **Group processes**—Cyclical and noncyclical spontaneous moment-by-moment shared experiences within the group
- **Group norms**—What behavior is desirable and undesirable

- **Group culture**—Traditions that the group develops
- **Group development**—Phases or stages through which the group proceeds

They list the following essential knowledge and skills for anyone seeking to establish an effective group:

- How to compose groups
- How to assist members to develop relationships with one another
- How to create norms that assist members to accomplish the objectives of the group
- How to utilize activities
- How to engage the group in problem solving

Group Process

In a group of older people the pacing is slower and modifications are necessary. The increased physical limitations of older persons and the

Table 6–2   AFFECTION IN GROUPS OF OLDER PEOPLE

Occasions for expression of affection to aged group members

1. During hellos	5. Assuage guilt	9. Alleviate grief
2. During good-byes	6. Ease forgetful moments, memory loss	10. Share happiness of leader or member
3. Congratulate over accomplishment	7. Intervene in loneliness	
4. Assuage embarrassment	8. Spontaneous reaction of leader	

Problems in giving affection

Leader	Group member	Staff or agency
1. Professional, reserved stance	1. Too lonely	1. Lack of role models in agency
2. Embarrassed by affectionate gestures	2. Grieving	2. Philosophy of agency inhibited
3. Lifestyle; not used to it	3. Lifestyle; not used to it	3. Hurried atmosphere; everyone always busy
4. Cultural background	4. Cultural background	4. Task-oriented physical care takes priority over psychosocial care
5. Aged person dirty; has bad odor, jaundiced, and so on	5. Depressed	5. Rapid turnover of staff precludes close relationships
	6. Embarrassed	
	7. Lack of significant others	
	8. Apathy	
	9. Dying	
	10. In pain	
	11. Angry	
	12. Paranoid state	
	13. Low energy level	

Problems in receiving affection

1. Embarrassed by affectionate gestures	1. Embarrassed by affection	1. Embarrassed by affectionate overtures: (a) staff/staff (b) staff/patient (c) patient/patient
	2. Barricades: bed rails, wheelchairs, walkers	2. Need to maintain a professional stance; discomfort in role

lower energy levels in very old people are particularly relevant:

- Members need to know when the group begins and ends
- Leaders should plan ahead the goals they have for the group and share them with agency administrators
- Leaders must plan well in advance whenever materials are needed for a group
- Confidentiality is one of the basic ground rules of the group
- Pregroup selection of members and a pregroup meeting are most important
- Homogeneity versus heterogeneity—Some groups may be homogeneous in terms of one characteristic—age, for example—but be heterogeneous in terms of culture
- Each member needs to feel important, worthwhile, and a valued member of the group

It is helpful for new group leaders to learn how other disciplines lead groups of older persons. The chapters in Part 5 on multidisciplinary perspectives will inform interprofessional coleadership. Various national and international organizations and publications report research and evidence-based practice insights from single- and multidisciplinary perspectives concerning the psychosocial care of older persons in groups. *Groupwork*, *Social Work with Groups*, and *Specialists in Group Work* are highly relevant journals. (See also the Resources section for information about relevant national organizations.)

Preventive Health Care

Many older people are increasingly interested in questions concerning the meaning of life and the part played by health, wealth, happiness, activity, and engagement in aging successfully (Moody, 2003). Preventive health care is a central concept in the field of health and aging (Laurie, 2000). The chief goal of social gerontology and geriatric medicine and related human service professions concerned with older people must be to work collaboratively to improve quality of life as much as length of life. Antonovsky (1987, 1994) suggested a salutogenic model that proposed that people strive to develop a sense of coherence that makes the world comprehensible, manageable, and meaningful. It is this sense of coherence that prevents breakdown when faced with life's stresses. Concepts of primary and secondary aging are relevant to working towards achieving these goals.

Primary aging is a steady decline in function even though the individual is in good health and disease free. Secondary aging is characterized by decline that is due to illness with aging. It will be helpful for leaders to know about normal aging changes, major illnesses of later life, and the influence of chronicity (see Chapter 12). Aging is an individual process, and this must be taken into account when working with older persons. The development of preventive health care programs for older persons is receiving increasing attention and is an area of both concern and debate among health care professionals. There is now wide support for programs designed to keep older people physically and mentally active as a means of promoting health and well-being. "If you want to keep it, use it," is a slogan that now attracts considerable multiprofessional support.

A study by Menec (2003) showed that greater happiness, better function, and reduced mortality were associated with levels of overall activity but that different activities produced different kinds of successful outcomes. Social and productive activities were positively related to happiness, better function, and mortality levels. More solitary activities such as handwork, reading, or hobbies only influenced happiness outcomes. These results suggest that different types of activities have different benefits. While social and productive activities may produce better functioning and increased longevity, more solitary activities may provide a greater sense of engagement in life.

These findings tend to suggest that opportunities for both group and individual activities may provide the best returns and that sociable and solitary activities contribute valuable but different outcomes.

Group modalities as interventions for older people can be categorized into primary preventive interventions, secondary interventions, and tertiary interventions. Group work, as a modality is relevant to intervention in all three of these categories. Each will be discussed separately.

Primary Prevention

When considering the relevance of group work to primary prevention it is important carefully to define the types of needs being considered, the content of the type of group work program being offered, and how its effectiveness will be evaluated.

In primary preventive interventions, attempts are made to avert problems before they occur. One of the broadest mechanisms of primary prevention is social policies that eliminate the problem at its source—for example, policies shaping income, health, and physical and social living arrangements. Primary preventions, of course, are preferable to secondary and tertiary interventions, because the goal is to prevent problems occurring. If primary prevention is to be effective, the professional should know what causes dysfunctional states. As our knowledge of the complexities of aging is incomplete, our efforts at prevention at the primary level can only be based on present knowledge with all its imperfections.

Examples of primary prevention groups could include: (1) groups focused on nutrition, exercise, or prevention of osteoporosis; (2) groups focused on preventing severe depression—for example, a group of newly widowed persons; (3) groups for providing cognitive and social stimulation; and (4) groups for caregivers of persons with dementia, with the goal of helping them maintain their own health.

Secondary Prevention

Secondary prevention interventions are planned during the first signs of problems, and the focus is on early diagnosis and prompt treatment. This stage of prevention focuses on two areas: avoiding the occurrence of further breakdown in a situation and helping people to develop coping strategies that can help them avoid similar situations in the future (Turner, 1996).

Support groups and psychoeducational groups implemented during this phase may help the convalescent older person and the family. While these are meant to be self-help groups, they frequently include education, advice, and information from professional practitioners who may present guest lectures. (See Chapter 17 on support groups.)

Support groups that concentrate on a specific condition can be implemented—for example, arthritis, diabetes, chronic pain, cancer, Parkinson's, early stage Alzheimer's (Yale, 1995), and poststroke. The group leader should have an in-depth knowledge of the disease and of some of the psychosocial complications that the older people and their caregivers face.

Tertiary Prevention

Tertiary prevention has a preventive element because there is intense treatment or rehabilitation, and the aim is to control the development of further disability. Deterioration in social functioning is to be prevented; the idea is to help the patient or client make the best possible use of available resources. In tertiary prevention, the goal is to limit disability, as, for example, in cardiac rehabilitation programs that combine information, advice, support, health checks, and exercise.

Chronic depression is one of the major causes of mental impairment in older people (Manton, Cornelius, & Woodbury, 1995). Cappeleiz (2000) reported significant improvements in older adults undertaking 10 weekly sessions of cognitive-reminiscence therapy in small groups of two to four people in day hospitals and long-term care facilities. Another dysfunctional or impaired group requiring special attention is people with dementia. The group modality, while appropriate for both groups, requires skilled leadership and careful consideration of size and program (see Chapters 11 and 12).

Summary

This chapter discusses both the physical and mental health needs of older adults and the implications these have for group workers. Although considerable advances have been achieved in the treatment of many disorders and disabilities many problems remain. The inexorable growth in the numbers of people reaching advanced old age and their rising expectations generally about health care and social well-being result in increasing demands for assistance from health and social care professionals. The number and type of psychosocial problems being recognized are inevitably leading to increased treatment demands, especially concerning mental disorders.

Mental health workers should learn how to give expert care, work with members of all disciplines, assume primary responsibility for a group of older people, and be able to instruct ancillary workers in group principles and practice. Training methods include classroom instruction involving teaching and discussion, student logs, experiential exercises, participation in a peer learning group, field experience requiring reflection with a supervisor or mentor, evaluation of leading a group, teamwork experience, writing case studies, and participation in research projects. This later point is important, as it is no longer sufficient for students to be consumers of research. They also need to become active participants, developing research skills in order to scrutinize their own practice and contribute to extending their professions' knowledge base (Choi & Dinse, 1998).

The ability to lead groups of older people is based on the leader's knowledge of psychology, group theory, group dynamics, role theory, systems theory, group work theory, psychiatry, and whether or not he or she has a background in social gerontology and geriatrics. Educational programs range from special short courses to bachelors and masters degrees and doctorates.

Understanding older people's needs for inclusion, control, and affection can help the group leader to meet the needs of each group member. Once each group member feels understood and accepted, he or she is more likely to remain within the group and to benefit from the group experience. Inclusion can consist of either verbal or nonverbal acknowledgment of individual members. Underinclusion of a member by the leader may lead to absenteeism. Some suggestions for achieving inclusion are giving personal attention before and after the meeting, frequent use of names, allowing every member a chance to speak, frequent touching, sitting close to an individual, and eye contact.

Encouraging older people to seize more control over their day-to-day situations and their lives in general is a difficult leadership task. Yet it is especially important for older people living in institutions who seem to have lost or relinquished their locus of control. Group membership can be important in restoring or increasing control, at least to some degree.

Affection is usually lacking in initial meetings, when everyone may be a stranger. Affection for the leader and between members usually increases as the group develops. The demonstration of affection should not overwhelm the group member or be experienced as unacceptably intrusive or inappropriate. The group leader can serve the group as a role model for giving and receiving affection.

Group leaders should be encouraged to flourish and develop their own style. Coleadership can be an important part of the learning process, for leaders can share their multidisciplinary accomplishments. New leaders need to be prepared for the expression of strong feelings even though they are doing group work, not psychotherapy. Meticulous preparation, communication, consistent scheduling, and attention to detail are important. Student leaders may encounter resistance from staff members or simply disorganization and inefficiency, but a well-run facility in which support for the new leader filters down from the top administrators and clinical managers can take group work in its stride. In any case, students or any group leader should have strong preceptor support while working with a group. Groups for primary, secondary, and tertiary prevention are also important interventions.

Exercises

EXERCISE 1

Three essential needs of group members have been identified as inclusion, control, and affection. In the following account of a group meeting identify one example of inclusion, control, and affection.

This is the twentieth meeting of a long-term, closed group that meets weekly in a retirement home. A baccalaureate student from a nearby college interested in reminiscence groups began the group. After the student completed the semester, the activity director continued the group. The group had been discussing important people in their childhood and had brought photograph albums to share with one another. One quiet woman had no photographs with her. The leader noticed and made a special effort to draw her out and to get her to describe some of the people in her early life. As she described them, she quietly explained that the family possessions had been lost when their home burned to the ground. She started to cry. The leader said, "Oh, let's be brave now," and quickly changed the subject. A woman sitting next to the crying woman reached over and took her hand. At that point, an older man stated that no one had listened to him when he talked about being a fireman in an earthquake in San Francisco. The leader ignored him and asked what the group would like to see in next month's activity programs.

EXERCISE 2

Lack of knowledge about what other disciplines do regarding groups hampers our understanding. Make a list of all the disciplines you think might conduct groups with older people, and then write a succinct description of the types of groups you think they lead. Double-check your answers with a peer or colleague.

Example: Choose occupational therapists. Write your list; then read Chapter 27 and ascertain how accurate your perceptions were.

EXERCISE 3

Write a paragraph about a group you would implement for people at each type of prevention: primary, secondary, and tertiary. State why it would be appropriate for each level of intervention.

References

Antonovsky, A. (1987). *Unraveling the mystery of health*. San Francisco: Jossey Bass.

Antonovsky, A. (1994). The sense of coherence: An historical and future perspective. In H. McCubbin et al. (Eds.), *Sense of coherence and resiliency*. Wisconsin: University of Wisconsin Systems.

Cappeleiz, P. (2002). Cognitive-reminiscence therapy for depressed older adults in day hospitals and long-term care. In J. D. Webster & B. K. Haight (Eds.), *Critical advances in reminiscence work: From theory to application* (pp. 300–313). New York: Springer.

Choi, N. G., & Dinse, S. (1998). Challenges and opportunities of the aging population: Social work education and practice for productive aging. *Educational Gerontology*, 24(2), 159–173.

Erikson, E. H. (1950). *Childhood and society*. New York: W. W. Norton & Co.

Erikson, E. H. (1982). *The life cycle completed*. New York: W. W. Norton & Co.

Gitterman, A. (2002). Reflections on dealing with group member's testing of my authority. In R. Kurland & A. Malekoff (Eds.), *Stories celebrating group work: It is not always easy to sit on your mouth* (pp. 185–192). Binghamton, NY: Haworth Social Work Practice Press.

Haulotte, S., & McNeil, J. (1998). Integrating didactic and experiential aging curriculum. *Journal of Gerontological Social Work*, 30(3/4), 43–57.

Laurie, N. (2000). Healthy people 2010: Setting the nation's public health agenda. *Academic Medicine*, 75(1), 12–13.

Manton, K. G., Cornelius, E. S., & Woodbury, M. A. (1995). Nursing home residents: A multivariate analysis of their medical, behavioral, psychosocial and service use characteristics. *Journal of Gerontology*, 50A(5), M242–M251.

Menec, V. (2003). The relation between everyday activities and successful aging: A six year longitudinal study. *Journal of Gerontology*, 58B(2), P574–P582.

Miller, J. F. (1992). *Coping with chronic illness: Overcoming powerlessness* (pp. 3–18). Philadelphia: F. A. Davis.

Moody, R. (2003). *Human values in aging newsletter.* Institute for Human Values in Aging. www.HRMoody.com (Retrieved August 6, 2003).

Reish, M., & Jarman-Rhode, L. (2000). The future of social work in the US. *Journal of Social Work Education*, 36(2), 201–204.

Rice, S. (2004). Group work with the elderly. In P. Ephross & F. Greif (Eds.), *Group work with populations at risk.* New York: Oxford University Press.

Safford, F., & Krell, G. (Eds.), (1997). *Gerontology for health professionals.* New York: NASW.

Scharlach, A., Damron-Rodriguez, J., Robinson, B., & Feldman, R. (2000). Educating social workers for an aging society: A vision for the twenty first century. *Journal of Social Work Education*, (3), 521–538.

Schutz, W. C. (1966). *Interpersonal underworld.* Palo Alto, CA: Science & Behavior.

Tolson, E. R., Reid, W. J., & Garvin, C. D. (2003). *Generalist practice: A task-centered approach.* New York: Columbia University Press.

Turner, F. J. (1996). *Social work treatment: Interlocking theoretical approaches.* New York: Free Press.

Yale, R. (1995). *Developing support groups for individuals with early-stage Alzheimer's disease: Planning, implementation and evaluation.* Baltimore: Health Professions Press.

BIBLIOGRAPHY

Association for the Advancement of Social Work with Groups/Council for Social Work Education. (1997). *Standards of social work practice with groups.* Author. New York: CSWE.

AASWG/CSWE. (1997). *Bibliography on group work.* Author. New York: CSWE.

Berman-Rossi, T. (Ed.). (1994). *Social work: The collected works of William Schwartz.* Itasca: IL: F. E. Peacock.

Mellor, M. J., & Ivry, J. (Eds.). (2002). *Advancing gerontological social work education.* New York: Haworth. Copublished as *Journal of Gerontological Social Work,* 39 (1/2), 2002.

Ragan, A. M., & Bowen, A. (2001). Improving attitudes regarding the elderly population. *The Gerontologist*, 41, 511–515.

Chapter 7

Group Goals and Contracts: Assessment and Planning

Faith Gibson
Irene Burnside

Key Words

- Agreement
- Anxiety
- Assessment
- Confidentiality
- Group objectives
- Information
- Verbal and written contracts

Learning Objectives

- Identify the four phases or stages in the life of a group
- Define the term *contract* and list its major components
- Discuss the importance of agreeing on group objectives.
- State the importance of confidentiality to group work
- Describe six secondary purposes of the screening interview

This chapter offers students, instructors, health and social care workers, and volunteers a discussion of stages of group development and emphasizes the importance of contracting.

Phases or Stages in the Development of Groups

All groups throughout their existence, regardless of where their objectives fall along a continuum of treatment to task, move through four different stages or phases. These stages apply overall and within each separate session. They are usually described as the preliminary or planning phase; the beginning phase; the work or middle phase; and the ending phase. Some writers separate out preparation and then refer to three other stages. This division provides structure to a group throughout its existence and within each separate session. The beginning phase is concerned with introductions, clarifying and agreeing on the contract, and helping people to feel sufficiently relaxed to begin work on the agreed agenda. The middle phase is characterized by increasing trust, commitment to task, and growing respect between members. The ending phase provides time for winding down, taking stock of accomplishments and disengagement (Berman-Rossi, 1993).

The length of each phase depends upon the number of sessions overall and the tasks to be accomplished. The dynamics and development of each group change over time and the behavior and emotions experienced by leaders and members also vary from phase to phase (Shulman, 1999). It is important for leaders to tune in to each phase overall and within each session, and to be aware of the associated feelings and work to be undertaken. Uncertainty, tentativeness, anxiety, and heightened expectations usually characterize beginnings (Northen & Kurland, 2001). By the middle phase trust, confidence, and engagement develops and endings are likely to evoke a mixture of pride in accomplishment, sadness that the group is ending, and regret that more was not accomplished (Kelly & Berman-Rossi, 1999; Northen & Kurland, 2001).

Written and Verbal Contracts

One of the most important tasks of the group leader is the formation of a contract with each aged group member and with the group as a whole. This aspect of professional performance in group leadership is often ignored by beginners. The foundation of a contract is laid in the preliminary or planning phase when a leader first meets a potential member and it is then carried forward into the early sessions of the beginning phase as well as sessional contracting taking place at the start of each separate session.

A *contract* is a "binding agreement between two or more persons or parties" (*Webster*, 1973). Sometimes students confuse the words *contract* and *contact*. To make contact with a person is not the same as to contract with the person. A contact can be just a casual encounter such as a greeting like "Good morning." But when planning group work a contact is the beginning of a discussion about the possibility of doing something together. It leads on to a contract that is built on the exchange of very specific information, and it contains a mutual agreement about a course of action, and the roles and responsibilities expected of group leaders and members.

A contract is considered to be voluntary for both parties and is explicitly agreed to by both. As Northen and Kurland (2001) explain, there may be wide disparities in what leaders and potential members expect from a group experience. "If they are to make good use of the group, the members need to know what rights and responsibilities they have in relation to each other and to the worker and what the basic rules are that govern their relationship with each other" (p. 312). The contract is a device for clarifying such concerns.

One can never simply assume that an older individual is eager to be in a group, so the leader must move gently and never assertively in the initiation and completion of the contract. This is especially true of frail and institutionalized older people, who have little control over their lives and are likely to feel they are in a subservient position concerning the staff and the group leader (Berman-Rossi, 1990, 1993) Older group members are too frequently selected on the basis of their ability to participate in a group (for example, mobility, hearing, social and cognitive functioning), rather than their explicit desire to attend. Because many older adults in institutions have little opportunity to say no, they may decline to join a group because a refusal provides a rare opportunity for them to assert themselves even though they may be quite interested in attending. A leader should suggest to all those who refuse an initial invitation that they attend the first meeting on a trial basis without commitment to see what it is like. A personal invitation often works well or an invitation made by a person who is well acquainted with and respected by the potential member. Respect for the client's wishes is important. There needs to be clarity about the purpose of the group, but too much information at this preliminary stage can be overwhelming or provoke anxiety.

In group work, a contract is an agreement between the leader and members regarding the group experience and should include a careful explanation of the objectives, and number, frequency, location, and duration of meetings. The older person should be encouraged to ask questions, especially if it is the member's first group experience. It is very important to give the potential member an opportunity to discuss the goals of the group as expressed in the original proposal. It is customary to distinguish between a preliminary contract initiated with each individual member which forms the basis for the group coming together and a group contract that emerges after full discussion in the early meetings and is agreed upon by the whole group.

Contracting takes time; it should not be rushed. Information usually has to be repeated both in and out of the group for a variety of reasons. It needs to be precise, not vague, and the leader should ensure that all members have an opportunity to ask questions and express their views. A concerted effort to communicate in simple direct ways to achieve understanding and cooperation is essential with all people, especially people who have dementia. Learning the skill of checking back with people to make sure they have understood what has been said is very important.

A contract may be verbal or written. If one is working with forgetful, disoriented older persons, it is best to summarize a verbal contract with a simple written statement. The contract, once discussed and finalized with the members, should include the following information:

1. Name of group   Name of member
2. Aims and objectives (or outcomes, including any anticipated tangible products)
3. Time
4. Place
5. Duration of group sessions
6. Lifetime of the group
7. Ground rules
8. List of other members (This information can be important because the presence of a peer or roommate on the list may serve as an incentive for a shy person to try the group.)
9. Name of the leader

In making the contract, the leader should keep the characteristics of the group members clearly in mind. (Group membership is discussed in detail in Chapter 8.) Essentially, the group leader should consider the following information about the prospective member:

- Age
- Race and ethnicity
- Physical and psychological problems
- Diagnosis
- Functional capacity
- Communication abilities
- Gender, sexual orientation, first language, and religion
- Amount of affect—depressed, sullen, giggly, and so forth
- Mobility
- Transportation
- Living arrangements
- Level of education

Nursing and care plans may be helpful as a source of some of this information. For example, a director of nurses in a Canadian nursing home keeps a small book entitled *Openers*, which contains a list of the interests, accomplishments, and talents of each resident. The lists give nurses' aides some leads for conversation during care. Bell and Troxel (1997, 2001) recommend keeping short summaries of the salient points in the life stories of day center members in a ring binder in the staff break room. Some facilities place short summaries on individual plastic-coated cards. The group leader can then readily gather up the cards of group members and use the summarized information as a basis for relationship building and contracting.

Reaching a mutual agreement does not mean that group leaders abdicate responsibility for leadership. Goal setting must begin with the leader's statements regarding the purpose and function of the group (Toseland & Rivas, 2001). This is especially true for students doing group work in agencies. Preceptors need to insist that students be very clear in their minds about the type of group they are leading and what they hope to accomplish. It is helpful if goal formation is clarified so the leader can focus on three sets of interrelated goals:

1. Group-centered goals—Proper functioning and maintenance of a group.
2. Shared goals—These goals focus on the mutual needs of all members of the group (Shulman, 1999).
3. Individual goals—Goals are focused on the particular needs of each group member (Shulman, 1999).

A leader must help each member to fulfill expectations and to achieve his or her desired goals. Group experiences may be new to some members, and they might not know what to expect. But if a group does not provide fulfillment for them, they may drop out. Coffee, tea, and other refreshments are often strong reasons for some members to stay, especially those in long-term care facilities. There are other considerations about groups in long-term care. Gitterman and Shulman (2004) emphasize that group goals must be achievable and in tune with the philosophy and objectives of the host establishment. It would be, for example, unethical to start a patients' rights group in a nursing home if it was obvious that the administrator did not seriously intend to implement its recommendations (Northen, 1998).

Goals for a group should be carefully balanced and need to include both process and outcome goals. There must be agreement about what the group will work on and how the group will conduct itself. Focusing exclusively on either tasks or process can cause the group to disband. Focusing on tasks can lead to undue competitiveness, conflict, and members relating only on an instrumental level. However, focusing only on the socioemotional needs of members can lead to frustration, because the group cannot accomplish tasks efficiently (Toseland & Rivas, 2001).

Goals can change during the life of the group and contracts may need to be renegotiated if they no longer command the allegiance of the members as demonstrated by their commitment to and engagement in the agreed work program. The leader can help the process by being positive and upbeat and by praising group members for their accomplishments; it is also important for the leader to state the obstacles individuals face (Northen & Kurland, 2001).

It is well known that relationships with older people begin on a one-to-one basis; this is also true in group work. The vis-à-vis encounter is of great importance while establishing the contract. The time spent making the initial contract gives the group leader a chance to assess the individual both physically and psychologically. If the group is to be co-led, both leaders should meet with the potential member and jointly, if possible, share the contract negotiation so as to model coleadership. This principle is especially important in egalitarian leadership. If in some situations there is to be senior-junior or teacher-student coleadership, it is important that the junior leader carries clearly defined responsibilities and is not viewed simply as an assistant. As the student's experience grows, he or she may rotate and increase responsibilities as it is widely accepted that leadership skills are best acquired by direct practice. If a prospective group is likely to consist of men and women of different ethnicity, it can also help to have leaders representing these differences (Brown & Mistry, 1994; Mistry & Brown, 1997). Coleadership with each person carrying carefully defined roles and responsibilities can be an effective means of developing future group work leaders, and role modeling is viewed as an excellent mode of learning for many students.

Group Member Selection

Assessment of the potential group member during the contact-making period is of crucial importance. It is better not to negotiate a contract if one has some doubts but rather just to visit with the older person for a while and secure more information.

A group leader should not take an individual into the group solely on someone else's advice—for example, the doctor, the family, the director of nurses. The leader should make the final decision about the appropriateness of the individual for a specific group (Northen & Kurland, 2001). After several inappropriate decisions, students will learn how to make the correct ones. Burnside recounts how she once accepted into a group a woman whose behavior was upsetting to everyone. She was agitated, restless, and ruined the refreshment period by drinking the cream and eating the sugar on the serving tray; it was necessary to remove her from the group. That is an action of very last resort.

The size of the group should be carefully considered, and few, if any, group leaders would now wish to emulate Linden's work (1953) with 40 to 51 regressed aged women on a geriatric ward; one wonders how he managed them all. Students often get carried away and feel that group work is like cooking potatoes—one more will not matter very much.

The frailties and physical status of the members should be carefully evaluated in considering a manageable group. If there are able, helpful, mobile members in the group, they will often be of great assistance to the leader. Also, if there are coleaders, a larger group can be planned, because there will be one leader available to handle the extraneous occurrences such as observing the non-included, the silent members, or the nonverbal cues that might otherwise be missed. It is also helpful to have someone to assist with the transportation problems that inevitably arise in both hospital-based groups and those conducted on an outpatient basis. In outpatient or day care groups, the receptionist or a volunteer is often most helpful with some of these logistics.

The leader should select a variety of persons, keeping in mind that two hard-of-hearing or three silent, withdrawn, depressed persons can make the work of a leader extremely difficult. If all group members are in wheelchairs, extra help will be needed. In an outpatient setting, the needs of the group members must be carefully analyzed. Subsequent poor attendance may be due to transportation difficulties that were not taken care of before the group began. If a group is specifically for people with sensory impairment, then specific knowledge and skills will be essential in order to meet the needs of the members. The size of the group will need to be adjusted to enable each person to participate and be able to derive satisfaction from belonging to the group.

The group leader needs to be prepared to work hard, plan ahead, and change plans as group needs emerge in the meetings. Staff members and other individuals often view group work as an easy intervention, but group work with older adults requires energy, spontaneity, organization, and tenacity.

Group Work Expenses and Payment

Cost must be carefully considered at the time of planning a group. Costs in terms of leadership, manpower, materials, supplies, refreshments, and staff time to assist in assembling group work can be an overhead expense for the leader—something Burnside learned from her own experience. She once had a weekly group in a facility far from her home, which involved a fair amount of traveling. When gasoline was rationed during the energy crunch, she had to discontinue the group because she did not have the necessary fuel. Similarly, it is unfair for students to carry the costs of all props and materials used. Costs should be budgeted for and hopefully shared by the agency. Volunteers may wish to contribute, but it should be their own choice. In one group Burnside led, the patients found out that she was furnishing the refreshments; they wanted to pay and would often share the expenses because they enjoyed the snacks that were served. Group psychotherapy in a private office and groups in an outpatient clinical setting would involve a cost to the aged person, but students usually work without pay.

Medicare is the major funder of geriatric group work and group work practitioners may be licensed to deliver these services. The Omnibus Budget Reconciliation Act (1987) Medicare Part B updates give information about reimbursement of clinical psychologists and licensed clinical social workers practicing as independent providers. State Medicaid offices or state welfare and social services offices determine the qualification and application processes for psychologists and mental health professionals who wish to become providers. Medigap coverage delivered through managed care is a supplemental source of payment for some people (Erwin, 1996).

Group Goals and Anxiety

Group goals should be explicit in the beginning, even though they may change as the group evolves. Most new leaders and the group members need some structure to reduce anxiety. It is to be expected that a group of strangers meeting together for the first time—both members and leaders—will experience some anxiety associated with newness and memories of prior experiences of group participation.

Toseland and Rivas (2001) remind us that the beginning of a group can be a stressful time for those who have decided to participate. Beginnings are characterized by caution and tentativeness as members attempt to find their place within the group while at the same time maintaining their own identities.

The goals of the group meetings may have to be restated frequently, as they are often unheard by anxious group members. Anxiety must be dealt with continually, first in the encounter of the contract making and later in the group meetings. The new group leader should begin to look for cues to anxiety during the contract making; these may be cues the leader will observe in later group meetings. Most groups, even familiar ones, tend to evoke anxiety in most people. The degree of anxiety is diminished with acquaintance and length of membership in it. No person, however, feels as comfortable in a group as he or she does with one individual. An individual is seldom as threatening as a group, where anxiety or ambivalence is always present. The leader may therefore see less anxiety in the initial interview than is observed in the same individual during later group meetings.

New leaders must also be prepared to deal with their own anxiety. Many of us who do group work with older people feel that we floundered when we began; we had no definite guidelines to follow and experienced high anxiety. Out of such floundering, however, came a sound rationale and an awareness of what to do and what not to do in group work.

Confidentiality

Group workers agree that it is essential to contract with group members about confidentiality. Members need to feel safe in the group. Not everyone, however, agrees on the means by which standards of confidentiality should be initiated and maintained. The crucial issue is whether the group leaders should structure the situation by making a ground rule about confidentiality or should wait for an agreement to come from the group itself. Stock Whitaker (2000) believes that agreement about confidentiality must emerge from the felt needs of the group. Yalom (1995) states that the rule about confidentiality can be raised by either the group or the leader and that a valuable discussion about trust, shame, fear of disclosure, and commitment to the group may arise when confidentiality is a matter of common concern. In groups of older adults who cannot verbalize well or have problems being articulate, the leader may need to provide the direction and formulate the rule about confidentiality and then seek agreement to it.

New group workers may feel diffident about dealing with confidentiality; they need to acquaint themselves with the existing policies and practices of the agency in which the group is located as well as being guided by their personal and professional values. Older people in institutions frequently suffer from lack of privacy and often fear punitive treatment by family or staff. For suspicious or paranoid persons, a ground rule of confidentiality stated by the group leader may offer some reassurance. Northen and Kurland (2001) argue that group members have a right to expect that the worker will use information constructively in their interests so that the best possible service can be provided. The agency is responsible to the clients it serves but also to the community which supports it. This double responsibility requires very careful negotiation concerning confidentiality matters. If problems arise that need to be discussed with staff members or doctors (such as talk of suicide by a group member, a sudden change in mood, or a drastic change in behavior), the leader can request permission of the group member to discuss the matter with the others concerned. Doing so can be seen as being an advocate for the older person in the group.

Prejudging the Members

New group leaders have a tendency to underestimate the potential of the individual members of a group of older people in an institutionalized setting (Berman-Rossi, 2004). Older persons living in the community are also often coping more creatively with their problems than health care workers realize. Positive, optimistic attitudes are important. Respect and trust for older persons and a belief in what they can still do rather than an emphasis on what they can no longer do are essential. In a world where underestimating the potential of older group members is unfortunately very common, a strengths approach is crucial (Fast & Chapin, 2000; Kivnick & Murray, 2001).

Summary

This chapter discusses stages of group development and emphasizes the importance of contracting. It suggests that the new group leader carefully consider group member selection, expenses and payments, anxiety, confidentiality, prejudgment of members, and underestimation of their capacities.

Initial interviews are needed to assess the potential group member and undertake initial contracting. Not everyone proposed for a particular group may be suitable for membership. The leader makes the final decision on whether a particular person is to be admitted to the group and should not be swayed by others.

A preliminary contract with each prospective group member is the first step in initiating a new group. The process of contracting is then addressed within the whole group in the early sessions and either a verbal or written (preferably both) contract is negotiated. This should include the following information: time, place, duration of group sessions, lifetime of the group, list of other members, purpose or objectives of the group, its name, and name of the leader.

In making the contract, the leader should assess the prospective member both physically and psychologically and make as sure as possible that the member understands and agrees to the contract. Size of the group, availability of assistance from staff and group members, transportation, and financial arrangements must also be considered.

The initial meeting may give the leader a clue to the prospective member's anxiety level and effective methods for reducing it. Giving structure to the group by carefully agreeing to objectives, membership, and meeting arrangements early in the beginning phase and systematically contracting at the beginning of each subsequent session concerning what is to take place within that session helps to reduce anxiety in both new leaders and group members.

Confidentiality in the group is more likely to be respected if negotiated as a ground rule of the contract and not imposed by the leader. Protecting the confidences of wary institutionalized older people is extremely important. It is well to remember that we often underestimate the potential of aged group members; they may delightfully surprise us with their ability, talent, and performance in a group.

Exercises

Exercise 1

1. Define *contract*.
2. List at least four important kinds of specific information that a leader should give to an older client while making a contract.
3. Suggest several steps a leader can take to reduce anxiety among group members.

Exercise 2

You have interviewed six older persons in the hope of forming a group. The answers are two "Maybes," one "I will think about it," and four "Yes, I'll attend." List the three steps you would take next with the persons who answered "Maybe" and "I will think about it." Give your rationale for each step.

Exercise 3

What is meant by phases or stages in the life of a group? What are they, and what is their relevance to leaders and members?

Exercise 4

The agency in which you plan to conduct a group requests a detailed plan. Write goals, objectives, and evaluation methods, and enclose a possible draft contract.

References

Bell, V., & Troxel, D. (1997). *The best friend's approach to Alzheimer's care*. Baltimore: Health Professions Press.

Bell, V., & Troxel, D. (2001). *The best friend's staff*. Baltimore: Health Professions Press.

Berman-Rossi, T. (1990). Group work and older persons. In A. Monk (Ed.), *Handbook of gerontological services* (pp. 141–150). New York: Columbia University Press.

Berman-Rossi, T. (1993). Tasks and skills of the social worker across stages of group development. In S. Wencur, P. H. Epross, T. V. Vassal, & R. K. Varghese (Eds.), *Social work with groups: Expanding horizons*. New York: Haworth Press.

Berman-Rossi, T. (2004). Institutionalized older people. In A. Gitterman & L. Shulman (Eds.), *Mutual aid groups, vulnerable populations, and the life cycle*. New York: Columbia University Press.

Brown, A., & Mistry, T. (1994). Group work and mixed membership groups: Issues of race and gender. *Social Work with Groups*, 17(3), 5–20.

Erwin, K. T. (1996). *Group techniques for aging adults*. Washington, DC: Taylor Francis.

Fast, B., & Chapin, R. (2000). *Strengths-based care management for older adults*. Baltimore: Health Professions Press.

Gitterman, A., & Shulman, L. (Eds.). 2004. *Mutual aid groups, vulnerable populations, and the life cycle*. New York: Columbia University Press.

Kelly, T., & Berman-Rossi, T. (1999). Advancing stages of group developmental theory: The case of institutionalized older persons. *Social Work with Groups*, 22(2/3), 119–137.

Kivnick, H., & Murray, S. (2001). Life strengths interview guide. *Journal of Gerontological Social Work*, 34(4), 7–32.

Linden, M. (1953). Group psychotherapy with institutionalized senile women: A study in gerontological human relations. *International Journal of Group Psychotherapy*, 3, 150–170.

Mistry, T., & Brown, A. (1997). *Race and groupwork*. London: Whiting & Birch.

Northen, H. (1998). Ethical implications of social work with groups. *Social Work with Groups*, 21(1/2), 5–17.

Northen, H., & Kurland, R. (2001). *Social work with groups* (3rd ed.). New York: Columbia University Press.

Omnibus Budget Reconciliation Act (1987). Amendments to title X1X of the Social Security Act, Sections 1819 & 1919, B.4

Shulman, L. (1999). *The skills of helping individuals, families, groups, and communities* (4th ed.). Itasca, IL: F. E. Peacock.

Stock Whitaker, D. (2000). *Using groups to help people.* New York: Brunner-Routledge.

Toseland, R. W., & Rivas, R. (2001). *An introduction to group work practice.* New York: Macmillan Publishing Co.

Webster's New Collegiate Dictionary. (1973). H. B. Woolf (Ed.), Springfield, MA: Merriam Webster.

Yalom, I.D. (1995). *The theory and practice of group psychotherapy.* New York: Basic Books.

BIBLIOGRAPHY

Kurland, R., & Salmon, R. (Eds.). (1995). *Group work practice in a troubled society: Problems and opportunities.* Binghamton, New York: Haworth.

Lindsay, J., Turcotta, D., & Hopmeyer, E. (Eds.). (2003). *Crossing boundaries and developing alliances through group work.* Binghamton, New York: Haworth.

Chapter 8

Membership Selection and Criteria

Faith Gibson
Irene Burnside

Key Words

- Agitation
- Catastrophic reaction
- Catharsis
- Group setting
- Initial composition
- Intergenerational
- Life cycle
- Safety

Learning Objectives

- List 10 potential settings for group meetings
- Describe four beneficial effects of intergenerational groups
- Define three principles for guiding the selection of people with cognitive or sensory disabilities for group membership
- Discuss the types of persons to exclude from groups
- State three factors to consider in regard to group size
- Analyze the possible consequences of mixing people with dementia and alert older people in a group

By the crowd they have been broken, by the crowd shall they be healed.

—*L. Cody Marsh (1935, p. 392)*

Older people comprise a fascinating, unique collection of individuals of disparate ages ranging from around 55 to 100 plus. Students or new group leaders may approach the assignment of older people to groups with dismay, reluctance, and trepidation or with excitement, interest, and enthusiasm, depending on their past experience with older people (Pillemer & Albright, 1996). This chapter is concerned with considering group settings, criteria for group membership, goals, and some cautions to consider when beginning group work.

Settings for Group Meetings

The places where group meetings can be held vary widely. They include:

- Agencies serving older people and their families
- Acute care hospitals
- Board-and-care facilities
- Churches
- Community arts organizations
- Community mental health centers

- Continuing care retirement communities
- Day care centers
- Domiciliary care by Veterans Administration
- Foster homes
- Hotel–apartment residences
- Hotels in geriatric ghettos of cities
- Industrial plants (for example, preretirement groups)
- Libraries
- Low-cost housing units
- Mobile home units
- Museums
- Nonproprietary intermediate care facilities
- Nonproprietary skilled nursing care facilities
- Nutrition sites
- Outpatient departments
- Prisons
- Private offices
- Private residences
- Proprietary intermediate care facilities
- Proprietary skilled nursing care facilities
- Recreation and park centers
- Rehabilitation hospitals
- Religious homes for retired persons
- Retirement homes and retirement campus communities
- School settings
- Senior centers
- State mental hospitals
- Veterans hospitals
- Volunteer centers

The setting for group meetings can give some indication of the individuals who may be available for group membership in that milieu. One can also make some assumptions about the age and physical condition of such individuals. For example, in nursing homes, one can expect to find very old people. Residents of skilled and intermediate care facilities can usually be expected to be old and frail and to have multiple diagnoses. See Chapter 12 for suggestions for working with people who are old and physically impaired. At a senior center, however, there may be participants who retired early and are in quite stable health who are viewed as young-old.

Because health care providers' involvement with the aged population is so widespread, it is conceivable they could be doing group work in any of the above settings. The most likely settings, of course, are acute care hospitals, rehabilitation hospitals, skilled and intermediate nursing care facilities, outpatient departments, day care centers, retirement communities, and senior centers. It has been well documented that only 3–4% of those treated at community mental health centers are older persons, so older people unfortunately have only limited opportunities to engage in either group psychotherapy or group work with explicit therapeutic objectives.

Group Member Selection

One of the most important planning phase responsibilities is selection of group members. Yalom's (1985) considerations for group membership are discussed here as they relate specifically to group work with older persons and are still relevant today. Yalom, although writing from the stance of a group psychotherapist, states a widely applicable general point:

> The fate of a group therapy patient and of a therapy group may, in large measure, be determined before the first group therapy session. Unless careful selection criteria are used, the majority of patients assigned to group therapy will terminate treatment, discouraged and without benefit. Research on small groups… suggests that the initial composition of the group has a powerful influence on the ultimate outcome of the entire group (p. 156).

Yalom (1985) describes the importance of ensuring that positive expectations and experiences are perceived as outweighing negative or ambivalent aspects of group membership. He believes:

> Members are prone to terminate membership in a therapy group and are thereby poor candidates when the punishments or disadvantages of group membership outweigh the rewards or anticipated rewards. When speaking of punishments or disadvantages of group membership, I refer to the price the patient must pay for group membership. This includes an investment of time, money, energy, as well as a variety of dysphorias arising from the group experience, including anxiety, frustration, discouragement, and rejection (p. 173).

When establishing a group, a major decision concerns the characteristics of the potential members. Should the group members share major characteristics and be homogeneous or should they be different or heterogeneous? The decision will be influenced by access to members, their availability and personal preferences, and what mix of membership is likely to best serve the group's intended objectives (Brown & Mistry, 1994; Mistry & Brown, 1997; Northen & Kurland, 2001).

Inexperienced group leaders should not overload themselves with too many potentially complex factors. As skill and confidence develop, leaders will be better able to assist groups to cope with more diverse membership in ways that are satisfying for the group as a whole and for each individual member. The need to respect and integrate differences refers to many characteristics including physical, sensory, cognitive, ethnic, class, sexual, and cultural characteristics.

Characteristics of Members

It is important to carefully assess the personality of the older person while negotiating the preliminary contract. (See Chapter 7 on contracting.) Group work requires the skillful selection of a variety of personalities. A well-balanced group should have both talkative and quiet persons, depressed and not-so-depressed persons. Mistrusting members need to be balanced with trusting persons. Calm, serene individuals can offset hyperactive individuals. Members will take on various roles and tasks in a group. Making an assessment during initial contract negotiation is possible and important because the leader has an opportunity then to observe the patterns of behavior in each individual.

Selecting people who have dementia for inclusion in a group requires particular care in order to avoid making excessive demands upon their impaired cognitive abilities. It is equally important not to underestimate their residual abilities. A catastrophic reaction is a term used to describe an extreme, sudden, and distressing reaction that sometimes occurs when an individual who has dementia finds he or she cannot perform a task requested or feels overwhelmed by the demands made upon them. The response may appear exaggerated but it is essential to try to appreciate the situation from the viewpoint of the person with dementia. A person who feels overloaded may weep or blush or become agitated, angry, or paranoid. The person may even strike out or get up and leave the situation. They may have little comprehension of why they are reacting this way, but they know they feel threatened. The best tactic for dealing with catastrophic reactions is, of course, prevention. Avoid making excessive demands on vulnerable people and learn to empathize with them, which means to see things as if you were in their shoes or sitting in their chair. When the interviewer or group leader perceives a slight increase in agitation or anxiety, the subject should be changed or the limelight removed from the group member. The leader can also avoid some catastrophic reactions by simplifying the demands made upon the individual and by assisting and supporting them through required tasks. Mace, Rabins, Castleton, McEwen, and Meredith (1999) in *The 36-Hour Day* give sound advice about preventing and handling catastrophic reactions.

The leader should be aware that the members do not have to be at the same cognitive level, but that to mix very cognitively impaired older individuals with alert and lucid persons is to court problems. In extreme cases, an impaired individual may be precipitated into a catastrophic reaction, as he or she will not be able to perform as well as some of the more alert members of the group. Also, the alert members may well perceive themselves to be slowed up and retarded if they are asked to attend such a group, and the experience could be harmful to their self-esteem. A small number of people with early stage dementia may, however, cope well in a mixed ability group in which they are stimulated by socializing with others who are willing to accept them. Similarly, it is unwise to overload a group with too many members who have sensory or speech difficulties and who require special assistance if they are to participate in and benefit from belonging to a group.

Educational level or present cognitive capacity alone cannot be used as an accurate tool for group selection. In one group in a skilled nursing facility, Burnside observed a man with a third-grade education and another with a college degree. They got along famously and had the utmost respect for each other; in fact, when the group was terminated, the men asked to be roommates because the bond of friendship between them was so strong.

Mobile persons should be included with persons in wheelchairs if the group is in an institutional setting, especially if there is to be only one leader. Seating arrangements are most important. A group consisting entirely of wheelchair patients is unwieldy—that is, the leader and the members cannot get close to one another in meetings. Wheelchairs will also require a larger meeting room and questions of transportation and access require careful consideration at the planning stage. The leader often may have to assist in seating arrangements, especially with people who are physically frail or seriously impaired. The number and mix of members with a disability and the sitting arrangements within a group session are closely linked to the number and deployment of leaders and helpers.

Persons to Exclude

Not everyone wishes to join a group and there are some people whose disabilities, personality, or behavior makes it improbable that they will benefit from membership. Their presence may also seriously detract from the benefits expected for other people. Generally it is considered wise to exclude the following, although there will always be exceptions:

- Disturbed, hyperactive, or aggressive persons
- People who are habitually tearful
- People with a psychotic depression
- People recommended solely by the staff
- People who indicate that they do not wish to participate
- Individuals diagnosed as having bipolar disorder
- Deaf people without adequate lip-reading skills
- Excessively hypochondriacal or obsessional people
- Exceedingly private individuals who resent intrusion by others

Medical Problems

It is important that the group leader be aware of the medical problems of each person in the group. Patients with emphysema, for instance, may need medication before group meetings to enable them to participate more fully. Arthritic patients may need aspirin before meetings so that they are not uncomfortable; patients with recent hip fractures may also need medication. It would be wise for the leader to check the medications of the members. Too many depressed withdrawn people are likely to be problematic for other members. Some people who have had a stroke cry habitually even if they are not unduly depressed. Sometimes over-medicated patients doze off in a group meeting, and their sleepiness has nothing to do with the quality of the meeting itself or with anxiety or withdrawal. New leaders may blame themselves for such behaviors. (See Chapter 12 for further information on physical limitations in members.)

Leaders also should be alert to the physical problems of group members. Edematous feet, for example, could be elevated during the group sessions to prevent severe stasis edema. Kidney problems are common in old age, and prostatitis or benign prostatic hypertrophy is a common problem in old men. Patients who have to urinate frequently may also need some special consideration; for example, perhaps they should sit near the door, so they can easily go to the bathroom and return to the group with a minimum of disturbance. Such individuals should also be advised to stop at the rest room en route to the group meeting.

Number of Group Members

The group leader decides the size of the group although new leaders often have trouble deciding how many persons to include. The number depends on such factors as who is available; the type of group, its objectives and program; whether there is a single leader or coleaders; available space (for example, wheelchair-bound persons require more space); whether it is an open or a closed group (an open group may allow for greater fluctuation of the membership and therefore may be a larger group); whether any members have a sensory loss; the degree of frailty of the members; and the past experience and confidence of the group leader. If the leader chooses to work with cognitively impaired or very frail individuals, two to four is usually a workable number. (See Chapter 11 on groups for people with dementia.)

One of the difficulties encountered in residential facilities is that the people who are not asked to join the group may feel offended. Older people often become jealous of their roommates who go off to group meetings (or "classes" as many older persons prefer to describe them). Sometimes they request to be put on the waiting list. Burnside recalled a 90-year-old man, Mr. H., who approached her in the hall one day when she was on her way to a group meeting. "Excuse me," he said, "but I would sure like to join that group of old people who meet with you every Friday." He joined the group after another member died. Mr. H. had taken the initiative to join, was readily accepted by the group, and seemed to get a great deal of pleasure from the meetings. In fact, he insisted his daughter attend a meeting and meet "the friends"; he told her she would have to change her visiting hours because he had to go to his meeting on the afternoon she usually visited.

There are three salient points to be drawn from this man's experience: (1) A request for membership should be honored if possible. If older people take responsibility for their own lives, and are observant about their own milieu, they should be rewarded for such behavior. It also says something about the importance of group work if the residents discuss it among themselves, and this is a justification for not making confidentiality guidelines too restrictive. (2) The importance of the group meetings to the member must be considered. This man even had his family change their visiting hours! (3) Families may resent the group if it interferes with their own schedule, and some work may have to be done with members of the family if they express displeasure or display anxiety about their relatives' participation (Toseland, 1995). There is probably no optimum size for a group, but in larger groups there is less opportunity for the members to interact with each other. In smaller groups, there will be greater demands on each member to participate (Kelly, 1999).

It is customary for mutual aid and therapy groups to have from six to ten members. Advocacy groups, however, can benefit from larger numbers of members because they can contribute their expertise and person power for selected projects and tasks. Gibson (2004) suggests that reminiscence groups usually have from 6 to 10 members and are very much smaller for people who have dementia unless members are paired with an equal number of leaders and helpers to permit considerable individual attention within a larger group. Leaders will soon discover not only the types of groups they are most skilled at leading, but the optimum size of the groups as well. As their experience grows and their skills develop, they will be able to confidently increase the size of the group.

Suggestions for New Leaders

The leader must decide whether to have an open or closed group (Toseland, 1995; Corey, & Corey, 2002). The merits of open and closed groups are summarized in **Table 8–1**. In open groups, members may come to meetings when they wish. The membership varies widely from meeting to meeting, with members joining and leaving at any time throughout the life of the group. This means that members will experience the group in different ways. While newcomers will be at the beginning phase, longer established members will be keen to progress through the work phase, and they may be retarded in experiencing the intimacy and mutual trust that develops in well-established groups with a stable membership. Closed groups have a stable membership, and new members are usually not added, or added only by a joint decision of leaders and members. In many closed groups, lost members are not replaced and the group dwindles in size. This is a particular hazard in older people's groups where illness and death may threaten the viability of the group (Orr, 1994). Therefore it is usually wiser to start off with more members than may first seem desirable so that the group may be sustained even with reduced numbers.

The leader also must decide on heterogeneity versus homogeneity in the group. **Table 8–2** summarizes the advantages and disadvantages of each. Brown and Mistry (1994) and Mistry and Brown (1997) consider how issues of diversity of race and gender affect both leaders and members of groups. Toseland and Rivas (2001) comprehensively discuss issues of race, class, gender, and ethnicity, and Cohen and Mullender (2003) explore the implications of gender in group work.

Some practice examples may serve as warnings for the new leader. Including two or more persons of the same minority group in the membership will facilitate the group process and avoid the risk of an isolated member being scapegoated. Once a student included in her group a full-blooded native American and a white man who hated native Americans. The native American dropped the group within a few meetings. In the Hawaiian Islands, the melting-pot islands, Burnside found that it was easier to include people from many ethnic groups because of greater tolerance for racial diversity and for different lifestyles there. In general, however, if a single minority person is included, he or she may drop out soon after the group has begun. This also applies to a lone man in an all women's group or a lone woman in an all male group. A single member risks being stereotyped or isolated by the rest of the group. Even if the lone person does not attract negative attention, he or she may nevertheless feel overwhelmed by being the sole representative of a minority.

Safety of Members

Another caution for the new leader concerns the unstable person who blows up frequently and is verbally or physically abusive. Just the verbal abusiveness can intimidate some group members. Even if obstreperous people behave well in the meetings, their reputations have probably preceded them, and group members will have heard

Table 8–1 OPEN AND CLOSED GROUPS

Open

Advantages

- Allows new resources and ideas to be brought to the group
- Ensures sufficient participation over the life of the group
- Leader may find it more challenging than a closed group
- Task completion may be more effective if newcomers complement existing members

Disadvantages

- Open, explicit sessional contracting is crucial
- May become difficult to lead if many new members attend. Adding new members can be disruptive to the group
- New members do not know previous experiences in group
- Phases of group process are different because of changing membership
- Instability may result from leadership and membership changes
- Lack of cohesion and reduced levels of trust and intimacy
- Need to review ground rules with each new member
- Continuity between sessions is difficult to achieve
- Interventions made need closure within each session
- Development of trust, intimacy, and cohesion is inhibited

Closed

Advantages

- Greater sense of cohesion, trust, and intimacy
- Greater stability of roles and norms
- Passage through group steps is more orderly, predictable
- Fewer variables for a neophyte leader to attend to because of stability of membership
- Leader can effectively deal with absences and terminations because they are fewer

Disadvantages

- When members drop out or are absent, group may become too small for effective interaction
- May become stale without ideas of new members
- Leader may become bored with the same members

Source: Adapted from Corey, M. S., & Corey, G., 1992.

enough hair-raising stories to be inclined to give such people a wide berth. Meetings can be strained if such an individual is included. New group leaders will eventually learn how to handle such a member. A tiny 95-year-old woman, for example, was knocked off her chair by another resident during a violent outburst in the dining room before the group meeting. She was badly shaken up; although not physically hurt, she was thoroughly frightened and avoided the other woman thereafter.

It is the responsibility of the leader to provide for the safety of the members and to protect the frail members of the group. Some people may be extremely frail and can be taken advantage of by stronger group members, by other members, and, unfortunately, by the staff.

Agitated Members

Agitation should not be confused with the initial anxiety members experience when they first enter

Table 8–2   GROUP COMPOSITION

Heterogeneity

Advantages

- Different types of personality characteristics enliven group interaction
- Allows for intergenerational groups
- The variety of skills and problem-solving abilities in a group can be educational for members and leader
- Members selected for diversity or expertise can enhance group movement

Disadvantages

- May be difficult for leader to deal with all the variables: age, culture, abilities, and personalities
- May be difficult for leader to combine affluent members with those who have been poor
- Potential members who are ambulatory may refuse to be in groups with persons in wheelchairs

Homogeneity

Advantages

- If members have dementia, they may function better with others at similar level of cognition
- Peer groups of about the same age will remember the same historical events and may experience similar health problems
- Members share similar levels of social or communication skills, even physical problems

Disadvantages

- May increase work of leader, for example, group of very frail or group of confused elders
- Leader may get bored or impatient if group and individual members move slowly

Source: Based on Toseland, R. W., 1990 and Corey, G., & Corey, M., 1992.

a group. Agitation is observable outside meetings as well as within the group. Initial anxiety is often seen in the resident who leaves the group. This problem is fairly common, and the leader will soon learn the most effective intervention for retaining such a member. Initial anxiety is also seen in chain-smoking, rapid talking, monopolization of the group, and nervous mannerisms of the extremities. Others handle anxiety by staring out the window or at the floor, avoiding eye contact with others—especially the group leader, and retreating into silence.

Confinement in a small circle at meetings seems to increase anxiety, especially in the early meetings. Because of the sensory defects usually apparent, however, the group has to be seated close together. It may take a while for members to adjust to such physical closeness, and they may pull back from the circle. Usually if they have hearing or vision problems, they will prefer to be in a small circle so they do not miss anything.

Agitated members can be very disruptive, so the leader should carefully investigate agitated potential group members. Is the agitation fairly constant, or is it vacillating and triggered by events or certain people? Will group membership really be beneficial to this person? Burnside once accepted a woman because the staff convinced her that group membership would help her. She disrupted the group so much that Burnside, as the group leader, finally had to ask her to leave; this is a regrettable action of last resort and difficult to handle constructively. Ideally, there would be a doctor available with whom the leader could discuss the severity of marked agitation evident in an individual and the medication regimen. Wherever possible, the leader should also seek advice from a mentor or supervisor before terminating any person's membership. Mixing former state hospital patients and non-state hospital members in a group may create problems for a new leader. If such patients are combined in a group, the leader should be prepared to deal with the resentment, hostility, and rejection that is often shown to these poor, shuffled-about human beings. Staff members are often afraid of expsychiatric patients. The anxiety of the staff may be lessened, and they may be more accepting of a person, when the leader shares with them the behavior observed in a group. Group behavior may be quite different from the usual behavior reported by staff who are often quite surprised at how well patients manage in group settings. Labels such as senile, violent, obstreperous, and suicidal may be on a patient's chart, and the staff latches onto the label even though it is no longer accurate.

Members with Religious and Political Preoccupations

If very religious or very politically minded persons are accepted in the group, the leader must be prepared to deal with the desires of such members to convert other members—either religiously or politically. If this is a problem within a group, it is possible as a last resort to suggest a ground rule excluding certain topics from discussion. Most groups, however, given support from a sensitive leader, are able to control dominating members and manage the group's meeting time in ways that address the agreed interests and concerns of members (Shulman, 1999).

Assessment

And finally, the importance of pregroup assessments must be underscored. Chapter 11 identifies the problems that can be encountered when failing to thoroughly assess the potential group members' ability to handle a group experience. A leader should not accept a client who is unlikely to be able to function appropriately in a group or who will be deleterious to the entire group. In a slightly different vein, Toseland and Rivas (2001)

discuss the importance of a needs assessment. They suggest that practitioners collect information from others to validate their perceptions of existing unmet needs. Team meetings could be one avenue, consultation with other agencies or a survey made by the practitioner of the population she or he intends to serve are all possible ways of obtaining the required information. If larger programs are being considered, a survey of the needs and resources in a community might yield a more accurate estimate of what is needed before decisions about setting up groups are made (Bertcher, Kurtz, & Lamont, 1999).

Intergenerational Groups

Intergenerational groups are increasingly recognized as a valuable means for increasing understanding between people of different ages and backgrounds. Perlstein and Bliss (2003) and Golden and Perlstein (2003) describe establishing groups designed to increase understanding between older and younger people, foster community solidarity, and intergenerational friendships by working together in artistic projects that use a large oral history component. The Center for Intergenerational Learning at Temple University, Philadelphia, uses many varied intergenerational group work projects to foster cooperation, friendship, and personal development between the generations, particularly in socially and economically deprived neighborhoods. Older people are recruited to group projects so that they can be experienced as models and examples to younger people who are helped to appreciate the long and courageous lives many have lived. Lutz and Haller (1996) provide guidelines for intergenerational work.

There are many examples of groups in which younger students befriend frail older residents in nursing facilities or in day care centers. There is universal agreement that all such successful projects require meticulous planning and preparation with careful attention to issues of time and pacing. Willing cooperation of older and younger participants rather than implicit or explicit coercion is essential. Most of these types of projects combine group sessions and dyad sessions which bring together pairs of older and younger people to spend time together sharing conversation about each other's life stories to date, and present circumstances and concerns. For example, an eight-week project might consist of the following:

Session 1: Group leader explains the purpose of the group. One member interviews another; later each member introduces the member interviewed to the group.

Session 2: Members consider their similarities and differences in pairs; then discuss them in the group.

Session 3: Discussion of factors that lead to personal strengths and ultimately personal happiness. Members are asked to choose strengths they would like to possess that they saw in the other age group.

Session 4: Older group members share photographs of themselves at different stages of their lives so they can talk about their perspectives on life.

Session 5: Members discuss how young and old people are depicted in the media; this is accomplished by sharing news articles.

Session 6: Members explore messages in music by comparing yesteryear's music with today's. Common themes are elicited, and events in the world occurring at time of music identified.

Session 7: Ethnic backgrounds discussed; older members share their heritage.

Session 8: The group divides into pairs to share what they learned from each other. Exchange names and addresses to keep in touch.

Gains from such groups showed that the young group members were less biased toward older people than they were at the beginning and that the older members reported increased self-esteem. Other identified benefits included the ability to understand better the various developmental phases of the life cycle, the chance to act out family roles. There are also opportunities for the older adult to give support and advice to younger group members, and the opportunity for both older and younger members to review their values and experiences.

Within a life cycle approach to group work, the following have been identified as positive outcomes of intergenerational group work:

- Amelioration of suffering
- Overcoming of disability
- The chance for new experiences of self-fulfillment and friendship
- The gift of personal legacy through recounting life experience
- Transmission and preservation of historical information
- Preservation of valued memories through recall, partial reconstruction, and the chance to verbalize the emotions associated with the memories by sharing them with others

Because intergenerational groups require such meticulous preparation, some writers believe that a neophyte group leader should probably exclude younger members from the first group led. The rationale is that the leader can focus on the problems of the older people, and exclusion of younger members should also decrease the number of variables for the leader to handle. Another reason is that some new group leaders do not have a basic grounding in the developmental tasks of each age group or have an incomplete understanding of a life span perspective. On the other hand, leading a mixed age group is an excellent way of building understanding about the different life stages and the developmental tasks associated with different ages within the life cycle (Erikson, 1982; Erikson, Erikson, & Kivnick, 1986).

Summary

This chapter discusses criteria for group membership. Yalom urges careful selection to prevent early termination by members. Goals for intergenerational groups are explored.

Settings for group meetings, which can range from acute care hospitals to prisons, may well indicate the competence and caliber of a potential group member although it is essential not to prejudge people or be unduly influenced by other people's points of view. In selecting members, the group leader should strive for a balance by including a variety of personalities. The leader is cautioned not to be too cavalier in mixing cognitively alert and nonalert members or including too many members with sensory disabilities. Leaders should remember, however, that educational level alone is not an accurate indicator of group potential. The meeting room needs to provide adequate space, especially if wheelchair users are to be included. The leader must consider the number of minority members to be included while trying to avoid a single representative and always provide a safe, nonthreatening milieu. The leader should be skilled in handling political or religious issues if very pious or politically minded individuals are included in the group.

Persons who should probably be excluded from groups are those who are agitated, hyperactive, habitually tearful, or aggressive. Persons diagnosed as psychotic, manic-depressive, hypochondriacal or obsessional also should be excluded, except for psychotherapy groups. The new leader needs to be wary of any individual enthusiastically recommended by the staff. Medical problems need to be assessed because they may affect group participation.

The size of the group will depend on the type of group, its objectives, whether there are coleaders, and whether it has open or closed membership. Open groups allow for fluctuation of membership from meeting to meeting. Closed groups have a stable membership and are likely to achieve a degree of intimacy not usually reached in a group with constantly changing membership. Closed groups are usually easier for a new leader to manage, but remember that confidence and skill will develop over time.

Exercises

EXERCISE 1

Describe four possible settings for group meetings, and, for each, indicate how the setting determines the types of older persons who may be available to participate in that group.

EXERCISE 2

The following is a list of older persons described by the staff as potential members for a group you are planning. Carefully screen out those you would not include if you were leading your first group. Give your rationale for not accepting them into your group.

1. Mrs. Loquacious is 90 years old, very stubborn and controlling, and talks incessantly. It is impossible to stop her, and she irritates both residents and staff by bawling them out for not listening to her.
2. Mr. Deaf is 78 years old and extremely hard of hearing but often pretends he hears by nodding his head or saying "Yes." He refuses to wear a hearing aid.
3. Mrs. Depressed is 88 years old and is now withdrawn, listless, and confused. Her husband died a month ago. She says over and over, "What's the use of living?"
4. Mr. Alone is 79 years old, a loner, and has been a heavy drinker most of his life. He never married, never had a steady job, and was a drifter. He does not mingle with any residents in the long-term care facility.

5. Mrs. Obnoxious is a 68-year-old with a behavior problem. She is aggressive, noisy, and scares other residents. She pushed Miss Frail off her chair in the dining room recently. Mrs. O needs help.

6. Miss Frail is 95 years old and has outlived all her friends. She is petrified of Mrs. Obnoxious and avoids her. Miss Frail is very paranoid; she thinks that the government took her house and that the nurses are having affairs with her brother.

7. Mr. Flirt is blind and 86 years old. He used to drink heavily, chased women, and was not a very good father. He is getting increasingly depressed and withdrawn and refuses to get out of bed.

8. Miss Learned is a 75-year-old former school teacher, sweet but terribly confused. She is especially confused at night. She keeps talking about her mother coming to visit. (Mother has been dead 20 years.)

9. Mrs. Old is a centenarian, physically frail but mentally alert. She loves to reminisce. She has become the pet because of her sweet disposition and sharp wit.

10. Mr. Sly is 86 years old and pretends to be out of it, but he bedevils the staff by hiding wheelchairs and linens; then he pleads innocence. When things get very boring, he pulls the fire alarm, turns up the thermostat, or calls the police department at 2 a.m. to tell them that the staff is beating up the residents and that they had better come down.

EXERCISE 3

You have just begun a small group in a nursing home. After the second meeting, other residents are waiting to talk to you. They want to know why they are not in your group. What will you tell them?

References

Bertcher, H., Kurtz, L., & Lamont, A. (1999). (Eds.), *Rebuilding communities: Challenges for group work*. Binghamton, NY: Haworth Press.

Brown, A., & Mistry, T. (1994). Group work with mixed membership groups: Issues of race and gender. *Social Work with Groups*, 17(3), 5–21.

Cohen, M. B., & Mullender, A. (2003). (Eds.), *Gender and groupwork*. New York: Routledge.

Corey, M. S., & Corey, G. (1992). *Groups: Process and practice*. Pacific Grove, CA: Brooks-Cole.

Corey, M. S., & Corey, G. (2002). *Groups: Process and practice*. Pacific Grove, CA: Brooks-Cole.

Erikson, E. H. (1982). *The life cycle completed: A review*. New York: Norton.

Erikson, E. H., Erikson, J. M., & Kivnick, H. Q. (1986). *Vital involvement in old age*. New York: Norton.

Gibson, F. (2004). *The past in the present: Using reminiscence in health and social care*. Baltimore: Health Professions Press.

Golden, S., & Perlstein, S. (2003). *Legacy works: Transforming memory into visual arts*. New York: Elders Share the Arts.

Kelly, T. B. (1999). Mutual aid groups with mentally ill older adults. *Social Work with Groups*, 22(2/3), 119–138.

Lutz, S. & Haller, J. (1996). *Seniors & children: Building bridges together*. Washington, DC: National Council on Aging.

Mace, N. L., Rabins, P. V., Castleton, B. A., McEwen, E., & Meredith, B. (1999). *The 36-hour day*. Baltimore: Johns Hopkins University Press.

Mistry, T., & Brown, A. (1997). Black/white co-working in groups. In T. Mistry & A. Brown (Eds.), *Race & group work* (pp. 26–42). London: Whiting & Birch.

Northen, H., & Kurland, R. (2001). *Social work with groups*. New York: Columbia University Press.

Orr, A. (1994). Dealing with the death of a group member: Visually impaired elderly. In A. Gitterman & L. Shulman (Eds.), *Mutual aid groups, vulnerable populations, and the life cycle* (pp. 36–84). New York: Columbia University Press.

Perlstein, S., & Bliss, J. (2003). *Generating community: Intergenerational partnerships through the expressive arts*. New York: Elders Share the Arts.

Pillemer, K., & Albright, B. (1996). Fostering intergenerational linkages now at risk because of mobility. In B. M. Westacott & C. R. Hegeman (Eds.), *Service learning in elder care: A resource manual* (pp. 99–106). Albany, NY: Foundation for Long-term Care.

Shulman, L. (1999). *The skills of helping individuals, families, groups, and communities* (4th ed.). Itasca, IL: F. E. Peacock.

Toseland, R. W. (1990). *Group work with older adults*. New York: New York University Press.

Toseland, R. W. (1995). *Group work with the elderly and family caregivers*. New York: Springer.

Toseland, R. W., & Rivas, R. F. (2001). *An introduction to group work practice*. Boston: Allyn & Bacon.

Yalom, I. D. (1985). *The theory and practice of group psychotherapy*. New York: Basic Books.

Leadership and Coleadership Issues

Faith Gibson

Irene Burnside

Key Words

- Absenteeism
- Entrée
- Hostile member
- Monopolist
- Roadblocks
- Sabotage
- Sensory deficits
- Silent member

Learning Objectives

- Discuss entrée into an agency
- List four techniques of group leadership
- List six categories of problems that may occur in a group
- Discuss depression in relation to the leader
- Discuss absenteeism
- Define sabotage as it relates to group leadership
- List 10 ways a leader may be sabotaged in an agency
- List five qualifications for a group leader
- State 15 simple techniques to promote a stable group of older persons

Experience is a wonderful thing; it enables you to recognize a mistake every time you make it.

—Anonymous

Leadership is defined by Toseland (1990) as "the process of guiding the development of a group through all stages of its life, from planning to termination" (p. 46). Furthermore, it is a shared function that is composed of a sequence of actions rather than a certain quality in one person. The group has a designated leader, but that leader helps the members to become indigenous leaders within the group. The designated leader, for example, helps the group and the members to achieve the goals they want to accomplish. (See Chapter 8 for a discussion of goals.)

Practitioners must be careful that they do not let the facility for which they work subvert group member leadership abilities. Capable older people can be undermined by ageism because they too readily adopt dependency roles in line with younger people's expectations. Ageism erodes their confidence and competence to accept leadership roles, which they are capable of performing if given encouragement and recognition.

The problems in maintaining a group of older adults are varied and unique, and in many ways they differ from those of leading a group of younger persons. In this chapter, students, health care workers, instructors, and volunteers are alerted to some of the common problems a new leader may encounter. One participant in a conference on group work with older people wrote on the evaluation form, "Why do groups get started and fall apart when we need them, and how can we make them more lasting?" The purpose of this chapter is to answer those questions.

Leaders need to keep in mind the developmental tasks of later life. Several authors especially Erikson (1982; Erikson, Erikson, & Kivnick, 1986) describe these tasks. An awareness of these developmental tasks helps the leader understand the group members better. Knowledge of group theory and process needs to inform practice.

Yalom (1995) believes that the curative factors in group therapy are mediated not by the therapist but by the members, who provide the qualities of acceptance, support, and hope, plus the experience of universality, interpersonal feedback, testing, and learning. Birren, Kenyon, Ruth, Schroots, and Svensson (1996) although deliberately not wishing to identify guided autobiographical writing groups as therapy, but rather as therapeutic, identified similar significant mutual contributions made by members to each other.

The leader works to reinstate independence in the older person by being clear about mutual roles and responsibilities within the group, valuing each person's contribution, and encouraging awareness of interdependence, each upon the other. The leader lends an optimistic vision of what it is possible to achieve. Impediments or blocks sometimes prevent such achievements in groups for older people. These road blocks include: the attitude of the leaders, who may have little belief in the creative potential of an older member; the difficulty leaders have in communicating their hopes and feelings; and leaders' over

concern about time—ignoring the timing and sense of time of older people.

Students struggle to develop their own personal style of leadership as they face issues of authority in the groups they establish. They have to develop sufficient security to be willing to share responsibility with the group members—the group belongs to the members, not the leader. Leaders should not see themselves as unchallenged authority figures or as laissez-faire equals where anything goes and nobody is responsible for what happens (Toseland & Rivas, 2001). The discussion in Chapter 8 about differential roles and tasks related to the stages of development within a group is also relevant.

Gaining the Cooperation of an Agency

One of the first tasks faced by the group leader is to gain entrance into an institution or agency. This may be difficult for both students and volunteers. Often, credentials are simply not enough. Students need to clarify their own and their educational institutions' roles and responsibilities in gaining access to learning opportunities in undertaking group work with older people. There are formal and informal aspects, both of which are important in securing permission, establishing a group, successfully working with it, and then withdrawing. Administrators, senior health and social care professionals, and direct care staff are likely to influence the decision about permission and the outcome of any group that is established. One way to elicit the support of the staff is to give them a short talk describing what your plans are for the group you hope to lead. The staff may, however, remain uninterested in group work until their curiosity is aroused by their observation of changes in the behavior of group members.

Some staff may feel ambivalent towards students leading groups and a few may be openly critical. Most are very welcoming providing students are conscientious and clear about their intentions. Reliability and dependability are crucial and it is most important to have a mentor or supervisor with whom to discuss the group work experience. Residential establishments of all kinds are complex institutions, usually with significant histories of staff–staff and staff–resident relationships. Students and new workers need to observe acutely, listen attentively, and proceed with sensitivity when seeking to introduce a new service or alter existing programs.

Activity programs in many facilities may fail to meet the needs of some individuals who may long for opportunities to discuss issues of personal significance, explore spiritual concerns, and pursue creative solutions to past and present problems in warmly accepting reciprocal groups. Some residents will be more interested in conversation than in diversional activities (Northen & Kurland, 2001). Chapter 21 is relevant to this discussion.

More is needed than bingo games and sing-alongs to combat the boredom, loneliness, and inactivity that many people are forced to endure in late life; participation in group work can be a rewarding and enriching experience for people who otherwise pass their days doing nothing. On the other hand, many activities can be used as part of the program within a mutual aid group (Basting & Killick, 2003). Creative activities may serve both as a bridge into supportive conversation and rewarding relationships as well as being valued for their own intrinsic artistic contribution to enhancing the quality of life (Shectman, 2000).

Multiple Problems of Older Adults

The group leader must juggle multiple problems simultaneously. Although this can be true in all group work, it is especially true in work with older people, who may experience socioeconomic, physical, and emotional problems simultaneously. Staff in gerontological services often find that they need to be generalists because of the multiple problems that beset older people.

The multiple health problems of older people are both physical and psychological. Although many experience heart disease, cancer, and other physical problems, dementia and depression are the real epidemics of late life (Grayson, Lubin, & Whitlock, 1995; Manton, Cornelius, & Woodbury, 1995). Both occur more frequently in people who live in residential facilities of all kinds than in those who live alone or with other family members in the community. Dealing with visual and hearing impairments also presents a challenge. The rate of visual impairments appears higher with increasing age. Hearing deficits are the most common type of impairment. Patients in institutions are often diagnosed as having five or six different problems. The leader has to be aware of that fact constantly. Deterioration will be observed in members if the group continues over a substantial period.

There will be vacillation between good and bad days, and the group experience may be very helpful in the maintenance of such persons. Often they become ill or have a crisis situation. Some group members may become very sick, stay in bed for a while, and eventually return to the group.

In a closed group it is important to always include absent members; that is, the leader sees those people at their bedside and finds out why they are absent and what is happening. Also, the leader reports to sick members what happened in the group session. Some new group leaders, however, are unaccustomed to working with older clients and do not seek out absent group members. It is not usually the role of a group leader of adults, but one needs to remember that the older people are actually incapacitated on some days. And, of course, forgetfulness on the part of group members plays havoc with any group. (Forgetfulness on the part of the group leader delights the group members.) Follow-up work is easy in an institution where one has a captive group; but if one is leading a group in a day care center, an outpatient clinic, or elsewhere in the community, the leader might have to make phone calls to absent members. At group sessions the leader should mention absent members and, while safeguarding confidentiality, report on their well-being or reasons for absence. In this way their continuing membership is acknowledged, and if they are able to return at a future time, their reentry is made easier.

Once the group is under way, the leader is, in essence, the glue that holds the group together. Groups fall apart when the leader is insensitive to the needs of the group members. (See Chapter 5 on the importance of inclusion in group work with older people.) Groups also fail if the leader is not conscientious about the group leadership role and is late, absent, cancels meetings frequently, and so on. Members soon sense when a leader is making every effort to keep the group intact. When concern is shown for an absent member, they are well aware that the same type of concern will be shown for them if they break a hip, have an embolus, or are so incapacitated that they cannot attend the group.

One woman in a group was bedridden due to a pulmonary embolus. When Burnside visited her, she expressed regret about missing the meetings but could not get out of bed even though she felt much better. Burnside rolled her bed into the meeting room, and the woman visited with the group for a portion of the meeting. She felt somewhat nauseated and did not want any coffee; she had ginger ale. When Burnside visited absent patients at their bedsides, she also brought them the refreshments the group was having that day. Such continual inclusion, whether or not the member attends meetings, is an important factor in the maintenance of a group and should be remembered by new leaders.

Another important way to maintain the group is for the leader to pay meticulous attention to the levels of discomfort or pain of the group members (McLean, 2003). The leader must also learn to handle the sensory deficits of the group members and how to maximize the vision, hearing, and understanding of each member in the group. One way to minimize deficits is to pay close attention to the environment itself and to the seating arrangements. Students can be sensitized to the problem of sensory deprivation with the use of experiential exercises in which sensory loss and its effects are simulated.

Group Concerns

There are several categories of problems that may arise in a group. The following list illustrates those common group concerns

1. Problems with coleader
   a. Nonacceptance of coleader by group
   b. Competitiveness between leaders
2. Problems with individual members— that is, individual problem members
   a. The monopolist
   b. The silent member
   c. The hostile member
3. Problems with the leadership role
   a. Leader's degree of directiveness or activity
   b. Leader's role in maintaining group— for example, problem of attendance
   c. Leader's role in establishing trust and confidentiality
4. Miscellaneous concerns
   a. Problem of inclusion
   b. Ground rules

The new leader should consider which problems might have to be dealt with, especially in the initial meetings. A list of common problems appears in **Table 9–1.**

Table 9–1 Problems Experienced by New Group Leaders

Type of problem
1. Monopolizers
2. Members forget about meetings
3. Absent members
4. Adding new members to group
5. Group members approaching leaders individually after meetings for further discussion
6. Anxiety and/or depression of leaders
7. How to handle a person who refuses to join the group
8. How to handle a situation when member does not wish to remember sad parts of the past
9. Members who leave group while a session is still in progress
10. Dealing with deafness, loss of memory, poor speech, soft voices, and so on
11. Interventions for withdrawn members
12. The one-to-one by the leader that occurs in early meetings
13. Touching during crying; is it helpful?
14. Leaders' worries about lessening self-confidence of members
15. How much discussion of past changes, such as death and moves, is helpful to members?
16. Dealing with leaders' feelings about losing group members or when the group members say meetings are not useful for them
17. What to serve for a snack
18. Getting members to feel more relaxed with leaders
19. Whether to pursue reality testing in a group in the face of massive denial
20. How does leader respond to low mood in members
21. Group members' problems hit close to leaders' own problems
22. Lack of support from staff
23. Topics to reminisce about
24. How to use props or triggers
25. Leader needs more professionalism and greater objectivity
26. Seating arrangements—continue same? Change?
27. Coleaders' attitudes and beliefs that conflict with older members' attitudes and beliefs
28. Coleader conflict about roles, styles of leadership, and so on
29. Closure of group meeting
30. How to include all members in topics being discussed
31. Topics to include in groups
32. Group members concerned about taping the meetings
33. Inclusion of staff and other visitors in meetings. Pros and cons?
34. Strategies for dialog when group member comments *after* meeting, "I want to be dead"
35. Termination: How to plan so members do not feel abandoned. Feelings of leader about termination
36. Leader needs to be better organized

Source: I. Burnside & M. G. Schmidt, 1994.

Problems in Coleadership

Problems in coleadership run the gamut from interpersonal squabbles to power struggles. **Table 9–2** lists coleadership's advantages and disadvantages. Preceptors can be most helpful in mediating some of these problems (Kurland & Malekoff, 2003).

Special attention must be paid to the location of coleaders in a group. The seating arrangements for the members and leaders must be carefully planned. Members should sit close to each other so that they can see, hear, and touch one another. Leaders should be dispersed throughout the group. Most older persons cannot be expected to plan how a room should be arranged; therefore, the leaders must plan ahead to have the chairs and tables in the best position. **Figures 9–1a, b, c** and **9–2a, b, c** show a variety of seating arrangements. The one shown in **Figure 9–2c** is the most successful positioning of clients and leaders.

Remember that although the leaders may be aware of the problems inherent in poor seating arrangements, an attempt should be made to include the members in planning and be sensitive to individual preferences. Group members should not be treated as if they were helpless or incapable of contributing meaningfully to such discussions. The leader may make suggestions or rearrange wheelchairs after they have moved into the group circle. If it is necessary to move a member, the leader should explain the reason why. "Mrs. Jones, I am going to move your chair over beside me so that I can hear what you say better. Is that alright?," or "Mrs. Anderson, may I move you over here so that the glare from that window will not be in your eyes? I know that bright sunlight makes you uncomfortable."

Feelings Experienced by Group Leaders

The new group leader should be warned that it is not uncommon to experience feelings of depres-

sion, and the leader should examine how this depression might affect the group. Is the leader more quiet and withdrawn? Is the leader aware of how depressing the frailties of members and all the people in wheelchairs or with canes and crutches can be? The leader may need to confront anxiety about their own or their parents' possible frailty and inevitable mortality. During this time, when some of the enthusiasm of the leader may be waning, strong peer support or preceptor support can be very helpful. Not all students will be able to immediately pinpoint their depression and may need some help from the instructor to identify it.

In the first group of older people Burnside led, she was struck with their sensitivity to her self. She was an inexperienced group leader, and at that time her husband was dying. In one meeting, the group wanted to talk about death and dying, but because of her own pain, she shied away from the topic. The group had immediately picked up on her reluctance. The logs she kept helped her to understand later. They waited until she was more comfortable about bringing up the subject. In another instance, a pregnant young leader was conducting a group of older persons. Their concern for her was obvious in each meeting, and they made concerted efforts to help her with the group-related tasks.

Problems in Attendance

Inpatient groups may or may not have problems with attendance. Once the group is established, the residents are usually there and eagerly waiting for each session to begin. The emptiness and boredom of institutional life may prompt a good deal of their receptivity. Boredom is an ever-present threat in such environments. As the atheist in a group once said when questioned about going to mass so regularly, "Sure I go. There's nothing better to do around here on Thursday afternoon."

The real problem with group work in institutions is handling the residents who are not in

Table 9–2 COLEADERSHIP

Advantages

- Greater sense of cohesion
- Assistance when working with frail older persons
- Assistance during demanding group activities
- Support during difficult group experiences
- Validation for one another regarding group dynamics and events in group
- Catalyst for professional development
- Another role model for effective communication and group participation
- An educational tool, especially for neophytes
- When one leader is on vacation or ill, group continuity is not lost
- With two leaders, larger group may be possible
- Can reduce burnout in a leader
- If intense emotions are expressed, one leader can interact with member while coleader scans group for reactions
- If one leader is strongly affected by session, other leader can be a sounding board
- If counter transference occurs with one leader, other leader may be better able to work with the member

Disadvantages

- Costlier than having just one leader
- Coleaders may not work well together
- Coleading is time consuming (need to debrief and spend time between meetings planning)
- Difficult to establish egalitarian relationship
- Members may attempt to play one leader against the other
- Experienced leader may resent having to explain and teach a new leader, which slows the leader
- A junior leader may resent not having the status of the senior leader
- Coleaders from different disciplines may have different perspectives about how to conduct the group, which may not be discussed or resolved
- Problems arise if coleaders rarely meet with one another
- Competition and rivalry can occur
- If they do not build trust, coleaders may not trust each other's interventions
- One leader may side with members against the other leader
- Coleaders involved in an intimate relationship may use the group to solve relationship struggles

Source: Based on R. W. Toseland, 1990 and M. S. Corey, & G. Corey, 1992. Adapted with permission.

groups. They may request that they be put on a waiting list. Sometimes relatives ask on behalf of their family member for a place in the group. One relative said, "I don't like to ask for special favors, but could my mother please be placed in one of the groups? I believe it would help her." Such interest in groups may spur the administrator or the activity director to find more activities for the residents.

Most group leaders find that they have a stable membership with inpatient groups, but that is because they have concentrated on making a cohesive group. Outpatient groups are different. For example, in rainy weather, many of the group members may call in with transportation problems and/or complaints of their arthritis. Older people are also afraid of falling during a rainy or snowy day.

Figure 9–1 RECTANGULAR TABLE SEATING ARRANGEMENTS

Because of its length, a rectangular table can present seating problems—for example, the inability of group members to see or hear the leaders or others in the group. The leaders should position themselves with care. In diagram (a) the coleaders are weighted at one end of the group and are unable to assist the four members at the opposite end of the table. In diagram (b) the coleaders weight one side of the group; the arrangement also makes it difficult for the leaders to interact—they must look over the head of the member sitting between them. Diagram (c) shows the best seating arrangement for coleaders if a long table must be used.

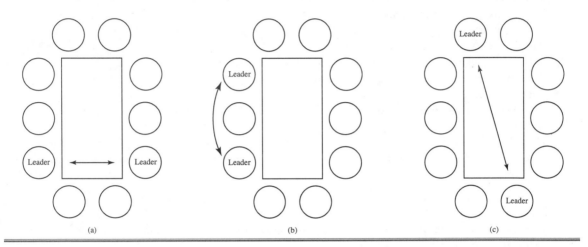

Figure 9–2 CIRCULAR TABLE SEATING ARRANGEMENTS

In the seating arrangement using a round table shown in diagram (a), in which the coleaders sit side by side, both authority figures are on one side of the table; the arrangement does not allow eye contact between the leaders or permit each of them to be close to two members. In the arrangement in diagram (b), the member seated between the coleaders may feel overwhelmed, and eye contact between the leaders is limited. Diagram (c) shows the ideal seating arrangement for a round table. It offers eye contact, and each leader can assist the member on either side. This is important when the group contains frail, confused, disoriented members or aged persons with severe sensory losses. A round table is always preferable to a rectangular or square table.

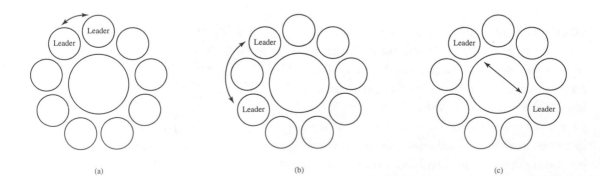

Administrative Support for the Leader

Sometimes groups fail because of lack of interest and support by the administration. It is of paramount importance that the leader have support from two directions: (1) from the administrative staff of the agency where the group is to be held, and (2) from a preceptor, supervisor, colleague, or whomever will be serving in that capacity.

Support from the administrator and the director of nurses is important, because they influence both staff and residents. Directors of senior centers similarly influence the staff and the seniors about coming to group meetings. Lip service is not enough; there must be active encouragement and support by the people in top positions. The following list includes examples observed in which the administration made the task of leading a group easier for volunteers and students.

1. One facility provided lunch for the volunteer group leader because the leader had a hectic schedule on that particular day and was skipping lunch to be at the group meeting on time.

2. One interested administrator sat in on several group meetings so that she could observe the behavior of patients in the group setting (which may be quite different from usual behavior on the ward). However, if the administrator chooses to sit in on a meeting, the leader must realize that there may be some resentment from the members, there may be some concern about the presence of an authority figure, and there may be reluctance to share experiences and ideas. Confidentiality is one important factor to consider when there are observers.

3. The same administrator always had a special goodbye cake for the group leader when she completed a group and left the facility.

4. One director of nurses was very conscientious about having the patients ready in the room when the student arrived. She made a special effort to dress the patients neatly that day. The men came in white shirts and ties; the women had their hair done nicely. The message to both the staff and the residents of such concern for appearance was "This is important for them; they must look their very best."

5. In one facility, the nursing instructor who began a new group was provided with an assistant because of the multiple handicaps of the members.

6. Photographers took pictures of group meetings and placed them on a bulletin board in the hallway, where the residents showed them to family members and friends.

7. An in-service class or two devoted to group work or group dynamics also shows interest in the efforts of the leader.

8. Training a coleader who can take over the group when the student or volunteer leaves is also a way of maintaining the group.

Sabotage

Sabotage is a negative term, but it is the word that keeps coming to mind when thinking of the many barriers with which leaders have to struggle. There are numerous ways in which persons can sabotage the work of a leader and make it difficult to maintain the group.

1. Constant criticism of the leader may occur, often in the form of negative feedback implying that the group work is incorrect, foolish, or bothersome.

2. Staff members may show no interest in the group, fail to report on the patients in the group, and ignore what is occurring in the group.

12. Capitalize on birthdays, holidays, current events, and changing seasons. Themes can help—for example, nature, travel, books, and friendships.

13. Elements of reminiscence are likely to intrude into most sessions regardless of the theme or topic.

14. Dealing with sad themes and memories is part of the leader's role.

15. Avoid changing meeting places or times; this has a tendency to disturb some members.

16. Never be late for a meeting. If you anticipate being late, notify the members.

17. Never fail to appear without an explanation or without providing a substitute leader.

18. Do not make promises you cannot keep.

19. Make a contract with each person in the group. Contracts are important; they alert the older person, particularly the forgetful one, to the time and place of the meetings and give the leader a chance to assess that individual for impaired memory, disorientation, and other disabilities, before taking him or her into the group.

20. Do not depend on the staff for a list of potential group members. They may list, for various reasons, people difficult to handle in a group or people who cannot benefit at all from the group experience.

21. Recognize the importance of hellos and good-byes.

22. Deal with all absences openly in the group, including deaths. If a member has died, be sure to try to handle the death in the meeting. (Some leaders leave an empty chair in the meeting after a death so that if the members do not hear what is said, at least they can see what has happened.)

23. Recognize that touching and closeness—both leader–member closeness and member–member closeness—are of crucial importance.

24. Mix men and women when possible and arrange the group seating pattern to achieve maximum participation.

25. Be meticulous in anticipating and meeting members' needs, as they cannot always verbalize them. Either say the words or allow the members to say what their needs are. Pain is one area to consider.

26. Use food and beverages to add surprise and atmosphere to meetings.

27. Recognize the importance of spontaneity and surprises. Do not let the surprise be, "Look, we are all moving to a new room today!" Jostling the group about is not helpful. Members who have dementia, for example, do poorly if moved about too much. Some surprises provide acceptable novelty and could include changing the food or beverages from week to week, adding an activity, occasionally having a guest leader take over the group, or changing the usual structure of the group.

28. Use the here and now. Talk about the weather, the seasons, or whatever to get started. The superficial is acceptable. You will also have to share things about yourself; older people will not often let you out of that.

29. Work on self-image. Praise and compliment whenever possible, but be sincere. Do not have confrontation groups.

30. Arrange transportation to help members get to meetings.

31. Consider, when possible, the era and the geographical areas in which the members lived and talk about them in the meetings.

32. Work with positive and negative feelings expressed by members and acknowledge your own feelings.

33. Use humor in the group and encourage others to do likewise.

34. Only mix individuals with dementia with alert people with great care; it can create problems for the alert people who

may in some circumstances lack patience with the limitations of the others.

35. Never promise what you are unable to deliver such as agreeing to continue to visit members after the group ends or extending the life of a group beyond the number of planned sessions.

It takes courage, stamina, creativity, and great patience to be a group leader, but there are results and rewards. The results may seem minuscule, but they are important. The rewards are an individual matter, what is rewarding for one group leader may not be so for another. As you continue to lead groups, you will discover your own style of leader-ship—one that is comfortable for you, therapeutic for the members, and always uniquely yours.

Most leaders of groups of older persons com-bine different leadership models to help meet the needs of the group members in the most effective way. There is not one single practice model that is effective in all situations. The leader needs to be very flexible to provide tailor-made strategies for each situation. In fact, the methods used by the leader should be founded upon a comprehensive assessment of the potential members of the pro-posed group. **Table 9–3** presents personal charac-teristics of an effective leader.

Table 9–3　Personal Characteristics of an Effective Leader

- Genuine respect for old people
- A history of positive experiences with old people
- A deep sense of caring for older people
- A respect for the elderly person's cultural values
- An understanding of the ways in which the individual's cultural background continues to influence present attitudes and behaviors
- An ability and desire to learn from old people
- An understanding of the biological aspects of aging
- The conviction that the last years of life can be challenging and developmental
- Patience, especially with repetition of stories
- Knowledge of the special biological, psychological, and social needs of older persons
- Sensitivity to people's burdens and anxieties
- The ability to get older people to challenge many of the myths about old age
- A healthy attitude regarding one's own aging
- An understanding of the developmental tasks of each period of life, from infancy to old age
- An appreciation for the effects that one period of life has on other stages of development
- A particular understanding of how one's ability to handle present life difficulties hinges on how well one deals with problems in earlier stages
- A background in the pathology of aging
- The ability to deal with extreme feelings of depression, hopelessness, grief, hostility, and despair
- Personal characteristics such as humor, enthusiasm, patience, courage, endurance, hopefulness, tolerance, nondefensiveness, freedom from limiting prejudices, and a willingness to learn
- An ability to be both gentle and challenging
- The sensitivity to know when it is therapeutic to provide support and when to challenge
- A working knowledge of group work theory along with the special skills needed for group work with the elderly

Source: M. S. Corey & G. Corey, 1992. Used with permission.

Summary

Leading a group of older persons is a demanding task that requires both generic and specific group work skills. The problems experienced by older people may stagger the new leader; they are multiple, complex, and often recurring. Locating a receptive facility in which to establish a group is usually the first hurdle. Sensory loss requires special attention by the leader. Careful attention must also be given to psychosomatic complaints and to pain and discomfort.

Conducting a group can be hampered by such problems as sabotage by the staff; nonacceptance of a coleader; and monopolizing, mute, or hostile members. Trust, confidentiality, inclusion, affection, and ground rules are also concerns. If absenteeism is a problem, the leader should consider possible reasons. Nursing home residents may be so bored that they welcome a group experience.

Qualifications and abilities needed for group leadership with older people include background in normal aging, background in the pathology of aging, experience in groups of any kind, tolerance for groups, ability to recognize dependent relationships, ability to handle directness and criticism, ability to handle one's own feelings, and ability to organize one's work schedule.

Suggestions for new leaders are given as guidelines to facilitate their own and the group's movement, to decrease anxiety, and to promote learning and development.

Exercises

EXERCISE 1

A leader's role can be active or passive. Which is preferable in group leadership with older people? State the reasons for your choice.

EXERCISE 2

Absenteeism is a common problem in groups of older persons and may be due to a variety of factors. List as many reasons as you can why older people might not attend a group meeting. For each reason, list interventions by the leader that might improve group attendance. When possible, document the sources of such information. The following is an example:

Reasons for absenteeism	Leader intervention
Example: Ill health	Leader visits resident at bedside (or phones home on day of meeting) and states that the member was missed at the group meeting; inquires about health problem. Uses active listening and is supportive and concerned.

EXERCISE 3

Obtain permission from the leader and a group of older persons to observe. Observe the leader's actions and interventions. Describe five different actions or interventions performed by the leader. Were they effective or ineffective? State why you think so.

EXERCISE 4

This is an exercise in self-assessment. Because there are different types of leadership, list some of your own characteristics as a group leader. Which ones would you like to improve?

References

Basting, A., & Killick, J. (2003). *The arts and dementia care: A resource guide.* New York: Center for Creative Aging.

Birren, J. E., Kenyon, G. M., Ruth, J. E., Schoots, J. J., & Svensson, T. (1996). *Aging and biography: Explorations in adult development.* New York: Springer.

Burnside, I., & Schmidt, M. G. (1994). *Working with older adults: Group process and techniques.* Boston: Jones & Bartlett.

Corey, M. S., & Corey, G. (1992). *Groups: Process and practice.* Pacific Grove, CA: Brooks/Cole.

Erikson, E. H. (1982). *The life cycle completed: A review.* New York: Norton.

Erikson, E. H., Erikson, J. M., & Kivnick, H. Q. (1986). *Vital involvement in old age.* New York: Norton.

Grayson, P., Lubin, B., & Whitlock, R. V. (1995). Comparison of depression in community-dwelling and assisted-living elderly. *Journal of Clinical Psychology, 51*(1), 18–21.

Kurland, R., & Malekoff, A. (Eds.). (2003). Stories celebrating group work: Its not always easy to sit on your mouth. *Social Work with Groups, 25*(1/2).

Manton, K. G., Cornelius, E. S., & Woodbury, M. A. (1995). Nursing home residents: A multivariate analysis of their medical, behavioral, psychological and service use characteristics. *The Journal of Gerontology, 50A*(5), M242–M251.

McLean, W. (2003). *Practice guide for pain management for people with dementia in institutional care.* Stirling, UK: University of Stirling Dementia Services Development Centre.

Northen, H., & Kurland, R. (2001). *Social work with groups.* New York: Columbia University Press.

Shectman, Z. (2000). A comparison of therapeutic factors in two treatment models: Verbal and art therapy. *Journal of Specialists in Group Work, 25*(3), 288–304.

Toseland, R.W. (1990). *Group work with older adults.* New York: New York University Press.

Toseland, R. W., & Rivas, R.F. (2001). *An introduction to group work practice.* Boston: Allyn & Bacon.

Yalom, I. D. (1995). *The theory and practice of group psychotherapy.* New York: Basic Books.

Teaching Resources

- The films, Erik H. Erikson: A Life's Work and Old Age I and II: Conversations with Joan Erikson, and a study guide to Erikson's life and work are available at **www.davidsonfilms.com/aging.htm**

- A compendium of resources and ideas about Erikson's stages of life span development is available at **http://facultyweb.cortland.edu/ ~ANDERSMD/ERIK/welcome.html**

- Tutorials and Web links about Erikson and his work are available at **http://college.hmco.com/psychology/ seifert/lifespan_dev/2e/students/ weblinks.htm**

- See also **www.ship.edu/~cgboeree/ erikson.html**

Part Three

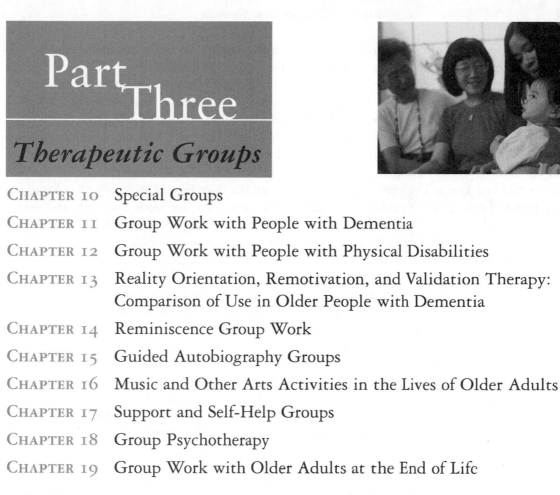

Therapeutic Groups

Part 3 has 10 chapters, each directed toward the treatment of specific issues or presenting specific therapeutic modalities that are helpful to older people. The first chapter, Chapter 10, discusses groups designed to help satellite clusters of workers, such as volunteers, staff, families, and the community in general. Working with older people presents new challenges to employees and this chapter, by Barbara Haight, provides vignettes of groups that have been helpful to families and employees in the past. Chapter 11, revised and updated by Faith Gibson, a social worker and dementia specialist in Northern Ireland, is key to helping workers as the number of older people with dementia increases. Originally written by Irene Burnside, this chapter presents many helpful approaches for dealing with the problems of dementia and offers new insights into care.

Chapter 12 looks at the difficulties involved in getting people with physical disabilities to a group and again, Haight looks at the adjustments needed to treat them. There is a very helpful table of the normal changes which physical aging brings, and a review of sensory losses that sometimes interfere with the group processes.

In Chapter 13 we look at specific therapies that have been helpful to older adults in the past. Elizabeth Williams discusses reality orientation and contrasts a reality orientation group with a validation therapy group. These two groups are at opposite ends of the continuum and make an interesting contrast as we continue to search for ways to communicate with people who have dementia.

Gibson, who has been directing and running reminiscence groups for over twenty years, shares her insights and wealth of experience on the conduct of reminiscence in Chapter 14. Her special expertise is running these groups for people with dementia and there is a section devoted to cognitively impaired people. Her work nicely complements the earlier work of Burnside.

Jim Birren and Donna Deutchman provide us with a masterful description of guided autobiography groups in Chapter 15. They present thrilling new insights into the field of written narratives by individuals working alone and in groups and provide a supplemental view to what we learned from Gibson's work on reminiscence groups.

Chapter 16 addresses creative and artistic groups. Barry Bortnick, who is very experienced in leading music groups with older people, gives a wealth of examples of how using the arts, especially music, transforms and enriches people's lives.

Carole Winston, a social worker and professor at the University of North Carolina in Charlotte, runs a support group for grandparents and offers her insights in Chapter 17. In Chapter 18, Robin Haight, a psychotherapist in Washington, DC, presents two kinds of psychotherapeutic groups that are helpful to older adults. She comments on the issues that may arise in such groups when dealing with older people and offers tips for addressing problem behaviors. Brian deVries, originally from Canada and now in San Francisco, and known for his work on death and dying, writes an insightful chapter on therapeutic groups for people at the end of life.

Many other authors contributed to the work of the third edition of this book but were either not available or could not be located to work on the fourth edition. We have retained some of their good work and ideas by incorporating them into newer, revised chapters for the fourth edition. Special acknowledgements go to Florence Safford, Mary Gwynne Schmidt, and Joan Parry, for their contributions made to the third edition of *Working with Older Adults*, some of which have been included in Chapter 10.

Special Groups

Barbara K. Haight

Key Words

- Community meetings/nursing facility
- Family groups
- In-service training groups
- Psychoeducational groups
- Single-session groups
- Grief
- Volunteers

Learning Objectives

- List three agency or nursing facility activities in which group process plays an important part.
- Contrast the use of structure in training groups for volunteers with in insight-oriented treatment groups.
- Tell why the psychoeducational group is especially suited for working with the families of mentally impaired residents.
- Describe the function of the community meeting in a nursing facility.
- State the role of the single-session group to meet crisis needs.
- Describe a single-session group as a means of coping with loss.

This chapter deals with group process as a powerful dynamic in social agencies and residential settings. The chapter discusses five situations in which attention to group process heightens effectiveness: (1) in-service training for staff, (2) programs for volunteers, (3) educational groups for families, (4) community meetings for nursing home residents, and (5) grief groups when a resident dies in a nursing home. Often these situations are not recognized as small-group activities, because their implicit purposes are educational or organizational or because the persons involved are not viewed as patients or clients.

These instrumental (or task) groups differ from expressive (or treatment) groups in purpose, structure, and emotional intensity. An example of an instrumental group is a work group with a defined purpose, understood role assignments and responsibilities, an agenda, and an emphasis on doing rather than feeling. An example of an expressive group is a therapy group having a degree of ambiguity that may conduce to anxiety and regression or become healing (see Chapter 18, Psychotherapeutic Groups). In between the polar opposites of instrumental and expressive groups is a whole range of groups with varied purposes.

Because structure contributes to group comfort, and flexibility leads to group creativity, many leaders of groups for the aged begin with structure and then ease up a bit as members make the group their own. This initially more structured approach is supportive not only to aged participants but also to new leaders, who become better able to accept detours in the agenda as they gain more confidence. For example, groups undertaking simple reminiscence, tend to be more structured than life-review groups: topics are announced, props are more likely to be employed, and participants are not encouraged to uncover feelings and memories that neither they nor their leaders are ready to deal with. Life-review groups entail more probing and more risk-taking by participants and leaders alike. The emotional level also may become more intense. (See Chapter 14, Reminiscence Groups.)

The kinds of group situations described in this chapter move along a continuum of purpose, structure, and intensity of feeling. For example, in skilled nursing facilities, there are required in-service programs focusing on technical skills. Staff typically must participate in these when hired and then repeat them annually (Roberto, Wacker, Jewell, & Rickard, 1997). The purpose of such groups is to teach staff a process or technique or to impart other information needed for job performance. Goals in the in-service training of staff may include a goal for attitude change as well as goals for learning skills.

Even when experiential learning is employed, there are occasions when the instructor must pull together and prioritize the content. By organizing the information through learning objectives, the educator is helping the learner retain the information (Dunlap, 1997). There are clear lines of authority in this teaching–learning situation. Attendance is rarely optional. The knowledge and skills gained through staff development can be transferred to practice and result in improved care of patients (Kaasalainen, 2002).

Groups for volunteers may share similar goals, but because volunteers are not employees, they should be treated differently. Training for them also has a how-to character. As adult learners, volunteers like organization in the educational process, prepared education materials, and an informal teaching–learning environment allowing for individual involvement (Davis & White, 2000). Yet, how they feel about the agency and its clientele, the educator, and one another is vital to ensuring their continuing engagement with the agency. Volunteers must receive emotional satisfaction from their work and affiliation. Often peer learning partnerships, which are voluntary reciprocal helping relationships between individuals who share closely related learning objectives, work well with volunteers (Eisen, 2001).

Like volunteers, family members of residents and patients usually embrace the educational aspect of any program. At the same time, emotions are the real barriers to their support of their aging relatives. Unless they can work through some of their feelings, any instrumental learning may be hobbled by pain, distress, and old hurts. Often, both resident and family members have difficulty adjusting to long-term care (Iwasiw, Goldenberg, Bol, & MacMaster, 2003). Caregiver depression is closely related to how well both the caregiver and the nursing home resident adjust to the nursing home environment (Whitlach, Schur, Noelker, Ejaz, & Looman, 2001). Of course the caregivers' own health needs can have a negative impact on the resident's adjustment to the institution (Bradley, 2003).

Family member groups often exist near the border between education and treatment and sometimes tip over into treatment. Thus the model of a prototypical program for families of residents with dementia takes into account the families' dual needs for emotional support and factual knowledge. Children who act as caregivers for those with dementia carry a heavy burden. Fortunately, caring for a family member in one's youth does not impact negatively on one's health in adulthood (Shifren, 2001).

In institutional settings where people live so close to one another and yet, in so many ways, are isolated and lonely, there is a strong need for residents to nurture community beyond shared recreation and shared meals. Friends are very important to the ongoing social support of people living in a nursing home (Lilly, Richards, & Buckwalter, 2003). Above all, very old people need to participate in a segment of group life in which they are responsible members, not patients with the recipient status that implies.

This chapter will describe a model for community meetings that was developed by the Live Oak Institute in Sobrante, California. Although that model evolved in a residential facility, it has been adapted for day care centers, senior centers, nutrition sites, and board-and-care facilities. The phrase "community meeting" in this chapter refers to these residents' groups, not to neighborhood get-togethers in the wider community.

When there is a death in an aged community, residents know it, feel it, and respond to it, but there is rarely a group that meets their need to talk about it. When death occurs in an institutional setting, such as a nursing home, it tends to be a negative experience for everyone. For families, the death may reawaken the ambivalence and pain they felt when they placed their relative in the facility. For residents, the death is both a preview and a taboo. If fellow residents ask about a dying or deceased resident, they receive an evasive answer. Perceiving the professional calm of their caregivers, they come to believe that staff will be indifferent to their deaths as well. Some staff members become close to the residents and, when they are dealing with their own anticipatory or unresolved mourning, they find it difficult to meet the emotional needs of families, other residents, or even the dying person. No one can turn to staff when staff members themselves have been schooled in avoidance. Family members of the deceased resident also need to deal with their grief (Davidson, Hsiao-Chen, & Titler, 2003).

But, the nursing home is associated with death. Once, nursing facilities sent many of their moribund patients to the hospital to die. Today, the hopelessly ill resident is often spared that journey, and the skilled nursing facility must cope with its own burdens of dying. Thus this chapter will close with the single-session grief group, the group that deals with death in a skilled nursing facility.

In-Service Training

In-service classes do more than educate. They can improve staff morale, encourage peer discussions, and keep staff members in close touch with one another. The latter is especially important when staff has little opportunity for daily contact even though they must build upon one another's work, shift after shift. This is as true in community agencies in which staff members may do much of their work away from each other in the field, as it is true in nursing homes, where everyone works in shifts. Getting to know one another better prepares staff for quick collaboration and substitution when either is required.

Because the staff are indeed a small group, certain identifiable roles are common: the expert, who is anxious to update the presenter; the yes-but-er, who takes issue with every point; the Scheherazade, who can provide a tale to illustrate—or challenge—every point; and the distractor, who comes in late, introduces irrelevancies, and otherwise impedes the process.

To a point, both the expert and the yes-but-er can be encouraged to expand their views further because they are often a reminder that the leader has been talking too long. If they are merely intrusive, the group itself will manifest impatience with them. When they are interrupting a sequence, they can be asked to wait. When the Scheherazade's tales are relevant, they can be powerful reinforcers of the instructor's point because they come from a member of the group. The late-entry distractor provides the speaker with a reason for recapitulating, which may be helpful for all. When the interruptions are disruptive, the speaker can be asked to tell the instructor afterwards or to prepare some written materials to share with the group.

Obstacles

Attendance may be compulsory, but attention is not. The leader may struggle against formidable odds if the administrator who mandated the in-service training is less committed to its learning goals than to merely documenting that it took place at all. Lack of true commitment is best typified by the nursing facility that schedules two consecutive 30-minute sessions around the 3 p.m. change of shifts. Bone-weary nursing assistants, who drowse or watch the clock, attend the first session. Just when they have convinced the leader that she or he should consider another occupation, these weary workers leave and a new crew appears, wide awake and enthusiastic.

Thirty minutes is not enough time to teach anything: Time for discussion and experiential learning is severely curtailed. The only solution lies in sharply limiting content. When the time given is inadequate, there often is equal inattention to the learning environment. Confused residents may be permitted to wander in and out, participants may be called out of the class to perform various tasks, and an intercom may break in at intervals.

The leader is further challenged when there are great educational disparities between participants, as when nursing assistants are included with licensed nurses and even advanced practice nurses (Ryden et al. 2000). Generally, all nurse groups are serving the same population, which does provide a common focus, but they are serving in different ways. The task is to make the content comprehensible to the less educated while acknowledging the expertise of the professionals.

The paraprofessionals are aided by frequent definition of terms and use of examples. The professionals can be engaged by invoking them as authorities and as helpers—and by reminding them privately that it is important for them to hear what their supervisees have been told so they can assist them with the material.

Often dedicated agency personnel are reluctant to waste time on staff meetings and in-service training because the needs of their clients seem more urgent. These are the very persons at risk of burnout. They need an intra-agency support system and the larger perspective that training can provide. The instructor should never feel diffident about requiring the staff's attendance but must demonstrate that the content is relevant to their work.

Techniques

A seating arrangement communicates the expected level of participation: Classroom rows call for passive listening; circles and roundtables call for taking part. Also, group process can be enlisted to promote active learning. Discussion often changes attitudes, and simply viewing videotape together may stimulate discussion. Nurses have always learned and grown in clinical nursing practice; thus, the educator should also consider action learning as a model for group learning (Daley, 2001). Role playing within the larger circle elicits another level of involvement. For example, you can have one participant be the patient and two others play nursing assistants pushing her wheelchair and talking over her head. Afterwards all parties can discuss how they felt, and the group will make your point for you. Finally, breaking the large class into smaller groups or pairs for problem-solving exercises provides training in teamwork. This also builds group cohesion and enables shy persons to speak up. Only irrelevance and time constraints are barriers to this kind of learning. When these exercises work well, they always take longer than expected. Because they foster fellowship, small-group approaches such as these are even more important for volunteers. The very flexibility of these approaches makes it essential, however, that the leader develop a learning plan. See **Table 10–1** for an outline useful for work with either staff or volunteers.

Group Processes in Working with Volunteers

Agencies and facilities serving the older adult benefit from the services of groups of volunteers who are often effectively recruited, managed, and retained as a group. Volunteering not only appeals to their altruism but also offers volunteers an expanded social network and an improved self-image. Older volunteers are replacing the younger housewives who used to be the daytime volunteers. By 1990, 41% of volunteers were over 65 (Chambré, 1993). Today, there are numerous Web sites offering volunteer opportunities for older people abroad as well as at home (Volunteers of America, 2004). Volunteers in an agency often make the difference between a Spartan existence for the residents and one that is full of stimulation and personal attention. But, the volunteers need to be encouraged and appreciated to feel their efforts are worthwhile (Volunteers for helping the elderly and disabled, 2004). Engaging some of the older residents as volunteers in their own facilities and retirement communities makes sense as well. They should receive the same screening, training, supervision, and recognition as nonresidents.

Table 10–1 LESSON PLAN

Learning needs to be addressed:	Why this lesson at this time?
Learners:	Consider what you know about their learning style and how they are likely to feel about this content. Will it seem relevant to their goals and work?
Time and place:	
Goal(s):	These can be more global than the objectives.
Objectives:	State these in specific, observable terms.
Content:	What you wish to cover
Method:	This should include:
	• Modalities: Lecturing, group discussion, experiential exercises, the case method, or any combination
	• Strategy: How you plan to get their attention, convey information, and help them retain it; how you intend to overcome attitudinal resistance to the content
	• Sequencing: How you plan to organize the material so they can integrate and retain it
Material and equipment:	Slides, overhead projector, handouts, chalk board, flip chart, and the like
Measurement of goal achievement:	Depending on the setting, this can be derived from quality improvement data, tests, charts, observation, questionnaires, and subsequent attendance figures. Stating your objectives in specific, observable terms makes measurement easier.

Hospice volunteers are a good example of the need for volunteer training because they often have to function on their own in difficult situations. One model training program for hospice volunteer group leaders includes: reading assignments and films, participation in a reminiscence group, peer group discussion, and an evaluation. Because volunteers go alone into the homes of the dying, hospices have a great need for screening and also for bonding their volunteers into a strong, mutually supportive group. Some hospices require all would-be volunteers to take three weeks of bereavement training, followed by a second interview. At this point, some screen themselves out or are counseled into less stressful programs. After the second interview, volunteers undergo intensive training designed not only to impart skills but also to build relationships within the group.

A very successful volunteer training program was held as a weekend retreat in a beautiful mountain setting. Staff members came and went, but volunteers and the coordinator remained overnight. Throughout the education process, the volunteer coordinator gave a higher priority to creating a climate of acceptance and warmth than the staff developer, whose chief focus was skills acquisition. Volunteers also need skills, but their staying depends on their relations with people.

Training Programs for Families

Peer group support is equally important for a second group of persons, more burdened than volunteers—the families. For example, family caregivers of dementia patients experience great amounts of grief whether caring for their loved one at home or in a nursing home (Rudd, Viney, & Preston, 1999). Safford and Schmidt (1994) developed a program to help families of residents deal with the devastating consequences of dementia. The program's goal was to provide families with the non-

technical knowledge about the causes and symptoms of mental impairment. The families also learned about the resources available, the skills they needed for responding to their relatives, and the skills needed for relating to the professional service system. The program was presented to families as an educational opportunity and is described here.

The group was opened to families caring for their relatives in the community, as well as families of nursing home residents. It was assumed that the community group and the nursing home group would benefit from the same knowledge and that each group's members would be mutually supportive through sharing experiences. This assumption proved correct. The community group learned about which factors lead to the decision to place a relative in an institution, while family members of the nursing home group were supported in their choice by the reminder of the ongoing nature of the problems in the community group.

A two-hour intensive program was offered once a week for six weeks. The first hour covered didactic material; the second hour was open to questions and discussion of participants' experiences. The program drew 48 participants from a radius of 200 miles. Despite the large numbers, there was a great deal of participant interaction, and by the middle phase of the program, group cohesion was evident, with many participants sharing telephone numbers. Refreshments that were served before and after the meeting facilitated this informal interaction.

Careful attention was paid to the learning environment, with the goal of establishing a climate of informality and warmth. A multipurpose activity room was selected that was large enough for comfort but not so large that the participants would lose a sense of intimacy. The chairs were arranged in three concentric semicircles, filling the room but not overcrowding it.

Session One

A large number of participants arrived a half hour early and sat quietly, looking tense and not talking to one another. When a huge urn of coffee and platters of pastries were brought in, conversation started. The session began 20 minutes late to put the participants more at ease by allowing them to become acquainted. During the break, there was much animated interaction among the participants. The first session ended a half hour later than scheduled, and many participants remained to talk with their newly found peer group.

From the outset, the program was presented as a problem-solving model, with the goal of providing the tools needed for more rational, satisfactory family and institutional relations.

The heightened emotional level of the group was evidenced frequently by the urgency with which problems were presented for discussion and the tears with which experiences were shared. Although the format was educational, the program turned out to be an equally therapeutic experience.

As the knowledge component was developed, the participants were invited to raise questions or make comments based on their personal experiences, which were then used to reinforce the more abstract learning. The following case example illustrates the process.

The project director identified the need to acquire new role behaviors, which would be difficult without prior experience and without the benefit of role models, One married daughter in her fifties commented that when she brought her parents for their initial interview to Isabella Homes, she recalled having the same feelings as when she registered her children for kindergarten. She also recalled her feelings as she helped her mother dress. The daughter was painfully aware of the difference in her emotions from when she had helped her own daughter dress. She said, with tears in her eyes, "I didn't want to be her mother—she had been a wonderful mother!"

The rest of the group nodded in agreement, most having experienced similar emotions at what seemed to be the strain of role reversals. The project director pointed out that it is not role reversal that takes place but the assumption of a new role, that of protective kin or helper. The psychological relationship between adult child and parent does not turn around because of the parents' impairment, although the incorrect concept of role reversal and second childhood is widely held.

The group was then introduced to the concept of filial maturity as the developmental task that confronted them, the need to assume dependable role behavior, appropriate to the level of their kin's impairment.

The problems most frequently expressed by the family group centered around their difficulty during visits and their frustrations in seeking help from the staff. To deal with the first set of problems, the leader emphasized the need to understand the nature of impairment and the meaning of their relative's behavior.

To deal with the second problem, the leader suggested that the group form the nucleus of a family council, which could bring their shared concerns to the administrators of the home. There was immediate interest. The project director discussed the mechanics of establishing such an organization with administration and reported back at the second session. Because many participants had internalized the myth that families abandon their own when putting them in institutions, serving on a family council to counteract the guilt-producing myth emerged as an unanticipated goal of the program.

A common theme was the need to change the behavior of the person with dementia, revealing a lack of knowledge of the neurological disorder by the family and a denial of the extent of the relative's impairment. Certain problematic behaviors and violence can become part of the behavior of the demented patient and family members need to be taught to handle these behaviors. Wilkinson

(1999) presents a helpful educational program for managing dementia-compromised behavior, and Gates, Fitzwater, and Meyer (1999) provide an in-depth look at the effects of violence on caregivers. Because the litany of heartbreaking problems was beginning to sound like a soap opera, the project director made conscious use of humor in the form of amusing anecdotes to release some of the mounting emotion.

GROUNDWORK FOR A FAMILY COUNCIL

Before the second session, the project director talked with the administration about the relatives' interest in establishing a family council. The administration welcomed the plan as a means of demonstrating a responsive stance to criticisms and openness to suggestions. In addition, an active family council was viewed as a potential partner. Communication was to be established directly with the administration through elected representatives of the council.

Session Two

The difference in mood of the group at the start of the second session was dramatic. There was already a sense of group cohesion, and animated discussion took place before the session began. Picking up the commonly held desire to change the behavior of their relatives, the project director suggested borrowing the Alcoholics Anonymous prayer: "Grant me the serenity to accept what cannot be changed, the courage to change what can be changed, and the wisdom to know the difference." This slogan was a psychological aid as the participants worked at the task of learning the nature of their relative's condition and at identifying when the condition might be ameliorated and when they had to accept irreversible decline. The participants gave examples which served as a springboard for clarification and discussion about learning to unravel the meaning behind much problematic behavior that sometimes is a nonverbal means used by people with dementia when their verbal skills deteriorate and they become increasingly frustrated by their condition.

The second half of the session was devoted to role playing, in which several participants were to enact the problem of the family whose impaired older relative could no longer be maintained safely in the community but who refused to go into a nursing home. The goal was to give participants a chance to practice new skills and to experience more effective decision making, but role playing was a fiasco with this population, because they could not transcend their current roles to handle the problem situation. The project director was forced to drop role play and to teach directly. Also, the report about the administration's cooperation in founding a family council was received enthusiastically. Some stayed afterward to work out plans for their new council.

Session Three

This session included another attempt at role playing, when a relative of a nursing home resident came to the nurse with a long list of legitimate complaints of neglect of the resident. When the role playing nurse responded to the complaints, "These things happen because your mother is so confused," the relative immediately retreated, saying, "I'm sorry I bothered you." When the project director tried to encourage other responses, a member of the group commented empathetically, "That's because nurses are so authoritarian that we're all intimidated by them."

This led to a fruitful discussion of the guilt-provoking behavior of many members of the staff in nursing homes and to the discussion of concrete methods relatives can use to present legitimate complaints. It was decided to drop other planned experiential techniques, because it was clear that this group was in need of more direct sources of information. Furthermore, it was evident that they were developing their new skills through interaction with their newly found reference group.

Sessions Four and Five

The most emotionally charged session was the fourth, when sexuality was discussed. There was absolute silence in the room as the project director discussed normal sexuality in old age and problems with some mentally impaired people. Case examples were presented of behavior resulting from damage to the part of the brain that controls sexual impulses. Examples of problems in the nursing home, as well as in the community, elicited personal experiences that had been too painful for participants to discuss until that point. The suppressed embarrassment and outrage were released with evident relief, based on the newly acquired knowledge that unexpected sexual behavior can be part of the normal process of deterioration caused by dementia or related mental impairments. Compared to residents and spouses, staff are much more accepting of sexual behaviors of residents in nursing homes (Gibson, Bol, Woodbury, Beaton, & Janke, 1999).

Session five's discussion of personal values regarding sexual behavior seemed particularly stimulating to the participants. The values of independence, egalitarianism, responsibility, family security, and self-actualization were discussed, revealing how these values might conflict with the relative's behavior and lead to anger and then guilt. Analyzing situations to uncover the underlying values that dictate choices in everyday behavior was a new experience for most of the participants. These values were then related to the earlier discussion of filial maturity and the need to find a balance of shared function with the formal organizations equipped to care for the person with dementia in modern society.

Session Six

The final session dealt with separation and the need for the group to dissolve on time as was planned before the group started. Most participants expressed the wish that the program would continue. One stated almost angrily, "I'm sure you said the program was going to last ten weeks!" Another brought a bouquet of flowers. A community relative gave a contribution to the home. One took pictures of the group. The project director had to submerge a powerful impulse to continue the program.

The participant most interested in establishing a family council reported that the group had decided to hold their first meeting the very next Saturday in order to lose neither their group identity nor the impetus of their meetings. The session ended with a spirit of activism and optimism that they would as a group continue to manifest concern not only for their own mentally impaired relatives, but also for all the residents of the home and for the aged in general.

The next step was to try 8-session and 10-session programs. Each time participants asked for more sessions. The common request for more time made it clear that the participants needed opportunities to talk out their feelings. As a result, a support group was formed later and met on a monthly basis. Support groups in this setting have become ubiquitous since the first ones were tried. They are especially helpful to caregivers who benefit from hearing other people's approaches to care (Waterhouse, Dietsch, and Francis, 2002) and who require frequent reassurance and support (Larrimore, 2003). There are multiple information sites on the Internet that can be helpful to support groups (Anderson & Olmstadt, 2003). Long-term care facilities still benefit through improved relations with residents' relatives when support group programs are offered as an integral service. These programs are now called psychoeducational, because of the multiple benefits of knowledge, skills acquisition, and opportunity for emotional release and repair (Hebert et al. 2003).

Group Process in the Community Meeting

Within the institutional walls it is important to foster a community that will nourish the individuality of residents and offer them meaningful roles. The latest attempt to do this is called Edenizing. The Eden Alternative was conceived by Thomas (1996) who looked to nature for an alternative to the sterile environment of the nursing home. He wanted a human habitat that included plants, animals, and children; he also wanted residents to be responsible for the plants and animals (Barba, Tesh, & Courts, 2002). Before Edenizing, the Barkans (1993) had devised a similar plan and took over a setting where residents were already socialized to institutional dependence. The Barkan's goal was to create a regenerative community that would support the individuality and potential of the elders who lived there. They developed a special ethos to counter the isolation and resignation of the residents and to help them see themselves in a context larger than their infirmity.

One of the Barkan's major tools was the daily community meeting, which provided a centerpiece for life within the facility. This section will describe those meetings and the memorial services, which also are critical components in the regenerative community approach. Although similar in size to the big groups often conducted in psychiatric settings, the purpose of community meetings is quite different: The purpose is to create a community in which group members can thrive through a sense of membership in a group that relates to them as multidimensional individuals. No one is put in the hot seat, as in psychiatric centers, and the group is not employed as a coercive instrument, as in the Synanon model of the 1960s.

The outline of the community meetings is provided in **Table 10–2**.

Table 10–2 brings into focus several notable features:

1. *There is a predictable order of events.* The dependable sequence not only provides the security of structure but also enables residents to use that structure to meet their individual needs. They may wander in after the exercises or leave before the closing song. No one is required to attend, but staff tries to make the meeting so interesting and relevant to their lives that everyone wants to come.

2. *Life within the environment is highlighted, and residents are actively involved in making decisions* about events affecting their lives as members of the group (Community news).

3. *They are intellectually challenged and encouraged to view themselves as part of the greater world* and to respond to issues and events that they find relevant to them as a community (World news and discussion of the day).

4. *Individuality is recognized, but connectedness also is nurtured* (Welcoming and community news).

5. *There is ongoing attention to cueing.* Participants in the group included the full spectrum of any nursing facility population, ranging from persons who are cognitively integrated to those suffering from Alzheimer's disease and other dementias. All have a right to be there and a part to play. The underlying concept is that all residents, even those who are severely impaired, have a part of them that is well. By staff's relating to them at their highest level of functioning, the well part is nurtured and expanded. The role of the leader is defined as that of a community developer. As managers, the

Table 10–2 STRUCTURE OF THE COMMUNITY MEETING

Exercises

Sitting exercises:
- Help participants become more alert for the meeting
- Increase health and well-being

Welcoming

Participating staff members go around the circle, greeting each member:
- Provides an opportunity to connect with the elders before the meeting
- Helps participants feel known and appreciated
- Lets participants know the meeting will begin soon
- Provides opportunity to introduce visitors and guests

Opening song
- Connects people to one another
- Builds group spirit and joy

Community news

Two kinds of announcements:
- Coming and past events in the life of the community
- Life events for participants and their families and the planning and decision making that arise from them

World news
- Stimulates and challenges participants
- Invites involvement in community affairs and current topics of national and world discussion

Discussion of the day
- Stimulates and challenges participants through talking, feeling, and thinking about a topic
- Helps participants get to know each other
- Provides a point of connection for future conversations

Closing song
- Lets people know the meeting is over
- Gives everyone a good feeling for and connection to the group

Barkan, & Barkan, 1993.

Barkans participated frequently, and all staff members were encouraged to drop by and make a contribution whenever possible.

6. *Memorial service.* The memorial service for deceased members is notable because it addresses an aspect of nursing facility life more often dealt with by denial. Instead, the memorial service seeks to turn an occasion of loss into an affirmation of the worth of the individual and a reaffirma-tion of community. **Table 10–3** illustrates the process.

The Live Oak approach fits the wellness model that offers an alternative to the medical model, with its emphasis on problems and pathology. It is consistent with the resident-centered position promulgated by the Nursing Home Reform Amendments, which call not only for more humane care but also for active rehabilitation that will enable each resident to achieve his or her highest potential.

Table 10-3   THE LIVE OAK MEMORIAL SERVICE

Preparing the community

During community meetings, members have discussed the memorial services and what they feel is appropriate. When a death occurs, members of the resident's family and other residents and staff who knew him or her best are consulted about the content of the service. Always, these services affirm that each person's life is precious and that he or she will be remembered by the community.

Introduction

The community developer or a resident welcomes community members and speaks a little about the deceased. For example, "We are gathered today to remember Joe Fraser. He came to the Home six years ago. Originally he worked as a tailor in New York, where he…"

Shared remembrances

Residents, staff, and family members share their memories of Mr. Fraser. Some may wish to bring poems or other appropriate readings.

Reflection

The community developer and others talk about what the community learned from Mr. Fraser. Usually embedded in these reflections is a message related to the community ethos.

Prayers

The community developer and/or others offer appropriate prayers for Mr. Fraser and his transition.

Well wishing

The community developer blesses the community, wishing its members healing from what ails them, health and joy for family members, and peace for the world.

Singing is added as appropriate

Barkan,& Barkan,1993.

Single-Session Grief Group

The memorial service reported at Live Oak leads coherently into a discussion of a single-session grief group in a skilled nursing facility (Parry, 1994). Little is known about the personal experience of death in a nursing home (Jones, 2002). Parry reports that the sudden death of a resident has a powerful effect on surviving residents, and she discusses the death of a resident called Janet. Janet was one of the more active, visible, and vital residents of a skilled nursing facility (SNF) in northern California. She passed away suddenly, on a Tuesday. Janet was 84 and died of a massive cerebrovascular accident. She had lived in the facility for 18 months. She was a widow with two children. Because she was a popular resident, her death profoundly affected many of the other resi-

dents of the facility. To deal with everyone's unease, the social worker suggested a single-session group meeting for residents and staff willing to participate in discussing Janet's death. Such a group would serve residents who did not participate also because they would know it occurred and know that the persons who operate the institution cared about the residents. The worker then visited the facility's units and talked with residents who appeared to be upset by the loss of Janet. The social worker particularly paid attention to Janet's room mate, Judith, thinking Judith would feel the loss of Janet the most. The administrator invited all of the facility staff to attend, as well as Janet's family, and the residents.

Group work with older persons like the above is a very useful way of helping residents to discuss and share their losses. Making residents feel they are not alone reduces their fear of death. This single-session group not only served the residents by reducing their anxiety about Janet's death, but also enabled the staff, the administrator, and the social worker to say good-bye to Janet. The single-session group helped to bring together people in crisis who otherwise would remain anxious, isolated, and hurting. Such groups can also help family members and others deal with their loss (Cutillo-Schmitter, 1996). To deal with grief, it is important to provide support and help as soon as possible after the event has occurred. The death in the above example occurred on Tuesday, and the group was held on Friday. Acute grief is almost always present as a result of sudden death and groups can help associates and families accept their grief (Kirk & McManus, 2002). The administrator in this case felt the need to respond rapidly, and the social worker was in agreement.

The social worker knew that frequently the single-session group provides worker, agency, and clients with their only possibility of engagement. The constraints of the agency, such as limited availability of staff social workers and inability to disturb work schedules, were in operation in this facility. Therefore, this would be the only group session offered to residents.

The social worker and the administrator knew how important it was for the members of the group to have a clear understanding of the purpose of the group and defined the purpose as: a way to say good-bye to Janet, an opportunity for the members to share memories of other losses or other deaths, an opportunity to express feelings about Janet's death, and to reduce anxieties about death for themselves.

The Group Process

As the group commenced, the administrator thanked the residents and staff for coming and expressed her own sadness at the death of Janet. Then the social worker, serving as group leader, articulated the purpose of the group and followed this by going around the circle, asking each person to state his or her name and tell in one word how he or she was feeling. The group leader felt that if all group members spoke, it would relieve some tension. The leader said group members could pass if they chose, but no one did. Some of the words were "sad," "lonely," "unhappy," and a couple of members said "fine."

The leader set up two rules for the group: one person talks at a time and things said remain in the group. The leader also stated that the purpose of the group was healing. The leader then gave the group background about Janet: her age, information about her bereaved family, and the length of time Janet had lived in the facility. The leader's goal was to review Janet's life in the facility, while helping the group members perhaps to review their own lives. The leader then opened the meeting for general discussion of losses the others had experienced and sharing of memories about Janet. The majority of the members were widowed women who had experienced multiple losses. The most severe loss had been the loss of a spouse, although there was one group member who had also lost a child, and reported that loss as the greatest loss. Some members talked about losses in business; some said Janet was out of her misery, suggesting their own feelings of misery. The theme was one of toughing it out. The staff talked about losing parents and how working in the facility meant seeing many deaths.

The group talked about ways to cope with loss. Many of the group members cried during the meeting, and this was accepted and encouraged. The group lasted about 75 minutes and ended with a minute of silence. Before the minute of silence, the leader requested an evaluation of the group by the group members. Members' comments were positive. They said they liked getting together as a group and that the leader had encouraged everyone to talk openly. They said that it didn't change anything, but it was nice to talk, and some members said the opportunity to acknowledge the loss reduced their own anxiety about Janet's sudden death.

Summary

Group process has always been an important element in staff and volunteer training and in general meetings for families and residents. Today, it is more consciously employed to foster the educational and developmental goals of the sponsoring agency or institution. This chapter has illustrated general principles and specific differences involved in working with staff, volunteers, families, and the resident community. The single-session grief group was very much a response to unmet needs. The group provided a sense of "we-ness" and helped group members to feel they were not alone. The sense of belonging and the feeling that everyone was "all in the same boat" provided for the start of the healing process.

Exercises

EXERCISE 1

Plan an in-service class for a nursing facility staff using the following format:

1. Goal
2. Objectives
3. Outline of content
4. Brief quiz on content
5. Reading list
6. Audiovisual or teaching aids
7. Supply list

Tell how you might adapt this if you were planning the class for volunteers.

EXERCISE 2

Go to your local Alzheimer's association and ask permission to attend a family support group, or call a nursing facility and ask to observe a family council meeting. Be sure to clear your attendance with members themselves as well as the sponsoring body. Do not take notes at the meeting, but

afterward prepare a short report describing the extent to which the meeting was devoted to business and the exchange of information and to what degree it was devoted to emotional catharsis and the expression of feeling.

References

Anderson, M., & Olmstadt, W. (2003). Providing systematic training for patient support groups. *Journal of Hospital Librarianship, 3*(3), 13–23.

Barba, B., Tesh, A., & Courts, N. (2002). Promoting thriving in nursing homes: The Eden Alternative. *Journal of Gerontological Nursing, 28*(3), 7–13.

Barkan, D., & Barkan, B. (1993, April). *The nursing home as community*. Presentation to the annual workshop of the organization of social service providers in long-term care, San Diego, CA.

Bradley, P. (2003). Family caregiver assessment: Essential for effective home health care. *Journal of Gerontological Nursing, 29*(2), 29–36.

Chambré, S. M. (1993). Volunteerism by elders: Past trends and future prospects. *The Gerontologist, 33*(2), 221–228.

Cutillo-Schmitter, T. (1996). Managing ambiguous loss in dementia and terminal illness. *Journal of Gerontological Nursing, 22*(5), 32–38.

Daley, B. (2001). Learning in clinical practice. *Holistic Nursing Practice, 16*(1), 43–54.

Davidson, K., Hsiao-Chen, J., & Titler, M. (2003). Evidence-based protocol: Family bereavement support before and after the death of a nursing home resident. *Journal of Gerontological Nursing, 29*(1), 10–18.

Davis, G., & White, T. (2000). Planning an osteoporosis education program for older adults in a residential setting. *Journal of Gerontological Nursing, 26*(1), 16–23.

Dunlap, R. (1997). Teaching advance directives: The why, when, and how. *Journal of Gerontological Nursing, 23*(12), 11–16.

Eisen, M. J. (2001). Peer-based professional development viewed through the lens of transformative learning. *Holistic Nursing Practice, 16*(1), 30–42.

Gates, D., Fitzwater, E., & Meyer, U. (1999). Violence against caregivers in nursing homes: Expected, tolerated, and accepted. *Journal of Gerontological Nursing, 25*(4), 12–22.

Gibson, M., Bol, N., Woodbury, M., Beaton, C., and Janke, C. (1999). Expressing sexuality in an institutional setting. *Journal of Gerontological Nursing, 25*(4), 30–39.

Hebert, R., Levesque, L., Vezina, J., Lavoie, J., Ducharme, F., Gendron, C. et al. (2003). Efficacy of a psycho educative group program for caregivers of demented persons living at home: A randomized controlled trial. *Journal of Gerontology B, Social Sciences,* 58B(1), S58–67.

Iwasiw, C., Goldenberg, D., Bol, N., & MacMaster, E. (2003). Resident and family perspectives: The first year in a long-term care facility. *Journal of Gerontological Nursing,* 29(1), 45–54.

Jones, J. (2002). The experience of dying: An ethnographic nursing home study. *The Gerontologist,* 47(Suppl. 3), 11–19.

Kaasalainen, S. (2002). Staff development and long-term care of patients with dementia. *Journal of Gerontological Nursing,* 28(7), 39–46.

Kirk, K. & McManus, M. (2002). Containing families' grief: Therapeutic group work in a hospice setting. *International Journal of Palliative Nursing,* 8(10), 20–24.

Larrimore, K. (2003). Alzheimer disease support group characteristics: A comparison of caregivers. *Geriatric Nursing,* 24(1), 32–35.

Lilly, M., Richards, B., Buckwalter, K. (2003). Friends and social support in dementia care giving: Assessment and intervention. *Journal of Gerontological Nursing,* 29(1), 29–36.

Parry, J. (1994). Another special group: The single-session grief grouping. In I. Burnside, & M. Schmidt (Eds.), *Working with older adults: Group processes and techniques.* Boston: Jones and Bartlett.

Roberto, K., Wacker, R., Jewell, E., & Rickard, M., (1997). Resident rights: Knowledge of and implementation by nursing staff in long-term care facilities. *Journal of Gerontological Nursing,* 23(12), 32–40.

Rudd, M., Viney, L., & Preston, C. (1999). The grief experience of spousal caregivers of dementia patients: The role of place of care of patient and gender of caregiver. *International Journal of Aging and Human Development,* 48(3), 217–240.

Ryden, M., Snyder, M., Gross, C., Savik, K., Pearson, V., Krichbaum, K. et al. (2000). Value-added outcomes: The use of advanced practice nurses in long-term care facilities. *The Gerontologist,* 40(6), 654–662.

Safford, F., & Schmidt, M. (1994). Special groups: Staff, volunteers, families, and residential groups. In I. Burnside, & M. Schmidt (Eds.), *Working with older adults: Group processes and techniques.* Boston: Jones and Bartlett.

Shifren, K. (2001). Early caregiving and adult depression: Good news for young caregivers. *The Gerontologist,* 41(2), 188–190.

Thomas, W. (1994). *The Eden Alternative: Nature, hope, and nursing homes.* Sherburne, New York: Eden Alternative Foundation.

Volunteers of America. (2004, May 16). Retrieved May 16, 2004, from *http://www.voa.org/xq/CFM/folder_id.118/qx/tier2_ka.cfm*

Volunteers for helping the elderly and disabled. (2004, May16). Retrieved May 16, 2004, from *http://www.positivelights.org/volunteers.htm*

Waterhouse, A., Dietsch, E., & Francis, K. (2002). All in the same boat: An investigation into the effects of a caregiver's support group. *Geriatrician,* 20(4), 5–8.

Whitlach, C., Schur, D., Noelker, L., Ejaz, F., & Looman, W. (2001). The stress process of family care giving in an institutional setting. *The Gerontologist,* 41(4), 462–473.

Wilkinson, C. (1999). An evaluation of an educational program on the management of assaultive behaviors. *Journal of Gerontological Nursing,* 25(4), 6–11.

BIBLIOGRAPHY

Johnson, D. R., Agresti, A., Jacob, M. C., & Nies, K. (1990). Building a therapeutic community through specialized groups in nursing homes. *Clinical Gerontology,* 9(3/4), 203–217.

Palmer D. S. (1991). Co-leading a family council in a long-term care facility. *Journal of Gerontological Social Work,* 16(3/4), 121–134.

Smyer, M., Brannon, D., & Cohn, M. (1992). Improving nursing home care through training and job redesign. *Gerontologist,* 32(3), 327–333.

Spitzer, W. J., & Burke, L. (1993). A critical-incident stress debriefing program for hospital-based health care personnel. *Health and Social Work,* 18(2), 149–156.

Resources

BOOKS

- *Unlocking the Secrets of the Effective In-Service: A Resource Manual,* by Janice C. Smith. This manual is addressed to inexperienced staff developers teaching nursing assistants. It comes with equipment for psychosocial bingo and other learning games. Psychosocial Consultants, 13506 Hike Lane, San Diego, CA 92129.

FILMS

- *Because Somebody Cares* (16 mm or video, 27 minutes). This film shows several real-life vignettes of volunteers, young and old, as they visit older persons who are homebound or in nursing homes. It shows the friendships that grow when people of all ages reach out to each other. Produced by Terra Nova Films, Inc., directed by James Van den Bosch. Purchase: $465 (16 mm), $295 (video); rental: $55.

- *Nurse's Aides: Making a Difference* (videocassette, 31 minutes, color) 1991. This film, highly praised by *The Gerontologist* reviewer, presents a panel consisting of three nursing assistants and an LPN discussing the management of behavior problems with accompanying vignettes. Producer and distributor: UT Southwestern ADRC Videos, Department of Gerontology and Geriatrics Services, P.O. Box 45567, Dallas, TX 75245; Purchase $85.

Chapter 11

Group Work with People with Dementia

Faith Gibson
Irene Burnside

Key Words

- Alzheimer's disease
- Aphasia
- Delirium
- Dementia
- Depression
- Flat affect
- Individualization
- Nonverbal communication
- Organic mental disorder
- Person-centered orientation
- Therapeutic nihilism

Learning Objectives

- Define person-centered work and suggest how this is relevant to group work
- Describe four common characteristics of dementia that make adaptations in group work essential
- Explain why it is important to take care of one's self when working with people who have dementia
- Analyze five inappropriate group member selections
- Discuss changes in behavior that might occur during the course of a group

- Discuss individualization within the group setting

Tell me, I'll forget. Show me, I may remember. But involve me, and I'll understand.

—*Ancient Chinese proverb*

The therapeutic nihilism, once so prevalent among health professionals involved in providing services for older people generally, and especially for people with dementia, is slowly being replaced by a more optimistic, person-centered, strengths-based philosophy of care. This new approach seeks to understand and to utilize people's remaining abilities and to provide opportunities for their continued involvement in daily life (Kitwood, 1997). Recent pharmaceutical advances are providing medication for some people, particularly in the early stages of Alzheimer's disease, and psychosocial supportive interventions are increasingly being valued. Research is increasing our understanding about the causes, treatment, duration, and individual variations of the various complex conditions loosely known as dementia (Harris, 2002). Dementia has grave implications for the person with the condition, their family, and the professional caregivers involved (Mace, Rabins, Castleton, McEwen, & Meredith, 1999). Stigma, although decreasing, still exists, and increasing isolation for the person with dementia and those with whom they live is still too common.

Although the social systems or structures within which we live and interact affect behavior, we do have an active influence on these systems. We are co-constructors rather than passive recipients of their influence, according to Kondrat (1999). But people with dementia have considerable difficulty in understanding their part in this co-constructive process and because of short-term memory impairment they need repeated opportunities for practicing and rehearsing social roles. Having opportunities to engage in social interactions within small nonthreatening groups can provide some of this essential practice for actively engaging in small social systems and for maintaining a continuing sense of identity and personhood when assailed by dementia (Kondrat, 2002).

The Nature of Dementia

Dementia is an umbrella term used loosely to refer to a syndrome or collection of characteristics associated with many different diseases, the most common being Alzheimer's disease. Collectively these conditions present one of the greatest public health challenges of the present age because the dementias are largely, but not exclusively, diseases of later life and populations throughout the world are markedly aging. (See Chapter 2 on the demographics and psychosocial aspects of aging.) Age is the single biggest risk factor for developing dementia. While increasing longevity increases risk, and people are being diagnosed sooner, there are also growing numbers of much younger people being identified. Approximately one in ten people over 65 years of age and nearly one in two of those aged 85 or over have dementia. Some four and a half million older Americans are now thought to have dementia. This is estimated as likely to increase to some 14 million by 2050 (Alzheimer's fact sheets, 2004). While most people with dementia are cared for by families and friends,

and many attend day care centers, over half of the 1.4 million people now residing in nursing homes have some degree of dementia and many also have depression (Lesnoff-Caravaglia, 2001; American Health Care Association, 2003). Many people living in assisted-living facilities also have mild or moderate dementia although they are unlikely to require the same level of assistance as occupants of nursing homes.

In this chapter the word Alzheimer's is used to refer to all types of dementia. Increasingly, what was once regarded as an organic brain condition is now seen as more complex. How an individual is affected depends on the interplay of neurobiopsychosocial dimensions linked to individual lifetime factors, present interpersonal supports, and the care environment. The major features of dementia include progressive, usually irreversible decline that affects cognitive, emotional, and social aspects of functioning (American Psychological Association, 1998; American Psychiatric Association, 2000).

While usually sparing physical health, memory, especially short term memory, is affected along with at least one other cognitive impairment such as impaired judgment, language, comprehension, and the ability to learn and recall new information. Speech can be affected, and in the later stages immobility and incontinence are common. Creativity, humor, and core personality characteristics are often retained and there are considerable individual variations in the nature and speed of people's decline (Sabat, 2001). Depression and anxiety are common accompaniments and caregivers need to provide a sense of security, affection, and constructive occupation based on a detailed knowledge of lifetime interests and in keeping with present abilities. Other types apart from Alzheimer's disease include vascular dementia, Lewy body dementia, HIV/AIDS related dementia, alcohol-related dementia, Huntington's chorea, Pick's disease, and Creutzfeldt-Jakob disease. A person may have more than one type of dementia simultaneously and some symptoms often resemble depression so that a differential diagnosis is essential. Behavioral problems may be associated with the particular part of the brain affected, particularly the frontal lobes, but may also be a response to present fears, frustrations, unsatisfactory environments, or unsympathetic management regimes. Behavioral problems may also be associated with nonverbal attempts to communicate present pain or other unmet needs.

Nurse's aides, in spite of the limited training, preparation, and support so many receive for their demanding work, are still the staff members most likely to have the greatest contact with people with dementia who live in residential facilities. Many aides do a remarkable job of relating to people with these complex conditions who need to be respected as unique individuals and whose life experience, present fears, frustrations, and hopes need to be understood.

Communicating with People with Dementia

Caregivers of people with dementia need to learn new ways of communicating. These new ways are based upon acute observation, attentive listening, imaginative reading of nonverbal behavior, empathy with expressed emotions, and creative responses informed by detailed knowledge of each person's unique life history. Here are some simple guidelines:

- Consider the message behind the behavior —is the person trying to tell you something?
- Speak directly to the person, do not talk down to them and never talk over them to someone else.
- Speak clearly and slowly, using only short sentences.
- Mirror the actions and words of the other person and use the same kind of communication that they are using.

- Let people set their own pace.
- Be still and calm, and do not fear silence.
- Use smiles, head nods, and humor.
- Use touch where appropriate and acceptable.

Communicating with older adults who have dementia is very demanding, but also highly rewarding; when words fail, they often speak through their actions. Group work demands that leaders attend to many different stimuli simultaneously so the complexities are multiplied when leading a group and coleadership is usually highly desirable. This chapter offers students, instructors, health and social care workers, and administrators guidance about how general group work principles need to be adapted for people with dementia. Three groups illustrate some of these important modifications. Group A illustrates the need for careful selection of group members, especially if some have behavioral problems; group B illustrates the importance of individualization within a group; and group C illustrates the significance of nonverbal communication. Group leading is much easier if the group is kept small, approximately four to six persons, particularly if there are members who also have speech, physical, or sensory disabilities (Orange, Ryan, Meredith, & McLean, 1995). All the group examples met on a weekly basis except during the termination phase, when meetings were spaced further apart. Experience indicates that groups that meet more frequently, say twice weekly or daily, may result in increased interaction between members.

Cautions for New Group Leaders

New leaders may still be faced with pessimistic attitudes from staff when wanting to establish a small group for people with dementia. If the leaders share such pessimism it will be difficult for them to reach out with hope, warmth, and affection to establish effective communication.

Leaders must grapple with their fears about dementia and be aware of how such fears limit the efforts they are prepared to make. Often there is a lack of information about the past lives of group members; this makes it difficult to appraise how much of present behavior is due to dementia, how much to present living circumstances, and how much reflects lifelong characteristics and past experience. It is essential to gather as much information as possible about the life history of potential group members. Family members and contemporary friends, if such are available, can be excellent sources of information (Dran, 2003).

All the usual courtesies concerned with invitations, contracting, and commitment to members' free choice about participation are important, with explanations given in simple, straightforward language (Post, 1995; Van Hooft, 1995). Giving the group or "club" a catchy title and writing details of meeting arrangements on a card can be helpful, but members may still need to be reminded about meetings. Careful observation by the leader for any cues of increased awareness (verbal or nonverbal) helps pinpoint progress, which is often slow and small in scale; momentary interactions can be of great significance. The leader must set realistic, ethical objectives, neither expecting too much or too little, and be comfortable with silences in a group (Bell & Troxell, 1997, 2001). Introducing humor, music, crafts, projects utilizing implicit procedural memory and nonverbal means of communication, reminiscence, and exercise may be necessary to sustain the leader as well as the group. Having fun together and capitalizing on people's retained abilities should be central objectives (Bruce, Hodgson, & Schweitzer, 1999; Clair, 1996; Erwin, 1996).

New group leaders should learn to take care of themselves. Some specific suggestions follow:

1. Use a support system; have one person available on the staff to whom you can talk in confidence about your group experiences.
2. Use staff meetings to explore feelings—not as a gripe session but as constructive catharsis with problem solving.
3. Practice more spontaneity. Don't get so bogged down in routine that you become bored and indifferent.
4. Assess your own reactions to the dependency and deterioration of the group members. Are the problems of the members hitting too close to those of your own relatives, for example? Consider whether you are conducting the right group for you.
5. Plan careful, individualized programs within the group so that participants have maximum support but continue to do as much for themselves as possible.
6. If you are a staff member, suggest a monthly morale booster meeting. At each meeting, look at positive approaches to what is happening, find something to feel good about in your work, permit no negative input, and reward everyone with something different—a surprise.
7. Examine your own patterns of coping with discouragement, depression, dependency, and deterioration. What will you do about the patterns?
8. Learn from one another. What people do you know who have unique and successful ways of taking care of themselves—people who have the "knack" (Bell & Troxel, 2001)?
9. Practice observing your members. Discover the person behind the dementia. How do older people you know take care of themselves? Older people are your best teachers; borrow from their wisdom.

Leaders also have to be willing to try varied approaches. Dementia care requires versatility, flexibility, and imagination. If one technique does not work, try another. Student leaders often get discouraged when their plans go awry, but creative problem solving is a learned leadership skill. An experimental approach is essential when working with people with dementia.

New solutions do have a way of backfiring, and the successful ones may even create new problems. If there is a change in a troubled resident who has been a member of a group, the staff may think the group leader can perform mini miracles—do not be seduced. Staff may want to hand over an especially difficult person and then sit back and watch the leader struggle with behavior that they can neither handle nor tolerate.

Curiosity is aroused when an outsider comes in to a residential facility and plans and prepares for the group. As a result, interest in the group members by the administrator and the staff often increases, and they begin to observe the members more closely. This curiosity and interest helps group leaders to contact the staff while planning the group. The cook may be involved if refreshments are to be served. Receptionists and office personnel can provide a great deal of help. Indeed, Burnside found that maintenance personnel often helped her locate missing members because the personnel knew where the patients hid out. The biggest spin-off Burnside observed was that friendships formed within the group continued to be very significant outside the group, especially when the group ceased meeting.

Group A: Membership Selection and Behavioral Problems

Group A met 30 minutes weekly for seven months. Members were seven older women who were hospitalized in a 68-bed dementia facility. Group A did not really get going until the sev-

enth meeting. Staff members had suggested potential group members who they felt would benefit from a group experience. Five individuals had to be removed from the group soon after it was launched because of disruptive behavior; each person was immediately replaced. Descriptions of the five individuals removed from the group follow. They were a colorful, albeit unmanageable, group and underlined the danger of inadequate assessments of potential group members.

Inappropriate Group Selections

Mrs. A.

Mrs. A. was in her mid sixties and was born in Warsaw. She rarely spoke, even in Polish. Though she seemed to understand English, her behavior cast some doubt on this. She attended five meetings and displayed unusually high anxiety. She frequently jumped up and left the room; when she did remain seated, she fidgeted and mumbled constantly. In the second meeting, with the leader's constant reminding she was able to sit still, but she continued to disrupt the group by drinking the cream from the pitcher on the coffee serving tray, snatching the sugar when the cream pitcher was empty, and grabbing the refreshments before they could be served.

After the fifth meeting the leader decided she could not cope with this woman because her behavior unnerved the leader so much at times that she focused on her instead of also attending to the entire group. Such over-individualization wears the leader down and leaves the rest of the group resentful. It was soon clear that her disruptive behavior impeded the group's progress. This example illustrates the dual responsibility leaders have, first to the group as a whole, and second to each individual group member. Sometimes these dual responsibilities confront the leader with irreconcilable demands (Dolgoff & Skolnik 1996). The lesson Mrs. A. illustrated is to obtain adequate data about behavior (and observe for a time if in doubt) before selecting a group member.

MRS. F.

Mrs. F. was in her mid seventies, religious—but more temperamental than religious most of the time. Her diagnosis was chronic brain syndrome with paranoia. Although she sat still, her tongue did not. She monopolized the conversation. She was constantly supercilious. She came to group meetings only sporadically but always with aloof, condescending behavior. By the seventh meeting, a close group was forming, but Mrs. F. was not interested enough to attend, although she gave no specific reason. Burnside did not encourage her to continue and finally terminated with her. Mrs. F. showed that paranoid individuals can be very difficult at times to keep in a group and may intimidate both leader and group members with their hostile ways.

MRS. H.

Mrs. H., age 72, attended only three meetings. She, too, felt the group was beneath her. Once after a meeting, she came up to the leader and said, "And how did you pick that motley crew?" In the second meeting, she flatly announced her dislike of men. Burnside learned later from the staff that she was a long-time lesbian. Because the leader often touched aged individuals, she realized she was inhibited while this woman was in the group. The leader was disinclined to touch her; thinking she might misconstrue the touching as having sexual connotations. Leaders must strive continually to lower their own anxiety in group work to be free to attend to the needs of members. The leader felt that her own reserve and inhibitions with this woman would ultimately influence her interactions with the entire group. Much to her relief, this woman voluntarily dropped the group after the third meeting. Mrs. H. illustrated that group leaders, although consulting with staff, should make their own assessment of potential members and gather background information, whenever possible, before issuing invitations.

MRS. M.

Mrs. M., age 78, was a retired nurse. She was very hostile; her verbal abuse was sometimes matched by physically striking out at other residents. She usually hit patients when the staff could not see her, so that particular behavior was observed only if a staff member unexpectedly walked into the room. The staff thought she might benefit by joining the group. It soon became apparent that she wanted to attend meetings only at her whim. The nurse began setting strict limits with her at about the time the group was forming. Because of her quick temper, hostile remarks, and the fear she engendered in other patients, she was asked to leave the group. Frail group members need to be protected, and the group milieu should be safe and secure. Mrs. M. highlighted the effects a hostile, abusive person can have on a group and the leader's responsibility for protecting very old and very frail members.

MRS. L.

Mrs. L. was 74 years old. She had been hospitalized for several years and spent most of her time in a wheelchair. She would not try to walk or talk. At the first meeting she stiffened her body and nearly slid out of the wheelchair. Her eyes became rather glassy, and she frothed a little at the mouth. The nurse helped the leader to return Mrs. L. to her room, adding that this was not uncommon behavior for her. She died suddenly two months after the trial group experience. Mrs. L. illustrated the necessity for investigating physical problems in greater detail and to interrogate several staff members about a resident's life history, behavior, and physical complaints.

No group should be overloaded with too many people whose cognitive and physical disabilities along with their present behavior presents such a challenge to the competence and confidence of the beginning leader that the well-being of other group members is jeopardized. These people might have benefited from a one-to-one relationship with a student, an interested staff member, or a volunteer, or one of them might have been absorbed into an already established, stable group (Zgola, 1999).

The Final Group Membership

The final group membership is shown in **Table 11–1**. The mean age of the group members was 79.7 years. Each individual in the group had a diagnosis of vascular dementia, and five of the women were diagnosed as having psychiatric problems.

There were several impressive things about this group. One was the lack of physical disabilities; there was a certain physical toughness about the members, which Burnside attributed to their many years of hard work. Lack of education was also a characteristic of the group; most completed eighth grade only. Another noticeable thing was the brevity of the diagnoses on the members' charts. There was no list of six or seven ailments, as is usually seen in an average older person's

Table 11–1 MEMBERS OF GROUP A

Patient	Age	Marital status	Diagnosis	Ambulation	Strengths in group	Problems in group
Mrs. L.M.	71	Married	CAS,[1] schizophrenic, paranoid	Ambulatory	Gentleness	Dependency, crying spells, depression
Mrs. T.	85	Widow (from age 63)	CAS, paranoid	Ambulatory	Warmth, loving ways, quick to praise	Forgetfulness
Miss H.	95	Single (never married)	CAS, paranoid	Ambulatory	Toughness, sharpness, observation ability, articulate	Hallucinations
Mrs. V.	78	Married	OMD,[2] degenerative arthritis, CAS	Ambulatory	Sense of humor, warmth, spontaneity	Forgetfulness
Mrs. H.	72	Widow	Legally blind, congestive heart failure, epilepsy, CAS	Ambulatory	Sense of humor, articulate, courage, acceptance of blindness	Monopolization of group
Mrs. S.M.	79	Widow	CAS, manic-depressive	Ambulatory	Sharpness, helpfulness, appreciative	Bitterness, constant carping
Mrs. D.M.	78	Widow (at age 34)	CAS, reactive-depressive state	Ambulatory (with assistance)	Gratitude, articulate	Crying spells, depression

[1] *Cerebral arteriosclerosis.*

[2] *Organic mental disorder.*

record. It is possible that the most fitting diagnosis was emphasized—that is, the one diagnosis that would gain fastest entrée into a dementia-specific facility and also pass the medical review team.

There were no aphasics in the group, no immobile persons, and no paralyzed persons. One woman, though legally blind, said one day, "I have ten eyes," and held up her 10 fingers to show the group. One reason for the lack of such impairments may be that to be admitted to this facility, most patients had to be able to care for themselves. Bedridden and wheelchair patients were not admitted.

Observed Changes

Improvements in behavior often make staff members more receptive to a resident. Behavioral changes in members of group A often followed a rewarding group experience. For example, Mrs. D.M. entered group A at the sixth meeting and was considered by the staff to be a problem patient. She refused to walk and had many psychosomatic complaints. She expressed guilt about her only child's suicide; her daughter had committed suicide while the woman was in a board-and-care home. Mrs. D.M. became so depressed and agitated that she was transferred to another facility. The director of nurses and the leader discussed the nursing care plan so that the staff's therapeutic regimen could be supported during group meetings. Specifically, it was agreed that Mrs. D.M. would be encouraged to walk, and that she would be offered an opportunity to express guilt (and other feelings) in group meetings, and her degree of depression would be observed from week to week.

The staff members were surprised at her rather sudden improvement. The day before Mother's Day, the group had weathered a difficult session. The leader's small, inexpensive gifts for each member caused visible sadness, especially in Mrs. D.M. She took her gift, cried openly, and said, "I don't deserve it. I am not a fit mother. And I don't even

have 10 cents to give anyone else a gift." The leader sat on the arm of her chair and put her arm around her. She served Mrs. D.M. tea, which she preferred to coffee. (Fixing a member's coffee or tea exactly as requested is one simple way to individualize care and is more important than the leader may realize.) The group talked about the daughter's suicide and the mother's guilt. Everyone acknowledged feelings they had had on Mother's Day. When the meeting was over, an aide and the leader helped her walk back to her room.

In the subsequent meeting, Mrs. D.M. was tearless, though obviously still depressed. A staff member had shaved off the hairs on her chin. (That had been in the nursing care plan—she hated the hair on her face.) She apologized for not having combed her hair before coming to the meeting. This time she said that coffee was fine ("if you would just put a little cold water in it"). She did not mention her stomachache, as she had done many times in the previous meeting. The leader sat close to her but touched her arm or shoulder only occasionally. During the sad expressions of loss during the Mother's Day session, the leader had suggested homework. Because coping with losses was a task all the members were facing, they were to recall how they had coped with a particular loss in their lives and share with the group what had been helpful to them. It was during such sharing that it was discovered that two members had lived very close to each other before their admission to the hospital. Such discoveries are important because they reveal information that helps members develop friendships outside the meetings. One should always capitalize on such serendipity when it occurs.

Summary of Group A

Seven women met weekly for seven months in a dementia facility. Conversation focused on feelings about being a woman, clothes, teas, social affairs, and the "prisoner's life" they now led (their description). Occasionally the group drew, but mostly the members talked. Each session ended with refreshments and the members demonstrated appreciation of involvement in the meetings.

Group B: Individualization Within a Group

Group B met weekly for six months in the small, cozy employees' dining room of a 91-bed extended care facility. (Group members are listed in Table 11–2). The lack of affect, spontaneity, and motivation in the group forced the leader to try various methods: (1) topics were assigned to discuss, (2) reminiscence sessions were tried, and (3) simple art sessions were instituted, using chalk, crayons, and so forth. The last was the most successful of the three techniques tried. Members were assigned a building, toy, pet, boyfriend, or girlfriend to draw—some thing or person out of their past. Only one art exercise was not successful.

Table 11–2 MEMBERS OF GROUP B

Patient	Former occupation	Age	Ambulation	Diagnosis	Visitors	Length of hospitalization	Restorative potential (by MD)	Strengths in group	Problems in group
Mr. D.M.	Automobile mechanic	75	Ambulatory	TBC (inactive),[1] malnutrition, dementia	None	2 years, 6 months	Fair	Sweet, gentle air, beautiful smile	Apathy, withdrawal, listlessness
Mr. S.	Railroad clerk	63	Ambulatory	Schizo-phrenic, simple type, marked deterioration	None	3 years, 6 months	Zero	Tried hard	Lack of social graces, sometimes inattentive
Mr. P.	Fisherman, construction worker	58	Ambulatory	CVA[2]	None	3 years	Poor	Sharp, improvement in self-care	Stubborn, cross, sometimes would not talk
Mrs. B.	Registered nurse	79	Ambulatory	Dementia secondary to Parkinson's (although she was extremely paranoid, not in diagnosis)	None	5 years, 8 months	Fair	Sharp, observing, enjoyed drawing	Hallucinating, high anxiety, would leave group abruptly, quiet
Mrs. M.	Journalist	90	Wheelchair	Dementia	Yes	2 years	Zero	Articulate	Anger at staff, monopolizing
Mr. D.	Gardener	88	Ambulatory	Dementia	Yes	2 years	Fair	Gentleness, obvious enjoyment of group, smile	Aphasic, difficulties in com-munication

[1] *Tuberculosis.*

[2] *Cardiovascular accident.*

Following a trip to Africa, Burnside asked the group members to draw an African animal. These people were never a wildly enthusiastic group at any time, but this day their enthusiasm reached a new low. In her eagerness, she had assigned something to meet her need, not theirs—a common problem in leaders who neglect to form an adequate sessional contract with the group. Neither had she reckoned with asking them to draw the unfamiliar—after all, elephants and giraffes may hold no interest for many older people.

Mr. D.M.

This man did a series of drawings over a six-month period. Severe chronic brain syndrome was his diagnosis. His ability to compose a neat likeness, especially after the scribbling of his first drawing, seemed remarkable, especially to a nonartist leader. His signs of therapeutic progress were slow and small. Mr. D.M. was easy to work with and was easily encouraged to draw. He was so quiet in the meetings that the leader wondered whether he understood. He smiled instead of answering her. (A way of conserving energy? A nonverbal way to handle unsure areas? A successful way to win over staff?) He attended the meetings consistently and in each one produced drawings with increasing clarity.

Mr. S.

Mr. S. had suffered a stroke in his late sixties while on a construction job. He was sullen, morose, and withdrawn before joining the group. He often wheeled himself out of the meeting, but he always returned. He smiled, almost with disdain, when drawings were introduced, but he worked carefully on them. His left hand was paralyzed, so he placed a heavy ashtray on the paper to hold it still as he drew. After several months, Mr. S. began to loosen up and started combing his hair and wearing a clean shirt to meetings. After the group was completed, he went out against medical advice and wheeled himself to the beach to live!

Mrs. B.

This 79-year-old woman suffered from Parkinson's disease and chronic brain syndrome. She also had severe paranoid ideation, which was not noted anywhere in her chart. She was very self-conscious about her crossed eye. She drew readily and with great concentration; she called the group "the drawing class." She showed her anxiety in early meetings by jumping up suddenly and leaving. During the drawing sessions, she was able to concentrate intently on the drawings and did not leave the meetings. She gradually deteriorated during the life of the group, a decline that was reflected in her drawings.

Summary

Members' problems included poststroke paralysis, aphasia, flat affect, and immobility. The most successful strategy was drawing and discussing the drawings. Perhaps the most significant aspect of this group was that it launched an entire group program in the facility, which later included current events groups, reminiscence groups led by students, practice groups for students, and a group composed only of residents over 90. That kind of ground breaking is one important aspect of the experimental groups described in this chapter.

Group C: Nonverbal Communication in a Group

Group C illustrates the importance of touch as a means of communication with people who no longer can efficiently use speech and how important it is not to underestimate people who have lost conventional speech. Group C (**Table 11–3**) could be described as experiencing "nonverbal living."

The closed group of six met weekly for 30 to 60 minutes in a nursing home for 14 months. Mrs. K. would always turn and wave or blow kisses as an aide wheeled her out of the meeting room.

Table 11–3 Members of Group C

Patient	Age	Marital status	Length of hospitalization	Diagnosis	Ambulation	Strengths in group	Problems in group
Mrs. K.	82	Widowed	1 year, 8 months	Dementia, fractured right hip with prosthesis, neurofibroma of scalp	Ambulatory and wheelchair	Affectionate ways, awareness, sense of humor	Aphasia, fidgeting, withdrawing by closing eyes
Mr. Z.	64	Divorced	2 years, 10 months	Dementia, arteriosclerosis, secondary polyneuritis, old TBC[1]	Ambulatory	Gentleness, kindly air, awareness	Inarticulate, listless, anxious at times
Mrs. S.	81	Single	5 months	Dementia	Ambulatory	Assisted leader, observed others in group, change gradual: increase in affect, increase in orientation	Forgetful
Mrs. S.T.	79	Widowed	1 year, 4 months	Dementia	Ambulatory, to wheelchair in thirteenth meeting	Sweetness, responsiveness, appreciative	Severe hearing loss, in wheelchair
Mr. B.	80	Single	10 months	Dementia, central nervous system lues (meningo-encephalitic type), blindness, anemia	Wheelchair	Sense of humor, openness, courageous, uncomplaining gratitude, gave feedback to leader	Overweight, in wheelchair (hard to push chair), blind, heavy personal loss, speech impediment
Mr. K.	86	Single	8 months (died 2 weeks after eighth group meeting)	Dementia	Wheelchair	Independent, sense of humor, observant, slowly responded to increased interaction contacts with leader	Withdrawn, depressed, nearly mute, fiercely independent (originally labeled as "stubborn")
Mr. J. (replaced Mr. K.)	68			Fractured right hip, CAS,[2] dementia secondary to alcoholism	Ambulatory		

[1] *Tuberculosis.*

[2] *Cerebral arteriosclerosis.*

Mr. B. and Mr. Z. would smile as they conversed in a French patois. The leader tried many different projects with this group, including exercises, music in the form of records, socializing and discussing the refreshments and what they meant, slides of themselves (an absolute fiasco), and bringing young people to group meetings. Her 20-year-old daughter once went to a meeting with her. Because she had worked in a nursing home and in a psychiatric hospital, she could relate to the group members with great ease. They also enjoyed the day her secretary played the banjo for them. But pervasive passivity was the outstanding feature of the total group.

Summary of Group C

Nonverbal communication was an important component of the group leadership. Mrs. K. especially had high affectional needs, which were obvious at the first group meeting. The single most pervasive characteristic of this group was their flat affect or apathy. Students often describe this as a wall they cannot get through.

Members as Resources to Others

In spite of severe dementia, some persons retain their conversational ability, creativity, their interpersonal skills, and their fabulous sense of humor (Killick & Allan, 2001; Basting & Killick, 2003). They often communicate far more directly and honestly than most of us and are particularly sensitive to how other people respond to them. They can find rare opportunities to assist each other within a small group. In one day center, Burnside described a spontaneous demonstration group she was to undertake for a group of students. Because she remembered that one lady had been a star in a previous group, she was glad when she agreed to be a member. There was also a psychiatrist suffering from dementia who still retained many of his social skills, and others suffering from either the primary disease of Alzheimer's or a dementia secondary to Parkinson's, stroke, or alcoholism. This vignette will give the reader the reason why these sparkling people facilitate a group.

Mrs. A., a sprightly lady in her eighties, fooled most people during the first meeting because of her meticulous dress, her outgoing, friendly ways, and her humor. During the demonstration group, Burnside was attempting to have members recount their memories of long ago, which she thought would not be too threatening for them. She asked them to sit for a few minutes and think about something they remembered very clearly from their childhood. It is so important to allow these thinking times as people with dementia take longer to recall and articulate their memories. This technique helps the members very much. It gives them a sense of slower pace, but it can also help the leader to assess what is happening in the group, what changes need to be made, and who has not actively participated.

Suddenly Mrs. A. became very excited and announced that she remembered something from when she was a little girl. She carefully and vividly told a story about following her brothers and their friend around until they were exasperated with her. Finally they went to the barn, and she traipsed along behind them. When they got to the haymow, they wanted to get rid of her, she said, and told her in emphatic terms to leave. She acknowledged that she was a pest, but she refused to budge. Then she said, "They sure did get rid of me all right." Burnside asked her what had happened. With a big smile she said, "They peed on me." She absolutely broke the group up, and there was no doubt that even the most disabled member of the group could enjoy her special brand of humor.

Combining Alert and Cognitively Disabled Members in a Group

When considering whether to combine people who are cognitively alert and those who have dementia in the same group the following questions should be considered:

1. What resident characteristics should be considered when planning integrated groups?
2. What are the likely advantages and disadvantages and for whom?
3. What types of activities are appropriate for integrated groups?
4. What special skills and techniques can the leader of an integrated group use?
5. How large should an integrated group be?
6. Are there persuasive reasons for using coleadership?

It is difficult to answer the question "Should one mix alert and cognitively disabled individuals in the same group?" The answer is "sometimes." A rule of thumb is not to mix very disabled people with very alert people. If a leader is conscientious about making contracts before the group meetings, they can get a sense of who is unlikely to accept more disabled people. It would be unacceptable to expose the person with dementia to insults, ridicule, and interactions that further lower self-esteem. Older people can be very outspoken; they do not always "draw a circle that draws others in."

It is also important not to overload the group with so many disabled members that there is no natural helper, no person vivacious enough to add spark to the group or to carry some of the understanding and conversation. In some circumstances an integrated group can work well if members are carefully selected. Doel and Sawdon (1999) cite a study of 25 separate time-limited reminiscence groups in which cognitively impaired people participated together with unimpaired people. In these groups aberrant behavior was rarely displayed. Wandering and hyperactivity were reduced, and relevant contributions reinforced, enjoyed, and generally appreciated.

Often individuals with dementia spontaneously team up with individuals who have a similar level of impairment. In one group, a person with early onset dementia (a man who had just turned 60) and a woman with Alzheimer's (who was in her seventies) developed a warm and close relationship in spite of the fact that both were aphasic. The staff also encouraged their kindness and devotion to one another. It is fortunate that the man's wife was quite understanding and felt that if she could no longer communicate with him, it was all to the good if there was someone else who could reach him. The group leader can also encourage such interactions by seating paired members next to one another in the group so that they can draw support from one another. Often they will walk to and from the group meetings together. While a group leader may not encourage subgrouping in other types of groups, it becomes important in dementia care. Subgrouping may contribute to attendance and encourage a person to become a part of the larger group.

Cautions

New group leaders must assess the capabilities of prospective group members so that they do not overload the group with persons who either have the same diagnosis (for example, all depressed individuals) or are grossly impaired. This particularly applies to visual and hearing impairments when it is easier to include no more than one blind person or one person who is hard of hearing. If the entire group is in wheelchairs, the burden on the group leader will be incredibly heavy—just transporting members to the meeting place will be an arduous and time-consuming task.

Regarding Alzheimer's disease, the leader should check potential members for apraxia (inability to distinguish and correctly use objects), because it can make participation in some tasks and crafts, and refreshment time, difficult (Junn-Krebbs, 2004). One man had to be helped each meeting simply to get the coffee cup to his mouth; he would wave it around in the air and yet be trying so hard to follow the leader's instructions. It is in situations such as these that a coleader or trained volunteer can help meet the specific needs of individuals.

It seems to be easier to draw in some of the withdrawn and quiet members than it is to curb the loquacious and noisy ones, at least for the student or the new group leader. One woman, who came to the group on her walker, sat at a separate table and refused to join the group in the early meetings. The student turned, sensitively addressed her, and served her coffee as though she was participating in the group. This courteous, skillful action helped the woman gain enough trust gradually to move into the group.

Seating in meetings should follow some of these guidelines:

- Place the more alert, helpful people next to disabled or anxious members.
- The leaders should sit between the two most disabled (either physically or cognitively impaired) members of the group.
- A blind person or one who is hard of hearing should sit next to someone who is willing to assist with explanations.
- Two members who are always together and seem to have a close relationship should sit next to one another.
- If there are two ethnic minority persons (and one should never take just one into the group), they should sit together. This strategy and the one above help to increase the "we-ness" of the group.
- Check crafts carefully to ensure that they are safe and within the capacity of the members.
- A very quiet area with no distractions should be used for group meetings. This is crucial for people with dementia, who can easily be overloaded and distracted by too many stimuli or competing noises.
- Push fluids in meetings to prevent dehydration and confusional states.

- Be careful not to pressure group members because of the potential for a catastrophic reaction.
- Be aware of your own boredom and ennui. Group leadership with older people can be a very draining experience; if you do not build in rewards for yourself, you may burn out.
- Save the refreshments until the end of the meeting. Older clients enjoy food and will often stay until they receive their share.
- If the group meeting is held on a ward that houses people with dementia, it is sometimes desirable to close, but never lock, the doors to the meeting area so that if someone wishes to leave, he or she can do so.
- An early easy, quick assignment to assess skills such as a simple drawing task can be helpful, providing it does not create anxiety or set people up for failure and embarrassment.
- Men in the group may not like some crafts. It is best to have an alternate project that they can do. Not all men will view the tasks as kid's stuff, but those who do will be adamant about not participating.
- Be prepared for strange things to happen to your supplies, props, equipment, food, and so on. One woman put the plum blossom stem in her coffee. Another woman stirred her coffee with an orange crayon. Another colored her banana with a green felt-tipped pen. When things such as this occur, check to see if you have overloaded the group with materials or instructions, a common problem for eager inexperienced leaders.
- A variety of approaches—use of exercises, music, reminiscence, crafts, food—helps make the group more interesting for both members and leaders.

- Do not expect to conduct psychotherapy groups with people with dementia although some will display insight, and in one-on-one situations may well be able to discuss their condition and its implications, and resolve old problems (Killick & Allan, 2000; Yale, 1995).
- Analyze all nonverbal behavior for possible meanings. This, of course, includes your own nonverbal behavior because when language is impaired, or people are stressed, they are even more likely to communicate nonverbally through their behavior.

Group Safety

Safety for the person with dementia is a common concern. A group leader who has members with dementia should assess the environment of the group meeting before launching the group. Such a careful assessment could prevent problems occurring after the group has begun. Persons with dementia experience confusion concerning place, space and time, and loss of judgment; therefore, the group leader needs to be extra cautious. Providing a safe, calm, comfortable, secure environment is crucial for members' well being (Brawley, 1997). There are three important principles to be remembered in regard to safety:

1. Think prevention.
2. It is more effective to change the environment than it is to attempt to change most behaviors.
3. By minimizing danger you can maximize independence, because the member can experience increased security and mobility.

Activities for Persons with Dementia

People with various diagnoses of dementia are able to enjoy group activities. The presence in a group of people disabled by dementia presents special challenges for group leaders because of their limited concentration, reduced ability to follow directions, slower reaction times, impaired communication and sometimes the presence of behavioral problems. The following steps may help a new group leader to introduce and sustain acceptable activities (Bell & Troxel, 2001).

1. Gather information about each potential member's past interests, activities, and hobbies and try to match these interests to present abilities.
2. Identify failure-free activities.
3. Build in structure and ritual to a group's program, possibly using the same opening and ending routines.
4. Offer support appropriate to each member to enable participation.
5. Look for familiar and favorite pastimes.
6. Plan carefully, but be prepared to be flexible.
7. Emphasize involvement—help the person to feel wanted and useful.
8. Focus on enjoyment, not achievement.
9. Be realistic and experimental.
10. Suspend judgment.
11. Adjust frequency, pace, and length of meetings.
12. Whenever possible work with a coleader or volunteer
13. Consider involving family members, volunteers, and other staff.
14. Ensure the program evokes long-established social skills and utilizes long-term implicit procedural memory.
15. Secure supervision, consultation, or mentoring for this demanding work.
16. Consider these specific activity areas to incorporate into group meetings:
    a. Painting, drawing, working with clay
    b. Exercise in a group
    c. Music, singing, movement, and dancing
    d. Albums and pictures

  e. Reading simple familiar stories,
     rhymes, and poetry
  f. Old movies (from 1930s or 1940s)
  g. Simple, improvised drama
  h. Gardening and excursions
  i. Reminiscence and life story work
     (see Chapter 14)

Universal Strengths

Effective group work depends upon the leader's ability to identify the positive characteristics and retained abilities of people with dementia. It is important to use knowledge of these strengths in planning a program of activities (Gibson, 2004):

- They retain primary motor function (strength, dexterity, and motor control), but they may need to break activities down into simple steps and may need help starting and stopping.
- They retain primary sensory function, and they experience sensations as pleasant, noxious, and so on.
- Their sense of rhythm and movement makes dancing, sawing, sanding, folding, and rocking appropriate activities.
- They can do things that are naturally repetitive but not boring such as kneading, sanding, mixing, turning, and pulling.
- They are emotional: they still experience positive and negative feelings, and they need outlets.
- They retain a sense of humor and react to the novel, the unusual, and the unexpected.

Summary

This chapter includes descriptions of three nurse-led groups of older people with cognitive impairments. Modifications to such group work are discussed. Group leaders must remember to supplement and/or complement the individualized nursing care plans. The quality of life of older people, whether in an institution or a day care center, can be greatly improved by membership in a group that meets regularly with a patient, empathic leader in a familiar, safe, structured context.

Three examples of groups are given. It was observed in all three groups that behavior does change and sometimes can improve rather suddenly and dramatically when the group process—for example, the "we-ness" of the group—is maximized. The leader's sensitivity, empathy, capacity to work at a feeling level, appreciation of the perspective of each member, and dedication are of paramount importance. The leader should also be skillful in nonverbal communication and prepared to use humor and informality. Leaders must slow their pace and be prepared to enter the time frame of the members. Group members can emulate normal behavior demonstrated by a leader, and they will gain in confidence and trust with a leader who treats them with warmth and respect. It is important to create situations that stimulate the long-established social skills of members.

The difficulties of doing group work with people with dementia include quick mood changes, passivity, short attention spans, extreme dependency, apathy, behavioral problems, and minimal information on each member. Long silences are common. Minuscule changes observed in group members can be discouraging for impatient or unrealistically ambitious leaders. The ability to discard techniques that do not work and try new ones proves to be one of the challenges and rewards of work with this type of group. Leaders of groups for people with dementia need to be willing to slow down, adjust their pace, adapt their demands, be willing to share the world of the person with dementia, empathize with feelings, and flexibly create imaginative opportunities for nonverbal and, to a lesser extent, verbal communication.

Exercises

EXERCISE 1

When group work is begun, staff members often notice a decrease in problematic behavior, as members are stimulated to engage in more appropriate social behavior. However, the staff has to try to maintain that gain and may become very discouraged with such continued responsibility. Staff members may feel that much effort is expended for little observable gain, or they may feel burned out—tired of the job, dismissive of residents' feelings, distancing themselves from the residents, and so on.

Consider ways that staff morale might be maintained or even improved during such discouraging times. Then list five suggestions for taking care of one's self, both as staff collectively and as staff members individually.

EXERCISE 2

Select one of the case histories from group A and write a one-page description of how you would have handled that person if you had been the group leader.

EXERCISE 3

Identify a person you know who has dementia. Write a brief summary of the person's life history. Suggest how you would use this information to involve this person in a group, and identify objectives and a possible program.

References

Alzheimer's fact sheets from the Alzheimer's Association. (2004). Retrieved March, 2004, from http://www.alz.org/Resources/FactSheets.asp

American Health Care Association. (2003). *OSCAR data reports: Patient characteristics*. Washington DC: AHCA.

American Psychiatric Association. (2000). *Diagnostic and statistical manual of mental disorders: (DSM-4-TR)*. Washington, DC: Author.

American Psychological Association. (1998). Guidelines for the evaluation of dementia and age-related cognitive decline. *American Psychologist*, 53, 1298–1303.

Basting, A. D., & Killick, J. (2003). *The arts and dementia care: A resource guide*. New York: Center for Creative Aging.

Bell, V., & Troxell, D. (1997). *The best friend's approach to Alzheimer's care*. Baltimore: Health Professions Press.

Bell, V., & Troxell, D. (2001). *The best friend's staff: Building a culture of care in dementia programs*. Baltimore: Health Professions Press.

Brawley, E. C. (1997). *Designing for Alzheimer's disease: Strategies for better care environments*. New York: John Wiley & Sons.

Bruce, E., Hodgson, S., & Schweitzer, P. (1999). *Reminiscing with people with dementia: A handbook for carers*. London: Age Exchange.

Clair, A. A. (1996). *Therapeutic uses of music with older adults*. Baltimore: Health Professions Press.

Doel, M., & Sawdon, C. (1999). *The essential groupworker: Teaching and learning creative groupwork*. London: Jessica Kingsley Publishers.

Dolgoff, R., & Skolnik, L. (1996). Ethical decision making in social work with groups: An empirical study. *Social Work with Groups*, 19(2), 49–65.

Dran, D. D. (2003, October). *The strangers we care for: Does it matter what aides know about the lives of nursing home residents?* Selected conference papers and proceedings (pp.63–78) from the International Reminiscence and Life Review Conference, Vancouver, British Columbia.

Erwin, K.T. (1996). *Group techniques for aging adults*. Washington, DC: Taylor & Francis.

Gibson, F. (2004). *The past in the present: Using reminiscence in health and social care*. Baltimore: Health Professions Press.

Harris, P. B. (2002). *The person with Alzheimer's disease: Pathways to understanding and experience*. Baltimore: John Hopkins University Press.

Junn-Krebbs, U. (2004). Group work with seniors who have Alzheimer's or dementia in a social adult day program. *Social Work with Groups*, 26(2), 51–64.

Killick, J., & Allan, K. (2001). *Communication and the care of people with dementia*. Philadelphia: Open University Press.

Kitwood, T. (1997). *Dementia reconsidered*. Philadelphia: Open University Press.

Kondrat, M. E. (1999). Who is the self in self-aware: Professional self-awareness from a critical theory perspective. *Social Services Review*, 73, 451–477.

Kondrat, M. E. (2002). Actor-centered social work: Revisioning "person in environment" through a critical theory lens. *Social Work,* 47(4), 435–448.

Lesnoff-Caravaglia, G. (2001). (Ed.). *Aging and public health: Technology and demography—parallel evolutions*. Springfield: C. T. Thomas.

Mace, N. L., Rabins, P. V., Castleton, B. A., McEwen, E. & Meredith, B. (1999). *The 36-hour day*. Baltimore: Johns Hopkins University Press.

Orange, J., Ryan, E., Meredith, S., & MacLean, A. (1995). Interventions for persons with Alzheimer's disease: Strategies for maintaining and enhancing communicative success. *Topics in Language Disorders, 15*, 20–35.

Post, S. G. (1995). *The moral challenge of Alzheimer's disease*. Baltimore: Johns Hopkins University Press.

Sabat, S. R. (2001). Surviving manifestations of selfhood in Alzheimer's disease. *Dementia, 1*(1), 25–36.

Van Hooft, S. (1995). *Caring: An essay in the philosophy of ethics*. Colorado: Colorado University Press.

Yale, R. (1995). *Developing support groups for people with early stage Alzheimer's disease*. Baltimore: Health Professions Press.

Zgola, J. M. (1999). *Care that works: A relationship approach to persons with dementia*. Baltimore: Johns Hopkins University Press.

RESOURCES

Finding Your Way: Explorations in Communication. Allan, K. (2003). Stirling, UK: University of Stirling, Dementia Services Development Centre. This is a unique learning and developmental tool designed to assist staff and students working with people with dementia to put communication and consultation at the center of their caring efforts. Available at www.stir.ac.uk/dsdc.

Chapter 12

Group Work with People with Physical Disabilities

Barbara Haight

Irene Burnside

Key Words

- Arthritis
- Chronicity
- Environment
- Hearing impairment
- Heart disease
- Mobility
- Old
- Oldest-old
- Quality of life
- Visual impairment
- Youngest-old

Learning Objectives

- Discuss the importance of the leader understanding common physical impairments in older adults
- List four limitations that may occur in older adults and one leader intervention for each
- List four of the top ten chronic conditions for people over 65 years of age
- Analyze two lifestyle characteristics of the oldest-old versus younger elderly persons

On a clear day you can see as far as you can look.

—*Anonymous*

Physical Impairments

This chapter is about common physical impairments that may occur in older adult groups. The limitations caused by these impairments have an effect on leadership, group attendance, and the group itself. Acute conditions were once a predominant pattern of illness for everyone, but now chronic conditions create the more prevalent health problems for older people. More than four out of five people aged 65 and older have at least one chronic condition, and multiple conditions are common among older people. The leading causes of death for older Americans are heart disease, cancer, and stroke. The group leader who chooses to work with older adults will have members who have chronic diseases, physical illnesses, and sensory losses. This will be true regardless of the group setting, but more so if the setting is the nursing home. In the nursing home, the physical limitations will be even greater, because members there tend to be older and often have multiple diagnoses. Even though older people are conscious of trying to improve their health through healthier living, such as eating healthier diets and participating in a less sedentary lifestyle, age and disability will take its toll (Federal Interagency Forum on Aging-Related Statistics, 2000). By the time people are age 65, 14% have difficulty performing some of the activities of daily living, and by age 80 the percentage is double that of the young-old (Haber, 2003).

Common Physical Impairments

ARTHRITIS

Almost all elderly people have one or more chronic conditions that they live with daily. Arthritis is one of those conditions that is debilitating because the associated pain is commonly severe, which in turn affects mobility. Over 50% of people 65 and older have arthritis that directly affects their function. Endurance and pain are two areas the group leader should assess when including people that have arthritis in a group because these parameters directly influence the ability of individuals to participate in group work. A single indicator for shortened endurance may be the person admitting to fatigue while performing ADLs. Pain is present in about 25–50% of community-dwelling elders, and in nursing homes the estimate rises to 45–80% (Ferrel, 2000). Because pain is the limiting factor in performing all functional activities and affects endurance, people with arthritis must be taught to respect their pain and to limit their activities accordingly (Osterweil, Brummel-Smith, & Beck, 2000). It is imperative that the group leader be alert to indications of each of these limitations in people with arthritis who are participating in group work.

HEART DISEASE

Heart disease remains the leading cause of death in people over age 65. Many patients who undergo surgery may participate in an educational group before surgery and again in a rehabilitation group after surgery. The leader needs to be aware of fatigue in the participants. There is also a high risk of pulmonary complications directly after surgery, thus alertness to changes in condition such as shortness of breath provide excellent clues to compromised health conditions. The group leader, who has an ongoing awareness of the risks and complications engendered by heart disease, will run a group within the capabilities of her patients (Ashton, 2000).

STROKE

Stroke is the third leading cause of death among older people (U.S. Department of Health and Human Services, 2000). People in poststroke groups often have difficulty understanding the concepts being discussed; they often have difficulty speaking, and they can suffer from lack of insight and require massive rehabilitation efforts. They may be aware of their difficulties, and their behavior may depend on the site of affliction in the brain (Kalra, 1998). Therefore it is essential for the leader to understand the differences and symptoms among stroke victims and to respond accordingly to each person's limitations.

CANCER

Many older people are cancer survivors; many others are in the recovery phase. The phase of recovery will often dictate the type of group that is appropriate. For example, support groups have been very successful with women who have breast cancer. Past victims of breast cancer often reach out to help those who are newly ill by sharing their own experiences and, for example, helping them to buy wigs before the debilitating effects of chemotherapy set in. Such groups have many settings: from those recovering in a nursing home to those becoming group members during chemotherapy appointments. End-of-life groups can also be of value to end-stage cancer patients who are anticipating death and leaving family and friends behind (Kayser-Jones, 2002). Universally, this group of cancer patients battles fatigue, and group leaders must consider fatigue when planning meetings.

Fatigue and inability to use services such as hospice, because the disease is so debilitating, often make it difficult to establish successful groups (Tang, 2003). The ten leading causes of death in older adults are found in **Table 12–1**.

Leadership

It can be overwhelming for a new leader of older adult groups to observe the many health conditions affecting the group members. The first step for a leader in handling the conditions is to be aware of them. The second step is to understand the various conditions and how they limit the members. The third step is to analyze how possible member limitations will affect leadership. The last step is to evaluate the effectiveness of various interventions to ascertain those that will encourage members to stay in the group, because attrition (especially in the early stages) can decimate a group.

Accepting the Health Conditions

It is probably not wise to include an individual in a group if the leader is really uncomfortable handling the individual's particular health condition. For example, a leader who has a close relative with Parkinson's disease may be constantly reminded of the relative or may compare the relative's disease progression to a member with Parkinson's. On the other hand, if the leader understands and accepts the effects of Parkinson's, the leader may have more empathy and may better understand how to intervene successfully.

All leaders must be introspective and aware of their biases; for example, health professionals may have great difficulty caring for alcoholics, because alcoholism exists in their own family. Yet, groups for aging alcoholics have been very successful. Eliason and Skinstad (2001) found that an educational presentation to a group of women vastly increased their knowledge of the dangers and interactions that occur with drugs and alcohol

and, in fact, served to prevent abuse of substances. The social support gained in these groups, and the knowledge learned that the abuse is more widespread than imagined, is often all that new drinkers need to begin their rehabilitation.

Alcoholics Anonymous is another well-known therapeutic group that has been extremely successful for older people, and they benefit even more if the group members are mainly older people like themselves (Gorecki-Scavetta, 1999). One needs to remember that all group leaders have their limitations in leading groups. Burnside recalled how difficult it was for her to work with an old man with dentures; he kept moving them about and clacking them, and she was not very accepting about this particular behavior. Though we may be professionals, we are also human and have our limitations.

KNOWING ABOUT THE HEALTH CONDITIONS OF MEMBERS

There are many fine medical texts that will help you better understand the various health conditions you will encounter. Being basically familiar with common diseases and related limitations will help the leader in several ways. Such basic knowledge should help with the formation

Table 12–1 THE 10 LEADING CAUSES OF DEATH

Cause
Heart disease
Malignant neoplasms
Cerebrovascular disease
Chronic lower respiratory disease
Accidents
Diabetes mellitus
Influenza and pneumonia
Alzheimer's
Nephritis
Septicemia

Source: R. Anderson, 2002. Reprinted with permission.

of the group; for example, if you are leading the group alone, can you handle transportation problems for those with limited mobility? Or the leadership problems inherent with the visually or hearing impaired? What about incontinence issues? What about shortness of breath and having members unable to carry on a conversation? Or a very low level of energy? Or a person prone to falling? Or a diabetic in the group? Any of these conditions will make more demands on the leader. You can glean some basic information by studying the members' charts (if they are in an institution) and through discussions with staff members. In nursing homes, nurse's aides can give much firsthand information because of their close daily contact. Your own observations during assessment are of the utmost importance. Burnside had a rule of thumb related to intuitive feelings: When in doubt, leave the person in question out.

When working with groups whose members are physically disabled, it is helpful to have two group leaders or a primary group leader and a helper. Group members may need help in getting to the site of the group, and they may need help with completing their dressing or toileting before they leave for the group, especially those living in a nursing home. Because the group meeting may be an outing for members, it is important to them that they look their best. Often staff is so overwhelmed with other duties, they find it difficult to help group members make special preparations that contribute to making the group meeting an occasion

The more physical conditions a member has, the more a leader needs to take that into account. This awareness should occur during the pregroup assessment to help the leader decide what he or she can handle in the group. If you have some basic knowledge about the disease, illness, or limitation, it can help you ascertain what you need to plan for in your group meetings. Simple interventions for group leaders can be found in **Table**

12–2. If you are in doubt about any of them, check with the staff members in the facility. Alternatively, an excellent assessment book that will help to determine a person's condition through the use of paper and pencil tests is the *Handbook of Geriatric Assessment* by Gallo, Fulmer, Paveza, and Reichel (2003). The book covers function, mental status, social status, and assessments for pain, among others, and can prove a valuable resource for those who do not have a medical background.

Sometimes the older member may be very proud and independent and thus resent any special attention. Or the member may love the extra attention and react accordingly. Or, for example, the member may be cunning and not admit to being a diabetic so that any sweets being served are not withheld. Or the member with some memory loss may go to great lengths to cover it up. Dr. Burnside discovered one member who refused to write pre- and posttests because "My arthritis is so bad," but the next day played the piano. That member rationalized her failing memory by using a physical complaint. Physical complaints also are common excuses for not attending groups. Sometimes the complaints are vague indeed. Making contact with the person and listening intently helps to get to the real issues, because sometimes there is something wrong about the group for that member. Exploration reveals true reasons similar to the following for members not attending group meetings:

- A group member or the leader hurt the member's feelings.
- The leader did not acknowledge the member's presence (see Chapter 6 for more details about the importance of inclusion).
- The member is waiting for someone (doctor, relative, or so on) or something (pain medicine has not been given) at an appointed time and thus cannot attend the group at that time.

Table 12–2 INTERVENTIONS TO CONSIDER WITH COMMON CONDITIONS

Condition	May cause	Intervention
Arthritis	Pain	• Can member take pain medicine prior to group meeting? Discuss with member best solution for getting to and from group. You may need help transporting members.
	Immobility	• Do not hurry them.
Dizziness	Fall	• Prevent falls by having member rise slowly; assist if he or she appears unstable. • Use assistive device, if member has one. • Use rails or furniture to help with balance. (Be sure that furniture is safe to hold on to. Folding chairs are treacherous.) • Do not hurry members.
Hearing impairment	Communication problems, suspiciousness, isolation	• Speak at a slow rate. • Keep your voice at about the same volume throughout. • Do not drop your voice at the end of each sentence. • Always speak as clearly and accurately as possible. • Articulate consonants with special care. • Do not mumble. • Pronounce every name with care. • Change to a new subject at a slower rate, making sure that the person follows the change to the new subject. A key word or two at the beginning of a new topic is a good indicator. • Do not cover your mouth with your hand. • Do not speak too rapidly. • Address the listener directly. Do not turn your head away. Keep good eye contact. • Do not get irritated if you have to repeat. Try not to repeat the same word; if they do not understand, try a new word. • Touch them when talking to them. • Have good light on your face. • Women: Wear bright red lipstick to help them read your lips. • Men: Keep mustache trimmed to help with lip reading. • Describe what's happening in the group. • If a member wears a hearing aid, check that batteries are working. • Do not speak while standing behind group members.
Glaucoma, cataracts, and visual impairments	Insecurity about environment, discomfort with glasses, night blindness; observers may believe the visually impaired person is confused	• Reduce glare. Do not hold meetings outside in bright sunlight. • Do not use glossy papers for group activities. • Be sure there is adequate but diffused lighting. Pull draperies or blinds over bright windows. • Do not schedule group meetings after dark. • Stairways must be well lit. Steps should be color-coded at edges. • If a member wears glasses, be sure they are clean. • Encourage use of magnifying glasses. • Describe what is happening in the group. • Use large-print newspapers, books, and magazines.

Table 12-2   INTERVENTIONS TO CONSIDER WITH COMMON CONDITIONS (CONTINUED)

Condition	May cause	Intervention
Deformity, orthopedic problems	Self-consciousness, transportation problems, use of accoutrements (canes, wheelchairs, etc.)	• Play down the deformity or problem. Offer assistance before actually doing anything. • Try to have transportation difficulties handled before group begins.
	Pain	• Request that members take medicine immediately before group.
	Unsteady gait	• Offer help as needed.
	Instability	• Offer help as needed; move slowly and do not rush them.
Hypertension and heart disease	Fatigue	• Do not call on members to perform if they are complaining of fatigue.
	Dizziness	• See above.
	Edema of feet	• Elevate feet on pillow or chair.
	Drug reactions (if on drugs)	• If a member seems different (begins to fall asleep, is very dizzy, etc.), report this to staff member. • A member may be on a low-cholesterol or no-salt diet; check if refreshments are served.
	Hypotension	• Change position slowly. • Avoid prolonged standing. • Do not have meeting right after meals (postprandial hypotension occurs then). • Have a safe environment, good lighting, grab rails, no clutter on floor.
Diabetes	Member to be on special diet	• If serving refreshments, check with staff about what members may have. Do not plan food that would not be on special diets.
	Diabetic retinopathy	• See intervention for visually impaired.
Parkinson's disease	Tremor	• Table will help hide trembling hands. • Do not fill cups or glasses full.
	Drooling	• Have tissues available to member.
	Difficult speech	• Other members may understand better than leader; learn from them.
	Instability	• Offer help as needed.
Chronic obstructive pulmonary disease (COPD)	Shortness of breath, fatigue	• Do not expect member to speak a great deal in group. • Try to include member by asking questions that can be answered briefly in lieu of "Tell me about…" • Allow ample time to get to meeting room. • Suggest resting before group meetings. • Do not hurry the individual. • Ask if he or she needs help getting to and from meetings.

- The member has been a loner all of his life and fears intimacy while the rest of the group is reaching cohesion.

The member, who had not complained before, may now assert physical ailments as an excuse to not attend. There may be other like reasons, of course. But the important point is that a physical complaint may seem safe, easy, and is rarely questioned.

When a group is truly cohesive, members will attend despite colds, fevers, and their aches and pains. Why? Simply because the group has great meaning for them, as one 86-year-old woman in a nursing home group said, "I'm just afraid I'll miss out on the gossip if I don't come." While enjoying gossip was not one of the leader's objectives, it was the group's. Members either came a bit early or stayed a bit later for the juiciest gossip of the day, night, or week, and they also reaped the real benefits of the group.

The primary function of cohesion is to support the other important processes occurring in the group that enhance members' self-esteem through validation and affirmation. Perhaps the need for that validation and affirmation is the reason members do attend. And, within the cohesive group, they may find a confidante, which is very important to their mood and personal life satisfaction.

The Environment

In Chapter 11, we offered suggestions for creating the safest possible environment. Many of those suggestions are also applicable for people with physical and mental impairments because the environment can be the factor responsible for dysfunction. For example, if there is a skylight in the roof with the sun shining through, the ray of sunlight is often mistaken for a puddle of water, causing the older person to walk around it, misstep, and fall. At the simplest level, the environment may produce hazards that lead to falls. At a more subtle level, the environment may require so much effort that the effort is decompensating. For example, an older person who is short of breath can manage in a meeting place on the ground floor, but if the group meeting takes place on the second floor, that same person would have difficulty traversing the stairs to get to the group.

The leader should assess the room in which meetings will be held and select the best possible room. Factors to consider are furniture, light, noise, accessibility, and temperature, to list a few. Chairs should have arms and be firm so that it is easy for the group member to get up and down. Lighting should be soft with no glare, and group members should not be facing a sunny window. A quiet room is a must. If some of the members suffer from presbycusis, they find extraneous noise a challenge to hearing and speech. Of course, the room should be easily accessible by wheelchair or for any handicapped member of the group (Ignatavicius, 2003).

People with hearing and visual impairments must be further considered, because the environment may determine how well they can function in the group. They may refuse to join a group because they are well aware of their limitations and prefer not to have their disabilities exposed (Bagley, 1995). Sensory losses of group members must be assessed prior to the group formation in order to plan strategies that take account of sensory losses. Additionally potential group members should be encouraged to talk about their feelings regarding any sensory losses before joining a group. They can then be assured that their losses will be considered when the group is formed. Often, groups are designed particularly for people with specific sensory losses. For example, a self-management intervention was taught to people with macular degeneration, which not only allowed them to manage better, but also resulted in reduced psychological distress caused by worry over the visual loss (Brody, Williams, Thomas, Kaplan, & Chu, 1999). Accommodating poor hearing is even more important than accommodating poor vision. People with poor hearing can make it to the group, but may have trouble participating after getting there. Dr. Haight once ran a group in the dining room of a nursing care center where spaces for groups were often at a premium. And though the space was large and sunny, the kitchen noise kept interrupting the group so that a few people could not hear what went on in the group due to the external noise. See **Table 12–2** for some of the possible strategies to consider.

Length of Meetings

It might be wise to plan shorter meetings with a group whose members have severe physical impairments. Because of such health considerations as limited attention span or poor circulation, sessions should be concise and short, at least initially. (The meetings can be increased in length gradually as the members are able to tolerate them both physically and psychologically.) The best sign that the group is filling a need occurs when members begin to linger and stay to talk either with the leader or with other members.

Accoutrements of Aging

Eyeglasses and hearing aids are common accoutrements of aging. A good group leader must be sure the eyeglasses are cleaned and the hearing aids are working. There will also be crutches, walkers, canes, and wheelchairs to consider. These items can be hazardous at times, and caution is advised. Crutches are difficult to set in place. If they fall down, someone can trip over them. It is preferable to find a windowsill or a table on which they can be placed. But remember, if they are placed too far from the user, that member cannot ambulate until someone fetches them. Likewise, wooden canes can fall down from a propped position. Because a cane can roll if stepped on, it can be extremely hazardous, as can be the user. Dr.

Burnside recalled a belligerent old man who used his cane almost as a weapon. Once he grabbed an attendant around the neck when the attendant did something he did not like. When he came to meetings, it was important to assure his cane was in a near, but safe, place. The metal three-pronged type of cane can remain safely upright. The three-pronged cane is usually readily seen, and the individual can keep the cane close at hand.

On the other hand, walkers on rollers are cumbersome. Like wheelchairs, they take up a great deal of space, especially when older adults want them kept close. When you are setting up chairs for the group, keep the walkers in mind and allow plenty of space for them. Wheelchairs also require lots of space. If a member gets out of a wheelchair, be sure that the foot rests are up and out of the way and that the brakes are on when the member is getting into or out of it. If you have a group of members all of whom are in wheelchairs, be sure you have adequate space in the meeting room to accommodate them. All of the above-mentioned devices should be labeled with the member's name. If some are not, request help from agency staff to avoid confusion when the meeting is over. A real brouhaha can result when one person has another's belongings.

There also might be a group member with a hook for a missing hand or an artificial limb. If the member has had the prosthesis for a long time, she or he usually has adapted well. If it is fairly new, the member may be self-conscious about it. The first inclination is to jump in and help the member, but it is better to wait and see how the situation is managed. If it seems to be a struggle, ask gently if the member wants some help. Always ask first, before you touch or do anything. Also keep in mind that group members are always observing your behavior. Your respect for efforts at independence will not be unnoticed. This is particularly important in the nursing home, where too much is done for residents and "excessive disability" develops.

Impact of Disease and Illness

The impact of disease and illness on the group leader's interventions has been noted in the suggested interventions listed in **Table 12–2**. However, physical ailments and related activities can also affect the group as a whole and the members as individuals. As noted before, physical complaints are sometimes offered by members as a reason not to attend meetings, leading to irregular attendance. Also the member may have a doctor's appointment at the time the group is scheduled. Or it could be an X-ray appointment, or a dental appointment, or a group member may be the caregiver for a parent. Burnside recalled having an 83-year-old in a group who went to the nursing home daily to feed the noon meal to her 103-year-old mother! It was necessary for her to rest a bit before she came to the group meeting. So physical problems related to the members can play havoc with attendance.

The special needs of older disabled people necessitate particular care. For example, groups should be scheduled during times when members are most alert. Very importantly, the leader should provide a comfortable physical environment with adequate access to bathroom and other facilities. Lastly, as stated earlier, the leader must be sensitive to the sensory deficits or other physical limitations of members.

Chronicity

The professional working with older people must be able to work with both chronic physical and chronic mental conditions. Although many older adults are in good health and lead active, busy lives, professionals employed in services for older people are likely to encounter many with multiple long-standing and long-lasting disabilities (Lechner & Neal, 1999). Chronic disabling conditions are generally those lasting longer than three months that will not be cured by a simple surgical procedure or brief course of medical treat-

ment. Group leaders should remember:

1. The person with a chronic illness experiences impaired functioning in more than one system—often multiple systems of the body, mind, and spirit are affected.
2. The illness-related demands on the individual are never completely removed.

Sometimes slow progress or even deterioration in a group may be related to the above two generalizations. The group leader in any setting should be cognizant of these two factors, but especially when conducting groups in hospitals, nursing homes, and day care centers.

Lack of control is a pervasive aspect of chronic illness—from the etiology of the disease to negative experiences within the health care system. Being a member of a group may help to empower an older person who is experiencing loss of control related to chronic illness and the changed life circumstances frequently associated with it. He or she can also learn in groups by listening to and observing how other members cope with the same or similar condition, and in these ways they may learn new ways of coping (Gitterman & Shulman, 1994).

The Oldest-Old

We talked about the oldest-old in Chapter 2. The oldest-old who have aged successfully are not independent; rather, the characteristics of their lifestyle are interdependence, reciprocity, and accessing helping networks. The interdependence allows activity and contact with friends. Such activities have long been considered important to successful aging. Interdependence benefits such as these are strong reasons for implementing groups with the oldest-old. The health of the oldest-old is the central concern underlying many other concerns and that is why group leaders of that age group must be sensitive to the health issues of the oldest-old. See **Table 12–3** for common health problems in those 85 and older.

The oldest-old have a rapid increase in functional disability as a result of chronic health conditions, often making nursing home placement the safe and desirable choice. The average nursing home resident is an 80-year-old white widow with several chronic health conditions. Because older women are twice as likely as older men to reside in a nursing home, the group you lead may be chiefly composed of women. Therefore, a group leader in a nursing home should expect frailty, the oldest-old, and larger numbers of women. **Table 12–4** should help the group leader better understand health in the oldest-old.

Gift Giving

The leader should be prepared to accept gifts, no matter how small, from the oldest-old. The ability to give gifts is important to them. Elderly people have a need to be needed; they will give as much to you—or more—than you give to them. Little gifts brought to you should be graciously accepted. This is important for a group leader to understand. Burnside reported how a member of a nursing home group saved a banana from his breakfast tray to give to her. Receive gifts graciously and quietly, because you do not want other group members to feel they should give you a gift also. Of course, there may be a policy in the agency about gifts, and you should know that policy.

Summary

This chapter provides the leader with some perspectives about group leadership with physically impaired older adults. Consideration of the physical difficulties of members helps leaders to implement a holistic approach to their leadership.

Table 12–3 MOST COMMON CHRONIC DISABLING CONDITIONS OF THE OLDEST-OLD

Condition	Common types
Bone and joint problems	• Osteoarthritis or degenerative joint disease; osteoarthritis may be a key factor in falls. • Osteoporosis, thinning of bones; it causes pain and restricts mobility. • Fractures can occur.
Cardiovascular disease	• Heart disease • Stroke • Arteriosclerosis (hardening of the arteries)
Vision problems	• Cataracts • Glaucoma • Macular degeneration
Cognitive impairment	• Dementia—Alzheimer's type • Secondary dementia
Depression and mental illness	• Reactive depression • Paranoia
High risk for disability	• Drug intoxication • Falls • Urinary incontinence

Table 12–4   HEALTH AND THE OLDEST-OLD

- Both acute and chronic diseases often go untreated in the very old, because they do not report symptoms to health providers.
- Common diseases of the oldest-old may have nonspecific symptoms, such as urinary incontinence, dizziness, acute confusion, refusal to eat or drink, weight loss, and failure to thrive.
- The oldest-old are likely to have more than one chronic condition.
- Most common disability conditions: bone and joint problems, osteoarthritis, degenerative joint diseases; osteoporosis; cardiovascular disease; vision problems; cognitive impairment.
- Other chronic disorders: depression and mental illness, drug intoxication, falls, urinary incontinence.
- Less disability for oldest-old: cancer, diabetes, and emphysema.
- The most likely causes of intractable disability are arthritis and Alzheimer's disease.
- Lifestyles are not characterized by independence, but rather by interdependence, reciprocity, and helping networks.
- An 85-year-old is 2 ½ times more likely to enter a nursing home than a 75-year-old.
- For the oldest-old, limited resources in one area will often mean limited resources in other areas as well.
- Among the oldest-old, women greatly outnumber men in institutions; the ratio is 4 to 1.
- Over half of those 85 and older report limitations in walking.
- Of those aged 85 and older, 54% need the help of another person in order to handle daily living.

Because there are common physical limitations and chronic diseases in older adults, suggestions for interventions are presented. The importance of preparing the environment, length of meetings, and accoutrements of aging are discussed. A discussion about health in the oldest-old is offered to help group leaders in the nursing home setting.

The chapter ends with a brief discussion on giving and receiving gifts.

Exercises

EXERCISE 1

Interview a 65-year-old regarding health problems; then interview a 90- or 95-year-old using the same interview questions. What differences did you note?

EXERCISE 2

Mobility is a problem for older adults, especially the oldest-old. Write a list of strategies a group leader might devise to help get these persons to group meetings.

EXERCISE 3

Assess a room used for group meetings with older adults (church, nursing home, day care center, senior center, and so on). List all the potential hazards or problems for older people that you observe.

EXERCISE 4

You have selected members for your group. What physical limitations have you assessed? You plan to serve coffee, tea, and snacks to the group. What precautions will you take that are directly related to the limitations in the group?

References

Anderson, R. (2002). Deaths: Leading causes for 2000. *National Vital Statistics Reports, 50*(16), 8.

Ashton, C. (2000). Preoperative assessment. In D. K. Brummel-Smith & J. Beck. (Eds.), *Comprehensive geriatric assessment* (pp. 349–380). New York: McGraw-Hill.

Bagley, M. (1995). The challenge to independence: Severe vision and hearing loss among older adults. *American Rehabilitation, 21*(2), 46–49.

Brody, B., Williams, R., Thomas, R., Kaplan, R., & Chu, R. (1999). Age-related macular degeneration: A randomized trial of a self-management intervention. *Annals of Behavioral Medicine, 21*(4), 322–329.

Eliason, M., & Skinstad, A. (2001). Drug and alcohol intervention for older women: A pilot study. *Journal of Gerontological Nursing, 27*(12), 18–24.

Federal Interagency Forum on Aging Related Statistics. (2000). *Older Americans 2000: Key indicators of well-being.* Washington, DC: U.S. Government Printing Office.

Ferrel, B. (2000). Pain. In D. Osterweil, K. Brummel-Smith, & J. Beck (Eds.), *Comprehensive geriatric assessment.* New York: McGraw-Hill. 381–398.

Gallo, J., Fulmer, T., Paveza, G., & Reichel, W. (2003). *Handbook of geriatric assessment* (Rev. ed.). Boston: Jones & Bartlett.

Gitterman, A., & Shulman, L. (Eds.). (2004). *Mutual aid groups, vulnerable populations and the life cycle.* New York: Columbia University Press.

Gorecki-Scavetta, M. (1999). Substance abuse issues. In S. Molony, C. Waszynski, & C. Lyder (Eds.), *Gerontological nursing: An advanced practice approach* (pp. 505–527). Connecticut: Appleton & Lange.

Haber, D. (2003). *Health promotion and aging* (Rev. ed.). New York: Springer.

Ignatavicius, D., (Ed.). (2003). *Geriatric patient education resource manual.* Aspen, CO: Aspen.

Kalra, L. (1998). Stroke: Clinical presentation and management. In R. Tallis, H. Fillet, & J. Brocklehurst (Eds.), *Brocklehurst's textbook of geriatric medicine and gerontology* (Rev. ed., pp. 499–532). Edinburgh, UK: Churchill Livingstone.

Kayser-Jones, J. (2002). The experience of dying: An ethnographic nursing home study. *The Gerontologist, 42*(special issue 111), 11–19.

Lechner, V. M., & Neal, M. B. (Eds.). (1999). *Work and caring for the elderly: International perspectives.* Philadelphia: Brunner-Mazel.

Osterweil, D., Brummel-Smith, K., & Beck, J. (2000). *Comprehensive geriatric assessment.* New York: McGraw-Hill.

Tang, S. (2003). Determinants of hospice home care use among terminally ill cancer patients. *Nursing Research, 52*(4), 217–233.

U. S. Department of Health and Human Resources. (2000). Census Data.

Resources

GENERAL

American Heart Association, National Center, 7320 Greenville Avenue, Dallas, TX 75231; (214) 750–5397.

National Arthritis and Musculoskeletal and Skin Diseases Information Clearinghouse, Box AMS, Bethesda, MD 20892; (301) 468–3235. Osteoporosis: Cause, treatment, prevention, Pub. No. 86-2226.

National Heart, Lung, and Blood Institute, National High Blood Pressure Education Program, U.S. Department of Health and Human Services, National Institutes of Health, Building 31, Bethesda, MD 20892; (301) 496-4236.

Osteoporosis: The silent thief. AARP Books/Scott, Foresman, 1865 Miner Street, Des Plaines, IL 60018; (800) 238–2300.

Understanding arthritis: The arthritis help book. Arthritis Foundation, Box 19000, Atlanta, GA 30326; (404) 266–0795.

VISUAL IMPAIRMENT

American Bank Stationery, 7501 Pulaski Highway, Baltimore, MD 21237; (301) 866-1900. Produces checks in large print and Braille.

American Foundation for the Blind, 15 West 16th Street, New York, NY 10011; (212) 620-2000. A nonprofit organization that provides information and sells aids and appliances; a catalog of products is available.

American Humane Society, P.O. Box 1266, Denver, CO 80201. Trains seeing eye dogs.

Bible Alliance, P.O. Box 1549, Bradenton, FL 33506; (813) 748-3031. Provides cassettes of Bible messages or the Bible free of charge; certification of need from physician or vision professional is required.

The Lighthouse, New York Association for the Blind, 111 East 59th Street, New York, NY 10022; (212) 355-2200. Provides information and some products.

HEARING IMPAIRMENT

Alexander Graham Bell Association for the Deaf, 1537 35th Street NW, Washington, DC 20007.

National Association of the Deaf, 814 Thayer Avenue, Silver Spring, MD 20910. Distributes information.

National Association of Hearing and Speech Agencies, 919 18th Street NW, Washington, DC 20006. Distributes information.

The National Hearing Aid Society, 20361 Middlebelt Road, Livonia, MI 48152; (313) 478-2610. Distributes information.

Reality Orientation, Remotivation, and Validation Therapy: Comparison of Use in Older People with Dementia

Elizabeth M. Williams

Key Words

- Confusion
- Dementia
- Behaviors
- Reality orientation (RO)
- Remotivation therapy (RT)
- Reality testing
- Validation therapy (VT)

Learning Objectives

- Define confusion
- Outline the historical development of reality orientation, remotivation, and validation therapy as modalities
- Distinguish between reality orientation, reality therapy, and reality testing
- Compare and contrast positive and negative research findings of these three modalities
- Describe at least three factors that are important to keep in mind when employing any of these modalities with older people
- Define and plan how any of these modalities can be incorporated into existing programs

Confusion is disorientation to person, time, place, or thing

—*Taulbee, 1978*

Three commonly used therapeutic techniques are used in group and individual work with people with dementia. The modalities utilize various communication styles and activities to encourage people to communicate, become involved in social experiences, and to change or reduce negative behaviors. These treatment modalities are: reality orientation (RO), remotivation therapy (RT), and validation therapy (VT). RO and RT are techniques thought to help bring people back to reality (Folsom, 1968; Bierma, 1998). VT is a communication technique designed to work with the individual from where they are in their confusional state and not to attempt to foist reality upon them (Benjamin, 1999; Feil, 2002; Warner, 2000).

Prior to attempting any of these techniques with a suspected confused person, a thorough assessment of their physiological and current and past cognitive status is imperative. Some confusional states are reversible with proper medical testing and treatment, such as those caused by infections, hormone deficiency, anemia, or drug interaction (Kahn, Gwyther, Frances, Silver, &

Alexopoulos, 1998). One should also assess the person's previous social, behavioral, mental, and coping skills employed in stressful situations; their spiritual work, and family background; as well as their hobbies (Grasel, Wiltfang, & Kornhuber, 2003). An assessment enables the provider to apply the appropriate treatment modality.

Definitions

Dementia is a degenerative brain process, caused by a disease, which leads to loss of cognitive abilities, especially memory, e.g., Alzheimer's, Parkinson's, and vascular disease (stroke) (Kahn et al., 1998).

Behaviors are an array of responses of a person to the environment, or to others, which reflects their ability to deal with stress. In this chapter, the therapies address negative behaviors in an effort to diminish, eliminate, or replace them with positive or desirable behaviors. Negative behaviors can be: acting out, complaining, blaming, verbal threats, hitting, biting, depression, or poverty of communication with others. Positive behaviors are: smiling, participation in care, activities and groups, positive self-concept, and decreased depressive symptoms (Babins, 1998; Babins, Dillon, and Merovitz, 1998; Feil, 2002).

Reality orientation, *reality therapy*, and *reality testing* are three terms that are often used interchangeably; however, the process and theory of each is different. *Reality therapy* is a confrontive therapy, developed by Glaser (1965), a psychiatrist, and was originally designed for mentally ill individuals who may be confused because of their mental illness, but not necessarily with dementia. The technique is an attempt to get the person to face the reality of their situation (Silverstone, 1976).

Reality testing may be undertaken by caregivers of people who have an acute confusional state (delirium), dementia, or a psychosis. It refers to the objective evaluation by another person of an emotion, thought, or event against their perception of real life. Normally people manage this reality testing process for themselves, but if a person is hallucinating, for example, the caregiver might say, "I know you hear voices, but I do not hear them."

Reality orientation is a specific treatment modality that usually occurs in a group setting, but it can be used on a one-to-one basis and is credited as the first psychiatric technique to bring older confused people back to reality (Schwenk, 1979).

Remotivation therapy (RT) is a structured group therapy originally designed for stimulating mentally ill people to be interested in the present and future. It is designed around reminiscing about discussion topics based on reality which includes use of visual aids (Dennis, 1994).

Validation therapy (VT) is a therapy that accepts the patient's view of reality as their reality and uses communication techniques that validate worth and caring, without attempting to bring the person out of their reality (Benjamin, 1999; Feil, 2002).

Literature Review

Reality Orientation

RO was developed by Dr. James Folsom between 1956 and 1965. The first stage began with a pilot project at the Topeka, Kansas, Veterans Administration Hospital on a geropsychiatric ward with patients who were given total care by nursing assistants. The nursing assistants were asked to initiate activities with the patients to encourage them to take responsibility for some of their own care. Folsom observed that the patients, who started to care for themselves, were more talkative with other residents, and were able to participate in activities off the ward (Folsom, 1968). While at the Mental Health Institute in Mt. Pleasant, Iowa, Dr. Folsom further developed specific RO guidelines out of an attitude therapy program.

These guidelines call for:

- a calm environment with a set routine.
- clear response to patient's questions, and the same types of questions should be asked of the patient.
- talking clearly to the patient, not necessarily loudly, and make requests of the patient in a calm manner, implying patient will comply.
- directing patients around by clear directions, if there is a need to guide them to and from their destinations.
- reminding them of the date, time, and so on.
- not allowing them to stay confused by rambling in their speech and actions.
- being firm, if necessary, and consistent.
- being sincere (Folsom, 1968, p. 299).

Patients were awakened by caregivers introducing themselves and calling the patient by name. Calendars were given to patients who had difficulty with time orientation, and they were assisted in marking off the day. Folsom states that after one year, 57% of the patients returned to their prehospital status, and some were able to leave the hospital.

The final stage of RO development occurred in 1965 at Tuscaloosa, Alabama, Veterans Administration Hospital and is the model for all RO programs used today. By that time, the process had been identified as consisting of three parts: basic classroom instruction, advanced classroom instruction, and 24-hour follow-through (Folsom, 1968). The basic class met twice daily for half an hour, and the advanced class met once a day five days a week. The class was held at the same time daily, and as much as possible the same personnel participated to give consistency. A specific attitude—active, passive, or matter of fact—was employed consistently with each patient. The use of an RO board with the name of the facility, month, day, and year, and other pertinent information was part of the basic class. Simple activities and games started in the classroom were

carried over through the 24-hour period following the class by all personnel coming into contact with the confused person. Twenty-four hour orientation used in conjunction with the structured classroom experience improved the orientation of the majority of the patients (Folsom, 1968).

Remotivation Therapy

Dorothy Smith, a college professor, is credited as the originator of RT. She worked as a hospital volunteer at the Pennsylvania State Hospital and introduced the technique while there (Dennis, 1994). The American Psychiatric Association formed a Remotivation Advisory Committee in response to interest in the technique and working with Smith, Kline and French Laboratories, remotivation programs were established throughout the country in mental hospitals (Dennis, 1994). In 1971 the National Remotivation Therapy Organization Inc. (NRTO) was formed. Remotivation at that time was called a therapy, not a technique with therapeutic effects, unless it was part of a treatment program or plan of care for a patient. NRTO's (2003) definition of RT is: "Remotivation is a small group therapeutic modality, objective in nature, designed to help clients by promoting self-esteem, awareness, and socialization."

RT is usually done as a group activity, but can also be done individually. The goal is to reach the part of the personality not harmed by mental or physical illness to encourage movement back to the reality that all humans share, rather than "I" only (Bierma, 1998). The group leader (remotivator) plans the topics, length of the group, and number of participants, assesses each participant for level of confusion and/or depression, and sets up a structured group format. The group leader acts and speaks in a nonthreatening and nonjudgmental manner, no matter what the participant's response to subject matter presented and to thank each member individually for their contributions. The theory is that with each contact the participant will increasingly feel that their contributions are worthwhile. This helps to decrease their feelings of hopelessness, helplessness, and sense of loss. In other words, focus on their abilities and not the disability (Sullivan, Bird, Alpay, and Cha, 2001). There are five structured components of an RT group:

Step 1: Climate of acceptance—Leader greets all and makes positive remark to each person.

Step 2: The bridge to reality—Several leading questions are asked to build up topic of discussion planned for the meeting.

Step 3: Sharing the world we live in—Topic is discussed in detail about things experienced by the five senses.

Step 4: An appreciation of the work of the world—The work or doing of the topic is discussed.

Step 5: Climate of appreciation—Leader summarizes session, announces the next meeting and time, and thanks all members for attending and contributing. (NRTO, 2003).

RT in facilities can be part of an activity program and is often led by activity personnel, social workers, nurses, or other trained staff. RT can also take place at the bedside for those who are too ill, disruptive, or not able to participate in a group for other reasons. The process, whether in a group or individually, serves as a part of the person's social circle within the nursing home, retirement facility, assisted-living center, day care center, or even in the person's home. The therapy can also be a useful way to educate about a disease process and self-care (NRTO, 2003; Sullivan et al., 2001). The content of the group or individual sessions is designed around the individual needs of each participant (NRTO, 2003). Sullivan et al. describe an RT program developed for hospitalized individuals with Huntington's disease, which was used at the bedside and in a group setting (see section on research).

Validation Therapy

VT was developed by Naomi Feil, MSW, between 1963 and 1980. She observed that her attempts and the attempts of others to reorient disoriented older people often led to further withdrawal and behavioral problems. She published her first book *V/F Validation: The Feil Method* in 1982, with revisions in 1992 and 2003; the last version is coauthored with Vicki DeKlerk-Rubin. A second book was published in 1993 and revised in 2002, *The Validation Breakthrough*. Over time, using verbal and nonverbal communication techniques that validate feelings and give support, Feil observed that behavioral outbursts, tension, withdrawal, and incontinence decreased, while speech improved, and desired behaviors that were positive, such as smiling and talking, were more evident (Babins, 1988; Babins et al., 1988; Feil, 2002). VT is based on "developmental theory that in old age, when controls loosen, disoriented very old persons need to express buried emotions in order to die in peace" (Feil, 2001).

VT views the confused person's thinking and behavior, as a means of coping with stress (Feil, 2002). The verbalization and behavior are a means of remembering pleasant things and retreating from those that are painful such as geriatric chairs, living alone, and losses built up over time. VT assumes that positive feelings and emotions from childhood determine the older disoriented adult's behavior. Recent memories begin to fade as early memories become more vivid and mental abilities decline. This leads to the end-of-life work of disoriented elderly people's expression of repressed emotions—this final phase is called resolution (Feil, 2002).

VT does not assume that the Alzheimer's person's thinking or behavior is wrong, just the opposite—that it is correct because that is their reality (Feil, 2002; Warner, 2000). Feil (2001) also claimed that disoriented older people were probably inflexible when dealing with stressors of life (death, job changes, moves, divorce, etc.) and used avoidance to deal with the losses when younger. VT does not force the disoriented person to "face reality" concerning their current situation or feelings. VT focuses on the person's emotional state, not the rational thinking that has been lost through brain damage. Benjamin (1999) wrote that nursing home staff can easily incorporate VT into daily interaction with moderately to severely confused patients to improve their quality of life and decrease stress for the caretaker. The caretaker's goal is to be convincing to the person who has dementia by validating their thoughts and feelings (empathy) and thereby molding the behavior to a positive outcome (Feil, 2002; Warner, 2000). To use VT effectively, the caretakers need to know the person's past work history, family relationships, hobbies, likes and dislikes, and so on to be able to interpret the topic about which the individual is talking or to which they are responding (Benjamin, 1999, Feil, 2002, Warner, 2000). This may mean taking their response, and asking further questions about the period or event they think they are living at the time (Benjamin, 1999; Feil, 2002). Feil (2002) has defined four stages of resolution and specific VT interventions for each.

FOUR STAGES OF RESOLUTION:

1. Malorientation—Individuals are oriented, occasionally confused, recognize their disorientation, are not mentally ill, are verbal, repeat untrue things, are anxious, tense, defensive, project frustration through accusing others, and hoard or clutch items.
   Interventions include allowing venting, listening with empathy, avoiding "feeling words," rephrasing key thoughts, reminiscing, providing routines, and not touching if the patient is averse to touch. Questions are aimed at getting more information, not confronting, getting people to further describe what they are feeling or their fears: who, what, when, and how, but never why.

2. Time confused—In very old people who are more physically disabled, present and past tense is often combined into one thought. They have no concept of current time, living on memories while attempting to resolve the past.
   Interventions include verbal and nonverbal techniques such as observing behavior, mirroring movements (such as pacing along with them when interacting), making eye contact, and matching their emotions.

3. Repetitive motion—These individuals have lost speech and depend on body movements in their attempts to communicate (lips, tongue, teeth, jaw, and body). Interventions include music, with childhood songs being especially helpful in this phase. The caregiver responds by picking up on the ambiguous pronouns and numbers spoken by the confused person.

4. Vegetation—These individuals are withdrawn and depressed, they shut others out and have given up.
   Interventions are few. Feil states that those in this stage are not easily reached, and the goal is to elicit some small response such as a smile.

Refer to **Table 13–1** for a brief comparison of the aforementioned therapies.

Research Literature

Reality Orientation

The last time this author conducted a literature review of RO thirty research articles were found, of which "ten RO studies demonstrated inconclusive or negative effects of RO" (Williams, 1994). The other twenty studies "conclude that RO was effective" (Williams, 1994). Only three new articles were located this time.

Table 13–1 Comparison of Reality Orientation, Remotivation Therapy, and Validation Therapy

Reality Orientation	Remotivation Therapy	Validation Therapy
Goal to reorient to present for any person with confusion	Goal to recreate interest in life for those who show interest or potential to return to reality	Goal to increase function and contentment by recognizing there's a basis behind the behavior and build validation and trust; looks at only the individual's reality—emotional focus Nonconfrontational, does not correct
Factual, confronts and corrects errors that are not factual in reality	Factual, not aimed at being confrontational, nor forcing individual to accept reality until ready to do so	Best for the moderately to severely demented
Used for all confused individuals, no matter the cause Probably best for the mildly confused	Best for mildly confused and with the mentally ill	
RO can be overused if cause of confusion is not taken into consideration		Individual or group; used 24/7
Individual or group use; in facilities used 24/7	Group or individual	Explore where person is and their reality; no attempt to bring to staff's reality; help reminisce and resolve their unfinished business
Provide repetitive information that is reality—date, time, place, role, who, what, why to stimulate the five senses	Uses objects to aid reminiscing and conversation; gets the person to talk and share	
The patient's response is corrected by providing the correct information; cues and prompting are used	All conversation is accepted unless inappropriate and not on the topic	

Spector, Orrel, Davies, and Woods (2000) analyzed six studies of randomly controlled trials (RCTs). The six RCTs (Baines, Saxby, & Ehlert, 1987; Breuil et al., 1994; Ferrario, Cappa, Molaschi, Rocco, & Fabris, 1991; Gerber et al., 1991; Wallis, Baldwin, & Higgenbotham, 1983; Woods, 1979) included data on 125 subjects (67 in experimental groups, 58 in control groups). The authors noted there was a significant effect on cognition and behavior, which demonstrated some benefit of RO with elderly patients with dementia. Classroom RO "had clear benefits to patients with dementia in both cognitive and behavioral domains, suggesting that RO techniques should be considered as an important component of dementia care" (Spector et al.). Spector et al. determined that long-term programs seem to help with continued sustained improvement. Further research was recommended to determine what features of RO are effective.

Koh et al. (1994) conducted an eight-week study on fifteen demented patients at a day care center to determine if RO, RT, and reminiscence therapy would improve scores on the Mental Status Questionnaire. Data was also collected on fifteen patients who received no therapy. All the study participants showed improved scores and twelve of the controlled group had deterioration in their scores. The authors concluded that the three therapies appeared to be effective on short-term mental stimulation.

Scanland and Emershaw (1993) used a quasi-experiential design to study RO and VT with 34 confused elderly people as to the effect on the level of depression and functional/cognitive status. Data analysis showed no significant differences between treatment and nontreatment groups on mental status or morale.

Remotivation Therapy

Sullivan, Bird, Alpay, and Cham (2001) tested the effectiveness of RT on 20 Huntington's patients on a neurological hospital ward, ranging in age from 26 to 85 years: 7 were male, 13 female, with lengths of stay of 3 weeks to 9 years. The participants received a series of 12 weekly sessions, lasting 30–60 minutes. Those not able to join a group because of behavior and or attention issues were treated individually. The authors discussed 6 participants' results in depth as the data was available and contained quality documentation which demonstrated the wide range of symptoms and complications the participants exhibited. An evaluation tool designed by the Bay State Remotivation Council, Inc. and later adopted by the NRTO to measure individual progress on interest, awareness, and attention span was used to collect data. A trained RT therapist, hired for the study, collected preassessment data on all subjects, determined appropriateness for the therapy, and provided RT for 12 weeks. The authors concluded that RT participants had improved scores in interest, awareness, attention span, frustration

tolerance, reading ability, oral communication, and overall participation in activities of daily living. Sullivan et al. concluded that RO was a successful intervention for this population. Positive effects on staff were also observed, such as more interest in the patients as individuals, increased participation in interdisciplinary meetings, and a decrease in one-on-one staffing (Sullivan et al., 2001).

Dennis (1994) discussed five early studies in Burnside's *Working With Older Adults: Group Process and Techniques*. These studies favored RT over no treatment. The studies indicated that confused older people who were treated with RT demonstrated increases in self-concept, higher levels of behavior, group participation, and interest in life. Dennis's study indicated nonpositive results that RT subjects were more depressed and less satisfied with life and showed no difference on behavioral ratings.

Validation Therapy

A literature review of available studies on VT found three articles describing the results of eight studies: Neal and Briggs (2003); Day (1997); and Finnema, Droes, Ribbe, and Van Tilburg (2000). Even though VT has been in use since the 1970s, no research appeared in the literature before 1990. Research conducted since the 1990s has shown promise in terms of affecting the negative behaviors of people with dementia by achieving more verbalization, and decreased agitation, but to date has not been replicated. All the studies have had methodological problems, including small sample sizes, no standardization of data collection instruments or instruments insufficiently sensitive to measure human behavior changes, lacked pilot studies, and there is no data indicating therapy should be an ongoing process. Refer to Table 13–2.

Two articles were located that discuss emotion-oriented care of which validation therapy is one type (Schrijnemaekers et al., 2003; Finnema et al., 2000). Schrijnemaekers et al. investigated the effects of emotion-oriented care on 151 cognitively impaired elderly and behavioral problems in 16 homes for the aged that had structured day care units. Subjects were randomly assigned to an intervention or control group. Measurements of participants and staff were performed at baseline, and three, six and twelve months. A multilevel analysis showed no statistically significant or clinically relevant effects in favor of the intervention group on the behavioral outcome measures. The authors indicated that there is insufficient evidence to justify the implementation of emotion-oriented care for residents (Schrijnemaekers et al., 2003).

Finnema et al. conducted a literature review on available studies of VT, emotion-oriented therapy, sensory integration/sensory stimulation/Snoezelen, simulated presence therapy, and reminisce/life review. They concluded despite the limited cogency of the studies, results of the VT studies are promising, but previously stated methodological issues make the comparison of studies and results not possible (Finnema et al., 2000).

Expanding RO: Cognitive Therapy

Other approaches being tried and researched, called cognitive-rehabilitation (Clare, 2005; Clare, Wilson, Carter, Roth, & Hodges, 2002), cognitive stimulation (Breuil et al., 1994), or cognitive-orientation (Zanetti et al. 2002), on older people with dementia, build on the strengths of RO, VT, and reminiscing (Woods, 2002) and incorporate principles from learning theory (Clare et al., 2002). These techniques focus on improving memory, retention, and learning, ensuring a respectful approach, and enhancing communication skills utilized in RT and VT. Cognitive rehabilitation works on the goals of the person to find ways to cope with the difficulties the person is experiencing by utilizing different memory and learning techniques (Woods, 2002). Cognitive therapies depend on the ability to verbalize and interact with others (Zanetti et al., 2002).

Little research has been done on the validity of these approaches. There is difficulty in applying the technique to more than one person at a time, and results don't indicate which level of cognitive deficit best benefits from the approach (Woods, 2002). However, some preliminary studies have shown some positive results on memory (Breuil et al., 1994; Clare et al., 2002; Zanetti et al., 2002). A study published by Zanetti et al. is described as a "revival" of RO by Woods. The Spector et al. (2000) meta-analysis on RO found that RO increases orientation and memory and is therefore effective in working with those who have mild to moderate cognitive deficits. Research by Clare et al. (2002) and Zanetti et al. (2002) indicated persons with mild to moderate cognitive deficits benefit from RO. Zanetti et al. also demonstrated that those individuals who were not euphoric prior to the study, did not benefit from RO. Zanetti et al.'s study included 38 outpatients, four subjects to a class, in a one-hour, five-day-a-week class for one month lead by an RO therapist. Content of the classes consisted of repetitive stimulation of the person's "autobiographical and semantic memory, attention, language and orientation" (Zanetti et al., 2002). This is an interesting finding as attention, concentration, and language that is impaired by dementia in the frontal area of the brain may interfere with cognitive rehabilitation. Therefore, cognitive rehabilitation may not be an appropriate intervention for individuals with advanced stages of these kinds of deficits. Clare et al. utilized errorless learning theory with groups of individuals in the early stages of Alzheimer's disease. These results were statistically significant in that the group scores improved with cognitive rehabilitation. And, the results were present at six and twelve months after the initial training. These studies are important in that the interventions were employed in a classroom setting, which means that the interventions may be transferable to settings where groups of older persons with dementia may be found.

Application of Modalities

Reality orientation has been on the decline in use, primarily because of the manner in which it has been improperly used, i.e., erroneous information on RO boards, and caregivers going overboard to get persons to accept reality without caution to how that affected them emotionally (Woods, 2002). As discussed under cognitive therapy, RO is being revived and incorporated into cognitive models of therapy. Therefore, application of RO, RT, VT, and cognitive therapies, which incorporate these three therapies, should only be undertaken after review of the literature, as to efficacy and results that best fit the population where the therapy is to be initiated. For example, Zanetti et al. (2002) suggested that those with euphoria (difficulties in the prefrontal and frontal

Table 13–2 COMPARISON OF VALIDATION STUDIES

Author	Sample Setting	Variable Studied	Design/Method	Results
Robb, S.S., Stegman, C.E., and Wolanin, M.O., 1986	Group	Social behavior Morale Mental status	Pre- and postintervention measurements Anecdotal	Inconclusive results for all variables Anecdotal notes reported negative behavior (more demanding) No affect on cognitive and social behavior
Babins, L., Dillon, J., and Merovitz, S., 1988	12 subjects in either stage two, time confusion, or three, repetitive motion of confusion	Cognitive Social Behavioral	22 sessions over 11 weeks (5 subjects). Control group, no treatment Comparison of data only from first 3 weeks and last 3 weeks of the sessions Scales not standardized	Increase in verbal and nonverbal expression with validation therapy (VT) Increase in irritability in one person with reminiscence, but decline with VT
Morton, I., and Bleathman, C., 1991	5 subjects Residential home	Mood Communication Behavior	10 weeks of no treatment (tx), then 10 weeks of tx with VT, then 10 weeks no tx., then 10 weeks with reminiscence therapy.	Two subjects with increased social interaction with VT, but decline with reminiscence. One subject with decreased social interaction

Table 13–2 COMPARISON OF VALIDATION STUDIES (CONTINUED)

Author	Sample Setting	Variable Studied	Design/Method	Results
Bleathman, I., and Morton, C., 1992	Moderately demented elderly in residential home 5 subjects	Communication, quantity and quality	Repeat of 1991 study	Increased interaction with VT and increased depth of interaction
Scanland, S. G., and Emershaw, L.E., 1993	Veterans Administration NHCU, 34 subjects	Depression Mental and functional status	RO and VFT group for 4 months, 5 times a week for 30 minutes Control group with no tx	No difference between groups on pre/post-measurements.
Fine, J. L., and Rouse-Bane, S., 1995	Residents of a dementia unit. 13 subjects in pretraining; 22 subjects posttraining	Behavior Psychological Medication	Quasi-experimental time series; study was on 1:1 intervention, not group intervention Pretraining data collected from staff and 13 subjects Posttraining data collected from staff and 22 subjects Staff completed recordings on interventions	Increase in staff selecting appropriate intervention Increased validation of technique for stage of dementia posttraining Problem behaviors decreased when appropriate intervention used for the appropriate stage of confusion
Nooren-Staal, W. H., Frederiks, C. M., and teWierik, M. J., 1998	Nursing home 10 patients 29 nurses	Behavior of patients Behavior of nurses	15 nurses trained in VT Patient behavior measured 3 times by nurses (prior to training, after training, and 4 mo after treatment)	Increased job satisfaction/attitude of the nurses Some improvement in patient behavior
Toseland, R. W., Diehl, M., Freeman, K., Manzanares, T., Naleppa, M., and McCallion, P., 1997	Sample size 88 Very demented nursing home residents	Psychosocial function Medication Physical restraints Positive behavior— verbal/nonverbal	Single blind study Group for 52 weeks, 4 times a week for 30 minutes: validation, social and no group Data collected at 3 months and 1 year	Less aggression and depression in validation group No difference with use of psychotropics and restraints VT did not decrease physical nonaggressive behavior

cortical areas that control inhibition, affect, and language) may not benefit from RO or other cognitive-oriented therapy. Prior to implementation of any approach in an outpatient or inpatient setting, the literature on the planning and implementation of the approaches and resources needed to start and maintain a program in any setting should be undertaken (Holden & Woods, 1995; Williams, 1994). Most proponents emphasize that the techniques need to be used on a 24/7 basis to be effective (Benjamin, 1999; Holden & Woods, 1995) and that RO and RT are best with people with mild to moderate confusion; they can be used in a group setting or one to one. RO is commonly employed with acutely confused patients admitted to acute care facilities. Often the baseline confusion is not known, or family members indicate that the confusion is new. RO may be effective then as the caregiver provides the patient orientation information with each con-

tact. As the confusion clears, reality orientation is a good tool for determining the patient's progress back towards their baseline level of functioning. VT interventions can be employed in any setting also, but the staff needs to be well trained in the interventions to use for each specific stage of resolution. The technique can be helpful in gaining the cooperation and trust of the older confused person with personal care and testing in an acute care hospital. Refer to **Table 13–3** for suggested items/themes to use.

Summary

Continued research into these modalities with older adults with dementia will provide caregivers with a number of interventions that are more appropriate for varied stages of cognitive functioning. The goal of caregivers should be to continue to preserve the cognitive and functional

Table 13–3   Suggested Tools for Reality Orientation and Remotivation Therapy

Memory boards/Calendars with date/time/season in patient rooms/group rooms, dining rooms—make certain *always* up to date
Current events—Using newspapers, magazines, etc. History discussions
Sensory testing—Smells, touch, vision, hearing, taste through cooking and eating of what was cooked
Observance of holidays
Group gardening
Bird feeders; outings to zoos, museums, etc.
Pets—Bringing animals to the facility, visiting the zoo, pictures
Family scrapbooks/photo albums, video- or audio-tape recording one's life history—All are good reminiscing tools
Flash cards—Games that stimulate conversation; large puzzles, crossword puzzles
Exercises/movement therapy in wheelchairs or other chairs
Music and dancing
Directional signs and nightlights in facilities
Radio, record players, videos, TV, and now computers
Computer games—great way for older persons to communicate with family members
Art therapy such as painting, drawing
World globes—Where they grew up, traveled, where they may have served in the military
Sports

abilities of the individual for as long as possible through RO, RT, and cognitive modalities. It is also important to preserve the integrity of the individual through respectful, empathetic approaches and communication techniques that are part of RO, RT, and VT. These therapies can be appropriate for all individuals with dementia as long as the caregivers are well trained in their theory and practice.

Exercises

EXERCISE 1

If you work in an acute care facility or a psychiatric unit for people with dementia, think about patients you are caring for or have cared for and identify ways that you can use one or all of these therapies. Describe what you need to know about dementia to determine which therapy to use. Outline how you would evaluate the effectiveness of your approach.

EXERCISE 2

If you work in a nursing home with confused elderly people, how can you assist yourself and other staff to deal with the angry, demanding, complaining, accusatory resident? With which of the three therapies would you start and why? Would you implement all three therapies? Why or why not? Plan how you are going to implement the technique in your routine care and teach others to use the technique.

References

Babins, L. (1988). Conceptual analysis of validation therapy. *International Journal of Aging and Human Development, 26*(3), 161–168.

Babins, L., Dillon, J., & Merovitz, S. (1988). The effects of validation therapy on disoriented elderly. *Activities, Adaptation & Aging, 12*, 73–86.

Baines, S., Saxby, P., & Ehlert, K. (1987). Reality orientation and reminiscence therapy: A controlled crossover study of elderly confused people. *British Journal of Psychiatry, 151*, 222–231.

Benjamin, B. J. (1999). Validation: A communication alternative. In L. Volicer & L. Bloom-Charette (Eds.), *Enhancing the Quality of Life in Advanced Dementia* (pp. 107–125). Ann Arbor, MI: Edward Brothers.

Bierma, J. (1998). *Remotivation group therapy: Handbook for the basic course.* Andover, MA: National Remotivation Therapy Organization.

Bleathman, I., & Morton, C. (1992). Validation therapy: Extracts from 20 groups with dementia sufferers. *Journal of Advanced Nursing, 17*, 658–666.

Breuil, V., De Rotrou, J., Forette, F., Tortrat, D., Ganansia-Ganem, A., Frambourt, A., et al. (1994). Cognitive stimulation of patients with dementia: Preliminary results. *International Journal of Geriatric Psychiatry, 9*, 211–217.

Burnside, I., & Schmidt, M. G. (Eds.). (1978). *Working with Older Adults: Group Process and Techniques* (1st ed.). Boston: Jones & Bartlett.

Clare, L. (2005). Cognitive rehabilitation for people with dementia. In M. Marshall (Ed). *Perspectives on reahbilitation and dementia* (pp. 180–186). London: Jessica Kingsley.

Clare, L., Wilson, B. A., Carter, G., Roth, I., & Hodges, J. R. (2002). Relearning face-name associations in early Alzheimer's disease. *Neuropsychology, 16*(4), 538–547.

Day, C. R. (1997). Validation therapy: A review of the literature. *Journal of Gerontological Nursing, 23*(4), 29–34.

Dennis, H. (1994). Remotivation groups. In I. Burnside & M.G. Schmidt (Eds.), *Working with Older Adults: Group Process and Techniques* (3rd ed. pp. 153–162). Boston: Jones & Bartlett.

Feil, N. (2001). Validation therapy. In M. D. Mezey, Editor in Chief, *The encyclopedia of elder care: The comprehensive resource on geriatric and social care.* New York: Springer.

Feil, N. (2002). *The validation breakthrough* (2nd ed.). Baltimore: Health Professions Press.

Ferrario, E., Cappa, G., Molaschi, M., Rocco, M., & Fabris, F. (1991). Reality orientation therapy in institutionalized elderly patients: Preliminary results. *Archives of Gerontology and Geriatrics, 2*, 139–142.

Fine, J. I., & Rouse-Bane, S. (1995). Using validation techniques to improve communication with cognitively impaired older adults. *Journal of Gerontological Nursing, 21*(6), 39–45.

Finnema, E., Droes, R., Ribbe, M., & Van Tilburg, W. (2000). The effects of emotion-oriented approaches in the care for persons suffering from dementia: A review of the literature. *International Journal of Geriatric Psychiatry, 15*, 141–161.

Folsom, A. (1968). Reality orientation for the elderly mental patient. *Journal of Geriatric Psychiatry, 1*(2), 291–307.

Gerber, G. J., Prince, P. N., Snider, H. G., Atchinson, K., Dubois, L., & Kilgour, J. A. (1991). Group activity and cognitive improvement among patients with Alzheimer's disease. *Hospital and Community Psychiatry, 42*(8), 843–846.

Glaser, W. (1965). *Reality therapy: A new approach to psychiatry.* New York: Harper & Row.

Grasel, E., Wiltfang, J., & Kornhuber, J. (2003). Non-drug therapies for dementia: An overview of the current situation with regard to proof of effectiveness. *Dementia and Geriatric Cognitive Disorders, 15*(3), 115–126.

Holden, U., & Woods, R. T. (1995). *Positive approaches to dementia care* (3rd ed.). London: Churchill Livingstone.

Kahn, D. A., Gwyther, L. P., Frances, A., Silver, J. M., & Alexopoulos, G. (1998). Agitation in older persons with dementia: A guide for families and caregivers. Expert consensus guideline series: Agitation in older persons with dementia [Special report]. *Postgraduate Medicine*, 81–88.

Koh, K., Ray, R, Lee, J., Nair, A., Ho, T., & Ang, P.C. (1994). Dementia in elderly patients: Can the 3R mental stimulation programme improve mental status? *Age and Ageing, 23*(3), 195–199.

Morton, I., & Bleathman, C. (1991). The effectiveness of validation therapy in dementia—A pilot study. *International Journal of Geriatric Psychiatry, 6*, 327–330.

Neal, M., Briggs, M. (2003). *Validation therapy for dementia.* Cochrane Database Systematic Review, Jan, 3. Oxford, UK: Cochrane Library.

Nooren-Staal, W. H., Frederiks, C. M., & teWierik, M. J. (1998). Validation: Its effect in residents and staff in a home for the aged. *Tijdschr Gerontology and Geriatrics, 26*(3), 117–21.

NRTO. Definition and structured components of remotivation therapy by the National Remotivation Therapy Organization, Inc. (NRTO). (2003). Retrieved 1 June, 2004, from *http://www.remotivation.com*

Robb, S. S., Stegman, C. E., & Wolanin, M. O. (1986). No research versus research with compromised results: A study of Validation Therapy. *Nursing Research, 35*(2), 113–118.

Scanland, S. G., & Emershaw, L. E. (1993). Reality orientation and validation therapy: Dementia, depression, and functional status. *Journal of Gerontological Nursing, 19*(6), 7–11.

Schrijnemaekers, V. J., van Rossum, E., Candel, L. M., Frederiks, C. M., Derix, M. M., Sielhorst, H. et al. (2003). Effects of emotion-oriented care on elderly people with cognitive impairment and behavioral problems in residential homes. *Tijdschr Gerontology and Geriatrics, 34*(4), 151–161.

Schwenk, M. (1979). Reality orientation for the institutionalized aged: Does it help? *The Gerontologist, 19*(4), 373–377.

Silverstone, B. (1976). Beyond the one-to-one treatment relationship. In L. Bellak & T. Karasu (Eds.), *Geriatric Psychiatry: A handbook for psychiatrists and primary care physicians* (pp. 207–224). New York: Grune & Stratton.

Spector, A., Orrel, M., Davies, S., & Woods, B. (2000). Reality orientation for dementia: A systematic review of the evidence of effectiveness from randomized controlled trials. *The Gerontologist, 40*(2), 206–212.

Sullivan, F. R., Bird, E. D., Alpay, M., & Cha, J. J. (2001). Remotivation therapy and Huntington's disease. *Journal of Neuroscience Nursing, 33*(3), 136–142.

Taulbee, L. (1978). Reality orientation: A therapeutic group activity for elderly persons. In I. Burnside (Ed.), *Working with the elderly: Group process and techniques* (2nd ed., pp. 206–218). North Scituate, MA: Duxbury Press.

Toseland, R. W., Diehl, M., Freeman, K., Manzanares, T., Naleppa, M., & McCallion, P. (1997). The impact of validation group therapy on nursing home residents with dementia. *Journal of Applied Gerontology, 16*, 31–50.

Wallis, G. G., Baldwin, M., & Higgenbotham, P. (1983). Reality orientation therapy: A controlled trial. *British Journal of Medical Psychology, 56*, 271–277.

Warner, M. (2000). Designs for validation therapy. *Nursing Homes, 49*, 6.

Williams, E. (1994). Reality orientation groups. In I. Burnside & M. Schmidt (Eds.), *Working with Older Adults: Group Process and Techniques* (3rd ed., pp. 139–152). Boston: Jones & Bartlett.

Woods, B. (2002). Reality orientation: A welcome return? *Age and Ageing, 31*, 155–156.

Woods, R. T. (1979). Reality orientation and staff attention: A controlled study. *British Journal of Psychiatry, 134*, 502–507.

Zanetti, O., Oriani, M., Geroldi, C., Binetti, G., Frisoni, G. B., DiGiovanni, G., et al. (2002). Predictors of cognitive improvement after reality orientation in Alzheimer's disease. *Age and Ageing, 31*, 193–196.

Resources

Alzheimer's Association. Selected list of resources.

- Alzheimer's Outreach.
  http://www.zarcrom.com/users/alzheimers
- Idyll Arbor, Inc. Books and activity items for RO. *http://www.idyllarbor.com*

- InterSign Corporation. RO information calendars. *http://www.intersigncorp.com*
- National Remotivation Therapy Organization, Inc. (NRTO).
- *http://www.charityadvantage.com/ remotivation/Skilled Nursing Homes.asp*
- S. & S. Product catalogs for Recreation and Activity Directors. *http://www.ssww.com*

- Validation Training Institute, Inc. *http://www.vfvalidation.org*

VIDEOS/TRAINING PROGRAM MATERIALS

- *http://www.healthprofessionspress.com/ CATALOG/LTC%20Books/ ValTrainmain.html*
- *http://www.brookespublishing.com/store/ books/feil-2564/*

Chapter 14

Reminiscence Group Work

Faith Gibson
Irene Burnside

Key Words

- Age appropriate
- Communication
- Life review
- Life story books
- Meaning making
- Recall and partial reconstruction of memories
- Reminiscence
- Themes and topics
- Triggers and props
- Traumatic memories

Learning Objectives

- Define reminiscence
- Differentiate between reminiscence and structured individual life review
- List Webster's eight empirically established functions of reminiscence
- Identify how to use long-term memory in reminiscence group work
- Define *triggers* or *props* and provide an example relating to the senses of sight, sound, touch, taste, and smell
- List 10 topics or themes appropriate for a reminiscence group

- Identify three reasons for undertaking reminiscence work with people with dementia
- List five ways in which group work needs to be adapted to enable people with dementia to participate in a reminiscence group.

Memory is much more than recall of past stimuli. It involves emotion, will, and creativity in the reconstruction of the past to serve present needs.

—*P. G. Coleman (1986, p. 2)*

The past exists only in memory and imagination; if accessed by means of reminiscence and recall, the past can become a rich resource for living in the present and anticipating the future. Since the early 1960s, reminiscence work has developed as a popular psychosocial intervention that is used by many different professionals, family caregivers, and volunteers. It is undertaken with individuals, couples, and small groups. It is suitable for people of all ages, not only older people. The places in which reminiscence work is practiced include health and social care facilities, schools, colleges, museums, libraries, arts organizations, and community service settings. Reminiscence is most often, although not invariably, enjoyable and is widely, though not universally, acceptable. While the outcomes of reminiscence are usually therapeutic, it is not strictly a therapy, although the term therapy is frequently used, especially in clinical settings. Reminiscence provides an easy pathway or bridge into other therapies and creative artistic activities. The term *reminiscence work*, not *therapy*, more accurately represents the distribution of power sought in reminiscence and life review relationships (Dunn, Haight, & Hendrix, 2002). The term *work* recognizes the expertise and authority of individuals when recalling accounts of their own life experience (Gibson, 2004). In reminiscence groups, leaders are primarily enablers or facilitators; they are not meant to be historical experts or teachers. The expertise lies with the person recounting their personal memories.

Reminiscence work should never be imposed, and careful selection of participants is essential. Just as group work does not suit everyone, so too reminiscence group work does not appeal to everyone. Some people are naturally future oriented and have no interest in looking back. Some are occupied with energetically pursuing various present activities. Some people with painful, problematic pasts do not wish to disturb their emotional equilibrium, usually hard won, by reawakening a past that they have struggled to contain or forget. Most people, however, relish an opportunity to revisit the past and to share their stories with appreciative listeners.

This chapter briefly reviews recent reminiscence literature, outlines definitions and characteristics, identifies types and functions of reminiscence, and considers various clinical applications. Essential modifications for doing reminiscence work with people who have dementia and sensory impairments are also discussed.

Literature Review

Readers wishing to understand the historical evolution and widening applications of reminiscence and life review will find the extensive literature reviews by Merriam (1980), Molinari and Reichlin (1984), Haight (1991), Haight and Hendrix (1995), and Hendrix and Haight (2002) invaluable. Even though reminiscence is a common phenomenon of old age, it is not exclusive to this stage of the life cycle. While almost everyone reminisces, younger and older people tend to reminisce more than middle-aged people (Webster, 1997) and the purposes served by recall vary across the life span (de Vries & Watt, 1996). Middle-aged people tend to draw on the past to solve present problems. Older people tend to engage in more comprehensive life review and evaluation as they search for meanings to life and to pass on their experience as a legacy to others (Cappelliez, Lavellee, & O'Rourke, 2001; Garland & Garland, 2001). Older people living in their own homes tend to think or talk about the past less than people of similar age who are socially isolated, in ill health, or living in institutions (Hansebo & Kihlgren, 2000). This suggests that some reminiscence is a response to boredom or lack of fulfillment in the present (Cohen & Taylor, 1998). Women tend to reminisce about children, friends, and partners while men usually recall memories related to employment. Young adults recall more issues concerning identity. Most studies examining the frequency of reminiscence report little difference between people of different ages. Webster & McCall (1999) and Cappeliez (2003) suggest that adults of all ages recall more memories related to their young adult life than to any other period. This "autobiographical memory bump" is possibly explained by the relatively greater number of significant life events that occur during this stage of life (Habermas & Bluck, 2000). Peuntes (2002) suggests that spontaneously occurring simple reminiscence that is triggered by present stress can be harnessed as a coping mechanism. Recall of past experiences is used to moderate present anxiety and equips the person to make judgments about the future.

Qualitative clinical, largely anecdotal reports of the effectiveness of reminiscence are consistently more positive than the results obtained from empirical quantitative studies. Spector, Orrell, Davies, and Woods (2000) and Webster and Haight (2002) have identified methodological shortcomings in many reminiscence studies. These include inconsistent terminology, failure to define objectives, inadequate sampling, including lack of randomization and controls, inadequate standardization of the methods and types of interventions used, thus preventing replication, and over-reliance on white aged subjects. Despite these limitations, steady progress in research is being made. Increasingly, qualitative methods, including single case studies of individuals and groups, as well as quantitative studies, are being reported (Brooker & Duce, 2000; Johnson, Beckerman, & Auerbach, 2001; Kazi, 1998).

Definitions and Characteristics of Reminiscence and Life Review

These two terms are sometimes used interchangeably, and at other times they refer to distinctive interventions. Butler (1963, p. 66) used both terms. He regarded reminiscence—"the act or process of recalling the past"—as the means for achieving life review. He also suggested that life review was universal, undertaken by all older people as they approached death, a viewpoint effectively challenged by Merriam (1993). Butler (2001, p. 9) emphasized the importance of listening, so central to reminiscence and life review, when he identified the contemporary challenge for professionals working with older people: "Along with helping to assuage pain, anger, guilt, and grief, health care professionals at all levels need to *listen* to their older patients. We must facilitate the opportunity for a person to achieve resolution and celebration, affirmation and hope, reconciliation and personal growth in the final years."

Spector, Orrell, Davies, and Woods (2000, p. 1) defined reminiscence therapy as "vocal or silent recall of events in a person's life, either alone, or with another person or group of people." Cappeliez, Lavellee, and O'Rourke (2001, p. 5) defined it as "the process of thinking or telling about past experiences."

We are all familiar with reminiscence, a seemingly ordinary everyday experience, but it is a complex process that consists of four interdependent component parts (Gibson, 2004). These are:

(1) Remembering—Becoming aware of or entertaining a memory
(2) Recall—Sharing the memory with others, either verbally or nonverbally
(3) Review—Evaluating the memory recalled, either alone or in the company of others
(4) Reconstruction—Representing the memory in a partially modified form.

Reminiscence may occur spontaneously or be purposely evoked. Memories may be retained as ideas, talked about, or translated into various tangible formats that often combine verbal and nonverbal aspects. Once the memories are externalized in whatever way, they become accessible to other people. Review refers to the process of thinking and thinking again about the recalled memories and reaching some evaluation of their significance. This may occur strictly in private, be shared with others, or often involves a mixture of both. Life review is the term often used to refer to this integrative, evaluative dimension which may be spontaneously set in motion as a consequence of reminiscence and recall even if not intended. This process is not restricted to late life as an intergenerational writing project involving elders and elementary school children demonstrates (Stelson & Dauk-Bleess, 2003).

Reconstruction of memories is usually only partial rather than comprehensive. All memories are modified to some extent each time they are entertained, and particularly when they are shared with others, they come to be understood in a new way before being consigned again to long-term memory.

The extent to which the review element occurs in planned reminiscence work varies according to the purposes or objectives agreed upon with the group members as part of the contract. It will, for example be a major objective in autobiographical and spiritual autobiographical writing groups (Cole & de Medeiros, 2000), now so popular with older people (see Chapter 15 by Birren and Deutchman).

Life review is also the term used to refer to a structured one-to-one planned intervention carried out in private and often guided by means of Haight's Life Review and Experiencing Form (LREF). In eight weekly, loosely structured sessions, the individual is guided systematically to recall life, from childhood to the present, and during the process comes to understand and to integrate past memories (Haight, Coleman, & Lord, 1995). Recall of personal memories and reminiscing about them with an empathetic listener are the means by which the person reviews or reevaluates the past and as a consequence integrates or comes to accept troubling memories in a reconstructed life story.

Reminiscence groups vary immensely in objectives, structure, program, process, and outcomes. Groups can be ranged along a continuum from simple diversion to explicit psychotherapy. Some may resemble oral history while others review unresolved conflicts and disabling memories of past traumatic events. In between these extremes there may be groups whose programs seek to achieve social and intellectual stimulation, reinforce personal identity, increase well-being, and preserve and transmit cultural heritage and personal and family history.

The Significance of Control

Control is recognized as a significant factor influencing the well-being and longevity of older peo-

ple, especially frail older people, including those with dementia, who live in health or welfare facilities. Control is closely allied with contemporary concerns about choice, empowerment, and anti-oppressive practice (Gwyther, 1999; Martin & Younger, 2000). Perceived control is associated with feelings of high emotional well-being. The opposite also holds. If others are perceived to exercise control, which is an inevitable consequence of living in a nursing home or similar institution, this is a potent threat to well-being. Voluntary participation in a reminiscence group is one means of reinvesting control and empowering members. In such groups each person freely chooses to attend, carries responsibility for recounting their own life story, and is recognized as the authentic authority on what is told.

The skills and experience of the leader need to match the needs of the group members, especially if some have cognitive or sensory disabilities or are severely depressed (Gibson, 2004). Training, supervision, consultation, or mentoring is essential because painful as well as happy memories may be recalled, and this may trigger disturbing memories in those who listen, including the leaders. The reminiscence worker needs to be able to encourage people to tell their stories and hold the group to hearing whatever is told. They need the ability to encourage people to talk and to listen, to connect with each other's stories and to value themselves and other members (Capuzzi & Gross, 1998). Reminiscence groups build on people's strengths; they promote personal growth and encourage group solidarity. Members are encouraged to locate themselves within a life span perspective, and in comparing lives common experiences are uncovered and trials and triumphs recognized. This sharing process helps individuals to develop a more kindly view of themselves and of other people, and to gain courage and hope for coping with the present and facing the future.

Reminiscence readily links with artistic activities, including music (Clair, 2001), dance, (Hill,

2001), exercise, movement, bibliotherapy, creative writing (Koch, 1977) and art (Rentz, 2002). These creative activities become vehicles for expressing memories and are also ways of encapsulating them in more tangible and durable forms (Sim, 1997). In some groups reminiscence may be combined with discussion of current events so that the conversation moves backwards and forwards between the past and the present. This enables members to make comparisons and evaluations and to examine discrepancies or dislocations between their past and present experience. In reminiscence groups as distinct from psychotherapy and structured life review groups, recall mostly involves selective aspects of the past rather than achieving a comprehensive recall of each stage of the life cycle.

Historical Changes in How Reminiscence Is Viewed

Long before neuroscientists began researching memory and the recall of memories, philosophers, artists, and writers explored this subject, and much can be learned from them about the power of reminiscence. Pear (1922) said that the mind never photographs, but paints pictures, thus anticipating contemporary concerns about the social construction of reality, the accuracy of memory, and how stories are influenced by time, context, hearers' reception and response, present mood, and the conscious and unconscious needs of the person reminiscing.

There has been a revolution in the way that clinician's view reminiscence in later life. Before Butler's historic 1963 article, reminiscence was regarded as pathological, escapist, rambling, and repetitious. No doubt, there are still some who believe that reminiscence is dysfunctional and should be discouraged, but most clinicians now regard recall of the past as a healthy activity that serves positive purposes for people as they age.

Sometimes group leaders may still not grasp the significance of talk about the past. Although reminiscing is about the past, it is actually a present, here-and-now experience. Some leaders may find reminiscence boring or have other priorities. This does not mean that every group for older people should be run as a reminiscence group. All leaders, however, should be alert to the importance of memories. When recall intrudes upon other activities, its significance needs to be understood so that rich opportunities for validating life experience and for appreciating that the past informs the present and shapes the future are not lost.

The popularity and acceptability of reminiscence groups have played significant roles in the overall development of group work with older people that originally was limited to isolated groups in medical institutions led by nurses or medics (Capuzzi & Gross, 1998). Now many groups are community based and are led by people from very varied backgrounds. Reminiscence group work with older people is greatly enriched when health, social care, and arts workers pool their expertise and share their skills.

Despite these developments, ageist stereotypes still abound and restrict the opportunities provided by younger people for older adults to remember their past and profit from doing so. Cappeliez, Lavallee, and O'Rourke (2001) caution young health workers to check with older people directly about the reasons why they might wish to use reminiscence in a group rather than imposing stereotypical views that may inadvertently curtail the type of opportunities young leaders make available to older group members.

Summary of Typologies of Reminiscence

Table 14–1 summarizes the major types of reminiscence identified by various writers. If reminiscence workers are to be effective then they need to be clear about the type of reminiscence they are intending to undertake, for what purpose, with what population, and in what context.

Table 14–1   TYPOLOGIES OF REMINISCENCE 1964–2003

McMahon and Rhudick (1964)
- Storytelling
- Material for life review
- Defensive reminiscence

Coleman (1974)
- Simple reminiscence
- Life review
- Informative reminiscence

Lo Gerfo (1980–1981)
- Informative reminiscence
- Evaluative reminiscence
- Obsessive reminiscence

Kaminsky (1984)
- Living history

Merriam (1989)
- Simple reminiscence

Watt and Wong (1991)
- Integrative reminiscence
- Instrumental reminiscence
- Transmissive reminiscence
- Escapist reminiscence
- Obsessive reminiscence
- Narrative reminiscence

Erwin (1996)
- Casual stories
- Relational
- Analytical—Life review
- Defensive
- Obsessive rumination

Webster (1997)
- Boredom reduction
- Death preparation
- Identity
- Problem solving
- Conversation
- Intimacy maintenance
- Bitterness revival
- Teach/inform

Bornat, Chamberlyne, Pavey, and Chant (1998)
- Formal and informal group
- Informal, individual, intimate
- Informal ad hoc with groups and individuals
- Reminiscence-related activities

Chandler and Ray (2002)
- Fixed
- Dynamic

Cappeliez (2003)
- Intrapersonal—Combines integrative, escapist, obsessive, and death preparation
- Interpersonal—Combines narrative, intimacy maintenance, instrumental, and transmissive

Webster's Reminiscence Functions

Webster (1993, 1997) and Webster and McCall (1999) identified eight separate reminiscence functions or objectives and produced a 43-item Reminiscence Functions Scale (RFS) applicable to all ages from young adulthood to late life (Webster, 1997, p. 140). The functions are:

- Boredom reduction—Having something to do: "Our propensity to reminisce when our environment is understimulating and we lack engagement in goal-directed activities."
- Death preparation—Valuing the life lived and becoming less fearful of death: "The way we use our past when thoughts of our own mortality are salient and may contribute to a sense of closure and calmness."
- Identity—Discovering and better understanding a sense of who we are: "How we use our past in an existential manner to discover, clarify, and crystallize important dimensions of our sense of who we are."
- Problem solving—Drawing on strengths and experience from the past for coping in the present: "How we employ reminiscence as a constructive coping mechanism whereby the remembrance of past problem-solving strategies may be used again in the present."
- Conversation—Rediscovering common bonds between old and new friends: "Our natural inclination to invoke the past as a means of connecting or reconnecting with others in an informal way."
- Intimacy maintenance—Remembrance of personally significant people: "Cognitive and emotional representations of important persons in our lives are resurrected in lieu of the remembered person's physical presence."
- Bitterness revival—To sustain memories of old hurts and justify negative thoughts and emotions: "The extent to which memories are used to affectively charge recalled episodes in which the reminiscer perceives themselves as having been unjustly treated."
- Teach/inform—Teaching younger people, including family members, about values and history: "The ways in which we use reminiscence to relay to others important information about life (e.g., a moral lesson). It is an instructional type of narrative."

The widespread use of Webster's framework would bring greater coherence and clarity to reminiscence practice and research. It could assist leaders to:

- Appreciate the various functions served by reminiscence.
- Recognize the type of reminiscence he or she wishes to elicit.
- Recognize the type of reminiscence that may be appropriate or inappropriate in a particular group.
- Be sensitive and responsive to the various ways in which individual members may be using reminiscence during group meetings.
- Contribute to research by evaluating the extent to which a group has met its objectives.

This summary of the many objectives or functions served by reminiscence is provided to assist group leaders to clarify the objectives for any group and to assist in planning a program that serves the agreed objectives; defining and evaluating outcomes will then be possible.

Leading Reminiscence Groups

It is not possible to become an effective reminiscence worker if you are uncomfortable with or unwilling to reminisce; therefore, it is essential that experiential reminiscence be included in any reminiscence leadership training. One such exercise undertaken in pairs invites participants initially to share memories (the suggestion of a topic or theme accelerates the process) and then to reflect upon this experience of recall within the larger group. This helps students to identify their own reactions and the feelings that are stimulated by reminiscence so they may better understand some of the meaning, significance, and possible obstacles reminiscence holds for older adults. It is important when learning to lead reminiscence groups that students have a supervisor or mentor (see Chapter 30). Students should be encouraged to keep a log and records of group process designed to encourage critical review and reflection of their group work experience.

Young group leaders doing reminiscence work may need to learn something about historical events related to the times through which group members have lived. Gibson (2004) provides a quick reference age chart and a time line of the 1900s that enables individual people's personal life experience to be mapped to corresponding public, social, and historical events. Making such connections enables people as they reminisce to locate themselves within a wider historical context and to appreciate how their lives are interwoven with the lives of other people, and national and international events.

Leaders need to take considerable care when planning reminiscence groups, bearing in mind that just like other groups, they move through preliminary, beginning, middle, and ending stages (Gibson, 1998). Time-limited closed reminiscence groups of approximately 10–12 members, meeting weekly for 8–12 sessions is the most typical. Allowing a two-hour time slot allows for members to gather, reminisce, enjoy refreshments, socialize informally, and disperse. Many variations are also used.

Whenever possible, leaders should meet potential members individually beforehand to collect background information and to undertake preliminary contracting. This means that the leader needs to consider whether the intended group will have open or closed membership, when, where, and for how long it will meet, and what are its objectives (Bender, Baukham, & Norris, 1999). Except for the first meeting when the leader chooses the theme on the basis of information gathered in the initial interviews, the ongoing program will form part of sessional contracting. Forward planning is undertaken as part of the ending work of each session. The responsibility of the leader is to ensure that the program is agreed to, and to lend assistance to ensure that what the group intends is carried through.

Themes and Topics

There is no single best way to structure a reminiscence group's program. The guiding principle is to begin with the life experience of the members and help them to identify what they would like to talk about, bearing in mind age, cultural, educational, ethnic, and gender differences. Themes or topics are often selected using a chronological life span framework, for example, childhood, adolescence, young adulthood, middle age, and old age as in a structured life review with an individual. An alternative approach concentrates on one period of life, as in childhood, and explores various related subjects, such as friends and family; toys and games; school; and special holidays and outings. School is usually a productive theme although not always remembered as the happiest days of our lives. People recall achievements and disappointments; teachers loved and feared; favorite and dreaded lessons; friends and enemies; escapades and triumphs. Themes may explore the seasons and related activities, hobbies, favorite or personally significant places, memorable trips, special days and events, cherished possessions, family sayings, poems, songs, clothing, meals, tools, homes and gardens, pets, and much loved cars.

Themes and topics need to encourage group members to reconsider, or think again, about both time and place as well as the people, events, and emotions aroused by these recollections (Chaudhury, 2003; Lawton, 2003).

Capuzzi and Gross (1998) recommend that chosen topics should explore both positive and negative aspects but that they should be sequenced to elicit happy memories in the early sessions, then in later sessions, once trust and confidence have developed, memories of conflicts, regrets, and sadness can be explored. In the beginning sessions, topics should be general, "safe," and likely to be within the known experience of all the members. By the middle stage of a group, members will feel sufficiently confident to share sad memories, and more reflective, evaluative discussion will take place.

All memories come wrapped in emotions, and acknowledging and validating the emotional component is as important as listening to the content of the stories told. Open ended topics need to be balanced with specific topics, as it is usually in the recollection of detail that the most personally significant integration of memories and social exchanges occur. As confidence and trust develop, the members will risk exploring more problematic experiences, providing they feel their stories will be accepted and they will be respected.

Props and Triggers

The terms *props* or *triggers* refer to anything that is used to elicit memories. A trigger may be anything that stimulates the senses of sight, sound, touch, taste, and smell. Visual and auditory triggers abound. Music is instantaneously evocative. Common everyday objects (do not use grand or valuable antiques) require members to interact with each other as they handle them and pass them around. Tastes and smells provide endless opportunities to recall associated circumstances and personally significant places and people. The more closely props and triggers reflect the life experience of the members, the more evocative they are likely to be. Personal cherished objects

brought to group meetings by members are likely to have spatial, temporal, and symbolic meaning for their owners. "Objects that represent relationships with others, particularly in the past, are more likely to be more meaningful to older women than to older men. Objects that represent a sense of self, and personal achievement are more likely to resonate with older men than older women" (Chapman, 2003, p. 104). All triggers should be:

- Age appropriate—The prop will be familiar to a certain age cohort.
- Culturally appropriate—The prop will be familiar to members of certain ethnic groups.
- Gender appropriate—The prop will appeal to the gender of the group, or if there are both men and women in a group, it will appeal to both.
- Geographically appropriate—The prop pertains to the geographic region, in which most of the group members live, lived, or visited.

Triggers are not essential, but they can speed up recall in the beginning phase and help members to participate in the discussion. We respond to sensory stimuli in different ways. Some of us will respond immediately to known preferred music (Clair, 2001), others respond more readily to smells, tastes, or touch; it is sensible to use various triggers in sequence. Pet animals and small children, especially babies, make excellent props and usually arouse curiosity, pleasure, and many personal memories.

Photographs can be projected or, providing they are large and clear, they can be held up or passed around a group one at a time so as not to fragment the discussion. If people have impaired vision, then it is obviously sensible not to rely on visual stimuli alone. Old photographs (and other props) may be highly treasured, and the leader will need to ensure that they are not lost or damaged. Many commercial trigger packages are also available.

If using modern information and communication technology and audiovisual equipment to project images, reproduce sounds, or record stories, make sure you have mastered the technology before the session begins. Always regard any technical aid, equipment, or trigger as a servant, not a master. Be prepared to turn the equipment off or not use a trigger, even if you have taken a lot of trouble to obtain it. As a leader you must be fully available to people. Your main role is to listen and facilitate exchange between the group members. It is not to tell, teach, show, or educate them.

Reminiscing in a group quickly becomes a cumulative experience. One person's recalled memories and actions help other members to recall. Whole poems, songs, hymns, rhymes, and games can also be recovered as each person's partial recall assists someone else to add a fragment so that the group experiences enormous satisfaction from their pooled memories. Questions such as "What were you doing when?" readily elicit recall. Pearl Harbor, the assassinations of President Kennedy or Martin Luther King, and 9/11 are all such iconic national events with related personal implications and associations. One commonly hears the phrase "That reminds me of ..." and the purpose of using triggers is to do just that.

Although it is important to have a plan, all plans can go astray or may need to be renegotiated, modified, or sometimes even abandoned. Flexibility is important. Possible reasons for a theme not eliciting reminiscence could be:

- The theme insufficiently reflects the age, background, gender, ethnicity, or experience of the group members.
- There is something urgent to discuss that takes priority over the selected theme (for example, a natural disaster, an important news item, or an unexpected happening near at hand).
- The leader may be uninterested, tentative, or ignorant about the theme and may have trouble stimulating reminiscence.

Recall of Sad Memories

The mood within reminiscence groups can quickly change from laughter to tears and from tears to laughter, depending upon the memories recalled and the associated emotions aroused. Painful recall will be inevitable. People are often surprised when very distant memories are evoked. Groups demonstrate their capacity for providing mutual aid and healing as past pain is shared and people feel that their experience is being heard. Telling, perhaps for the first time, and surviving the telling and hearing strengthen everyone present. The leader does not carry the burden of listening alone. The group becomes the source of support and assistance, providing the leader is sufficiently confident to let the stories be told and heard, and sufficiently skilled to encourage the members empathetically to connect with one another and with their own past experience.

Reminiscence Groups for People with Dementia

Reminiscence is an enjoyable and accessible intervention for people with early and moderate dementia (see also Chapter 11). Groups need to be very small, often with two to four members unless multiple helpers make considerable individual attention possible (Bruce, Hodgson, & Schweitzer, 1999). The program should favor nonverbal communication and use relevant multisensory triggers. Careful selection of members and detailed preparation is essential. Practice experience suggests that it is wise to exclude habitually aggressive, hyperactive, tearful, deeply depressed, or hostile people. They may, however, benefit greatly from individual work. Obsessional reminiscers who constantly rehearse the same memory may be better helped by diversional activities. Because long-term memories survive relatively intact long after short-term memory is impaired, reminiscence can assist communication, preserve relationships, and provide a sense of achievement, pleasure, and camaraderie. The major objectives should be to provide pleasurable opportunities for social and intellectual stimulation, and shared participation, pitched within the range of competence of the members. Reminding people who they used to be and the past roles they fulfilled may assist identity preservation.

Some adaptations are essential. The length and frequency of sessions will probably need adjusting to match mood and energy levels. Warm, uncritical acceptance is preeminent. No one should be set up to fail, so it is crucial to use themes and props that are relevant to the life experience of members of the group. The same guidance about issuing invitations, seeking consent or assent, and treating people with respect, courtesy, and warm appreciation applies.

More time may be needed in the beginning phase to allay anxiety and establish trust. Structure and ritual provide security, so the beginnings and endings of all sessions should use the same format. Leaders should seek to respond to the emotional content of a contribution and be less concerned with establishing factual content, veracity, or correct chronology. Respond to the expressed mood of communications and give opportunities for people to show what they can still do and enjoy, rather than emphasizing what they have lost and can no longer do.

Reminiscing with people with dementia and their family members either as couples or in small groups can remind people of past good times. It can preserve relationships, provide present enjoyment, lessen isolation, and assist communication (Parker, 1995, 1999; Kurokawa, 1998; Bruce, Hodgson, & Schweitzer, 1999; Haight, Bachman, Hendrix, & Wagner, 2003).

Workers must set realistic goals, slow down to mirror the group's pace, and anticipate that there will be variable performance by individuals within sessions and between sessions. They must actively initiate conversation and action. Triggers that appeal to more than one sense are most effec-

tive and need to be used sparingly so that people will not feel overloaded. They are used for cueing responses and as a means for achieving inclusion of all members. The entire program should provide ample opportunities for engagement in varied activities that utilize long-term implicit procedural memory and residual cognitive-linguistic skills (Gibson, 2004; Harris & Norman, 2002).

Practice Examples

Reda, a graduate student (Soltys, Reda, & Letson, 2002), described a group for four men whose ages ranged from 82–87. The 10 decades of the last century provided the structure for 10 weekly sessions and elicited recollections of wartime interests, major sporting figures, presidents—their legislation and achievements—and favorite automobiles. Reda reported that the group was fun, that it provided social stimulation, and achieved intergenerational communication. Perlstein and Bliss (2003) and McCrea and Smith (1997) describe other projects in which reminiscence and the arts are used to address intergenerational, personal, and community concerns.

Informal reminiscing in natural groupings in residential facilities also has a valued place (McKee, Wilson, Elford, & Goudie, 2003). Older people reported how much they appreciated conversations that occurred spontaneously with staff. Such informal exchanges, often but not invariably with reminiscence content, are too readily dismissed as "just chatting." Owners and managers of residential facilities must recognize the importance of caregivers having time to talk. Talking affirms each person's individuality and confirms their membership in a vibrant living community.

Death preparation is an important reason for reminiscing for many isolated or very old people or younger people whose health status is seriously threatened. Reminiscence also plays a large part in bereavement support groups. Participants often bring photographs, videos, music, artwork, and other memorabilia to meetings to share memories of their lost person with other members (Huart & O'Donnell, 1993).

Soltys, Reda, and Letson (2002) described using telemedicine conferencing via a two-way audio and video link (Perednia & Ace, 1995) to conduct reminiscence groups with patients, some with mild or moderate dementia, in a rural community hospital and a health clinic. The elders had no difficulty in sharing their life stories in this way, and the tapes of sessions were much appreciated by the families after their relatives' deaths. Soltys et al. also used reminiscence as a vehicle for encouraging groups of seven to nine African-American nursing home elders to explore with health providers and family members their life experiences, belief systems, values, and concerns related to end-of-life issues. "The group structure provides a method for members to put into perspective important events in their lives, to bring closure to many issues, and often brings gratification and resolution concerning past events" (Soltys et al., 2002, p. 60). The tapes became sources of information to assist decision making in lieu of advance directives. Identified gains for people participating in these groups were improved self-esteem, improved perceived quality of life, social support, changed perspectives on how individuals see their lives, and closure. Soltys et al. believed the groups were cost effective and that facilitators improved their professional skills as agents of social change, and acquired enhanced appreciation of history.

General Characteristics of Reminiscence Group Work

1. Some residential and day service facilities have created special reminiscence rooms furnished and decorated in the style of the forties, fifties, or sixties. These are comfortable, secure, and friendly spaces, free from noisy distraction, in which reminiscence is readily stimulated. Patients, residents, staff, and visitors all find them interesting and attractive spaces in which to spend time. Reminiscence gardens are also popular.

2. Reminiscence groups are relatively easy and inexpensive to implement. Refreshments are very important, and triggers and equipment may need to be purchased. When planning a group, identify potential expenses, prepare a budget, and identify funding sources.

3. Reminiscence is an excellent tool for learning how to relate to older people as unique, intriguing individuals. It is an excellent way of challenging ageism in students and stimulating their curiosity about aging processes and older people.

4. Using triggers related to past times and places can enhance the process. They can also be a means for involving families in sharing recollections. Triggers which stimulate personal recall provide a focus for conversation which enriches family visits.

5. Reminiscence can contribute to assessment and care planning because it identifies lifetime behaviors and the values and priorities that people believe are important.

6. Elders can be superb teachers. Learning history directly from people who have lived it brings history alive. Leaders must be willing to accept the learner role and help the older person to feel comfortable in the teacher role. This role reversal challenges the established power relationships that customarily exist in health and social care professions and the facilities that employ them.

7. New leaders often get preoccupied in trying to determine if the memories being shared are actually true. This should not be a concern as there are many versions of the one story and all memories, including our own, are partial reconstructions. Appreciating the significance to the teller is more important than challenging veracity.

8. There are innumerable ways of turning reminiscences into tangible products that are greatly valued by the people who create them as well as by others (Gibson, 2004). This allows for continuing enjoyment and stimulates other people to reminisce.

9. Reminiscence provides an easy bridge into other creative activities (Perlstein & Bliss, 2003).

10. Young group leaders may experience countertransference. Sometimes the youthful leader is inhibited in their role because "The person reminds me of my grandmother and I feel I should be respectful." Or the group member may treat the leader as a grandchild, niece, or nephew.

11. Reminiscence groups for people with dementia require effort, patience, and a need to settle for small but rewarding gains.

12. The benefits and rewards of listening to reminiscences are often ignored. People who are prepared to listen are enriched in many ways. They gain knowledge and understanding about the older person and the period in which they lived. It connects the past with the present and the generations with each other.

Summary

This chapter presented a brief literature review and historical perspective on reminiscence group work. It outlined various formulations of the functions served by reminiscence, including Webster's Reminiscence Functions Scale. It described how to work with a reminiscence group and the modifications required to enable people who have dementia to participate. Multisensory props, triggers, and themes, important adjuncts to reminiscence groups, were suggested and the importance of triggers being appropriate in terms of age, geographical location, gender, culture, and ethnicity was emphasized. Reminiscence group work is widely—although not universally—acceptable, usually very enjoyable, and is an excellent means for linking older people with others of various ages, and developing and preserving relationships with staff and family members.

Exercises

EXERCISE 1

Close your eyes. Think about a memory that is important to you. Then analyze all the senses that are involved in this memory. Which sense do you think is the most important? Do the same exercise with an older person and compare and contrast your memory of the senses involved with those the older person describes to you.

EXERCISE 2

Plan a small reminiscence group for residents of a nursing home who are physically frail. When you have listed ideas concerning the why, what, how, when, where, and with whom concerning this group, identify how you might adapt this plan for a group of residents who have dementia. Similarities and differences are more easily identified if you present your work in two parallel columns, one for each group. Identify what you have learned from this exercise.

EXERCISE 3

Establish a small reminiscence group and try out the following: Ask members in turn to walk you through the house where they grew up (or a significant place where they once lived). Ask them to explore a room at a time, identifying familiar furniture, noticing views from the windows and remembering where they slept or where food was prepared. The above exercise can be extended or modified in many ways to suit the interests of the group members. It could be focused on remembering what was on a shelf or in a cupboard in the kitchen, what was kept in the garage, what the yard contained. The recall of place intersects with the recall of associated time past and occurs in time present. This exercise could be developed into an outing or excursion where a visit to a school, church, graveyard, or the local shops might be undertaken and opportunities provided for talking about similar places of past personal significance. Reflect on what worked best and for whom and what difficulties were encountered.

References

Bender, M., Baukham, P., & Norris, A. (1999). *The therapeutic purposes of reminiscence.* London: Sage.

Berman-Rossi, T. (2002). My love affair with stages of group development. *Social Work with Groups, 25*(1/2), 149–152.

Bornat, J., Chamberlyne, P., Chant, L., & Pavey, S. (1998). *Redefining reminiscence in care settings.* London: Open University and University of East London.

Brooker, D. J. R., & Duce, L. (2000). Well–being and activity in dementia: A comparison of group reminiscence therapy, structured goal-directed activity and unstructured time. *Ageing & Mental Health, 4,* 356–360.

Bruce, E., Hodgson, S., & Schweitzer, P. (1999). *Reminiscing with people with dementia: A handbook for carers.* London: Age Exchange.

Burnside, I. (1995). Themes and props: Adjuncts for reminiscence therapy groups. In B. K. Haight & J. D. Webster (Eds.), *The art and science of reminiscing: Theory, research, methods and applications* (pp. 153–163). Washington, DC: Taylor & Francis.

Butler, R. (1963). The life review: An interpretation of reminiscence in the aged. *Psychiatry, 26,* 65–76.

Butler, R. (2001). The life review. *Journal of Geriatric Psychiatry, 35*(1), 7–10.

Cappeliez, P. (2003, October). A theory on the contributions of reminiscence to self-concept maintenance, emotional regulation, and experience-based coping (pp. 58–62). Selected conference papers and proceedings of the International Reminiscence and Life Review Conference sponsored by the University of Wisconsin-Superior and held in Vancouver, BC.

Cappeliez, P., Lavallee, R., & O'Rourke, N. (2001). Functions of reminiscence in later life as viewed by young and old adults. *Canadian Journal on Aging, 20*(4), 577–589.

Capuzzi, D., & Gross, D. R. (1998). *Introduction to group counseling.* Denver: Love.

Chandler, S., & Ray, R. (2002). New meanings for old tales: A discourse-based study of reminiscence and development in late life. In J. D. Webster & B. K. Haight (Eds.), *Critical advances in reminiscence work: From theory to application* (pp. 76–94). New York: Springer.

Chapman, S. A. (2003, October). Aging well: Cherished objects as windows on meaning (pp. 103–104). Selected conference papers and proceedings of the International Reminiscence and Life Review Conference sponsored by the University of Wisconsin-Superior and held in Vancouver, BC.

Chaudrey, H. (2003). Quality of life and place-therapy. In R. J. Scheidt, P. G. Windley (Eds.), *Physical environments and aging: Critical contributions of M. Powell Lawton to theory and practice* (pp. 85–103). Binghamton, NY: Haworth Press.

Clair, A. (2001). *Therapeutic uses of music with older adults.* Baltimore: Health Professions Press.

Clarke, A., Hanson, E. J., & Ross, H. (2003). Seeing the person behind the patient: Enhancing the care of older people using a biographical approach. *Journal of Clinical Nursing, 12,* 697–706.

Cohen, G., & Taylor, S. (1998). Reminiscence and ageing. *Ageing and Society, 18*(5), 601–610.

Cole, T. R., & De Medeioros, K. (2000, October). Elder writings: The making of stories and souls (pp. 26–31). Selected conference papers and proceedings of the International Reminiscence and Life Review Conference sponsored by the University of Wisconsin-Superior and held in Vancouver, BC.

Coleman, P. G. (1974). Measuring reminiscence characteristics from conversation. *International Journal of Aging and Human Development, 5,* 281–294.

Coleman, P. G. (1986). *Ageing and reminiscence processes: Social and clinical implications.* New York: Wiley.

De Vries, B. & Watt, D. (1996). A lifetime of events: Age and gender variations in the life story. *International Journal of Aging and Human Development, 42*(2), 81–102.

Dunn, P. H., Haight, B.K., & Hendrix, S. (2002). Power dynamics in the interpersonal life review dyad. *International Journal of Geriatric Psychiatry, 35*(1), 77–93.

Erwin, K. T. (1996). Group techniques for aging adults. Washington, DC: Taylor & Francis.

Garland, J., & Garland, C. (2001). *Life review in health and social care: A practitioner's guide.* Washington, DC: Brunner-Routledge.

Gibson, F. (1998). Reminiscence and recall (2nd ed.). London: ACE Books.

Gibson, F. (2004). *The past in the present: Using reminiscence in health and social care.* Baltimore: Health Professions Press.

Gwyther, L. P. (1999). The perspective of the person with Alzheimer's disease: Which outcomes matter in early to middle stages of dementia. *Alzheimer's Disease and Related Disorders, 11*(1, Suppl. 6), 18–24.

Habermas, T., & Bluck, S. (2000). Getting a life: The emergence of life story in adolescence. *Psychological Bulletin, 126*(5), 749–769.

Haight, B. K. (1991). Reminiscing: The state of the art as a basis for practice. *International Journal of Aging and Human Development, 33*, 1–32.

Haight, B. K., Bachman, D. L., Hendrix, S., Wagner, M. T., Meeks, A., & Johnson, J. (2003). Life review: Treating the dyadic family unit with dementia. *Clinical Psychology and Psychotherapy, 10*, 1–10.

Haight, B. K., Coleman, P. G., & Lord, K. (1995). The linchpins of a successful life review: Structure, evaluation and individuality. In B. K. Haight & J. D. Webster (Eds.), *The art and science of reminiscence: Theory, research, methods and applications* (pp.179–192). Washington, DC: Taylor & Francis.

Haight, B. K., & Hendrix, S. (1995). An integrated review of reminiscence. In B. K. Haight & J. D. Webster (Eds.), *The art and science of reminiscing: Theory, research, methods, and applications* (pp. 3–9). Washington, DC: Taylor & Francis.

Hansebo, G., & Kihlgren, M. (2000). Patient life stories and current situations as told by carers in nursing home wards. *Clinical Nursing Research, 9*(3), 260–279.

Hendrix, S., & Haight, B. K. (2002). A continued review of reminiscence. In J. D. Webster & B. K. Haight (Eds.), *Critical advances in reminiscence work: From theory to application* (pp. 3–29). New York: Springer.

Harris, J. L., & Norman, M. L. (2002). Reframing reminiscence as a cognitive-linguistic phenomenon. In J. D. Webster & B. K. Haight (Eds.), *Critical advances in reminiscence work: From theory to application* (pp. 95–105). New York: Springer.

Hill, H. (2001). *Invitation to the dance: Dance for people with dementia and their carers.* Stirling: University of Stirling, Dementia Services Development Centre.

Huart, S., & O'Donnell, M. (1993). The road to recovery from grief and bereavement. *Caring, 12*(11), 71–75.

Johnson, P., Beckerman, A., & Auerbach, C. (2001). Researching our own practice: Single system design for group work. *Groupwork, 13*(1), 57–72.

Kaminsky, M. (1984). *The uses of reminiscence: New ways of working with older adults.* Binghamton, NY: Haworth Press.

Kazi, M. A. (1998). *Single case evaluation by social workers.* Brookfield, VT: Ashgate Press.

Koch, K. (1977). *I never told anybody.* New York: Random House.

Kurokawa, Y. (1998). Couple reminiscence with Japanese dementia patients and their spouses. In P. Schweitzer (Ed.), *Reminiscence in dementia care* (pp.108–112). London: Age Exchange.

Lawton, M. P. (20003). Chance and choice make a good life. In J. E. Birren & J. F. Schoots (Eds.), *A history of geropsychology in autobiography* (pp. 185–196). Washington, DC: American Psychological Association.

Lo Gerfo, M. (1980. Three ways of reminiscence in theory and practice. *International Journal of Aging and Human Development, 12*(1) 39–48.

Martin, C. W., & Younger, D. (2000). Anti-oppressive practice: A route to the empowerment of people with dementia through communication and choice. *Journal of Psychiatric Mental Health Nursing, 7*, 59–67.

McCrea, J. M., & Smith, T. B. (1997). Types and models of intergenerational programs. In S. Newman et al. *Intergenerational programs: Past, present and future* (pp. 81–93). Washington, DC: Taylor & Francis.

McKee, K., Wilson, F., Elford, H., Goudie, F., Chung, M C., Bolton, G., et al.(2003). *Evaluating the impact of reminiscence on the quality of life of older people.* ESRC Report. University of Sheffield.

McMahon, A. W. & Rhudick, P. J. (1964). Reminiscence: Adaptational significance in the aged. *Archives of General Psychiatry, 10*, 292–298.

Merriam, S. B. (1980). The concept and function of reminiscence: A review of the research. *The Gerontologist, 20*, 604–609.

Merriam, S. B. (1989). The structure of simple reminiscence. *The Gerontologist, 29*(6), 761–767.

Merriam, S. B. (1993). Butler's life review: How universal is it? *International Journal of Aging and Human Development, 37*(3), 163–175.

Molinari, V. & Reichelin, R. (1984). Life review reminiscence in the elderly: A review of the literature. *International Journal of Aging and Human Development, 20*, 81–92.

Parker, R. G. (1995). Reminiscence: A continuity theory framework. *The Gerontologist, 34*, 515–525.

Parker, R. G. (1999). Reminiscence as continuity: Comparison of young and older adults. *Journal of Clinical Geropsychology, 5*, 147–357.

Pear, T. H. (1922). *Remembering and forgetting.* London: Methuen.

Perednia, D. A., & Ace, A. (1995). Telemedicine technology and clinical applications. *Journal of American Medical Association, 273*(6), 483–488.

Perlstein, S., & Bliss, J. (2003). *Generating community: Intergenerational partnerships through the expressive arts.* New York: Elders Share the Arts.

Puentes, W. J. (2002). Simple reminiscence: A stress-adaptation model of the phenomenon. *Issues in Mental Health Nursing, 23*, 497–511.

Randal, W., & Kenyon, G. (2001). *Ordinary wisdom: Biographical aging and the journey of life.* Westport, CT: Praeger.

Rentz, C. (2002). Memories in the making: Outcome-based evaluation of an art program for individuals with dementia illnesses. *American Journal of Alzheimer's Disease, 17*(3), 175–181.

Sim, R. (1997). *Reminiscence: Social and creative activities.* Bicester, UK: Winslow Press.

Soltys, F. G., Reda, S., & Letson, M. (2002). Use of the group process for reminiscence. *Journal of Geriatric Psychiatry, 35*(1), 50–61.

Spector, A., Orrell, M., Davies, S., & Woods, R. T. (2000). *Reminiscence therapy for dementia.* The Cochrane Library, 1

Stelson, C. B., & Dauk-Bleess, R. (2003, October). Lasting memories: An intergenerational writing project in the elementary classroom with implications for reminiscence and life review work with elders (pp. 40–45). Selected conference papers and proceedings of the International Reminiscence and Life Review Conference sponsored by the University of Wisconsin-Superior and held in Vancouver, BC.

Watt, L. M., & Wong, P. T. P. (1991). A taxonomy of reminiscence and therapeutic implications. *Journal of Gerontological Social Work, 16*(1/2), 37–57.

Webster, J. D., (1993). Construction and validation of the Reminiscence Functions Scale. *Journal of Gerontology, 48*(5), 256–262.

Webster, J. D., (1997). The Reminiscence Functions Scale: A replication. *International Journal of Aging and Human Development, 44*(2), 137–148.

Webster, J. D., & Haight, B. K. (2002). *Critical advances in reminiscence work: From theory to application.* New York: Springer.

Webster, J. D., & McCall, M. E. (1999). Reminiscence functions across adulthood: A replication and extension. *Journal of Adult Development, 6*, 73–85.

Wong, P. T. P., & Watt, L. M. (1991). What types of reminiscence are associated with successful aging? *Psychology of Aging, 6*(2), 272–279.

Activity and Training Products

Memories in the Making, a manual and 8-minute video and lesson plans are available from the Alzheimer's Society of Orange County, California. Shows how to encourage creative art expression for people with Alzheimer's and related disorders. (714) 283-1984, ext. 42. Available at *www.alz.org*

Reminiscence: Finding Meaning in Memories. The program trains volunteers to use memory recall, communication, and visiting skills to help older adults get in touch with meaningful, significant past experiences and improve their feelings of self-worth. For more information, contact Program Coordinator, Social Outreach and Support, American Association of Retired Persons, 601 E Street NW, Washington, DC 20049; (202) 434-2260.

Reminiscence Trainer's Pack. Gibson, F. (2000). London UK: Age Concern Books. The pack contains 12 lesson plans, photocopiable trainer's and student's notes, slides, and detailed experiential exercises suitable for training students, health and social care staff, museum workers, librarians, arts workers, volunteers, and family caregivers in reminiscence work with individuals and small groups. Covers training for reminiscing with people from various cultural and ethnic backgrounds, and those with learning disabilities, dementia, and sensory and speech impairments. Available at *www.ageconcern.org.uk/shop*

FILMS

Life Stories is a film about writing workshops for older people. It is available from New River Media at *www.nrmedia.com*

The Joys and Surprises of Telling Your Life Story is a 40-minute educational video. It is available from International Reminiscence and Life Review Institute, c/o John Kunz, 102 Main, Center for Continuing Education/Extension, Belknap & Catlin, PO Box 2000, University of Wisconsin-Superior, Superior, WI 54880; (715) 394-8529. *jkunz@staff.uwsuper.edu*

Chapter 15

Guided Autobiography Groups

James E. Birren
Donna E. Deutchman

Key Words

- Adaptation
- Autobiography
- Developmental exchange
- Generativity
- Integration
- Intergenerational programs
- Legacy
- Life review
- Older adults
- Sensitization
- Thematic approach

Learning Objectives

- Understand the value of the autobiographical process, particularly for older adults
- Distinguish *guided* autobiography from other forms of reminiscence
- Design a guided autobiography group around a chosen purpose
- Understand the importance of the group process in guided autobiography, and list ways to promote the developmental exchange
- List themes that are most salient for autobiographical review, and describe the sensitization process

Guided autobiography is designed to promote successful adaptation to old age and to assist persons in life transition to make positive choices. In an intergenerational context, it promotes *generativity*, a key developmental need of older adults. It combines individual and group experiences with autobiography, incorporating group interaction and leadership to sensitize people to recall the most salient issues of their lives and expand their private reflections. It requires the writing of two-page reminiscences or life stories on selected life themes, and reading these life stories and sharing thoughts about them in a mutually encouraging group, moderated by a group leader.

Guided autobiography creates an environment that provides the social support and mental stimulation for older adults to review their life stories and share them with others. Using strategies to both ensure positive group experiences and to sensitize group members to the significant themes of life, leaders can help older adults develop a heightened sense of self-awareness, social acceptance, and self-esteem. Through the process of guided autobiography, older adults can integrate their experiences and come to terms with their lives as they have been led. As a result, they become better prepared to meet changes and new demands with increased confidence and competence.

Everyone needs to feel important in some way, and older adults search for evidence that their lives have mattered, that there has been some purpose or impact on the world. From a human development viewpoint, there is little of greater importance to each of us as we age than gaining an insightful perspective on our own life story, to clarify, deepen, and find meaning in the accumulated experience of a lifetime (Butler, 2002; Birren & Deutchman, 1991; Shaw, 2001). Guided autobiography is an effective way to help older adults build greater understanding and self-worth. "The strength of life review lies in its ability to help promote life satisfaction, psychological well-being, and self-esteem" (Butler, 2002).

In guided autobiography, participants typically write and share with the guided autobiography group nine separate two-page autobiographical life stories. Themes are chosen that elicit powerful recollections of experience and related feelings. A prototypical array of themes is as follows:

- History of the major branching points in life
- History of the family
- History of career or major life work
- History of the role of money in life
- History of health and body image
- History of loves and hates
- History of sexual identity, sex roles, and sexual experiences
- History of experiences with death and ideas about dying
- History of aspirations and life goals and the meaning of life

Additional themes may be added or used as replacements depending on the nature and major purpose of the specific autobiography group, particularly for groups brought together on the basis of similar history or current life crisis.

The typical guided autobiography group meets a minimum of 10 times for at least two hours each time. Meetings consist of the members reading and discussing the theme assigned for that day's meeting and a discussion of the theme that forms the writing assignment for the next meeting. Because the sharing of life stories at the group meetings stimulates further recall and interaction, each written story is restricted to about two pages. This allows enough time for each member to read his or her statement and permits the opportunity for group feedback. Also, the two-page limit is a device to get the participants to focus on key elements of their life stories.

Benefits of Guided Autobiography

Guided autobiography is an efficient program for older adults to review their lives, using a proven series of themes and questions. The group leader uses these themes and sensitizing questions to create a road map, guiding persons interested in developing greater self-awareness toward recovering and integrating the memories and emotions most relevant to future decisions, the development of greater self-esteem, and the transmission of family history. Guided autobiography can make a positive difference in the quality of older adults' remaining years. Also, when it results in a written account, it can create an important legacy for others in the individual's family.

There is a rich literature base that grows out of research conducted to assess the consequences of life review, reminiscence, and the autobiographical process, a form of which is guided autobiography. This research has helped to clarify important outcomes and to highlight benefits for mature adults. The method of guided autobiography is designed to optimize these potential outcomes of life review. **Table 15–1** summarizes some of this research.

Integration, Fulfillment, and a Sense of Competence

In keeping with the developmental theories of such scholars as Buhler and Massarik (1968),

Figure 15–1 A POTENTIAL GROUP FOR AUTOBIOGRAPHY

This photograph portrays some of the guidelines offered in this chapter: (a) refreshments shared, (b) written accounts by members to share, and (c) use of a table. All of these factors are important to a guided autobiography group.
© Keith Brofsky/Photodisc/Getty Images

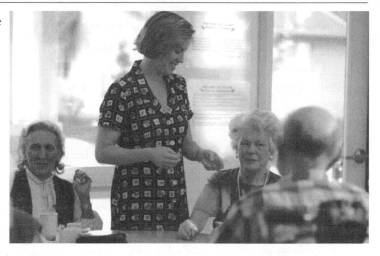

Erikson (1963), and Levinson (1978), later adulthood is viewed as a time for integration—resolution and acceptance of one's identity being key to mental and emotional well-being. Guided autobiography can play a vital role in this process. Research by Butler (2002); Porter (1998); Shaw, Westwood, and deVries (1999); and Schroots (1996) supports this view. A positive relationship has been found between the amount of reminiscence and the degree of ego integrity (or self-integration) achieved. *Reminiscence* is defined here as the process of recalling past events, a process on which the more structured guided autobiography is built. It is important to note that the relationship between reminiscence and ego integrity, and the positive outcome it implies for self-acceptance, is found even when memories of past experiences are painful or negative.

It is important to an older adult to be able to resolve old conflicts and feelings of ambivalence and to integrate his or her life as it is perceived to have been lived in relation to what was once possible or expected. The older adult must reconcile the past with present expectations and goals; this is particularly important in later life, as opportunities for altering the life course may be limited. Guided autobiography offers a chance for the older adult to reconcile the past and the legacy he or she will leave behind, modify future plans, and reaffirm past and present values and goals, deriving a feeling of completeness, of fulfillment in life (Birren & Deutchman, 1991; Shaw, 2001; Shaw, Westwood, & deVries, 1999). The group of older people in Figure 15–1 would benefit greatly from participating in an autobiographical group.

The guided autobiography process is not designed as a form of therapy. It is not problem centered. It is not actively directed toward the cure or amelioration of particular diseases or particular problems. Its therapeutic value is a by-product of that which occurs naturally and should only be purposefully harvested by the seasoned professional therapist.

In guided autobiography, older adults relive and recall a wide range of personal experiences. A feeling of significance is generally derived from reviewing the life course as a whole. In summing up the experiences of a lifetime, people are frequently surprised by their own ability and how much they have survived and transcended. Reactions of the group often support a person's perception and provide a sense that the ability to adjust or overcome the hardships of life is a formidable accomplishment. Insights of the group leader and other members can facilitate this process and smooth the road to greater understanding of the

Table 15–1   BENEFITS OF LIFE REVIEW: AN OVERVIEW OF RESEARCH FINDINGS

Area of benefit	Focus of study/article	Authors
Acceptance of death	Dying persons	Butler, 2002 Masai-Jones, 2001
Coping/adaptation	Older adults	Tabourne, 1995(a) (b) Wink & Schiff, 2002
	At-risk students (youth)	Cochrum-Murphy, 2001
Depression relief	Older adults Nursing home residents	Gatz et al., 1999 Cappeliez, 2002 Haight, Michel, & Hendrix, 2000
	Persons with AIDS	Erlin et al., 2001
Generativity	Older persons	Coleman, Hautamaki, & Podolskij, 2002

Integration	Older adults	Haight, Coleman,
		  & Lord, 1995
		Porter, 1998
		Schroots, 1996
		Shaw, Westwood,
		  & deVries, 1999

	All ages	Erikson, 1963
Interpersonal connections	Persons with early to moderate dementia	Godley & Gatz, 2000
Meaning in life	Dying persons	Masai-Jones, 2001
Reconciliation and resolution of past	Middle-aged women	Hartman, 2001
Role clarity	Older adults	deVries, Birren, & Deutchman, 1994 Gaden, 1996
Self-esteem	All ages Older adults	Allport, 1942 Porter, 1998 Tabourne, 1995(a) (b)
	Nursing home residents	Haight, Michel, & Hendrix, 2000
Self-actualization	Older adults	Kenyon, Clark, & Phillip, 2001
Spiritual well-being	Older adults	Eliason, 2001 McFadden, Brennan, & Patrick, 2003
Well-being	Older adults	Peck, 2001 Richeson & Thorson, 2002

self. Renewed confidence in one's adaptive capacity and increased understanding of one's personal agenda often form the basis from which successful future choices can be made.

Related to the subject of planning is the perception of the role of chance in a person's life. Just as an inventory of successful strategies can provide increased confidence in one's ability to meet new demands, an understanding of how chance events have helped to shape the life course can have a freeing quality. Insight into the influencing factors that have been outside of our control can help focus attention on adaptive capacities and strength in the face of hardship.

Adaptation to Old Age

The ability to take an inventory of the adaptive strategies used successfully over the life course is an important resource in late life as people are faced with many changes. Guided autobiography helps in coping with problems of old age as well as integrating early life experiences. As research points out, guided autobiography may: (a) help maintain self-esteem and allay anxiety provoked by physical and intellectual decline (Peck, 2001); (b) lead to a reorganization of personality and a fuller acceptance of one's life cycle (Birren, Kenyon, Ruth, Schroots, & Svensson 1996); (c) further interpersonal relationships and provide a means by which older people can share their knowledge of the past (Gaden, 1996; Tabourne, 1995a); and (d) help old people cope with grief and depression resulting from personal losses and achieve a heightened sense of subjective well-being (Peck, 2001; Porter, 1998; Richeson & Thorson 2002).

If a person is able to affirm and accept the contents of life and the continuity of his or her identity, the late life task of integration is advanced. In addition to highlighting the capacity for adaptation, guided autobiography reveals ways in which a person has maintained continuity throughout life. This continuity, particularly as it concerns a person's belief system and related patterns of behavior, reaffirms and supports a coherent sense of self, a grasp of the fabric of one's life.

Reducing Isolation for the Older Adult

A problem facing older adults is often a diminishing social network of friends and relatives. This becomes increasingly challenging in our society as older persons are set in a new family context, often defined by distance. Physical distance, along with the impact of increasingly complex family groups, presents older adults with new challenges. Role definition, particularly post-retirement, is more difficult in an increasingly isolated society where the traditional family tree has been replaced with a more complex diagram that accommodates family losses and additions linked to divorce and other social factors. There is a need for role definition, a continuing sense of one's self-esteem, and the development of a sense of continuity and meaning across the life span.

The development of new late life friendships and confidant relationships is often a by-product of participation in a guided autobiography group. Sharing life stories in groups is ideally suited to this purpose, because they build social networks and develop relationships among group members. Enduring friendships are often created as a result of the group process. Intergenerational groups offer unique benefits in terms of opportunities to mentor and to engage in intergenerational roles.

Homebound persons who are often highly isolated experience profound benefits from engaging in autobiographical exercises. These individuals are at high risk of depression due to living in relative isolation. More and more frequently, the homebound are cared for by third party caregivers (i.e., paid individuals outside the family). In certain regions it is common for care providers and the elderly frail individual to have limited communication caused by language differences.

For nursing home residents and others in institutional care, the move to the institution can symbolize separation from home and society. Newly institutionalized persons may further separate themselves due to depression, feelings of isolation, and fear of developing new emotional ties. The interactions afforded in guided autobiography groups have proven to have positive outcomes for such persons (Cappeliez, 2002; Haight, Michel, & Hendrix, 1995b, 2000).

Because life review is a developmental task of the later years, older adults are likely to engage in some form of life review whether or not there is an opportunity to do so in a group. Yet the role of trusted listeners, or confidants, is particularly helpful at this point in life, as many older adults engage in an unsupported life review during periods of loss (such as a personal disability or loss of a spouse). Losses result in decreased life satisfaction and can lead to depression. A negative worldview, invoked by loss and depression, can elicit a preoccupation with exaggerated memories of defeat or failure. However, such distortion of a life may remain unidentified in the absence of persons with whom to share such thoughts. The support and perspective provided by the guided autobiography group and other confidants can assist people in viewing their losses from the perspective of the entire life span, helping the older adult to achieve a balanced view (Peck, 2001).

The Family Context

In reviewing life, models of role change and exchange emerge as the person reconstructs the history of evolving relationships with children, parents, and grandparents. Guided autobiography evokes memories of family episodes and can assist people in working through earlier stages in life and gaining a sense of continuity (Byrd, 2001; Gaden, 1996).

There are symbolic and emotional benefits that accrue to family members as a consequence of the guided autobiography process. The interpretation of life as it has been lived provides the older adult as well as younger generations with a perspective on the past. This expanded perspective gives new shape to the current context and provides a basis for a confident approach to the future. Intergenerational contact afforded by sharing autobiographical writings can provide family members with bridges to historical times they may have not otherwise known or understood. Such connections can assist younger persons in synthesizing their own identities. Thus, older persons can represent living stories, their presence being a sign of tradition and transcendence. Sharing the family history provides a common ground, instilling a sense of belonging and continuity. Life review also appears to be linked to generativity, the need to make an intergenerational connection that can leave a legacy that integrates one's life and the past to the present and the future. Here, life review can be a critical tool for one's own family and others in generations to follow (Coleman, Hautamaki, & Podolskij, 2002).

Understanding the continuity of the family can free the person by (1) exposing the roots of family successes, failures, conflicts, and hardships; (2) identifying similarities among family members, helping a person come to terms with family issues that in the past might have been viewed as a fault of another person or oneself; (3) helping the person reconcile the anger or anxiety that are the residue of past events; and (4) making sense of the common themes of one's life.

The Guided Autobiography Method

A person can review his or her past from a variety of viewpoints: for example, recalling events as they happened chronologically in time, reviewing diaries, or focusing on specific facets of life or personality. We believe that exploring one's autobiography is most fruitful for older adults when done as part of a guided process that directs attention to major life themes. Guided autobiography is based on the conviction that certain common themes of life elicit the most salient memories, are most relevant to the issues and needs of older adults, and therefore are best suited for use. The individual is guided along productive themes to make the search of personal history effective and efficient.

It is important to design and conduct the guided autobiography group according to your purposes and expertise. Nonprofessionals should keep in mind that they are offering an opportunity for older adults to explore their personal histories and begin to integrate their life stories—they are not offering group psychotherapy. With this in mind, nonprofessionals should be cautioned not to probe into the feelings and emotions of group members beyond those that emerge spontaneously from the participants and are shared easily. Group leaders also must protect their members by guarding against probing by other group members. However, group leaders should not discourage the expression of emotions that are a natural part of interpersonal sharing. Guided autobiography may bring to the surface many of the emotions of the past, and participants may laugh or cry as they tell their stories. Unless a group member is demonstrating signs of depression or is in emotional danger, a hands-off philosophy may be best—allowing emotions to emerge naturally, but not soliciting them. Should a person show signs of depression, he or she should be referred immediately to a professional counselor.

Goals for the Group and Group Norms

It is important to develop group goals that encompass the purposes of conducting the guided autobiography. General group goals are:

- Become acquainted with the other members.
- Share life stories.
- Explore similarities and differences among the life experiences of group members.

- Share life strategies.
- Encourage the elaboration of each person's life story.
- Ensure confidentiality.

Other goals are derived from the purposes that determine the composition and nature of a specific group. For example, more specific goals might be adopted if guided autobiography is being used to begin to integrate group members into a new residential setting (e.g., retirement community or nursing home life); to explore life strategies that might be applied to new demands or life transitions (e.g., widowhood, disability, or retirement); as part of later life education in senior centers; or to begin to come to terms with impending death.

Such group goals are in addition to the personal goals of the individual members. Personal goals may vary and be as different as the group members themselves. Regardless of each member's personal goals, however, it is important that the group's goals be identified and agreed on to ensure a spirit of camaraderie and sharing.

The group leader creates a subculture for the group, establishing the norms that govern its conduct and helping to guide the development of relationships among members. The leader must describe and, most important, *model* the game rules that govern group interactions, creating a nonjudgmental atmosphere of acceptance, empathy, and support. Group norms are established relatively early in the life of a group and are difficult to change later. Therefore, in advance of the first meeting, it is essential for you to carefully consider what norms should be developed in the group and to discuss these norms with potential group members prior to their joining the group.

Group members are often strangers before the first meeting, so the group leader serves as a transitional object, a home base from which relationships with others in the group can be explored and to which a person can return with trust and acceptance. An important function of the group leader is to maintain the stability of the group. The group leader plays an important role in facilitating the members' connecting with each other, promoting interaction, trust, and social bonding. This can be achieved by commenting about similarities among group members and facilitating interaction. It is important to remember, however, that the process may be slow, particularly with older adults who are facing new demands and may be experiencing crises in maintaining a sense of self-worth. Such adults may be slow to develop feelings of trust with other group members or may have a strong competing desire to be validated by the group leader. The group leader can best facilitate the process by making all members feel that they are equally important to the group and by focusing group members' attention on their own capacity to support and validate each other. The growth of the group usually becomes evident by about the third session as shown by members coming early and staying afterward to chat.

Group Design

Because groups of older adults, particularly those who are experiencing social isolation or the need to adjust to age-related declines, require time to sort through their memories and emotions, it is recommended that group size be kept small, about five to six members. Too many members will result in an unmanageable group. People may be cut short or not have an opportunity to read their life story or provide insight into the life story of others. Too few members may result in a group that does not have enough content, limiting your potential to draw similarities and contrasts. Most important, too few members at the beginning can result in dissolution of the group should one or two members become ill, travel, or choose to leave.

The nature of the guided autobiography group should be decided by the group leader, and members should be chosen to meet that purpose. Members will take on various roles and tasks in a group, so the leader may want to take into account backgrounds and personality types when combining people into a group. In addition, the leader should discuss with each member the importance of maintaining the stability of the group and should request a commitment to completing the process to the degree possible.

Although anyone *can* participate, group leaders should consider the effective functioning of the group when choosing members. Our experience indicates that diversity is strength as compared to homogeneity. A diverse group may take somewhat longer for the group to form, but once it does, it is much stronger. The diversity appears to free individual members of many of the cultural, religious, or cohort-related concerns about what is expected of oneself. Burnside (1986) suggests that the following be excluded from groups of this type:

- Disturbed, active, wandering persons
- Patients with psychotic depression
- People who do not participate on their own recognizance, for example, who are coerced by others to attend
- Individuals diagnosed as having bipolar disorder
- Persons who are unable to communicate effectively with other group members due to a physical or cognitive disability
- Hypochondriacal persons

To this list might be added persons with paranoid personality disorders and persons suffering from delusional states.

The prototypic group has been made up of individuals from a wide age range and diverse ethnic backgrounds and careers. Heterogeneity provides a rich experience that focuses attention on not only the differences among people but also the similarities and the universalities of emotion and experience. Other groups have consisted of cohorts, people of the same generation with a common connection in the history of a community or culture. This type of group can provide an opportunity for exchanging memories of shared events. Common memories can stimulate further recall and provide the opportunity to view major life influences from the perspective of others. This type of group is particularly suited to the environment of a nursing home or senior center in that it promotes camaraderie and the opportunity for sentimental reminiscence. Individuals living in close association may initially be slow to divulge their life stories but will share as confidence in the group grows.

New members may be resistant or anxious about joining a group. Simple strategies can promote participation and enhance the group experience. For example, snacks have been found to increase attendance at most group meetings. After this is established, the group members may wish to rotate the responsibility for bringing snacks. This has proven to be an effective strategy for enhancing commitment to the group and for preventing member attrition, because members are brought back into the group when it is their turn to bring a snack. In addition to the enticement of snacks, opportunities can be created to show family photographs or to listen to music from the past as ways to attract and sustain participation. This also can help to prompt memories. Events and persons forgotten can be brought to mind by old photographs, and the emotions experienced can be heightened by such tangible stimulation.

During the time span of the guided autobiography group meetings, the leader may be called upon to deal with absenteeism, tardiness, and attrition. It may be necessary to intervene if a member frequently arrives late, is absent, or does not prepare a written statement to share with the group. Members may need to be reminded of their initial commitment, or it may be necessary to discuss the impact of inconsistent participation on the group process. It is useful at times to remind members of their important role in creating the group and how vital their full participation is to developing an atmosphere of mutual acceptance and sharing.

If a member has been absent, he or she should be asked to prepare the written autobiographical statement for the meeting that was missed and should be encouraged to briefly summarize and share this statement with other group members at the next meeting or upon his or her return. This is important because the guided autobiography process is a cumulative one that explores increasingly sensitive subject matter.

It is not recommended that new members be added after the second session, as this will disrupt the natural progression of the developmental exchange and the formation of a cohesive group. Should a new member be added, he or she should be asked to complete the previous life stories prior to entry into the group. The new member should summarize the content of these life stories at the first meeting he or she attends.

Meeting Times and Length

The guided autobiography group usually meets 10 times, including one meeting for each life story theme plus an introductory meeting. The process can be completed in an intensive experience of meeting every weekday for two weeks, or it can be extended over 10 weeks, meeting once a week, or any combination of times that is suitable for your purposes. Particularly in nursing homes and senior centers, group members may decide to continue to have meetings after the structured process is complete.

Each meeting should be scheduled for a minimum of two hours, as it must include both the sensitizing discussion of the next topic and the exchange of autobiographical statements. The individual reading time is typically 15 to 20 minutes. More than two hours will be needed if the group number increases beyond five or six, or if the process is part of a course that includes discussion of developmental issues. Sessions longer than two hours also have to schedule restroom and coffee breaks.

Autobiography groups frequently want to have reunions. They want further contact with each other, which evokes the creation of additional themes to be explored. It is a benefit for them to self-determine future themes and meet again to explore them in accordance with their own group dynamic.

Meeting Content

At each meeting, approximately a half hour should be devoted to discussion of the sensitizing questions that will guide the writing of the thematic life story for the next meeting. The group leader should distribute and read aloud a description of the topic and a sampling of the sensitizing questions (for a complete list of these sensitizing questions, see Birren and Deutchman, 1991). The group leader might share some personal thoughts and experiences related to the topic as a way to initiate group discussion. In addition, he or she might ask the group some prompting questions derived from the sensitizing material. Discussion of the topic at this point should be kept brief and moderated by the group leader. The goal is to stimulate thinking and expand members' perspectives regarding how a topic might be approached. As necessary, members should be made aware of this goal and of the fact that they will have the opportunity to write about the topic and share their experiences at the next meeting.

Approximately 1 ½ hours should be devoted to the reading of that day's life stories, allowing about 15 minutes for each person. This usually takes the form of 10 to 15 minutes of reading and 5 minutes of group interaction. The leader should moderate interactions to ensure that the group remains nonjudgmental and that each member has a turn of nearly equal length to tell his or her story.

The Importance of the Group

The exchange of life stories in a group is an important feature of the guided autobiography process. As each group member reads his or her thematic life story in the small group, intimate exchanges of her or his past with other persons reinforces and sustains the motivation to further review her or his life. This also provides the context for the development of new friendships and greater self-esteem. In addition, it is believed that the confidence and trust built in the small group experience enhance both recall and the ease of condensing experience on a written page.

A key feature of the guided autobiography process is the *developmental exchange*, the mutual sharing between members of where and how they grew up and personally important historical and emotional events. People involved in developmental exchange during the guided autobiography process move from tentatively and guardedly alluding to important features of their lives toward an increasingly open sharing of personal material. In the process, people implicitly take into account the affective importance of shared information. They trade personal information equivalent in affective value, though not necessarily similar in content. As time together increases and more of each life is shared, the developmental exchange leads to an increased willingness to self-disclose. Affective bonds are built among group members, and mutual respect and trust grow.

Increased confidence and trust among group members lead not only to greater willingness to share, but also to greater courage to explore. This exploration can lead to a clarity of one's identity and an understanding of the self that might otherwise not have been possible. The developmental exchange goes much like a poker game in which each player increases the ante on his or her turn. If a player does not want to proceed further, the last player's ante is simply met or the player passes and withdraws. By meeting the ante, the player remains part of the group but does not expand the emotional stake.

The group leader can promote the developmental exchange through the use of three primary strategies:

1. Link group members who have discussed similar stories by utilizing good listening skills and by alluding to connections between personal experiences.

2. Share your own thoughts or questions about what has just been said, thus demonstrating that you are not only hearing what they have to say, but also are genuinely interested in their life stories.

3. Use self-disclosure: It is recommended that the group leader facilitate interactions *between and among group members as a primary role*. This involves careful moderation of your own involvement in the group process of sharing life stories. When a group leader writes or shares excessive personal autobiographical statements, it may compete with his or her role as moderator and cause a feeling of inequality among members. However, it is important for members to feel that the group leader is an ally and to experience a sense of reciprocity. To accomplish this and to promote the developmental exchange, group leaders can engage in a limited use of self-disclosure by interjecting a *brief* personal vignette or sharing an emotion. It is best used when it is designed to highlight similarities between human experiences or universalities in human emotions. It is particularly important in situations in which a member feels alone or isolated in the group. It can be an effective antidote in instances in which group norms have been breached or privacy has been invaded.

Related to the developmental exchange, a benefit of sharing one's autobiography with a group is that cues to recall may arise from the discussion. Other people's experiences become reminders of feelings and events that have been set aside or forgotten. In addition, the distribution of attention among group members has the effect of reducing pressure on any one person and providing support in dealing with painful memories. One role of the group is to assist other members who become stuck at some painful point in the past, providing the stimulus to move on to new territory.

The Importance of the Written Form

Although the group experience holds rich potential and is a valuable component of the guided autobiography process, writing one's autobiographical statements is the basis of the process. The sensitization process that begins in the group is a first step in a person's journey into a review of the self and the personal past. Personal, private reflection and the motivation to delve deeply into the banks of the memory are summoned by the task of writing down one's recollections. In addition, the writing process itself is a stimulus to further recall. As thoughts are put on paper, rearranged, and read, related memories are elicited. In addition, by writing his or her thoughts down prior to sharing them with the group, a person can sift out what will be shared with the group, focusing on the experiences he or she perceives as most important. Without this opportunity, memories might ramble in a desultory manner, and the person's time to share with the group might be taken up by less productive recall. Similarly, a person has the opportunity to review his or her autobiographical statements on a particular life theme and determine what will and will not be shared with the group. This protects the individual's right to monitor the developmental exchange and not to share what he or she feels is too personal or painful.

Finally, without the written document, one would have difficulty reconstructing the flow of information in the group in order to expand later the autobiographical statement. It would also reduce both the potential of sharing one's autobiographical life stories with persons outside the group and the capacity of guided autobiography to help create a family legacy to pass on.

The Thematic Approach and the Use of Sensitizing Questions

The guided autobiography process is based on the conviction that there are certain common themes that provide the threads on which the fabric of human life is woven. The specific themes employed in guided autobiography are the result of many years of construction and refinement. These themes are described fully in Birren and Deutchman (1991) along with the sensitizing questions used to evoke memories and guide the participants in addressing the most meaningful, productive aspects of the themes. The themes and sensitizing questions have been chosen for four reasons. First, they are salient issues that underlie the life course. Second, review of one's life in this framework is believed to be beneficial in guiding the next steps and in transcending difficult transitions. Third, the thematic approach enhances the group process by providing a context in which common feelings and circumstances are explored collectively, and, perhaps most importantly, the sensitizing questions "prime" memories to be shared. Last, these themes represent life experiences and issues that are likely to be most relevant to individual development in other generations, thereby forming a meaningful legacy.

Potential Obstacles in the Guided Autobiography Group

Problems may arise in conducting guided autobiography groups. These can range from problems with a specific group member's behavior to lack of support from the institution. There are many ways to manage such problems, and the best will be based on the group leader's own judgment of the situation and personal style. It is important, however, to recognize the warning signs of such problems. Birren and Cochran (2001) draw attention to ten counterproductive group members,

and offer excellent troubleshooting tips for managing them in the group context. These are:

- Participants who dominate the discussion
- Participants who go off on tangents
- Participants who do not write their two pages
- Shy or reticent group members who slow the energy of the discussion
- Group members who make negative or judgmental comments
- Participants who are experts on every topic
- All group members speaking at once
- Participants who withdraw from the group, looking displeased
- Participants who share very serious material at an early session (disturbing the developmental exchange)
- Participants who act as therapists

Ensuring Institutional Support

The success of the guided autobiography group depends in part on the commitment and support of the institution in which it is conducted. Particularly in sites such as nursing homes, the cooperation of the administrative staff and caregivers is essential to ensure that group members are able to attend each session and that there is positive reinforcement for continued participation. Without this support, group members may feel they are being forced to choose between activities or that their relationship with staff will be harmed by participation in the guided autobiography group.

In most cases, such support comes easily. Generally, families and personnel of senior care facilities are enthusiastic about the potential of guided autobiography and welcome the availability of such groups. In some instances, however, staff may be wary of new or outside persons. Key to engaging their support is enlisting the cooperation and support of the top administrator and, where applicable, the head of nursing. These people will greatly influence the degree of cooperation provided by direct care providers. Without such cooperation, difficulties may arise.

Summary

This chapter has provided a brief guide to how effective guided autobiography groups can be conducted. Guided autobiography is an efficient way for older adults to review their lives by following a proven series of evocative themes and responding to questions designed to promote reflection. It provides an opportunity for older adults to strengthen their identities, increase their sense of competency, make new friendships, and create a legacy for their families.

There is a growing interest in autobiography, personal documents, and narratives of many sorts. This may reflect the fact that modern society gives little opportunity for personal exchanges during the work life. It also may reflect the transient atmosphere created by a society in which interpersonal relationships, jobs, and the structures of institutions are rapidly changing. Social change may make it difficult for older adults in particular to be able to integrate their lives and find durable meaning in their histories. In this context, guided autobiography has a place in raising the quality of life of the aged. The process is by no means fully explored in applications, and research will lead to further insights. Enough is known to encourage others to explore its use in helping the aged to find meaning in the way their lives have been led and to find companionship through sharing their stories.

Exercises

EXERCISE 1

Following the themes and sensitizing questions in Birren and Deutchman (1991), write your own guided autobiography.

EXERCISE 2

Design a guided autobiography group by developing a list of potential members and group goals.

EXERCISE 3

Solicit members and conduct a guided autobiography group. Develop a questionnaire and evaluate the group's effectiveness after the tenth session.

References

Allport, G. (1942). *The use of personal documents in psychological science.* Bulletin 49, New York: Social Science Research Council.

Birren, J. E., & Birren, B. A. (1996). Autobiography: Exploring the self and encouraging development. In J. E. Birren, G. M. Kenyon, J. E. Ruth, J. J. Schroots, & T. Svensson (Eds.), *Aging and biography: Explorations in adult development* (pp. 283–299). New York: Springer.

Birren, J. E., & Cochran, K. (2001). *Telling the stories of life through guided autobiography groups.* Baltimore: Johns Hopkins University Press.

Birren, J. E., & Deutchman, D. E. (1991). *Guiding autobiography groups for older adults: Exploring the fabric of life.* Baltimore: Johns Hopkins University Press.

Buhler, C., & Massarik, F. (1968). *The course of human life.* New York: Springer.

Burnside, I. M. (1986). *Working with the elderly: Group process and techniques* (2nd ed.). Boston: Jones & Bartlett.

Butler, R. N. (2002). Age, death and life review. In K. Doka, *Living with grief: Loss in later life.* Washington, DC: Hospice Foundation of America.

Byrd, M. (2001). Elderly individuals' reminiscences about the life-span development of their family. *International Journal of Aging and Human Development,* 52(3), 253–263.

Cappeliez, P. (2002). Cognitive reminiscence therapy for depressed older adults in day hospital and long-term care. In J. D. Webster & B. K. Haight (Eds.), *Critical advances in reminiscence work: From theory to application* (pp. 300–313). New York: Springer.

Cockrum-Murphy, L. (2001). Stronger at the broken places: Heuristic inquiry. *Dissertation abstracts: International Section A* (Humanities and Social Sciences), 62,1A, 75.

Coleman, P., Hautamaki, A., & Podolskij, A. (2002). Trauma, reconciliation, and generativity: The stories told by European war veterans. In J. D. Webster & B. K. Haight (Eds.), *Critical advances in reminiscence work: From theory to application*. New York: Springer.

deVries, B., Birren, J. E., & Deutchman, D. E. (1994). Adult development through guided autobiography. *Family Relations*, 39, 3–7.

Eliason, G. (2001). Spirituality and counseling of the older adult. In A. Tomer (Ed.), Death attitudes and the older adult: Theories, concepts and applications. New York: Brunner-Routledge.

Erikson, E. (1963). *Childhood and society*. New York: Norton.

Erlin, J., Mellors, M., Sereika, S., & Cook, C. (2001). The use of life review to enhance quality of life of people living with AIDS: A feasibility study. *Quality of Life Research: An international journal of quality of life aspects of treatment, care and rehabilitation*, 10(5), 453–464.

Gaden, C. (1996). The meaning and value of grandparenting in later life. *Dissertation abstracts: International Section B* (Sciences), 56, 12B, 7062.

Gatz, M., Fiske, A., Fox, L. S., Kaski, B., & Kasi-Godley, J. E., et al. (1999). Empirically validated psychological treatments for older adults. *Journal of Mental Health and Aging*, 4(1), 9–46.

Godley, J. K., & Gatz, M. (2000). Psychological intervention for individuals with dementia: An integration of theory. *Clinical Psychology Review*, 20(6), 755–782.

Haight, B., Coleman, P., & Lord, K. (1995). The linchpins of a successful life review: Structure, evaluation and individuality. In B. K. Haight & J. D. Webster (Eds.), *The art and science of reminiscing: Theory, research, methods and applications* (pp.179–189). Philadelphia: Taylor & Francis.

Haight, B. K., Michel, Y., & Hendrix, S. (2000). The extended effects of life review in nursing home residents. *International Journal of Aging and Human Development*, 50(2), 151–168.

Hartman, P. S. (2001). Women developing wisdom: Antecedents and correlates in a longitudinal study. *Dissertation abstracts: International Section B* (Sciences), 62, 1B, 591.

Kenyon, G., Clark, P., & de Vries, B. (Eds.). (2001). *Narrative gerontology: Theory, research and practice*. New York: Springer.

Levinson, D. J. (1978). *The season of a man's life*. New York: Knopf.

Masai-Jones, A. C. (2001). The life review: A narrative analysis of the stories of hospice clients. *Dissertation abstracts: International Section A* (Social Sciences), 6, 12A, 4897.

McFadden, S., Brannan, M., & Patrick, J. H. (2003). *New directions in the study of late life religiousness and spirituality*. New York: Haworth Press.

Peck, M. (2001). Looking back at life and its influence on subjective well-being. *Journal of Gerontological Social Work*, 35(2), 3–20.

Porter, E. (1998). Gathering our stories; claiming our lives: Seniors' life story books facilitate life review, integration and celebration. *Journal on Developmental Disabilities*, 6(1), 44–59.

Richeson, N., & Thorson, J. (2002). The effect of autobiographical writing on the subjective well-being of older adults. *North American Journal of Psychology*, 4(3), 395–404.

Schroots, J. (1996). The fractal structure of lives: Continuity and discontinuity in autobiography. In J. E. Birren, G. M. Kenyon, J. E. Ruth, J. J. Schroots, & T. Svensson (Eds.), *Aging and biography: Explorations in adult development*. New York: Springer.

Shaw, M. (2001). A history of guided autobiography. In G. M. Kenyon, P. Clark, & de Vries, B. (Eds.), *Narrative gerontology: Theory, research and practice* (pp. 291–309). New York: Springer.

Shaw, M., Westwood, M., & deVries, B. (1999). Integrating personal reflection and group-based enactments. *Journal of Aging Studies*, 13(1), 109–119.

Tabourne, C. E. S. (1995a). The life review program as an intervention for an older adult newly admitted to a nursing home facility: A case study. *Journal of Therapeutic Recreation*, 29(3), 228–236.

Tabourne, C. E. S. (1995b). The effects of a life review program on disorientation, social interaction and self-esteem of nursing home residents. *International Journal of Aging and Human Growth and Development*, 41(3), 251–266.

Wink, P., & Schiff, B. (2002). To review or not to review? The role of personality and life events in life review and adaptation to older age. In J. D. Webster & B. K. Haight (Eds.), *Critical advances in reminiscence work: From theory to application* (pp. 44–60). New York: Springer.

Chapter 16

Music and Other Arts Activities in the Lives of Older Adults

Barry Bortnick

Key Words

- Multiple modalities
- Life review
- Intergenerational programming
- Dementia
- Music therapist
- Musical intervention
- Sense of competence

Learning Objectives

- Describe four major kinds of musical activities that involve seniors
- Describe five major developmental, motivational, and/or behavioral functions of musical activities for seniors
- Demonstrate the use of three specific activities, of which one involves music and another art form
- Identify major areas of research that are being carried out to help quantify the value of music for seniors
- Discuss ways in which music can enhance or expand the process of reminiscence and life review
- Discuss the role music can play in enhancing an intergenerational program

The pianist looked out over the sea of faces in the packed dining room of the Jewish Home for the Aging. Many were alert with anticipation and attention. Others were staring into space without apparent awareness of what was transpiring around them. He began playing a Niggun, the wordless melody he had written in the style of older music with which many members of this audience were familiar. The singers entered from the rear humming the melody and fanning out across the room, handing out an assortment of bells, tambourines, miniature drums, and other percussion instruments, inviting the residents, all of them, to join in, to be part of the music making (Hurwitz, Wolfe, Bortnick, & Kokas, 1975).

This chapter is an overview of the major uses and functions of music and musical activities involving older adults, the effects of these activities, and the reasons for these effects. In addition, the chapter addresses three areas of considerable interest today: music in relation to life review, intergenerational programming, and dementia. A final section provides suggestions for future directions in the use of the arts, particularly music, with older adults.

Having occupied a relatively low role in this country's priorities for the well-being of our older population, the arts and humanities are slowly but steadily emerging from the shadows. The increased number of arts-related presentations at national conferences of the American Society on Aging is but one such example. This emergence is due in part to three factors: (1) the increased interest in the "whole" individual and not just his or her physical condition or medications, (2) the successes of those who have made an impact on the lives of seniors through the arts, and (3) the growing body of positive research results. The range of these programs is diverse, from activities that elders attend in the community to those brought into institutions; from groups whose prime objective is performing for seniors to those that involve seniors in virtually every step of the creative process. Music is the focus here, but because music is often combined with other forms of cultural expression, the discussion includes occasional references to other art forms as well as the creative process itself. The main purpose of such references is to suggest the broader context of which music is a part (and the broader value of the arts in general for older adults). Clearly, each art form has its own unique characteristics and deserves a separate and detailed discussion on its own terms in relation to its uses with seniors.

The intention throughout this chapter is to be illustrative, not exhaustive. The goal is to stimulate ideas and interest and to suggest areas worth further exploration or study. The intended readers are those working with older adults, students interested in future roles in this field, researchers, and others interested in the potential value of music for this increasingly prominent part of our population. It should be emphasized that the target audience—older adults—includes a wide variety of individuals from healthy active seniors to frail seniors in institutional settings.

The work of music therapists (defined in this chapter as professionally trained, board certified therapists) is central to much of the discussion. The certification board for music therapists (2004) defines *music therapy* as "The specialized use of music and the materials of music by a professional music therapist to restore, maintain, and improve skills, adaptation, and/or performance in one or more of the following domains: cognitive, psychological, affective, social, physical, physiological, sensory, sensory motor, communication, and behavior." In addition to music therapists, the scope of this chapter also extends to the work of other professionals as well as paraprofessionals and nonprofessionals whose actions and activities may contribute to the improvement of an individual's health. The chapter is also concerned with a broad spectrum of activities not necessarily designed with therapy or health explicitly in mind but nonetheless with valuable outcomes for improving the well-being of people.

Finally, in the ensuing sections, examples are introduced that draw from the author's personal experiences writing for and directing a musical group, From Healing to Hallelujah!, that performs for seniors, along with other examples from the literature.

Overview of Activities and Functions

> Following the opening Niggun, the male singer taught the audience hand and body movements to express in gesture the meaning of the lyrics. Then: "Build, build, build a sukkah together, bring fruit and gladness inside" the singers sang while the audience in gesture "built" and "filled up" the shelter associated with the ancient Jewish harvest holiday of Sukkot—and followed this with a discussion of what this re-creation means for people today (Bortnick, 2004).

Music enhances the lives of older adults in a variety of ways—ways that mirror the many musical activities that are possible and the many underlying modalities that can be involved. Activities include: singing, reading, listening, clapping, tapping, sequencing, expressing, communicating, finding meaning, praying, reaching out, going inside, moving, shaking, making connections and associations, relating to others, transposing, transmuting, developing, shaping, *and* improvising. These examples pertain to music per se; adding in the element of lyrics or other art forms opens up the possibility of yet more forms of engagement. A few key ways in which musically related activities can be categorized, accompanied by a few selected examples are:

Listening and Witnessing

Individuals and musical groups—amateur, professional, and combinations of the two—that specialize in concerts for older adults are available across the country, each offering its own blend of musical material, format, and style. There are also the beginnings of something long needed: a networking system, being developed by the National Center for Creative Aging, to help senior groups and organizations and music and arts organizations find each other.

Creating Rhythm

Given the elemental nature of rhythm and the fact that it takes nothing more than a pair of hands or sticks to create it, it is not surprising that many senior activities are connected with expressing musical beat and rhythm—through clapping, tapping, foot beating, playing drums, and other percussion instruments. Seniors constitute an important part of those who join drumming circles and the many activities that these offer. (See in the Resource section the reference to workshops conducted by *Health*RYHTHMS.) In these drumming one-hour recreational music making sessions participants play the rhythm of their names on drums, and have the other participants repeat it as they go around the circle.

Singing and Song Writing

Like playing a percussion instrument, the act of singing can touch a deep place within an individual, beginning with the breath itself. Judith-Kate Friedman and Songwriting Work™ take this aspect of the experience to another level by offering seniors the chance to participate in all aspects of songwriting, to whatever degree they are able, in a collective process facilitated by a professional. They also have the chance to perform their songs (or songs by other elders) for audiences ranging from immediate friends, family, staff and peers (i.e., at care facilities), and the general public. Elder songwriters have also been involved in all aspects of recording a CD from selection and arrangement of songs, to adding narrative vignettes, and having input into mixing the recording and designing the CD booklet featuring their original artwork.

In between being invited to be part of an audience and part of a group of songwriters are a range of other possibilities. For example, seniors can join in the chorus or in a recurring line of a song or sing entire songs. They can harmonize a song or suggest lyrics for one moment in a song, which they then sing each time that moment comes around. Other examples are given later in the chapter.

Songs and Storytelling

Songs and other kinds of music are often intertwined with storytelling activities (beyond the story told in the song itself). The creative approaches used by Heather MacTavish and the New Rhythms Foundation, for example, incorporate stories with cues from classic popular songs presented by the facilitator. The facilitator together with the audience might improvise stories around the theme "How I met the partner of my dreams." The stories are interspersed with classic popular songs with which seniors are familiar—"Ain't She Sweet," for example—to represent a person's first reaction on meeting the future partner. The leader introduces the songs and then the group joins in. As the group becomes more familiar with this approach, the group itself suggests other story and song themes and improvisations.

Figure 16–1

Lenore chudd and a group of elders about to take part in a concert with the group "From Healing to Hallelujah!", written and directed by Barry Bortnick.

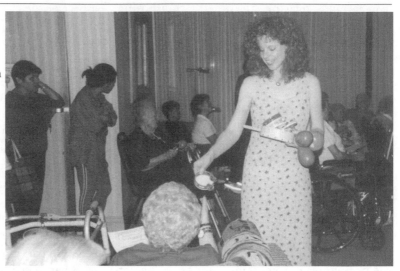

Used with permission from Cheryl Weiner.

Multiple Musical Activities — Music and Other Art Forms

Many programs and individuals offer not one but a range of activities. This range certainly characterizes the work of music therapists. Also included in the resource section are a few examples of the rich ways in which music is combined with painting and drawing, dance, and drama including musical theater, poetry, and other arts. Music can also enhance other activities ranging from daily exercise to the act of prayer. For example, listening to music can make dining more pleasant and contribute to improved health by increasing the nutritional intake and enjoyment of the meal (Ragnesgkog, 1996).

Effects

Much of the discussion about the value of musical activities and groups for seniors is couched in the context of challenges people face as they grow older and the ways music can help people respond to these challenges. Many of the values cited can as easily be described in terms of a more positive view of the aging process (Cohen, 2000).

Given the multidimensional nature of a musical experience, it is not surprising that writers focus on a wide range of specific developmental outcomes, which can include, among many possibilities: improved fitness levels through movements stimulated by music (Berryman-Miller, 1986); increased coordination of responses by participating in activities requiring temporal sequencing in singing, reading, or clapping to music (Aldridge, 1994); and the effects movement with music may have on balance and gait speed (Hamburg & Clair, 2003). Summarizing his own detailed analysis of the potential of the arts, Lindauer (2003) notes the "variety of behavioral, psychological, and social skills promoted by the arts" (p. 245).

Additional Values

EMOTIONAL ENGAGEMENT

Emotional engagement is defined as bringing people "out" of themselves, connecting inner and outer worlds. Rosling and Kitchen (1992) frame the discussion of the value of listening to music and art for an audience of institutionalized elderly in terms of emotional engagement:

> Our personal development is based on what happens to us in the two worlds in which we live. One is the external world of things and events; the other is the inner world of senses, feelings, and meanings. Art activities are important because they form a bridge of communication and interaction between these worlds (p. 27).

This sense of connectedness is particularly important in light of the external and internal isolation potentially faced by many seniors (Chavin, 2002). Stated in the context of a more positive view of aging, however, the value of the arts in keeping someone active in the world of emotions and ideas is an essential element of being human, regardless of whether one has specific "problems." If, as some argue, the nature of inner experience takes on added importance as one grows older, the arts can serve a particularly significant role in helping provide meaning, texture, richness, and integration to the quality of the later years.

RELATING TO OTHER INDIVIDUALS

Apart from connections made with the piece of music or aesthetic experience itself, music and the other arts can help seniors relate positively to those around them. As part of a group creating and/or singing a song, rehearsing together, sharing the triumph of a concert, sharing an enjoyable musical performance by others, or being part of a drumming circle, seniors have many opportunities to build or deepen positive interpersonal relationships. Some experiences—for example, being a member of one half of a room that is alternating with the other half in singing a recurring part of a song—are ideal in heightening this sense of working together to bring about something positive and rewarding.

Other forms of connectedness are discussed in the sections on life review and cross-generational programming.

IMPROVING SELF-ESTEEM, SENSE OF COMPETENCE, MASTERY, AND PURPOSE

The variety of uses to which music can be put and the variety of modalities that can be drawn on provide a wealth of opportunities for people to achieve a sense of mastery and self-esteem. For those who experience a problem with verbal expression or spatial memory, the musical experience can create another "way in" for a therapist, activity director, or friend to reach them, or for people to experience something positive on their own. Such experiences can be particularly important in light of the challenges to self-esteem faced by many seniors (e.g., loss of role upon retirement; diminishing physical capacity).

SELF-IDENTITY, EXPRESSING AND REINFORCING "WHO I AM"

The very act of creating, of putting oneself "out there," can reinforce a sense of identity for the senior. Additional activities can further reinforce that identity and one's positive sense of it. In a parallel way to the drumming noted earlier, Maria Genne, artistic director of the Kairos Dance Theater, involves participants in an exercise where each individual creates his or her own distinctive arm and hand gesture when they speak their name and the rest of the group repeats it.

FINDING MEANING

For many older adults, the above benefits become linked with having a sense of meaning for one's life. In addition, some writers, for example, some of the contributors to Campbell's (2002) *Music and Miracles* note the association of music with spiritual, religious, and other endeavors that can involve finding or deepening one's sense of meaning.

MUSIC AS ITS OWN VALUE

Lest we forget: music can be important simply for the reward inherent in listening; its capacity to move or delight, to experience something about the nature of being alive. Echoing not only this theme but several of the others just described is Twyla Tharp's answer when asked why creativity matters:

> "So that you walk out the door believing in yourself a little bit more. So you believe that in any given day you've made of it more than it might otherwise have been. So that you do not take things for granted. Creativity, ultimately, is a way of saying thank you." (Kulman, 2003).

General Research

A good deal of literature is available confirming the potential that older adults have for retaining their creativity and responsiveness to the arts well into the later years of life (Abba, 1989; Cohen, 2000; Cohen, Bailey, & Nilson, 2002; Dohr & Forbes, 1986; Kastenbaum, 1991, 1992; Lindauer, 2003; Simonton, 1990, 1991). Although this may seem obvious to many, the issue is critical particularly in terms of responding to a long-existing controversy about the nature and quality of creativity in the senior years (Abba; Lindauer). While this chapter does not take up this issue per se in any detail, it is important to note the key work of Cohen, Lindauer, and the others cited above in reinforcing the idea that the arts can continue to be a vital and accessible area for people in their senior years. Further, as discussed shortly in looking at those with dementia, for many seniors it is music and the other arts that continue to hold out the chance for continued cognitive involvement and emotional stimulation when other modalities become problematic (Basting & Killick, 2003).

Research into the effects of music and musical activities has run a wide gamut in terms of both dependent and independent variables. Professionally trained music therapists have been among those most interested in documenting the results of musical interventions, both their own and those of other board certified therapists who practice music therapy as a profession. (For information on forms of therapy involving the other arts, see the *National Coalition of Creative Arts Therapies Associations* in the Resources section.)

Adler (2004) has compiled an extensive annotated bibliography of research on the impact of music therapy on improvements in a wide range of patterns involving cognition, behavior, communication, vision, mood, quality of life, and functional status. Research into effects of music therapy is also often rich in suggestions about uses of particular kinds of music and other conditions for achieving various therapeutic objectives and other positive results (Burack, Jefferson, & Libow, 2002). The research literature includes studies of the positive results of musical interventions by others besides music therapists, e.g., nurses (Sanbandham & Schirm, 1995). Many of the broader themes posited in the previous section are also addressed in the research literature, whether measuring the results of the work of music therapists or that of other contributors to musical activities. For example, Fisher and Specht (1999) looked at the potential of the arts to foster a sense of competence, purpose, and growth. Chavin (2002) focuses on the value of music as communication and, in turn, its influence on mood, behavior, and other variables.

Some findings have practical implications for those working with older populations in broader capacities than the arts. Kramer (2001), for example, looked at implications for the role of the geriatric nurse in providing musical activities to improve a patient's food intake, sleep, language function, and mood. Shifting the focus from older adults themselves to long-term care workers and how music can help them do their job, Bittman, Bruhn, Stevens, Westengard, and Umbach (2003) found reduced burnout and improved mood states in long-term care workers who participated in a protocol focusing on building support, communication, and interpersonal respect utilizing group drumming and keyboard accompaniment.

In his own review of the research literature, Coffman (2002) identified outcomes not only of the work of music therapists but also of other activities, both music making and music listening, e.g., volunteer participation in wind bands. Other researchers have focused on special populations, e.g., older adults with disabilities (Katz, 1993; Barret & Clements, 1997), and those with Parkinson's disease (Tufts University, 2001).

A sense of competence is an essential factor in the framework underpinning one of the most significant research efforts currently being undertaken in this area: a research study by Cohen (2003) entitled "The Impact of Professional-Conducted Cultural Programs on Older Adults." This study is measuring the general health, mental health, and social functioning of older adults who are involved in structured, creative arts programs conducted by professional artists. The average age of the sample, all of whom lived independently, was 80 years. Of the several groups in different parts of the country studied, one group took part in a community-based music program for older adults run by the Levine School of Music in the Washington, D.C. area. Cohen hypothesized that such involvement provides a heightened sense of mastery or control and feeling of empowerment, which in turn is associated with positive health outcomes.

Preliminary results show significant differences between the arts groups and control groups with the arts groups reporting higher morale, fewer doctor visits per year, better self-reported health, fewer fall and hip fractures, reduced use of medications, and fewer vision problems. As measured by psychological scales, the arts groups also scored significantly lower with respect to level of depression and loneliness, and higher with respect to overall level of activity.

Music, Reminiscence, and Life Review

> Following the song "If I were a tree," the singers invite the audience to share a favorite memory of a tree or some other growing thing and how it played a role in their life. (Wakefield, 1990).

With the many approaches to and recognized value of reminiscence, life review (Butler, 1973, 1995), and autobiography (Birren & Cochran, 2001; Birren & Deutchman, 1991; Gibson, 2004) come new possibilities for bringing in activities involving other modalities besides the written and spoken word. Wakefield's (1990) exercise of drawing a favorite room from childhood and the many efforts to fuse drama and storytelling with reminiscence stand out as examples. There are at least three major ways in which music and the other arts can take on a role in reminiscence and life review.

Tapping into Memories

In several general reminiscence programs, workshop leaders have played several kinds of music as background to relax the individual and make it easier to draw on past memories. Karras (1987) and Kartman (1990, 1991) each provides examples of the use of nostalgic music in nursing homes to help stimulate memory and discussion. Music is also sometimes combined with photographs, dance, and other activities to stimulate reminiscence (Thorgrimsen, Schweitzer, & Orrell, 2002). In light of music's potential to help stimulate recall, it will also come as no surprise that research into the positive effect of music on patients with dementia have included musically related reminiscence activities (Ashida, 2000).

Music may be similarly used with all kinds of populations in more structured autobiography group settings. A leader's bringing in selections of various musical selections associated with different time periods in the participants' lives can provide another basis for sparking memory and sharing with others.

Duffey, Lumadue, and Woods (2001) have developed an approach that not only uses music to trigger memory but also provides a way to help people resolve issues that may come up through reminiscence. Their "musical chronology" approach uses songs and the discussion between therapist and client that is stimulated upon hearing those songs to help clients gain insights into their experiences and reframe past narratives.

Additional Mode of Expression

Participants in a guided autobiography class can bring in *their own* song that has a special meaning for them and play it for the rest of the class. This exercise has the benefit of allowing them not only to share something about their experience with the rest of the group, but also to have the added satisfaction of feeling that someone else (i.e., the writer of the song) has had a parallel experience. Other art forms can be similarly used, as Magee (1988) suggested regarding the use of poetry. Music and song can also be brought in as reference or metaphor in conjunction with autobiographical exploration. Examples for using music from the movies this way are given in an application exercise at the end of this chapter. Finally, participants can be encouraged to create their *own* song or song fragment (music, lyrics, or both) to express something about their past experiences.

Providing Social Context

Susan Perlstein (1988, 1991) in describing the method of life review, storytelling, and communal theater used by "Elders Share the Arts" discussed ways in which storytelling can connect people to a larger community, helping them see themselves as part of a continuum in time. She related this to Barbara Myerhoff's view of continuity as "Essential for psychological well-being and personal integration, for an individual to experience him/herself as one person, despite change and disruption throughout the life cycle" (Myerhoff & Simic, 1977, p. 164). As Butler (1973) noted, this sense of continuity can be of special import in later years given the challenges many experience with respect to isolation and depression.

One of the most powerful ways in which people maintain this sense of continuity is through

music, especially given its central role in shared popular culture. What may be shared is not only the music they buy or listen to but also music associated with movies, television shows, commercials, and other contexts. Music's connection to other aspects of people's identity—ethnicity, for example, or religious affiliation—opens up yet another way in which musical recall can help people relate to each other's backgrounds and past experiences (Durham & Whitmore, 1993).

Kartman (1990, 1991) looked at music's role not only in helping people recall, but in helping them share with others. An example is the use of song to allow people to share what it was like to live in an era in which a song about an Oldsmobile was part of the collective experience or what it was like to go through a particular life passage event (songs involving music played at weddings). (See also Karras' [1987] examples of bringing in songs around various other themes.)

How songs are used and the ways in which they are effective depends partly on the extent of homogeneity of the group. However, even with a heterogeneous group, music can be used to highlight the experiences people have in common. My own concerts have included songs I have written around the cycle of the seasons, with discussion about how this cycle resonates with rich connotations and meaning for all people, even if the particular forms that are used to express these meanings vary.

Music and Intergenerational Programs

Herb and Pauline, two of the residents in the Jewish Home who had practiced with the cast earlier that day, were introduced to the audience as two surprise guests who will take part in the next number. To the delight of the audience (and their own) they joined in a song inspired by a passage in the Bible, in which they played Abraham and Sarah, with two of the younger cast members playing their modern day descendents. The song itself was about handing down a legacy from generation to generation (Bortnick, 2004).

The arts lend themselves beautifully to the possibilities of intergenerational programming. The resource section lists a few of the opportunities for taking part in intergenerational dance, drama, and music groups. These groups, in turn, perform before younger audiences, older audiences, or intergenerational audiences experiencing an arts event together. In these cases, of course, the focus shifts from recall to shared group experience, with many of the values mentioned earlier coming into play. These include the chance to experience going outside oneself—or in the case of residents of an institution, *literally* going outside—as well as strengthening one's own sense of identity. An intergenerational program can also stimulate a heightened interest in the act of living through offering the chance for individuals to experience together something more about the richness of the human experience across peoples.

Music and the other arts can play a key role in making that experience more vivid or real or simply more enjoyable. When people bring in their favorite songs for an autobiography group, the experience can be very different if the group involves people of different ages. For example, if the assignment is to bring in songs from one's teenage years, the music might spark a discussion about what the messages of teenage songs in different decades say about the values of each period—as well as ways in which teenagers across time may share certain challenges and responses in common.

Music and Dementia

Music has long been viewed as having a special way of reaching persons with dementia. As defined by the Alzheimer's Association, *dementia* is an umbrella term for several symptoms related to a decline in thinking skills. "Common symptoms include a gradual loss of memory, problems with reasoning or judgment, disorientation, diffi-

culties in learning, loss of language skills, and decline in the ability to perform routine tasks (Alzheimer's Association, 2004). Much of the research discussed in this section pertains to Alzheimer's disease but the discussion includes dementia from other causes as well.

Three areas of research are of particular interest: (a) the extent to which musical memory often continues after people have experienced other memory loss or other kinds of cognitive, affective, or behavioral problems, (b) the extent to which positive musical interventions can still occur even in the presence of such problems, and (c) the extent to which such interventions not only occur but have additional positive effects particularly outside of music, e.g., strengthening self-esteem.

Studies are confirming positive results or building solid foundations for future research in all three of the above areas—whether it be increased neurological understanding of how the brain operates or further research studies of music's effect on levels of relative memory impairment (Ashida, 2000). A wide range of interventions are being examined, from playing someone a Mozart sonata (Johnson, Cotman, Tasaki, & Shaw, 1998; Johnson, Shaw, Vuong, Vuong, & Cotman, 2002) to engaging in drumming (Kelleher, 2001), to music combined with other activities, for example, social dancing (Palo-Bengtsson & Ekman, 2002). In some of the cases in which research has involved music and *another* intervention, musical activity seems to be important in helping to make the other activity possible or accessible.

Researchers are looking at many kinds of sensory-cognitive and behavioral responses as well as effects on mood, agitation (Jennings & Vance, 2002), verbally disruptive behavior (Cohen-Mansfield & Werner, 1977), motivation, communication, and language functioning (Brotons & Kroger, 2000). Researchers are also looking beyond these specific measures to more general effects that music can have, citing some of the same overarching themes described earlier: for example, the potential of music to help people communicate with others (Aldridge, 1995, 1996; Clair, 1996) or develop or maintain a sense of well-being (Kydd, 2001).

As in the case of research on healthy active seniors, the literature with respect to those with dementia also provides many suggestions about what conditions can maximize the positive impact of music (Christie, 1992; Whitcomb, 1994). Koger, Chapin, & Brotons (1999) discussed a number of variables that either have been studied or need to be further addressed in future research with respect to determining specific types of therapeutic treatments, amount and kind of training needed by those providing the musical activity, length of treatment, and other factors. In addition to looking at the role of the music therapist, other studies have looked at variables with respect to the effectiveness of the caregiver: the comparative value of in-service musical training for activity aides (Matthews, Clair, & Kososki, 2000) and the ways and conditions under which a caregiver's singing can have a positive effect on dementia patients (Gotell, Brown, & Ekman, 2002). Finally, Halpern and Bartlett (2002) looked at variables within the senior population itself, such as past experiences.

One last area of promise needs to be noted: recent research has studied the possible impact of involvement in musical and other activities on lowering the *risk* of dementia in the elderly (Katz, 2003).

In sum, as is the case with respect to research for the general population of older adults, the field is offering highly promising possibilities for better understanding of the relationship between music and dementia and valuable suggestions for future research.

The Future

Lest anyone start celebrating too soon:

> The artistic director of another music group that performs at nursing homes reported how difficult it is to get the nursing home staff to bring residents to a concert. There always are residents left sitting in their rooms or in the corridors because no one has bothered to bring them to the shows. She also mentioned her experience of arriving at a nursing home to find that all the chairs for the audience had been turned away from where the performance would take place because the person coordinating arrangements for the home thought there would be more room that way (Bortnick, 2004).

Increased recognition of the value of music and other arts does not mean the struggle for broader and deeper understanding and recognition is over, or that funding for these services is not going to remain an urgent challenge. Continued efforts to conduct research in this area are crucial in helping make the case for the arts and to convince others of their value.

In addition, I would offer the following comments and suggestions. Considerable attention has been paid by those working in the field to differences among the various approaches and roles—between the work and role of music therapists and others, for example—and there is certainly value in trying to clarify the best use of various approaches in relation to the outcomes that are desired. On the other hand, there is also value in recognizing the legitimacy of a wide range of activities and looking for common ground between them, especially given the common challenges faced by all those working in the field. While acknowledging that the value of approaches by those who are not music therapists in relation to health-related outcomes can be a matter of some controversy, Kelleher (2001) sees the need for greater openness to having a *range* of programs and activities available. This openness is particularly important given the difficulty many senior settings encounter in affording professional music therapy services—and, one might add, given some of the promising musical approaches for working with seniors that have been developed by people who are not music therapists.

Can music therapists, those running music activity programs at residential facilities, and others offering various musical programs work together more effectively in terms of the overall musically related services the facility or community is providing, or find other grounds for cooperative endeavors? Can the results of new research on one kind of musical intervention provide ideas and suggestions for those using another kind?

As already illustrated, there can be many activities that involve seniors as *both* audience and cocreators of the experience. By being open to developing these hybrid models, activity directors and others can provide further opportunities for engagement by older adults in music and other arts activities. Other potentially valuable hybrids for which there are interesting models involve combining music with other art forms, for example, drawing a picture to a piece of music, or conversely, coming up with a musical reaction or lyric to a drawing.

There are opportunities relatively untapped to prolong or deepen the impact of an *individual* concert or other supposedly one-time event. A series of concerts can be planned over the course of the year on a given theme, even if by different groups, and be interspersed with discussion groups between the concerts. (See the second application exercise below).

The potential of music to provide an added dimension to an everyday experience can be used more fully. The occasional use of music to accompany dining is one such example. Music can also provide a bridge between the potentially passive role of watching television and something more active. (See the third application exercise below.)

It may be valuable to explore further ways in which various modalities can be used in musical activities. Some of the methods of teaching music to children may be instructive here. For example, the Kodaly Method (Chosky, 1998) of music education is a highly sequential music program in which singing, moving, listening, musical reading and writing, improvising, and composing are the means through which children develop skills and acquire knowledge about melody, harmony, rhythm, form, tempo, timbre, and dynamics. The approach translates, for instance, the relationships between and among musical pitches into many kinds of relationships involving different modalities: hand signals, moving the body up and down, having people of different heights stand next to each other in different orders, and so on.

Are there aspects of musical experience shared particularly by people in the early and later years of life—the importance of a sense of wonder, for example? Could identification of such commonalities help in the selection of materials (songs, formats) that could be used in intergenerational musical programming?

What are the best practices? As suggested earlier, continued and sustained research is needed to understand what there is about a particular activity or group that makes it effective. How much is the effect due to the musical material itself, the way it is presented, the size of the group, the frequency with which it is presented, whether or not it involves material already familiar to listeners, or whether it is coupled with another art form or activity? How integral to an activity's success is the way that it is structured and whether or not it is offered under the guidance of a trained leader? Are some of these variables more important and effective in relation to particular kinds of goals, audiences, and groups?

Concluding Note

The concert is over and the hall is now empty. As the performers and I pick up our things and walk out, we hear a sound that stops us in our tracks. We look back and see several of the residents gathered in the outside hall. We listen more carefully. They are humming the Niggun that opened and closed the concert.

The singers and I look at each other with a quiet unspoken sense of what each of us is at that moment feeling. Twyla Tharp is right: creativity is about being grateful (Bortnick, 2004).

Exercises

EXERCISE 1

In an autobiography group, in relation to "Who am I and what has my life been about?" pose the question: "If your life were a movie, describe the kind of musical score that it would have. The mood? The style? Or: "Is there a particular song that sums up a major insight you have had in your life?"

EXERCISE 2

In scheduling an individual concert in a senior center, nursing home, or other senior setting, plan a workshop to take place in the facility approximately a week before the concert. The workshop would be on a theme or principal song used in the concert. For example, at a concert featuring a song about trees, there might be a preconcert workshop that discusses what kind of tree individuals would be, "if they were a tree" as well as their favorite memories of trees and the role of various aspects of nature in their lives. They might then draw a favorite tree. The drawing would be shown at the concert itself, which, along with the song, might stimulate further discussion about the topic of trees and what trees meant and still mean to those in the room. Finally, following the discussion, performers might ask audience members to suggest a theme that might form the basis both of a song performed at a future concert—and of a preconcert workshop, e.g., rivers and other bodies of water, traditions, or seasons of the year.

EXERCISE 3

Seniors in residential facilities might listen to selections of famous songs from movies and television shows and take part in a group experience of naming the song or the show from which the song comes. Conversely, they might be invited to assume the role of film scorer. They might be given the name of the show (or a character from the show or famous moment in the show) and a chance to come up with a musical fragment to capture that element—in a rhythmic pattern, perhaps, or a short melody.

Acknowledgements

The author would like to thank Cassandra L. Martin-Himmons for her invaluable assistance with the research and many other aspects of this article. I would also like to thank the talented performers of my musical group Paul Buch, Lenore Chudd, Zena David, and Rebecca Varon, and my invaluable artistic consultant, Cheryl Weiner, for helping shape, in such a creative and enjoyable way, my experience with working with seniors.

This chapter is dedicated to all those like them who give in so many ways to ensure and enlarge a place for the arts in the lives of seniors. It is also dedicated to my aunts Mae Bortnick and Eva Koffman whose continued pursuit of a life of activity and engagement has been inspiring, and to the memory of my parents Rose and Phil Bortnick whose interest in music was the original spark for my own interest and whose experiences and life-long values shaped and reinforced my interest in contributing to the quality of life of others.

References

Abba, J. (1989). Changes in creativity with age: Data, explanations and further predictions. *International Journal of Aging and Human Development*, 28(2), 105–126.

Adler, R. S. (2004). *Music therapy assessment and treatment planning: Annotated bibliography of research supporting the inclusion of music therapy on the MDS 3.0*. Unpublished monograph prepared for the American Music Therapy Association.

Aldridge, D. (1994). Alzheimer's disease: Rhythm, timing and music as therapy. *Biomedicine and Pharmacotherapy*, 48(7), 275–281.

Aldridge, D. (1995). Music therapy and the treatment of Alzheimer's disease. *Clinical Gerontologist*, 16(1), 41–57.

Aldridge, D. (1996). *Music therapy research and practice in medicine: From out of the silence.* London: Jessica Kingsley.

Alzheimer's Association. (2004). *What is Alzheimer's?* Retrieved June 27, 2004, from Alzheimer' Association Web site: *http://www.alz.org/AboutAD/WhatIsAD.asp*

Ashida, S. (2000). The effect of reminiscence music therapy sessions on changes in depressive symptoms in elderly persons with dementia. *Journal of Music Therapy*, 37(3), 170–182.

Barret, D. B., & Clements, C. B. (1997). Expressive arts programming for older adults both with and without disabilities: An opportunity for inclusion. In T. Tedrick (Ed.), *Older adults with developmental disabilities and leisure* (pp. 53–64). Binghamton, NY: Haworth Press.

Basting, A. D., & Killick, J. (2003). *The arts and dementia care: A resource guide.* New York: National Center for Creative Aging.

Berryman-Miller, S. (1986). Benefits of dance in the process of aging and retirement for the older adult. *Activities, Adaptation, & Aging*, 9(1), 43–51.

Birren, J. E., & Cochran, K. N. (2001). *Telling the stories of life through guided autobiography groups.* Baltimore: Johns Hopkins University Press.

Birren, J. E., & Deutchman, D. E., (1991). *Guiding autobiography groups for older adults: Exploring the fabric of life.* Baltimore: Johns Hopkins University Press.

Bittman, B., Berk, L., & Felton, D. L. (2001). Composite effects of group drumming music therapy on modulation of neuroendocrine-immune parameters in normal subjects. *Alternative Therapies in Medicine*, 7(1), 38–47.

Bittman, B., Bruhn, K. T., Stevens, C., Westengard, J., & Umbach, P.O. (2003). Recreational music-making: A cost effective group interdisciplinary strategy for reducing burnout and improving mood states in long-term care workers. *Advances in Mind-Body Medicine*, 19(3/4) 4–15.

Bortnick, B. (2004). personal communication.

Brotons, M., & Koger, S. M. (2000). The impact of music therapy on language functioning in dementia. *Journal of Music Therapy*, 37(3), 183–195.

Burack, O. R., Jefferson, P., & Libow, L. S. (2002). Individualized music: A route to improving the quality of life for long-term care residents. *Activities, Adaptation, & Aging*, 26(1), 63–76.

Butler, R. N. (1963). The life review: An interpretation of reminiscence in the aged. *Psychiatry*, 26, 65–76.

Butler, R. N. (1995). Life review. In G. L. Maddox, (Ed.), *The encyclopedia of aging* (2nd ed.). New York: Springer.

Campbell, D. (1992). *Music and miracles: A companion to music: Physician for times to come.* Wheaton, IL: Quest Books.

Chavin, M. (2002). Music as communication. *Alzheimer's Care Quarterly*, 3(2) 145–156.

Chosky, L. (1998). *The Kodaly Method I: Comprehensive music education.* Upper Saddle River, NJ: Pearson Education.

Christie, M. E. (1992). Music therapy applications in a skilled and intermediate care nursing home facility: A clinical study. *Activities, Adaptation, & Aging*, 16(4), 69–87.

Clair, A. A. (1996). *Therapeutic uses of music with older adults.* Baltimore: Health Professions Press.

Coffman, D. D. (2002). Music and quality of life in older adults. *Psychomusicology*, 18, 76–88.

Cohen, A., Bailey, B., & Nilson, T. (2002). The importance of music to seniors. *Psychomusicology*, 18, 89–101.

Cohen, G. D. (2000). *The creative age.* New York: HarperCollins.

Cohen, G. D. (2003). *The impact on older participants of professionally conducted cultural programs.* Washington, DC: National Endowment for the Arts, Center of Aging, Health and Humanities.

Cohen-Mansfield, J., & Werner, P. (1997). Management of verbally disruptive behaviors in nursing home residents. *Journals of Gerontology Series A, Biological Sciences and Medical Sciences*, 52, M369–M377.

Dohr, J. H., & Forbes, L. A. (1986). Creativity, arts and profiles of aging: A reexamination. *Educational Gerontology*, 12, 123–138.

Duffey, T. H., Lumadue, C. A., & Woods, S. (2001). A musical chronology and the emerging life song. The Family Journal: *Counseling and Therapy for Couples and Families*, 9(4), 398–406.

Durham, P. R., & Whittemore, M. P. (1993). Memory recall and participation levels in the elderly: A study of golden age radio. *Educational Gerontology*, 19, 569–575.

Erikson, E. (1959). *Identity and the life cycle.* New York: International Universities Press.

Fisher, B. J., & Specht, D. K. Successful aging and creativity in later life. *Journal of Aging Studies*, 13(4), 457–472.

Gibson, F. (2004). *The past in the present: Using reminiscence in health and social care.* Baltimore: Health Professions Press.

Gotell, E., Brown, S., & Ekman, S. (2002). Caregiver singing and background music in dementia care. *Western Journal of Nursing Research*, 24(2), 195–216.

Halpern, A. B., & Bartlett, J. C. (2002). The impact of music therapy on language functioning in dementia. *Journal of Music Therapy*, 37(3), 183–195.

Hamburg, J., & Clair, A. A. (2003). The effects of movement with music program on measures of balance and gait speed in healthy older adults. *Journal of Music Therapy*, 40(3), 213–226.

Jennings, B., & Vance, D. (2002). The short-term effects of music therapy on different types of agitation in adults with Alzheimer's. *Activities, Adaptation, & Aging*, 26(4), 27–33.

Johnson, J. K., Cotman, C. W., Tasaki, C. S., & Shaw, G. L. (1998). Enhancement of spatial-temporal reasoning after a Mozart listening condition in Alzheimer's disease: A case study. *Neurological Research*, 20, 666–672.

Johnson, J. K., Shaw, G. L., Vuong, M., Vuong, S., & Cotman, C. W. (2002). Short-term improvement on a visual-spatial task after music listening in Alzheimer's disease: A group study. *Activities, Adaptation, & Aging*, 26(3), 37–50.

Karras, B. (1987). Music and reminiscence: For groups and individuals. *Activities, Adaptation, & Aging*, 10(1/2), 79–91.

Kartman, L. L. (1990). Fun and entertainment: One aspect of making meaningful music for the elderly. *Activities, Adaptation, & Aging*, 14(4), 39–44.

Kartman, L. L. (1991). Life review: One aspect of making meaningful music for the elderly. *Activities, Adaptation, & Aging*, 15(3), 45–52.

Kastenbaum, R. (1991). The creative impulse: Why it won't just quit. *Generations*, 15(2), 7–12.

Kastenbaum, R. (1992). The creative process: A life span approach. In T. R. Cole, D. D. Van Tassel, & R. Kastenbaum (Eds.), *Handbook of the humanities and aging*. New York: Springer Publishing.

Katz, E. (1993). Art, aging, and developmental disabilities. *Activities, Adaptation, & Aging*, 17(4), 11–15.

Katz, M. (2003). Leisure activities and the risk of dementia in the elderly. *New England Journal of Medicine*, 348(25), 2508–2516.

Kelleher, A. Y. (2001). The beat of a different drummer: Music therapy's role in dementia respite care. *Activities, Adaptation, & Aging*, 25(2), 75–84.

Koger, S. M., Chapin, K., & Brotons, M. (1999). Is music therapy an effective intervention for dementia? A meta-analytic review of the literature. *Journal of Music Therapy*, 36(1), 2–15.

Kramer, M. K. (2001). A trio to treasure: The elderly, the nurse, and music. *Geriatric Nursing*, 22(4), 191–195.

Kulman, L. (2003, October 13). The habits of highly creative people. *U.S. News and World Report*, 50.

Kydd, P. (2001). Using music therapy to help a client with Alzheimer's disease adapt to long-term care. *American Journal of Alzheimer's Disease and other Dementias*, 16(2), 103–108.

Lindauer, M. S. (2003). *Aging, creativity, and art: A positive perspective on late life development*. New York: Kluwer Academic/Plenum.

MacTavish, H. (2003) *Rhythms, rhymes and reasons: A guide to enrich the lives and animate the spirits of individuals dealing with issues of aging and disability*. Unpublished manuscript.

Magee, J. J. (1988). Using poetry as an aid to life review. *Activities, Adaptation, & Aging*, 12(1/2), 91–101.

Matthews, R. M., Clair, A. A., & Kososki, K. (2000). Brief in-service training in music therapy for activity aides: Increasing engagement of persons with dementia in rhythm activities. *Activities, Adaptation, & Aging*, 24(4), 41–49.

Myerhoff, B., & Simic, A. (1977). *Life's career-aging: Cultural variations in growing old*. Thousand Oaks, CA: Sage.

Needler, W., & Baer, M. A. (1982). Movement, music, and remotivation with the regressed elderly. *Journal of Gerontological Nursing*, 8(9), 497–503.

Pacchetti, D., Mancini, F., Aglieri, R., Fundaro, C., Martigoni, E., & Nappi, G. (2000). Active music therapy on Parkinson's disease: An integrative method for motor and emotional rehabilitation. *Psychosomatic Medicine*, 62(3), 386–393.

Palo-Bengtsson, L., & Ekman, S. L. (2002). Emotional response to social dancing and walks in persons with dementia. *American Journal of Alzheimer's Disease and other Dementias*, 17(3), 149–153.

Perlstein, S. (1988). Transformation: Life review and communal theater. *Journal of Gerontological Social Work*, 12(3/4), 137–148.

Perlstein, S. (1991). Elders share the arts: Life review as a creative, therapeutic, and empowering tool. *Generations*, 16, 55–57.

Ragnesgkog, H., Brane, G., Karlssoc, I., & Kihlgren, M. (1996). Influence of dinner music on food intake and symptoms common in dementia. *Scandinavian Journal of Caring Sciences*, 10(1), 11–7.

Rosling, L. K., & Kitchen, J. (1992). Music and drawing with institutionalized elderly. *Activities, Adaptation, & Aging*, 17(2), 27–38.

Sambandham, M., & Schirm, V. (1995). Music as a nursing intervention for residents with Alzheimer's disease in long-term care. *Geriatric Nursing*, 16(2), 79–83.

Simonton, D. K. (1990). Creativity in the later years: Optimistic prospects for achievement. *The Gerontologist*, 30(5), 626–631.

Simonton, D. K. (1991). Creative productivity through the adult years. *Generations*, 16(2), 13–16.

Thorgrimsen, L., Schweitzer, P., & Orrell, M. (2002). Evaluating reminiscence for people with dementia: A pilot study. *The Arts in Psychotherapy*, 29(2), 93–97.

Tufts University. (2001). Music therapy: One key for people with Alzheimer's or Parkinson's disease. *Tufts University Health and Nutrition Letter*, Medford, MA.

Wakefield, D. (1990) *The story of your life: Writing a spiritual autobiography*. Beacon Press

Whitcomb, J. B. (1994). I would weave a song for you: Therapeutic music and milieu for dementia residents. *Activities, Adaptation & Aging*, 18(2), 57–74.

Bibliography

Basting, A.D. (2001). *The Stages of Age: Performing age in contemporary American culture*. Ann Arbor, MI: University of Michigan Press.

Brotons, M., & Koger, S. M. (1997). Music and dementias: A review of the literature. *Journal of Music Therapy*, 24(4), 204–245.

Cole, T., Van Tassel, D. R., & Kastenbaum, R. (Eds.). (1992). *Handbook of the humanities and aging*. New York: Springer.

DiGiammarino, M., Hanlon, H., Kassing, G., & Libman, K. (1992). Arts and aging: An annotated bibliography of selected resource materials in art, dance, drama, and music. *Activities, Adaptation, & Aging*, 17(2), 39–51.

Lehrman, L. (1984). *Teaching dance to senior adults*. Springfield, IL: Thomas Press.

Lynch, L. (1987). Music therapy: Its historical relationships and value programs for the long-term care setting. *Activities, Adaptation, & Aging*, 10(1/2), 5–15.

Perlstein, S., & Bliss, J. (1994). *Generating community: Intergenerational partnerships through the expressive arts*. New York: Elders Share the Arts.

Weisberg, N., & Wilder, R. (1985). *Creative arts with older adults: A sourcebook*. New York: Human Science Press.

Resources

See also the Resources Appendix

- Alzheimer's Disease Support Center (ADSC) is an online resource. Its Web site offers a selected list of resources compiled by the National Alzheimer's Association including sections on articles, books, and videocassettes dealing with Alzheimer's Disease and music, art, and dance/movement. Available at *http://adscmain.ohioalzcenter.org/Information/Reading/rtrlactiv.htm*

- ARTSeniors Web site is available at *http://www.artfaces.com/artseniors/index.htm*. This Internet gallery features senior citizen artists from around the world and from all walks of life.

- Arts for the Aging, 6917 Arlington Road, Suite 352, Bethesda, MD 20814; (301) 718-4990. Available at *http://www.aftaarts.org*. Provides artistic outreach services to psychologically and physically impaired seniors in senior day care centers and not-for-profit nursing homes in the metropolitan Washington, DC, area.

- The Bridge: An Intergenerational Exploration of the Arts, 4750 Woodward, Detroit, MI 48201; (313) 833-1300, ext 35. Features music and visual arts to help stimulate dialogue between children and elders.

- Cabaret, E-mail: *loislane3@earthlink.net*. A group of professional singers, instrumentalists, and dancers founded by Rena Dictor LeBlanc that performs for residents of 12 nursing homes in the Los Angeles area, with plans for expansion to other parts of the country.

- Center for Elders and Youth in the Arts; (415) 447-1989, ext. 534. E-mail: *ceya@ioaging.org*. Teams youth and elders in collaborative, educational programming under the instruction of professional visual and performing artists.

- Creative Growth and Creativity Explored, 3245 16th Street, San Francisco, CA 94103; (415) 863-2108. Available at *http://www.creativityexplored.org/*

- Creative Growth Art Center, 355 24th Street, Oakland, CA 94612; (510) 836-2340. Available at *http://www.creativegrowth.org/*. Provides creative art programs, educational and independent-living training, counseling, and vocational opportunities for adults who are physically, mentally, and emotionally disabled regardless of age.
- From Healing to Hallelujah, E-mail: *Barrybortnick@msn.com*. Musical group that performs multiparticipatory musical programs, interlaced with drama, movement, and the visual arts for senior residential communities, nursing homes, and other facilities in Southern California and other locations, as well as for intergenerational audiences.
- Healing and the Arts, C. Everett Koop Institute at Dartmouth, 7025 Strasenburgh, Hanover, NH 03755; (603) 650-1450. Available at *http://www.dartmouth.edu/dms/koop/programs/healing.shtml*. A joint activity by the Dartmouth Medical School and the C. Everett Koop Institute to explore the use of the arts and humanities to enhance medical education and support the process of healing.
- *Health*RHYTHMS, Division of Remo Drum Co., 28101 Industry Drive, Valencia, CA 91355; (661) 294-5655. Available at *http://www.remo.com/health/*. Develops and provides materials, programs, training, and research supporting the use of drumming as an effective means for promoting and maintaining health and well-being.
- Hospital Audiences, Inc., 548 Broadway, 3rd Fl., New York, NY 10012; (212) 575-7676. Available at *http://www.hospitalaudiences.org/hai/*. Provides access to the arts to culturally isolated New Yorkers.
- International Centre for Applied Imagination, E-mail: *dahlberg@highstream.net*. Available at *http://www.appliedimagination.co.uk/*. Has information on creativity and aging.
- International Foundation for Music Research, 5790 Armada Drive, Carlsbad, CA 92008. Available at *http://www.music-research.org/*. Supports scientific research to explore the relationship between music and physical and emotional wellness, with particular attention to the elderly population.
- Kairos Dance Theater Foundation, 4524 Beard Avenue South, Minneapolis, Minnesota 55410; (612) 927-7864. Available at *http://www.kairosdance.org/*. Intergenerational dance company whose work is informed by modern dance, folk dance traditions from around the world, movement, and storytelling improvisation techniques. Kodaly method. For references, see *http://trip.tripod.com/kodalybooks.html*
- Liz Lerman Dance Exchange, 7117 Maple Avenue, Takoma Park, Maryland 20912; (301) 270-6700. Available at *www.danceexchange.org*. Professional company of dance artists that creates, performs, teaches, and engages people of all ages in making art.
- Museum One, Inc., (800) 524-1730. Available at *http://www.museumoneinc.org/index.html*. Arts and educational outreach service which brings art appreciation and other art forms such as music, dance, and poetry to the community, with a special emphasis on the older adult and aging population.
- National Coalition of Creative Arts Therapies Associations, 93 Edwards Street, New Haven, CT 06515. Available at *http://www.nccata.org*. An alliance of

professional associations dedicated to the advancement of the arts as therapeutic modalities. Its web site also provides contact information for six associations: American Art Therapy Association, American Dance Therapy Association, American Music Therapy Association, American Society of Group Psychotherapy and Psychodrama, National Association for Drama Therapy, and National Association for Poetry Therapy.

- New Horizons Band, (607) 962-1125. Available at *http://www.newhorizonsband.com/*. Band program for adult beginners to allow them to fill their lives with music, new friends, fun, and accomplishment.

- New Rhythms Foundation, PO Box 1070, Tiburon, CA 94920; (415) 435-4870. Creates interactive programs involving percussion, storytelling, and song at nursing care facilities, adult day service programs, and programs working with the developmentally disabled.

- Senior Adult Theater Program, University of Nevada, Las Vegas, 4505 S. Maryland Parkway, Box 455084, Las Vegas, NV; 89154; (702) 895-4673. Available at *http://www.seniortheatre.com/html*. Offers the only Bachelor of Arts in Senior Theatre in the country and includes the bringing together of traditional and nontraditional

students for performances on the UNLV campus and in the Las Vegas community.

- Senior Theatre League of America, Educational Theatre Association, 2343 Auburn Avenue, Cincinnati, OH 45219; (513) 421-3900. Available at *http://www.seniortheatreleague.org*. Promotes and nurtures the growing senior adult theater movement by providing leadership, advocacy, and opportunities for its members.

- Society for the Arts in Healthcare, 1632 U Street NW, Washington, DC 20009; (202) 299-9770. Available at *http://www.societyartshealthcare.org/*. Not-for-profit organization dedicated to promoting the incorporation of the arts as an integral component of health care.

- Songwriting Works, PO Box 606, 2625 Alcatraz Avenue, Berkeley, CA 94705; (510) 548-3655. Available at *http://www.songwritingworks.org*. Develops avenues through which elders can be widely heard through their own words and music.

- Stagebridge, 2501 Harrison Street, Oakland, CA 94612; (510) 444-4755. Available at *http:///www.stagebridge.org*. The nation's oldest senior theater company. Provides opportunities for older adults to use theater and storytelling to bridge the generation gap and to stimulate positive attitudes toward aging.

Chapter 17

Support and Self-Help Groups

Carole A. Winston
Jane B. Neese

Key Words

- Common goal
- Coping
- Empathy
- Mutual affirmation
- Self-help
- Support group

Learning Objectives

- Define support group
- Define self-help group
- Discuss the role of professionals in support and self-help groups
- State five interventions a practitioner might introduce in sponsoring a support group
- Describe how you would evaluate the effectiveness of a caregiver's support group

It is estimated that more than 25 million people of all ages have participated in some type of self-help or mutual support group at some time in their lives (Kessler, Michelson, & Zhao, 1997). As a mode of intervention in working with older adults, support groups and self-help groups have the broad purpose of increasing the satisfaction of older persons' socioemotional needs. Group members are encouraged to actively interact. Self-disclosure is expected to be high and proceedings kept within the group. Typically, self-help and support groups are formed by individuals who share a similar problem or concern. The group members have common experiences that promote a sense of support and connection. There are support groups and self-help groups for persons with dementia, older adults with severe psychiatric disorders, cancer survivors, stroke patients, substance abusers, and persons with other serious medical conditions. There are support groups for the spouses, adult children, and paid caregivers of persons with Alzheimer's disease; for "partners" of those with visual impairments; for persons who have lost a spouse, and those older adults caring for family members infected with the human immunodeficiency virus (HIV).

Support groups have been particularly effective in the areas of health and mental health. Support groups help members cope with life stressors by fortifying and enhancing a variety of coping skills in order to more effectively adapt to life events. Some groups provide peer support, others provide education on specific topics, and most combine social support with opportunities to learn about specific issues (e.g., bereavement, late life sexuality).

Many self-help or mutual aid groups include professionals in an advisory or facilitating role (Compton & Galaway, 1999, p. 399). There are several roles professionals can play if they sponsor peer-led groups: help peer leaders with material support, provide the meeting place, help with supplies, serve as guest speakers; provide information, consultation, or supervision; serve as brokers by referring prospective members to the group; and plan for the development of new groups.

Support Groups for Older Adults

Support groups help older adults cope with stressors by revitalizing coping skills to more effectively adapt during some of life's difficult transitions. Additionally, older adults often suffer from conversation deprivation. To be encouraged to share and relate with others in a group setting has therapeutic value in itself (Toseland & Rivas, 2001). Older people often need support and encouragement more than they need confrontation. Therefore, support group work is oriented less toward personality reconstruction and more toward making life in the present more meaningful and enjoyable. However, never to challenge or confront older people could be seen as patronizing and may be based on the distorted belief that they cannot change (Corey & Corey, 2002).

Types of Support Groups

SELF-HELP GROUPS

People come together in self-help groups to share a common concern and to help one another cope with or resolve problems related to that concern. The common concern may be recovery from substance abuse, preparing for retirement, or coping with the stress of a particular illness. Group members rather than a professional usually lead self-help groups.

EDUCATIONAL SUPPORT GROUPS

Educational groups have the primary purpose of helping the group members learn about themselves and their roles and relationships in society. Along with imparting new knowledge, educational groups provide support and acceptance for the members who share common concerns and characteristics. Reissman (2000) writes that older adult patients often reach out to doctors, not out of medical necessity, but for emotional or social support to ease their loneliness. Such demands for emotional and social support disguised as medical queries, can be better met by connecting patients to one another in educational support groups. The informal, empathic environment created in the group setting and the group members' propensity to become helpers after being helped themselves enhances the effectiveness of such groups. Participants have been known to focus on what they can do for one another, rather than on their medical condition.

Educational support groups provide information about long-term chronic medical conditions such as coronary heart disease, diabetes, asthma, cancer, and illnesses that affect people as they age. Support groups for survivors and persons newly diagnosed with breast cancer and prostate cancer provide information about treatment options. Members learn what to expect from surgery, radiation, and chemotherapy (Breast Cancer Support and Prostate Cancer Discussion Group, 2004). There are also multiple types of groups that support older people who are well.

WELL-ELDERLY SUPPORT GROUPS

Healthy Aging. In working with well elderly, the social support mechanisms of a group help members understand the universality of their struggles. Many older adults have problems coping with the aging process. These people have to deal with the many losses associated with advancing age in addition to the pressures and conflicts that younger generations experience, and they can profit from personal-growth groups that serve people of all ages. Support group programs for the well elderly include: exercise programs, congregate meals, health club and wellness programs, abuse prevention services, retirement planning groups, and prayer groups.

Friendship Groups. Professional service providers in settings such as community mental health clinics, senior centers, older adult housing, home care agencies, and nursing homes have organized short-term support groups for older women to explore the significance of friendship in later life. In collaboration with the group leaders, group members determine weekly topics that explore the importance of friendship across the life cycle (Greenberg, Motenko, Roesch, & Embleton, 1999).

Grandparent Groups. There are 4.5 million children under 18 growing up in grandparent-headed households with approximately one-third of these children having no parent in the home. While the majority of grandparents raising grandchildren are between ages 55–64, 20–25% are over age 65 (Administration on Aging, 2000). Among the first interventions to assist grandparent caregivers were support groups, begun in the 1980s by the grandparents themselves. Some of the first were small groups in rural communities, meeting in the home of a grandparent who had just assumed full responsibility for one or more grandchildren. Other groups were convened in churches, schools, hospitals, or senior centers of larger cities, facilitated by a volunteer health or social service worker who had noticed the increasing number of young children in the care of older clients (Vakalahi & Khaja, 2000).

By 1998, over 500 parenting grandparent support groups were operating across the country (Roe & Minkler, 1999). Support groups offer crucial short-term emotional informational and material support to older people facing the challenges of raising children. The activities of grandparent support groups, even those with the most modest resources, often extend beyond simple mutual aid. Groups frequently invite speakers to discuss various aspects of parenting, including dealing with grief and loss, discipline, helping with homework, nutrition, and talking with teenagers about sex. Support groups have produced newsletters and developed local resource guides; have established clothing, toy, and furniture banks; and have offered children's programs and holiday celebrations or sponsored intergenerational activities (AARP Grandparent Information Center, 2004; Burnette, 1998; Roe & Minkler, 1998–1999).

BEHAVIOR MODIFICATION SUPPORT GROUPS

Some groups, such as Alcoholics Anonymous (AA), Narcotics Anonymous (NA), and Overeaters Anonymous (OA), focus on behavior modification. AA was the original self-help group. It was begun in 1935 in the United States as a twelve-step program, offering alcoholics a way to develop a satisfying life without alcohol (Information on Alcoholics Anonymous, 2004). For some older adults, alcoholism has been a part of their lives, yet there are growing numbers of older adults who are being diagnosed with alcohol dependence for the first time. According to the Epidemiologic Catchment Area Study conducted in the 1990s, there is an increasing trend in first-time occurrence of alcoholism in older adults (who are 65 and older) (Helzer, Burnam, & McEvoy, 1991). Blondell (1999) found that approximately 1–3% of the older people in the United States suffer from the consequences of excessive alcohol consumption, while many more drink amounts of alcohol that place them at risk for alcohol-related problems. Alcoholism is thought to be a significant contributor to the etiology of self-neglect among older adults. Affected individuals can suffer from malnutrition, develop chronic health problems, acquire unintentional injuries, become depressed, neglect their health care needs, and isolate themselves from friends and family

(Blondell). Therefore, alcoholism, whether it has just begun or has been an ongoing disease process, is occasionally present in older adulthood.

DOMESTIC VIOLENCE SUPPORT GROUPS

Brandl, Hebert, Rozwadowski, and Spangler (2003) interviewed 34 professional facilitators of support groups for older abused women. Based on those interviews they determined that support groups could provide information, friendship and hope to older women who may feel isolated. Wolf (2001) identified support groups for older victims of domestic violence sponsored by domestic violence programs and aging services programs. Wolf notes that group leaders found that older adults resisted the group experience. Major barriers to attending were: inaccessibility of the meeting sites and inadequate resources for recruitment. Recommendations for increased group participation included:

- Ensuring accessibility of the meeting site
- Using a leader and a coleader, at least one of whom is older or familiar with aging issues
- Allocating resources for recruitment
- Seeking a steady source of funding

CAREGIVER SUPPORT GROUPS

Spouses, family members, and other persons who care for the frail elderly, persons with dementia, and older adults with severe mental illness often report high levels of burden and stress. Support groups offer one option to help these caregivers. Although caregivers generally report satisfaction with support groups, the benefits are often modest and of short duration (Lavoie, 1995). More recently, however, programs have been developed to improve the ability of caregivers to cope with the stressful demands at the core of caring for older adults whose relational capacities are diminished by infirmity, progressive dementia, or mental illness, rather than focus on the task-oriented aspects of caring (Levesque et al., 2002). One of the coping strategies identified by the researchers was

"reframing" the thoughts, feelings, and expectations of the caregiver in the following ways:

- Interpreting dysfunctional behaviors as a consequence of infirmity, dementia, or mental illness rather than as deliberate behaviors
- Replacing dysfunctional thoughts with more helpful and rational thoughts
- Looking at the enrichment of caring rather than only the burdensome aspects
- Focusing on the reality and the acceptance of daily losses

Williams and Barton (2003–2004) described a caregiver support group sponsored by a chapter of the Philadelphia Alzheimer's Association that provides a constellation of programs and services for individuals with dementia and their families, including caregiver support groups. Over time, this chapter has developed a number of support groups to meet the particular needs of African-Americans who often do not participate in traditional family caregiver support programs. Often African-American caregivers assume they will be the lone minority group member and their understanding of the disease and management style might be misunderstood by other members of the group. Group members learn what to expect during the course of the disease and about the changes that will occur as the disease progresses. They learn how the disease affects them and other family members in an environment that allows them the freedom to express their emotions without guilt, and they have an opportunity to receive positive reinforcement from peers.

Obstacles to Self-Help and Mutual Aid

One potential obstacle to self-help and mutual aid support is the apparently divergent interests each group member brings to the engagement. Even in a group with a narrow, clearly defined purpose, some group members may perceive their sense of urgency differently from the others. Various group members may feel their concerns and feelings are unique and unrelated to those of the other members. In many ways the group is a microcosm of the larger society, and reflects the individual social encounter in society. As the group develops, individual members understand that they can learn and grow by giving help as well as receiving it (Shulman, 1999).

Practical and Professional Considerations for Group Work with Older People

Corey and Corey (2002) provide examples of practical issues to consider when thinking about forming specialized groups for older adults:

- *Developing a proposal for a group*—Many good ideas for groups are never put into practice because they are not developed into a clear and convincing plan. These five general areas form the basis of a sound and practical proposal:

  –Rationale—Do you have a clear and convincing rationale for the group?

  –Objectives—Are you clear about what you most want to attain and how you will go about doing so? Are your objectives specific, measurable, and attainable within the specified time?

  –Practical considerations—Is the membership defined? Are meeting times, frequency of meetings, and duration of the group reasonable?

  –Procedures—Have you selected specific procedures to meet the stated objectives? Are these procedures appropriate and realistic for this population?

  –Evaluation—Does your proposal contain strategies for evaluating how well the stated objectives were met? Are your evaluation methods objective, practical, and relevant?

An example of a support group: Grandmothers Support Group

Some groups were started for the purpose of offering mutual support and developing group strength through the process of empowerment. One of the authors of this chapter, Winston (1999), had occasion to observe a self-help support group of African-American grandmothers who were parenting their grandchildren because one or both parents had died of AIDS-related illnesses. The women lived in New York City's central Harlem community. The group facilitator utilized an empowerment model of social work practice epitomized by Solomon (1999) in her seminal work on strategies that social workers and other professionals can employ to strengthen families that have been marginalized because of skin color. While these women initially came together because of idiosyncratic difficulties they experienced in their new roles as parenting grandmothers, they soon identified common obstacles to the acquisition of resources for their grandchildren in the public school system, medical care facilities, court systems, public housing, and public assistance agencies. The group's facilitator helped them to recognize that they were not entirely or even primarily responsible for their problems, but they should take responsibility for their solutions. Problem resolution required the collaboration of the members and the group facilitator to develop strategies that capitalized on their individual and collective strengths in order to foster both independence and interdependence. The mutual aid group served as an appropriate model to address the grandmothers' need for expressive and instrumental support (Winston, 1999).

The grandmothers support group met regularly, and through informal discussions they began to develop an agenda that underscored concerns they had about accessing resources that would assist them in caring for their grandchildren. Working with the group facilitator, the women began to develop an empowerment training group whose tasks included strengthening their parenting skills so that they would be better able to cope with the many challenges they faced in their homes and within society. The facilitator of the group developed an empowerment curriculum to: help the grandmothers achieve a sense of personal power, become aware of connections between individual and community problems, develop helping skills, and develop the capacity to work collaboratively towards social change.

The "classes" consisted of 12 three-hour sessions, held twice weekly. Participation was mandatory. Missing two or more sessions meant the person was dropped from the training. At the end of each class, the grandmothers completed brief evaluations describing how much they felt they had learned. Homework assignments were given as a means of reinforcing the learning. With the completion of the training, the grandmothers began their ongoing task of reaching out to other grandparents in the community. They were responsible for giving presentations to groups at schools, senior centers, churches, tenant associations, and in other settings where grandparents and other caregivers were located. Follow-up training sessions were scheduled periodically to review the presentations and provide further assistance.

The majority of the women in the grandmothers' empowerment group were warm, friendly, assertive women who usually had a lot to say during the sessions, and when they met in the support group. One group member in particular often took the floor and had great difficulty relinquishing it to other members. On those occasions, the facilitator would use humor to gently chide her into allowing someone else to "jump in." Because it was a closed group, and the women had known one another for several years, it was a rare instance when the facilitator had to redefine limits. On occasion, a group member would refuse to take part in an exercise or would be uncharacteristically critical of another member. At those times, one of the other group members would raise her

concerns in the next support group meeting in the hope that the problem could be discussed in a supportive, nonthreatening environment.

The following guidelines are offered when organizing support groups for older people (also see **Table 17–1**):

- *Screening and selection issues*—Carefully consider the purposes of the group in determining who will or will not benefit from the experience. The decision to include or exclude members must be made appropriately and sensitively. For example, to mix regressed older persons with relatively well-functioning older adults is to invite fragmentation. There may be a rationale for excluding people who are highly agitated, delusional, or have severe physical problems that could inhibit their benefiting from the group. They display behaviors that are likely to be counterproductive to the group as a whole.
- *Confidentiality*—Older adult group members may be suspicious when they are asked to talk about themselves, and they may fear some sort of retaliation by fellow members. Take great care in defining boundaries of confidentiality to ensure that confidences will not be broken and to provide a safe nonthreatening environment.
- *Labeling and prejudging group members*— In working with older people, it is important not to be influenced by what you hear or read about a given member. Remain open to forming your own impressions and be willing to challenge any limiting labels imposed on your elderly clients.
- *Visitors to groups*—Visitors and other staff members may wish to attend a particular group session. A good practice is to announce visitors in advance of their attending a session and again at the beginning of the session. In addition, the purpose of their visit should be mentioned to lessen suspicion.

- *Values differences*—A good understanding of the social and cultural background of your group members will enable you to work with their concerns in a sensitive way. You may be younger than the members, and you may belong to a racial or ethnic group that is different from that of some or all of the members. Thus age, race, or ethnic difference may signal significant differences in values. For example, a group leader in her early 20s might consider living together as an unmarried couple an acceptable norm, whereas a member in her mid-70s might suffer guilt and shame for doing so. In another instance, a white group leader might address members by their first names, while some African-American elders could easily experience this familiarity as a sign of disrespect.

- *The issue of touching*—Aging people often have a special need to be touched. Many older people live alone and you and others in their group may be their only source of touching. Your own comfort level with touching will be a vital factor in determining how free members feel to exchange touches. It is also critical that you not misinterpret the touch of an older person.

- *Difficult group members*—You may encounter many types of difficult members in this age group. Some may refuse to speak or make a contract, some may never stop talking or interrupting, and some may be highly agitated and hostile. Learn to set firm limits, and deal with these members nondefensively. Members who display problematic behaviors should not be labeled or categorized. The challenge is to understand the broader meaning of the behaviors that these members are manifesting in the group, rather than simply labeling them "resisters."

Table 17–1   DOS AND DON'TS IN GROUP WORK WITH OLDER ADULTS

- Do not treat people as if they are frail when they are not.
- Avoid keeping members busy with meaningless activities.
- Affirm the dignity, intelligence, and pride of elderly group members.
- Do not assume that every elderly person likes being called by his or her first name or a pet name.
- Make use of humor appropriately. Avoid laughing at your members for failing to accomplish tasks, but laugh with them, for instance, when they have created a funny poem.
- Avoid talking to them as if they were small children, no matter how severely impaired they may be.
- Allow the members to complain; even if there is nothing you can do about their complaints. Do not burden yourself with the feeling that you should do something about all of their grievances; sometimes venting can be sufficient.
- Avoid probing for the release of strong emotions that neither you nor they can handle effectively in group sessions.
- Determine how much you can do without feeling depleted, and find avenues for staying vital and enthusiastic.

Source: M. S. Corey and G. Corey, 2002. Adapted with permission.

Summary

This chapter is about support groups and self-help groups for older adults. Support groups help members cope with life stressors by fortifying and enhancing their coping skills so they may more effectively adapt to life events. Self-help groups are groups that are led by nonprofessionals who are struggling with the same issues as members of the group. Professionals can consult with, facilitate, or sponsor support groups and self-help groups. An example is given of a self-help group that moved beyond mutual aid group empowerment for a cohort of parenting grandmothers. Suggestions are given for developing and maintaining groups for older adults.

Exercises

EXERCISE 1

Attend a meeting of some type of support group. List five reasons why you think it is a successful group and defend those reasons. Students are advised that it is essential to check with the leader(s) of self-help groups before going unannounced to observe the meetings.

EXERCISE 2

Attend a support group for families. List and explain four themes that you heard expressed by family members in the group meeting. See the note above about seeking permission to observe a group meeting.

EXERCISE 3

Select one support group that was started or aided by a professional. Study the history of the group, and write a two-page paper on the role the professional had in the formation of the group.

EXERCISE 4

Think about a time in your life when you would have appreciated a support group. Describe the group and say why you would have liked to have had it available.

References

Blondell, R. D. (1999). Alcohol abuse and self-neglect in the elderly. *Journal of Elder Abuse and Neglect,* 11(2), 55–75.

Brandl, R. Hebert, M., Rozwadowski, J., & Spangler, D. (2003). Feeling safe, feeling strong: Support groups for older abused women. *Violence against Women,* 9(12), 1490–1503.

Burnette, D. (1998). Grandparents rearing grandchildren: A school-based small group intervention. *Research on Social Work Practice,* 8(1), 10–27.

Compton, B. R., & Galaway, B. (1999). *Social work processes* (6th ed.). Pacific Grove, CA: Brooks/Cole.

Corey, M. S., & Corey, G. (2002). *Groups: Process and practice* (6th ed.). Pacific Grove, CA: Brooks/Cole.

Grandparent Information Center of the American Association of Retired Persons (AARP). Retrieved October 29, 2004, *http://www.aarp.org/life/grandparents/helpraising/Articles/a2004-01-20-supportgroups.html*

Grandparents raising grandchildren: US government's Administration on Aging fact sheet.

Greenberg, S., Motenko, A. K., Roesch, C., & Embleton, N. (1999). Friendship across the life cycle: A support group for older women. *Journal of Gerontological Social Work,* 32(4), 7–23.

Helzer, J. E., Burnam, A., & McEvoy, L. T. (1991). Alcohol abuse and dependence. In L. N. Robins & D. A. Regier (Eds.), *Psychiatric disorders in America: The epidemiologic catchment area study* (pp. 81–115). New York: Free Press.

Information on alcoholics anonymous. Retrieved April 3, 2004, from *http://www.alcoholics-anonymous.org/*

Kessler, R. C., Mickelson, K. D., & Zhao, S. (1997). Patterns and correlates of self-help in the United States. *Social Policy,* 27(3), 27–46.

Lavoie, J. P. (1995). Support groups for informal caregivers don't work! Refocus the groups or the evaluations? *Canadian Journal on Aging/La Revue cannadienne du vieillissement,* 14, 580–595.

Levesque, L., Gendron, C., Vezina J., Herbert, R., Ducharme, F., Lavoie, J. P, et al. (2002). The process of a group intervention for caregivers of demented persons living at home: Conceptual framework, components, and characteristics. *Aging & Mental Health,* 6(3), 239–247.

Reissman, F, (2000). A demand-side cure for the chronic illness crisis. *Social Policy,* 30(3), 14–19.

Roe, K. M., & Minkler, M. (1998–99). Grandparents raising grandchildren: Challenges and responses. *Generations,* 22(4), 25–32.

Shulman, L. (1999). *The skills of helping: Individuals, families, groups and communities* (4th ed.). Pacific Grove, CA: Wadsworth.

Solomon, B. B. (1999). How do we really empower families: Strategies for social work practitioners. In B. R. Compton & B. Galaway (Eds.), *Social Work Processes* (6th ed., pp. 351–353). Pacific Grove, CA: Brooks/Cole.

Support groups for grandparents raising grandchildren: What you should know, a report from the American Association of Retired Persons, Retrieved May 20, 2004, from *http://www.aarp.org/life/grandparents*.

Toseland, R.W., & Rivas, R. S. (2001). *An introduction to group work practice* (3rd ed.). Boston: Allyn & Bacon.

Vakalahi, H. F., & Khaja, K. (2000). Parent to parent and family to family: Innovative self-help and mutual support. In A. Sallee, H. Lawson, & K. Briar-Lawson (Eds.), *Innovative practices with children and families* (pp. 271–290). Dubuque, IA: Eddie Bowers.

Williams, E., & Barton, P. (2003–2004). Successful support groups for African American caregivers. *Generations, 27*(4), 81–83.

Winston, C. A. (1999). Self-help for grandmothers parenting again. *Journal of Social Distress and the Homeless, 8*(3), 157–165.

Wolf, R. (2001). Support group for older victims of domestic violence. *Journal of Women & Aging, 13*(4), 71–83.

Resources

- Breast cancer support is available at *http://bcsupport.org/*
- Prostate cancer discussion group is available at *http://www.pcasupportsm.org/homepage.htm*
- The American Self-Help Group Clearinghouse offers a guide that has been developed to act as a starting point for exploring real-life support groups and networks that are available throughout the world and in local communities. Available at *http://mentalhelp.net/selfhelp/*
- Directory of Online Resources offers annotated lists of other online support groups and resources. Available at *http://psychcentral.com/resources*

Chapter 18

Group Psychotherapy

Robin Stull Haight

Key Words

- Group process
- Transference
- Holding environment
- Group roles
- Roles
- Boundaries
- Acting out
- Psychoeducation
- Cohort beliefs

Learning Objectives

- Identify three key factors of psychodynamic group psychotherapy
- Identify four key factors of cognitive-behavioral group psychotherapy
- Discuss rationale for choosing either a psychodynamic group or a cognitive-behavioral group
- Describe what is meant by group as microcosm

Minor depression is almost an epidemic among the older age group. Because of the stigma older adults attach to mental health services, they tend not to seek traditional psychiatric care (Lyness et al., 2002). Group psychotherapy may be a good alternative for them because group psychotherapy provides a supportive space for older adults to explore their inner selves and their relationships. Group work offers older adults both a sense of relief knowing that other seniors share similar thoughts, and a sense of hope that they can feel better in the future. Often, in their isolation and distress, older people may think they are crazy and that they are the only ones who have negative thoughts. Group psychotherapy can bridge the sense of isolation through group support and offers the knowledge to group members that their situations are not uncommon. A well-run group creates a safe place for elders to express intense emotion and thus bring about healing through catharsis.

Older adults face many obstacles to getting psychological treatment. These fall into the general categories of cohort beliefs, physical limitations, situational stresses, and family stresses. Several cohort beliefs inhibit this population from seeking support. One is the belief that they are less valuable members of society and that their problems are less important than those of younger people. Older people may believe that anxiety and depression are signs of character weakness or spiritual failure. They may subscribe to the "understandability phenomenon" (Laidlaw, Thompson, Dick-Sisken, & Gallagher-Thompson, 2003), which states that elders are understandably depressed because old age is difficult (p. 36). Additionally, they may hold steadfastly to the role of caretaker as a way to avoid their own care needs (Laidlaw et al.). Physical obstacles to joining a group are general disability, chronic pain, chronic illness, and sensory loss. Situational and family stresses from care giving, substance abuse, and bereavement are yet more impediments to engaging in therapy groups.

Leaders of psychotherapy groups should give serious consideration to making accommodations that address these unique problems of older adulthood. It is true that group psychotherapy is well suited to older people. However, because of the high comorbidity of chronic health problems and depression in this group, older adults typically present to their physician with co-related physical problems rather than to mental health professionals (Haley, 1996). Furthermore, physicians are not well prepared to spot or address such problems or to make appropriate referrals. While it may seem "understandable" that those with chronic health problems are depressed, it should not be assumed. Depression stems from many sources, but for older adults it is common for depression to emerge from experiencing adjustment difficulties, inadequate support, and cumulative losses of various kinds.

This chapter is about the key elements of psychodynamic and cognitive-behavioral group psychotherapy and how to use these therapies in ways that accommodate older adults. The reader will learn the basic tenets of each mode of group psychotherapy and learn to establish a therapy group that adheres to the methodology of the selected approach.

Psychodynamic Group Psychotherapy

Psychodynamic group therapy has a different focus than other methods of conducting a therapy group. It is this focus that defines psychodynamic work. A psychodynamic therapy group's tasks are to observe and explore: (1) relationships between members, (2) relationships between members and leader(s), (3) patterns that emerge in the group as a whole (this is known as group process), and (4) the internal processes occurring for each member. The psychodynamic group is perhaps better understood by what it is not. It does not set out to educate members about the typical course of common difficulties elders face, such as disability, bereavement, and depression. This would be a psychoeducational focus. Instead, psychodynamic groups work to help members attain insight into their difficulties and the impact these difficulties have on their relationships and themselves. In the process, members do become educated about the course of their individual problems. Furthermore, they gain an understanding of how they contribute to these problems or fail to contribute to their solutions. This last part of self-understanding, or insight, is what sets apart psychodynamic therapies from others. The following sections describe three key features of psychodynamic groups.

The Individual's Inner World

Psychodynamic group therapy is interested in the individual's inner world One's inner world becomes manifest in behaviors, thoughts, and feelings. Thus, the psychodynamic therapy group is interested in behaviors, thoughts, and feelings because they are ways through which the individual gives expression to his or her interior being. A premise of psychodynamic group therapy is that symptom relief occurs when patients begin to understand how their inner conflicts affect their current functioning.

While behaviors, thoughts, and feelings are the tableau on which the work is done and through which changes become manifest, we can know changes occur inside the individual as well. How can we know this? Young and Reed (1995) describe an example of such inner change in their concept of "self-transcendence." This term, similar to ego psychology's concept of "ego strength," incorporates "inward expansion," or increased internal resources and capacities for intense affect and "outward expansion," which is an increased capacity for meaningful and rewarding relationships. In a group setting members initially talk about how vulnerable they feel. In time, they show vulnerability through expression of intense emotion and feelings of connection. Leaders will understand then that inner change has taken place. Intense affect expressed early on must not be confused with this inward expansion that occurs only after some time has elapsed. Increased tolerance for intimacy is the hallmark of inner growth.

Transference and Interpersonal Processes

The psychodynamic group attends to transference and interpersonal processes. Transference is an important concept in psychodynamic group work. Moore and Fine (1990) define transference as "the displacement of patterns of feelings, thoughts and behavior, originally experienced in childhood, onto a person involved in a current interpersonal relationship" (p. 196). Psychodynamic group work brings the focus onto patterns of relating in the here and now and to the immediate experience of being a member of a group. Ways of relating can be subtle or obvious, but the attuned therapist calls attention to these and helps members become better observers themselves. Taking a position of curious observer, the therapist helps to bring awareness to processes of which members were previously unaware. Members may sit silently week after week or monopolize sessions week after week for "urgent"

concerns. These are roles members take on unaware of their impact on the group. Transference helps explain such behaviors. For example, the silent member may feel undeserving or ashamed. The one who takes the spotlight each week may feel that others are not as important or, alternatively, may need to feel in the spotlight to feel important.

Transference becomes manifest not only in behaviors but also in members' feelings toward each other or toward the leader. Leaders must be on the lookout for evidence of transference in what members say or do not say, what they do and do not do. The therapist will become attuned to subtle communications. Older adults tend to be less outspoken than their younger counterparts, so paying attention to body language will give clues. It is helpful to attend, not only to the member who is speaking but also to what other members are doing. The leader will then ask others "what it was like" to hear their fellow member share their thoughts or feelings. Members' responses give clues to how connected they are with one another: Do they identify with the speaker? Do they see the other member as a victim or a complainer? Do they wish the leader would offer a solution and are annoyed when he or she does not?

In the psychodynamic group, cohesion builds not through a focus on solving problems and working together on tasks (though problems do get solved with group feedback) but through experiencing oneself in relation to others and then studying these experiences. Group relationships are "processed." This means the individual interactions between and among group members or between group members and group leaders become the focus of the work. A clinical example from Rutan and Stone (2001, p. 262) illustrates this point:

Orin: My mom's not feeling too good. Today she is going to the doctor to have her cancer measured to see if it's grown. Then Mary (his wife) is going to have surgery on her thumb; she has a big cyst.

Ralph:	I found out at church that one of the men I knew had cancer. It's pretty far advanced, and we talked a lot. I'm going to miss him. [pause]
Bruce:	[to the therapist] I was curious about Joan. You said she was on vacation for two weeks. Is she still on vacation?
Therapist:	I didn't hear from her today. So that's another relationship—here in the group.

This vignette illustrates how members' verbalizations about their experiences with others outside the group being damaged and absent are related, transferentially, to the feelings experienced within the group about an absent member and how fractured it feels. The leader will listen for verbalization about events, people, and situations outside the group for evidence of how members feel inside the group. This is group transference.

No Prescribed Structure

Psychodynamic groups do not have a prescribed structure Other than general guidelines given during screening, there are few clues for members about how to proceed in a psychodynamic therapy group. The beginning phase is stressful because it is an ambiguous situation where members, in their characteristic fashion, try to figure out whether this is a safe place and whether the other members are trustworthy. Members react to the situation differently depending on how they usually meet their needs for safety. A member, for example, soothed her discomfort in an early group session by instituting a practice of everyone, in turn, stating her "high and low" of the week. This ultimately became a regular practice in the group, or a group norm. Furthermore, it provided some information about this woman's way of handling the ambiguity of the situation.

Members often test group boundaries by coming in late or missing sessions, using their actions to ask the question, "Is this a reliable and safe environment?" When the leader allows the members to develop the group's structure, members will create a structure that is representative of their typical patterns of relating with others. Leaders then can use this opportunity to comment, as tactfully as possible, that the members are resisting engagement in the group as a way to protect themselves from feeling vulnerable.

How to Proceed

The ambiguous nature of a psychodynamic therapy group, where the focus is on transferences, group processes, and the individuals' inner life, requires a skilled leader to help the group develop and to manage or contain the strong feelings that inevitably emerge. There are three important areas to consider in preparing to run a psychodynamic group: (1) leadership, (2) group culture and norms, and (3) roles adopted in the group. By understanding the way these elements work together the therapist can train his or her eye to observe and respond to previously unexamined processes. The leader, then, will help members become aware of and explore subtle patterns of relating or lifelong patterns of thinking about the world and about oneself. This is a major therapeutic factor in psychodynamic group work.

LEADERSHIP

There can be one or two leaders for a psychodynamic group. Leaders assume several roles within the group, and these roles may be different depending on such variables as the stage of the group, the group's composition, and the group's overall purpose. One important leadership role is establishing the group's boundaries. Leaders do this in concrete ways by determining the place, time, and duration of the meetings. Leaders create boundaries also by: (1) restricting the membership to a limited range of concerns, physical limitations, or level of impairment or even gender, (2) making clear group rules, such as prohibition of group members against socializing outside the group, and (3) protecting therapeutic boundaries by appropriately managing intense affect or conflict that arises in the group. Over time, members in open-ended groups assume parts of this role from the leader. In time-limited groups leaders continue in the role of protectors of boundaries.

Leaders use their expertise and authority to define viable therapeutic boundaries, but the leader will be a follower of group process rather than directing group processes. This does not mean the leader is a passive observer, but that interventions are purposeful and tend to be interpretive or reflective of the process rather than educative, directive, or an attempt to reinforce behavior. The following clinical examples illustrate two different responses by a leader.

Example One: Active, but following the group process

Mary:	I noticed I didn't feel as guilty when I told my daughter I couldn't babysit last Saturday. I was working in my garden and I thought, "I need to clean out the weeds, and I just don't want to chase my grandson around the yard."
Bill:	I love spending time with my grandkids. I never turn down an opportunity to babysit.
Therapist:	Mary, how does it feel to hear Bill take a different stance?

Example Two: Active, but more directive and reinforcing of behavior

Mary:	I noticed I didn't feel as guilty when I told my daughter I couldn't babysit last Saturday. I was working in my garden and I thought, "I need to clean out the weeds, and I just don't want to chase my grandson around the yard."
Therapist:	You didn't let your guilty feeling change your plans. That's real progress for you Mary!

The first position requires the therapist to contain and internally process the affect that emerges in the group and reflect back to the membership what he or she observes. The second position is supportive and reinforces Mary's decision but does not foster a dialogue or more exploration into the feelings.

Older adults may have a hard time expressing feelings about another member directly. Instead, they express their criticisms by taking a "friendly disagreement" attitude. The therapist helps members understand the feelings beneath their divergent opinions. It takes time to get at the feelings, especially for seniors who value politeness and civility, discretion and decorum. One of the stumbling blocks to productive group psychotherapy for this population is their aversion to airing their "dirty laundry" in public. To state feelings openly may be uncomfortable for this reason.

The therapist's role in protecting boundaries creates, for older adults, a sense of safety that their feelings will be taken seriously and be met with respect. In the above example, it is possible that Mary's statement evoked a sense of guilt for Bill that he had to cover over with his enthusiastic wish to be always available to his children. Perhaps Bill too has experienced not wanting to babysit but does not feel ready to say no. Alternatively, Mary may feel anger that her daughter assumes she is always available but is not ready to address such a powerful feeling. In the vignette she spoke only of guilt, a familiar state for her and one she prefers to grapple with at this stage of her therapy. Bill's comment might energize her to get in touch with her angry feelings ("Well, I do not always love spending time with the grandkids!") or might inhibit her further ("You're right, I could have done the weeding some other time."). Whatever the feelings, it is the therapist's interventions that create an opportunity for acknowledging and grappling with them.

Another role leaders adopt is to teach by modeling and using reflective statements about how members communicate their inner world. This does not imply that psychodynamic group therapy is psychoeducational. External expressions of internal processes are common and often unconscious. For example, in reviewing the group rules the leader might state that expressions will be in words instead of behaviors. The therapist's curiosity when a member acts out reinforces this value. So, the leader takes a nonjudgmental and interested position when a member uses behavior to express something that is going on internally. A common occurrence is the member who is late or absent, especially repeatedly. With older adults, especially, where illness, transportation problems, caregiver responsibilities, and so on provide real impediments to attendance, it is tempting to allow these reasons to get in the way of further exploration of what might be happening internally with the member. There are many explanations for missing sessions beyond logistical impediments. Discomfort with direct confrontation may inhibit this member from stating dissatisfaction with some aspect of the group experience or a negative feeling toward the leader or another member. A sense of vulnerability or embarrassment may prevent a member from admitting to feeling hurt by another's comment during a meeting.

Another internal process that is often obscured by acting out is a sense of isolation within the group. Because loneliness is a common complaint in their everyday lives, older adults may be particularly sensitive to the experience of isolation in the therapy group. Individuals may express such feelings by missing meetings, being silent, or perhaps by monopolizing the group's time. The point is, unless the leader looks beyond the action to the deeper internal meaning of the acting out, group participants are not able to address these feelings or thoughts directly. These abilities are related to a final point about psychodynamic leadership.

Leaders help members begin to understand that their experiences in the group are similar in important ways to their experiences outside the group. This is the "microcosm" view of group therapy. The leader is curious about how feelings and thoughts that get activated in the group setting are similar to situations the client has experienced before. Because the leader has some background information gained during assessment of the client he or she can help the group members connect current and past experiences. Members also help each other by sharing experiences that are similar or contrast with each other. This "experiential" learning is a powerful therapeutic tool in the psychodynamic leader's repertoire.

GROUP CULTURE AND NORMS

Every therapy group develops its own culture and norms. Many things contribute to this: what the leader establishes as the group's focus, how long the group has been together, what are the concerns and personalities of individual members, to name only a few. Group culture is not static; members' ways of interacting with one another can be expected to change over time. The culture sets the stage for what members can and cannot do and creates a sense of belonging that fosters group cohesion. Culture in this sense is a large part of the holding environment. Donald W. Winnicott (1987) the noted child psychiatrist first used the word *holding* to apply to "All human holding wherein one's basic needs, the most salient of which is for safety, are met" (p. 37).

Leaders exert a powerful influence on group culture. Rutan and Stone (2001) pointed out that, "a dichotomy exists between therapists who emphasize transferences to the leader, thereby helping individuals learn of their inner fantasies, and therapists who focus on peer transaction, which highlights the learning of social skills and the giving and receiving of feedback but diminish exploration of the unconscious" (p. 32). Thus, behavior that is normative in one group, such as eliciting transference reactions, may be alien to the norms of a group where the individual's experience of the leader is not a topic for exploration. Norms that are appropriate for older adult groups may not be useful for a younger population. For example, leaders of older adult groups may repeat comments to assist with hearing loss, use metaphors or vocabulary that are familiar to their cohort, provide factual information, or support group members socializing outside of the group.

Saiger (2001) reported that modifications to psychotherapy groups with older adults are required to build and maintain cohesion. He states, "cognitive reframing, general supportive measures, and accommodations for problems in mobility, hearing and other disabilities" (p. 135) are useful tools that communicate to older patients that the group culture can meet their needs. This expression of openness and accommodation is especially important for those who have never before participated in a therapy group, or for those who struggle with physical disabilities or with mild to moderate dementia (Leszcz, 1996). Saiger described experimenting with a problem of older adults remembering each other's names (p. 138). He established a round of introductions to start the meetings wherein each person would introduce someone else. The results were illustrative. A man said:

John:	I want to introduce the lady on my right. She makes delicious Christmas cookies. She lives with her daughter, but she may have to go to assisted care. She is a real dynamo in this group.
Therapist:	[prompting] And say her name.
John:	[pause] I don't know your name.

What the above example shows us is that whether or not older adults remember some details, a culture has developed that supports meaningful relationships. The gentleman has a good sense of this woman and her place in the group. Therapists of psychodynamic groups of older adults will take into account such lapses of memory or learning difficulties. Learning through multiple modalities (for example, using auditory means such as spoken introductions and visually using name tags), using repetition, and incorporating an experiential component are accommodations that are appropriate for older people. This idea will be further developed in the cognitive-behavioral group therapy section of this chapter. What the group psychotherapist must keep in mind and be respectful of is the variety of ways individuals connect with one another. This may look different with groups of seniors, and psychotherapists need to adjust their group leadership style accordingly.

ROLES

Members assume roles within groups that are characteristic for them or that serve a purpose for the group. A psychodynamic therapy group creates a setting for examining these roles. Some roles aid the group in working on its task, that is, helping members to explore their thoughts, feelings, and behavior. Other roles serve to inhibit the group from achieving its goals. The push and pull between these forces serve to manage the intensity of affect, conflict, and intimacy in the group. Early in the group's life it is common to see one or more members acting as "host" to facilitate introductions and fill up silences. Another role is the member who plays "devil's advocate." The member who takes on this role may be viewed as rebellious or oppositional and risks being scapegoated and emotionally expelled from the group. For the group that always wants to "make nice" and values "polite dishonesty" in the service of civility, this member is experienced as irritating or even dangerous. That is because he or she is expressing for the group oppositional emotions or ideas that are uncomfortable for many to experience so directly.

Commonly, therapy groups with older people will contain several group members whose self-assigned role is that of the caretaker. Group therapists of younger adult populations will see this as a potential resistance to acknowledging their own needs and vulnerabilities. Seniors are not immune to this kind of resistance, but those who suffer from a disability, dementia, or chronic illness, for example, can regain some of their former self-esteem by becoming useful to others in the group (Bonhote, Romano-Egan, & Cornwell, 1999; Saiger, 2001). They may bring home-baked cookies to the meetings or rearrange chairs to make room for a member's wheelchair, for example. The therapist will take these opportunities to reflect to the group the benefits of taking care of others who are less able. Such an intervention enables both the caregiver and the recipient of the care to verbalize their experiences of being the "healthy" one or being the one who is dependent. These moments in the group can be profoundly healing since the relationships are not burdened by the angry ambivalence experienced with family or paid caregivers.

Unfortunately, as Saiger points out, the fear of disability or diminished capacities may cause seniors to "act as if they believe that proximity to disability will cause you to catch it" (p. 140). Even when group members use walkers or wheelchairs, it may be difficult to get them to discuss their disabilities, and if they do the impairments are minimized. The more able-bodied fear and distance those who are seen as less able-bodied in this way. This distancing maneuver may temporarily halt meaningful interaction. Therapists who can address both the fear and the complex emotions of being the afflicted one will contribute immensely to the group work experience of these older adults.

The group leader will observe more roles than those presented here of host, devil's advocate, and caretaker. Other common roles are that of the "comedian" or "socializer." These roles are not unique to seniors, but may manifest in ways that are particular to this population. It will be easier for seniors to digest therapeutic interventions about the roles that get played out in the group if the therapist provides enough time for them to

develop fully and then adopts a respectful and curious position in making comments.

Cognitive-Behavioral Group Psychotherapy

Group psychotherapy based on a cognitive-behavioral theoretical framework seeks to bring about change through dismantling dysfunctional thoughts that lead to negative feeling states. Because understanding the individual's dysfunctional thought patterns are the focus of the work, a thorough assessment of each member is required. Thompson et al. (2000) asserted that cognitive-behavioral group therapy (CBGT) is "particularly well-suited for elderly individuals who are experiencing numerous or substantive losses...[because] the experience of loss per se does not necessarily lead to depression; rather it is how that experience is perceived and what its meaning is to the individual..." (p. 237).

One's perception and the meaning one applies to a given circumstance create the links between thoughts and feelings. Cognitions, or thoughts, are dysfunctional when they are overgeneralized ("I am a worthless person because I can no longer take care of all my needs"), overly rigid ("Things are never going to get better"), or overly negative ("My children hate me"), among others. Burns (1980) outlined the variety of ways thoughts can be dysfunctional. CBGT directs its focus to uncovering participants' thought patterns and seeing how they affect behavior, mood, and self-esteem. The next sections describe the four key features of CBGT that distinguish it from psychodynamic group therapy.

The Collaborative Relationship Between Group Leader and Members

The relationship between the therapist and group members is collaborative versus the more hierarchical relationship of the traditional psychodynamic psychotherapy group. While the leader maintains the position of "expert," the feel is one of a joint process of learning. This approach may be more comfortable for older people as they are long accustomed to having a sense of control over their daily lives. Thus, an attitude of equality may reduce anxiety associated with vulnerable feelings that often emerge as individuals prepare to enter a group. The experience in CBGT may be similar to that of taking a class. This implies some level of self-motivation on the part of group members and may inform therapists whether or not this type of group therapy is indicated for an individual. CBGT is most successful for participants who show a minimal level of initiative. Leaders will focus initially on developing a viable working rapport as this is the foundation upon which members will invest in the work. This working rapport builds through implementation of the remaining three elements of CBGT.

Structured Course of Treatment

Time-limited and ongoing CB therapy groups are structured and unambiguous for the participant. There are treatment manuals (see Resources) wherein the entire course of therapy is transparent to the group from the beginning, akin to giving students a syllabus for a class. Even when not adhering to a manual, during screening and assessment therapists may present an outline of the overall focus of the group as well as the focus of each session. In an open-ended group, the leader may not have an agenda for each session but will list skills to be learned and how these skills will address each member's needs. Therapists using cognitive-behavioral techniques are clear about what individuals can expect of their group experience: (1) feedback from the leader and from peers, (2) homework assignments, (3) expected results, and (4) progress. Older adults often appreciate the solution-oriented approach offered by CBGT.

Focused Assessment and Goal Setting

When an individual presents for group therapy the therapist conducts a thorough assessment to establish appropriateness for treatment, an exercise needed for every group treatment. What separates CBGT from some other types of group therapy is that the therapist and patient together settle on specific goals that will be linked to a specified agenda and homework assignments. The therapist conducts the initial assessment and the group member supplements the assessment with data gathered during a period of self-monitoring.

During this phase the group member will identify patterns he or she wishes to alter. Homework may be prescribed (see the cognitive-behavioral exercises at the end of the chapter for examples) to help members think through their habitual patterns. Therapists can assist members in this task by taking a thorough history with an ear trained to the individual's pattern of bolstering self-esteem throughout life. Women typically will have gained a sense of self through interpersonal relationships and men though work and achievements (Laidlaw et al., 2003). Older adults are particularly vulnerable to losing such sources of self-esteem in retirement and widowhood. Part of goal setting will be defining new ways to achieve self-validation. After members collect data about themselves they can work to replace unhelpful patterns with patterns that are more in line with their goals. The group setting is ideal in that members can challenge one another about dysfunctional thoughts and beliefs. In behavioral terms, the group can "shape" behavior that is more adaptive by reinforcing even the smallest gains. Defining specific goals enables members to give each other feedback that has an immediate effect and fosters a sense of being heard, understood, and accepted. In this way, goal setting is one of the building blocks to self-esteem and group cohesion for older people (Link, 1997).

Psychoeducational Component

The emphasis in CBGT is on changing thoughts, feelings, and actions through experiential learning and psychoeducation. In other words, the focus is on acquiring information that will be therapeutic and useful in one's daily life. For example, cognitive-behavioral groups often learn about normal processes of aging, how chronic illness can lead to depression, the various ways anxiety manifests, how substance use may be a way of self-medicating, or about care-taking strategies for adult children. The psychoeducational component is simple to adapt as a more open-ended treatment by adjusting the pace to the needs of the group rather than adhering to the timetable established by the group or recommended in a manual. During initial stages of treatment, some participants respond favorably to psychoeducation. Quick improvements in symptoms and mood are usually a result of the increased sense of agency, or control, gained from having new information about one's situation. Improvements gained from psychoeducation bode well for building self-esteem.

How to Proceed

After determining the general rationale for establishing a therapy group and deciding on using a cognitive-behavioral approach, the therapist must select group members who will best benefit from such a group. CBGT may be contraindicated for individuals who: (1) are diagnosed with bipolar disorder or other major mental illness, (2) are currently abusing substances, (3) report active suicidal thinking, or (4) are suffering from moderate to severe dementia. Older adults who live independently, who reside with family, or who live in assisted-living settings will present with different problems than those residing in nursing homes or those with a debilitating illness. Adapting the goals to the specific population will go a long way toward achieving success for members and the

leader. It can be discouraging for therapists who aspire to restore members to a level of functioning that may not be attainable. Modest successes, however, can be achieved with even the most impaired individual regardless of age. Along with screening for appropriate group members, the leader must make clear the expectations for membership (Gallagher-Thompson & Thompson, 1996). Leaders will state up front that members are expected to discuss their concerns openly, to attend regularly, to complete homework assignments, and provide constructive feedback to one another.

Obstacles to attendance, such as transportation, family responsibilities, or illness must be considered in the selection process. How serious are these obstacles? Should potential members be screened out when such obstacles loom too large? These are important questions for the leader to consider because a group fractured by erratic attendance by even one of its members will interfere with the development of cohesion and a sense of trust. Other considerations that can make it difficult for older adults to fully participate are severe hearing impairments, language difficulties (due to either paralysis or foreign-born status), or low motivation or lack of time to complete written assignments.

During the early phase of the group the leader will directly address cohort beliefs that might interfere with group process. Specifically, the leader will comment on the common beliefs among seniors that mental illness is a sign of weakness or spiritual rift, that one should keep personal business to oneself, and that loneliness is a "fact" of old age (Laidlaw et al., 2003). It is often a relief to members to hear their inner fears spoken out loud. This goes a long way toward normalizing their silent feelings. Leaders should elicit members' thoughts and feelings about joining the group. Their experiences are varied: excitement, shame, a sense that this is their "last resort," fear, "too needy," "hope," and "sadness." The therapist understands members' feelings. Self-attributions about joining a group may fuel or inhibit their progress toward attaining their goals. In CBGT it is not necessary to work through these feelings, but simply to acknowledge the cognitive "spin" members put on their participation in the group. Identifying self-attributions can be a useful early homework exercise to assess aspects of participants' dysfunctional thinking.

Cognitive-behavioral strategies will work best with older adult groups when the leader remains flexible. The pace of the work may be substantially slower than for younger people (Gallagher-Thompson & Thompson, 1996). Initially, older adults are much less likely than younger people to ask questions when they do not understand a point (Thompson et al., 2000). It is the responsibility of the leader to repeat and review concepts and techniques that are presented and to cite examples offered by other members. An added benefit of CBGT for older adults is the reinforcement members receive hearing others respond successfully to treatment (Zeiss & Steffen, 1996). Leaders may have to explain how the techniques have produced such successes, however. The expectation should be for success by approximation, not for complete mastery of skills. Finally, therapists will use multiple sensory modalities for covering issues—talk about it (verbal and auditory), assign homework (visual and kinetic), use written agendas during sessions to stay on task (visual)—all used in an effort to make it easier for older adults to draw on their strengths to achieve their goals.

The overall purpose of CBGT is to identify dysfunctional thought patterns, self-statements, and beliefs about oneself and the world. The members work to collect data about themselves (in the session and through homework assignments) that can be discussed and explored in a group setting. The interpersonal element of group therapy provides countless opportunities for members to observe one another and to confirm or question each other's perceptions and beliefs about themselves. CBGT does not have to

incorporate a direct behavioral component for change to occur. Cognitive restructuring can take place using supportive measures within a group. For example, Ogrodniczuk, Joyce, and Piper (2003) pointed out that when an individual experiences a significant loss or death he or she assesses how much support is available to help with coping. It is one's assessment, or perception, of what support is available that can separate those who become depressed from those who do not. Those who assess their support as adequate believe they are able to cope with their grief and adjustment to the loss. CBGT is especially helpful for individuals who are experiencing multiple losses in understanding their perceptions of support, their sense of their ability to cope, and their capacity to acquire new coping strategies. The supportive element of the therapy group gives members the experience of being cared for. For many older adults, being able to tolerate receiving care can enable them, then, to turn to supportive resources in their everyday lives.

COGNITIVE-BEHAVIORAL EXERCISES FOR THE PATIENT

1. Daily record of dysfunctional thoughts (Burns, 1980; Free, 1999). The participant keeps a journal as he or she notices overly generalized, overly rigid, and overly negative thoughts. This exercise builds on itself as group members become better observers of their thought patterns. It is a simple yet powerful tool for gaining mastery over one's cognitions and moods. Leaders may describe and assign this exercise during the first meeting to help members develop agency over their personal and group experience.

2. ABC exercise (Free, 1999). Participants use this after keeping their daily record of dysfunctional thoughts for a few weeks. It helps link behaviors, thoughts, and feelings in an easily understandable way (**Table 18–1**).

Table 18–1   ABC RECORD

Activating event	Belief or thought	Emotional consequence
Death of a loved one	"I can't go on"	Helplessness
Fail driving test	"I'm incompetent"	Depression
Move to assisted living	"I will not have friends"	Anxiety

Summary

This chapter presents psychodynamic and cognitive-behavioral methods of conducting group psychotherapy with older adults. While the two methods are very different, both are especially useful in addressing the needs of this population. The psychodynamic therapy group lends itself to a focus on feeling experiences and interpersonal relationships. Cognitive-behavioral group therapy tends to be more solution focused and psychoeducational. Both methods can be used for time-limited or open-ended groups. Time-limited groups typically offer members the opportunity to focus on a particular problem, such as, bereavement, care-giving difficulties, or adjustment to chronic illness. These groups can meet for as little as six weeks and often not longer than twelve weeks. Session length should be tailored to the requirements and capacities of the membership. Smaller groups can cover the material in sixty minutes, while larger groups may require up to 90 minutes. Open-ended therapy groups can meet weekly for six months or longer. These groups may be open to admitting new members, not to exceed a certain group size, usually not more than 8 to 12 members, depending on whether there are one or two leaders. Open-ended groups allow for addressing a wider range of concerns among the membership. Using either method the therapist will conduct a thorough assessment and establish specific goals with group members.

One of the main differences presented between the two methods is the amount and type of structure the leader imposes on the group. In psychodynamic group therapy the leader establishes the group's boundaries by providing a reliable and safe space for the work. In CBGT leaders may establish an agenda for the entire course of the therapy group or use a manual as a guide for treatment. Both types of groups offer the older adult a vehicle to increase self-esteem through providing and receiving support, enhancing a sense of agency, and gaining useful information about themselves and their relationships.

Exercises

EXERCISE 1

Think about someone you care for in the nursing home. Identify the proper group therapy for that individual and tell why it is the best choice.

EXERCISE 2

Create a plan for running a cognitive behavioral group for older people

References

Bonhote, K., Romano-Egan, J., & Cornwell, C. (1999). Altruism and creative expression in a long-term older adult psychotherapy group. *Issues Mental Health Nursing,* 20(6), 603–17.

Burns, D. D. (1980). *Feeling good: The new mood therapy.* New York: Avon Books.

Free, M. L. (1999). *Cognitive therapy in groups: Guidelines and resources for practice.* New York: John Wiley.

Gallagher-Thompson, D., & Thompson, L. W. (1996). Applying cognitive-behavioral therapy to the psychological problems of later life. In S. Zarit & B. Knight (Eds.), *Effective clinical interventions in a life-stage context: A guide to psychotherapy and aging* (pp. 61–82). Washington, DC: American Psychological Association.

Haley, W. E. (1996). The medical context of psychotherapy with the elderly. In S. Zarit & B. Knight (Eds.), *Effective clinical interventions in a life-stage context: A guide to psychotherapy and aging* (pp. 221–240). Washington, DC: American Psychological Association.

Laidlaw, K., Thompson, L. W., Dick-Sisken, L., & Gallagher-Thompson, D. (2003). *Cognitive behavior therapy with older people.* New York: John Wiley & Sons.

Leszcz, M. (1996). Group therapy. In J. Sadavoy, L. W. Lazarus, L. F. Jarvik, & G. T. Grossberg (Eds.), *Comprehensive review of geriatric psychiatry.* (2nd ed., pp. 851–879). Washington, DC: American Psychiatric Press.

Lyness, J. M., Caine, E. D., King, D.A., Conwell, Y., Duberstein, P. R., & Cox, C. (2002). Depressive disorders and symptoms in older primary care patients: One-year outcomes. *American Journal of Geriatric Psychiatry, 10*(3), 275–282.

Moore, B. & Fine, B. *Psychoanalytic terms and concepts.* New Haven, CT: Yale University Press.

Ogrodniczuk, J. S., Joyce, A. S., & Piper, W. E. (2003). Changes in perceived social support after group therapy for complicated grief. *Journal of Nervous & Mental Disease, 191*(8), 524–530.

Rutan, J. S., & Stone, W. N. (2001). *Psychodynamic group psychotherapy.* New York: Guilford Press.

Saiger, G. M. (2001). Group psychotherapy with older adults. *Psychiatry, 64*(2), 132–145.

Thompson, L. W., Powers, D. V., Coon, D. W., Takagi, K., McKibbin, C., & Gallagher-Thompson, D. (2000). Older adults. In J. R.White & A. S. Freeman (Eds.), *Cognitive-behavioral group therapy for specific problems and populations* (pp. 235–261). Washington, DC: American Psychological Association.

Winnicott, D. W. (1987). *Babies and their mothers.* New York: Addison-Wesley.

Young, C. A., & Reed, P. G. (1995). Elders' perceptions of the role of group psychotherapy in fostering self-transcendence. *Archives of Psychiatric Nursing, 9*(6), 338–347.

Zeiss, A. M., & Steffen, A. (1996). Behavioral and cognitive-behavioral treatments: An overview of social learning. In S. Zarit & B. Knight (Eds.), *Effective clinical interventions in a life-stage context: A guide to psychotherapy and aging* (pp. 35–60). Washington, DC: American Psychological Association.

BIBLIOGRAPHY

Abouguendia, M., Joyce, A. S., Piper, W. E., & Ogrodniczuk, J. (2004). Alliance as a mediator of expectancy effects in short-term group psychotherapy. *Group Dynamics: Theory, Research, & Practice, 8*(1), 3–12.

Atholtz, J. (1994). Group psychotherapy. In I. Burnside & M. G. Schmidt (Eds.), *Working with older adults: Group process and techniques* (pp. 214–224). Boston: Jones & Bartlett.

Clark, W. G., & Vorst, V. R. (1994). Group therapy with chronically depressed geriatric patients. *Journal of Psychosocial Nursing in Mental Health Services, 32*(5), 9–13.

Kaas, M. J., & Lewis, M. L. (1999). Cognitive behavioral group therapy for residents in assisted-living facilities. *Journal of Psychosocial Nursing in Mental Health Services, 37*(10), 9–15.

Kennedy, G. J., & Tanenbaum, S. (2000). Psychotherapy with older adults. *American Journal of Psychotherapy, 54*(3), 386–407.

Klausner, E. J., Clarkin, J. F., Spielman, L., Pupo, C., Abrams, R., & Alexopoulos, G. S. (1998). Late-life depression and functional disability: The role of goal-focused group psychotherapy. *International Journal of Geriatric Psychiatry, 13,* 707–716.

Kleinberg, J. L. (1995). Group treatment of adults in midlife. *International Journal of Group Psychotherapy, 45*(2), 207–222.

Link, A. L. (1997). *Group work with elders: 50 therapeutic exercises for reminiscence, validation and remotivation.* Sarasota, FL: Professional Resource Press.

Ogrodniczuk, J. S., Piper, W. E., Joyce, A. S., McCallum, M., & Rosie, J. S. (2003). NEO-Five factor personality traits as predictors of response to two forms of group psychotherapy. *International Journal of Group Psychotherapy, 53*(4), 417–442.

Phoenix, E., Irvine, Y., & Kohr, R. (1997). Sharing stories: Group therapy with elderly depressed women. *Journal of Gerontological Nursing, 23*(4), 10–15.

Travis, L. A., Lyness, J. M., Shields, C. G., King, D. A., & Cox, C. (2004). Social support, depression, and functional disability in older adult primary-care patients. *American Journal of Geriatric Psychiatry, 12*(3), 265–271.

Wood, A., & Seymour, L. M. (1994). Psychodynamic group therapy for older adults: The life experiences group. *Journal of Psychosocial Nursing in Mental Health Services, 32*(7), 19–24.

Resources

- American Psychological Association. (2004). Guidelines for psychological practice with older adults. *American Psychologist,* 159(4), 236–260.
- Free, M. L. (1999). *Cognitive therapy in groups: Guidelines and resources for practice.* New York: John Wiley & Sons.

Group Work with Older Adults at the End of Life

Brian de Vries

Marvin Westwood

John Blando

Key Words

- Death
- Dying
- Ethical decision making
- Grief
- Bereavement
- Guided autobiography
- Group enactment

Learning Objectives

- Describe the issues facing people at the end of life
- Evaluate the need for decision making by the dying person
- Analyze the value of decision-making groups for the family
- Understand how group enactment works
- Synthesize a group reenactment scene

"We are born alone and we die alone." While we do not intend to undermine the emotional valence and agentic intention of this oft-repeated sentence reflecting the deeply personal nature of dying and death (and birth), we propose that the end (and the beginning) of life also may be broadly and importantly construed as deeply social. Others, for example, of various identities escort the dying through decision making and care delivery while expressing their grief over time both before and after the physical death (e.g., de Vries & Blando, 2000). The dying themselves make decisions and call for care, in part, with an awareness of the consequences of their decisions on others. Moreover, all of the participants in formal and informal social roles in the end-of-life journey are influenced by social norms, societal expectations, and culture(s).

In the pages that follow, we wish to focus on life's end in this social context. Such a context neatly suggests the interpersonal environment within which this takes place and some of the group dynamics and processes that might be engaged during this salient period of the life course. We conclude with some examples of our work with older adults in group settings, the guided autobiography, and dealing with issues of life's end.

The Social Dimensions of End of Life

End of life and old age are familiar bedfellows. It is worth noting that old people do not hold the market on death, although the correlation between age and death is significant and impressive (and perhaps disproportionately linked in the minds of too many—perchance evidence of a pervasive ageism) (Butler, 1969). Almost three quarters of all deaths in the United States are of persons at least 65 years of age (US Bureau of the Census, 1990). Such statistics have rendered the death of older persons as "normative," expected, and timely (Moss & Moss, 1989).

Such was not always the case. At the beginning of this century, death in childhood was more common (Teno, McNiff, & Lynn, 2000). Home deaths were the norm in the United States as recently as 1949 (Lerner, 1970). Today, almost two thirds of all deaths occur in institutional settings (Hays, Gold, Flint, & Winer, 1999) serving to screen and deritualize death behind hospital and nursing home walls with dramatic implications for the dying as well as for those providing care and those who grieve (de Vries & Rutherford, 2004).

Dying and Death

The end of life is complex and multifaceted (e.g., de Vries, 1999), encompassing numerous spheres of influence with state, event, and process characteristics that evolve over time in ways not yet fully understood. For example and notwithstanding the legal and biological definition and determination of the event of death, dying is a process that takes place over time and may also be described by psychological and social dimensions of experience (Bradley, Fried, Kasl, & Idler, 2000). Such a distinction begs the provocative question of when dying and end of life actually begin.

Bradley et al. (2000) offer three perspectives on this issue. A medical perspective proclaims that when a patient displays the medical signs consistent with imminent death, the patient may be said to be at the end of life. The health system offers a second perspective, frequently quantified as six months or less of expected life, organized around financing and access to current systems of care (e.g., hospice) for those individuals in the last stage of life. A third perspective, arguably more relevant to particular choices and decisions made, is that of the patient and his or her family or social support system. Within this perspective, Kastenbaum (2004) suggests that dying usually begins as a psychosocial process initially observed by a physician who communicates (verbally and/or nonverbally) such facts to a person who then realizes and personalizes them and subsequently communicates them (verbally and/or nonverbally) to the others in their surrounding psychoemotional sphere in recursive fashion.

For example, dying persons are treated differently—often as if they are already dead. This has been noted with both community samples (e.g., Lester, 1993) as well as professional nursing samples (LeShan, 1982). Kastenbaum (2004) cites poignant examples of how dying individuals felt that the way in which they lived with the knowledge of their dying trajectory differed significantly from how they lived before. Kastenbaum makes the social and interactional point that the lives of those intimates surrounding the dying individual are affected by their awareness of the impending death, which further affects the terminally ill person.

Decision Making at Life's End

The interactional complexities of the dying and their intimates have frequently been discussed in the context of end-of-life decision making. Many opportunities now exist for individuals to actively participate in and direct their end-of-life care, including living wills, advance directives, and requirements brought about by the Patient Self-Determination Act of 1990. Still, given these opportunities and evidence that individuals want control over medical decisions (as well as evidence that up to 75% of patients lack decision-making capacity when life-sustaining choices have to be made), surprisingly only a small percentage of individuals have actually completed advance directives (Braun & Kayashima, 1999).

Many of the reasons offered for the low completion rates of such documents include fear of the process and concerns that one's preferences might change, but most prominently a preference for leaving the decision to family members (Cicirelli, 2000) with whom such discussions may or, more probably, may not have taken place. Those who completed advance directives cited such issues as not wanting to be on life support, not wanting to suffer, avoiding the high cost of care and, again more prominently, not wanting to burden the family with such decisions (mentioned by over 40% of respondents in studies reviewed by High (1993a).

The important role of others and the family in particular was similarly evident in the decisions made by women with Stage IV breast cancer in the Hays et al. (1999) study. Among the reasons women provided for preferring home-based terminal care included issues related to symptom control and functional capacity and the intense desire not to burden their families, either physically with role expectations of caring for a terminally ill person or psychologically with fear of what the terminal decline might do to the emotional well-being of the caregiver. Those women preferring institution-based terminal care voiced many of these same reasons, but primarily the protection of children and others in the home environment from the trauma of seeing a loved one die. In all of the instances, the importance of the social context of these end-of-life decisions is noteworthy.

Grief, Mourning, and Bereavement

Bereavement is a social network crisis (Vachon & Stylianos, 1988); the death of a network member may draw the entire group into distress. Each year, over 8 million Americans experience the death of an immediate family member (Osterweis, Solomon, & Green, 1984) and many millions more experience the death of a member of their extended family, a lover, a friend, a companion animal, or another intimate. Responses to these losses reflect characteristics of both the grieving and bereaved individuals themselves as well as the mourning rituals of their cultures (Ashenburg, 2002). These responses reveal the intense emotional and cognitive efforts expended by the bereft and the social pressures of their environments as they cope with and try to make sense of their loss; this is the "work" of grief (de Vries, 2001). After all, as Deck and Folta (1989, p. 80) observed, the study of grief "is the study of people and their most intimate relationships."

This latter point in particular underscores the frequently neglected perspective that death marks the end of a life, not the end of a relationship (Anderson, 1970). The finality and unchanging nature of death have to be considered in the context of the ongoing nature and the fluidity of connections with the deceased (Silverman & Klass, 1996). In this perspective, grief is not only the response to what once was (i.e., the relationships individuals had—both before and after the death), it is also evidence of what persists (i.e., struggling to find the place in an individual's life for a deceased loved one).

Grief is even more complex, however. Manifestations of grief may be evident in the expressions of the dying as they say good-bye to those around them and as they say good-bye to those aspects of themselves rendered inaccessible through terminal decline. Similarly, those providing care to the dying are cognizant of the declining abilities of their loved one and the aspects of the persons they love seeping away and those parts of themselves lost in the same process. This recognition of grief and these expressions of grief are rarely studied and infrequently considered (de Vries, 2001).

More recent explorations have identified the accounts of loss described by bereft individuals that contain references to continuing bonds. These include: the experiences reported by partners of "checking in" and wondering what the deceased would think or do at a particular occasion (e.g., Jones, 1985); the claims of bereft adult children that the essential qualities of their relationship with their deceased parent continues, that "the child continues to hear echoes of the parent's voice, which may be carried over a lifetime" (Moss & Moss, 1989, p. 101); the empty historical tracking of bereaved parents and the ongoing role of deceased children in the parents' inner world (Klass & Marwitt, 1989, p. 41); the empty mirror or missing referent of bereaved friends (de Vries & Johnson, 2002). For those whose professional and personal practices bring them into contact with the bereaved, it is important to recognize these continuing bonds and these important reflections of intimacy (de Vries, 2001).

Group Process

The many social issues of life's end, some of which are referenced above, are naturally amenable to consideration in groups as suggested by previous work building upon the psychoeducational and social support functions of groups. Certainly the bulk of this work may be seen in the extensive efforts of bereavement mutual support (often referred to as self-help) groups. This particular group environment encourages sharing grief-related feelings, the opportunity to learn coping styles and skills from other members, and recognizing some of the universal manifestations and characterizations of grief. Support groups also can help strengthen informal support networks, address issues of loneliness and social isolation, and foster a sense of belongingness (Gottlieb, 1988; Lieberman, 1993). Bereaved individuals have reported that the most valuable features attracting them to bereavement support groups were the chance to meet people and make new

friends as well as to alleviate some of the loneliness they experience (Hopmeyer & Werk, 1994; Nash, 1992).

Many of these same ameliorative features function in groups operating outside of bereavement-specific contexts yet with direct relevance to the end-of-life issues referenced above. For example, in investigations of end-of-life decision making, and particularly the completion of advance directives, several authors have reported that individuals respond more favorably (i.e., they report being more comfortable with the subject and more likely to complete an advance directive) when engaged in more intensive discussions with people they trust (Heffner, Fahy, & Barbieri, 1996; Luptak & Boult, 1994). High (1993b), in a study comparing interventions aimed at improving the rates of completions of advance directives, reported that participants who received a moderate level of print material and attended a group educational meeting were the ones most likely to have completed such a document. The application of this social support process with those who are dying is less familiar, although may be seen in work with groups of individuals diagnosed with AIDS and groups of those suffering in the early stages of dementia (e.g., Yale, 1989) and is the subject of the discussion to follow.

Ethical Decision-Making Groups

Establishing a group where the dying person can be with others of his or her choice not only offers the opportunity for the provision of support, it also may become the place for them to begin to speak about things which previously were not possible—in the medical setting or even among friends or family, for example. One of the reasons that group-based interventions may be so helpful at this time and provide a structure for conversation is because of the conspiracy of silence that pervades such salient and emotionally charged topics as dying and death and family dynamics—some of the "toxic" issues of social life and family development (Magee, 1988). Breaking this silence, taking the risk to speak about what is truly important in life (and death) can be achieved in the inclusive, respectful, and trustful climate created by an effective group.

Kuhl (1999) has developed a client-centered decision-making group model to ensure that the needs of the dying client are more fully met across both the physical and psychosocial domains. This model, based on the Ethical Grid developed by Jonsen, Siegler, and Winslade (1992), proposes four quadrants (medical indications, patient preferences, quality of life, and contextual features) which focus the group conversations for decision making. The ethical decision-making group involves the direct application of specific group processes and communication competencies to facilitate the process, the intent of which is to enhance a sense of safety and comfort in the group. These processes and group leading skills are particularly important given that the anxiety surrounding end of life may aggravate and exacerbate "family dysfunction" at these times (Kuhl, 1999). Group members represent some of the various psychoemotional spheres in which the dying individual is embedded. That is, a typical group comprises the client, members of his or her care staff, and members of his or her family and friends network.

In addition to quality decision making in this group context, there are other benefits which include the support of the client by the group, member-to-member support, the letting go of regrets, making amends, saying those things that have been left unsaid or need to be said so the person can more easily move to personal integration versus despair at the end of life (Erikson, Erikson, & Kivnick, 1986). In such ethical decision-making groups, we have observed an increase in the quality of patient care, as the team collectively understands the needs of the patient and therefore can work more cooperatively to meet these.

Benefits also accrue for the health care providers; just as the family and friends need a place to express their thoughts and feelings, so too is this frequently the case for the health care team. Health care workers who are permitted to acknowledge and express their reactions, feel more integrated and resolved around their reactions to this person with whom they have become closely associated.

Setting up such a group may not feel like a natural intervention when a more common response to those who are dying is to move away, allegedly to give the person time and privacy and frequently in response to our own death denial; in many cases, however, the absence of the opportunities offered by such group interventions may well contribute to the pain and suffering of the person in an isolated state. It is worth remembering that even though a person may be physically in the presence of others, they are not necessarily *with* others in an intimate way. That is, the codes on how individuals speak to each other at times like this are the same codes with which individuals grew up in their own family context: e.g., don't talk about what you are feeling or thinking as it is either too upsetting for you or would certainly upset the other! Interestingly, Kuhl and Westwood (2000) found the opposite to be true, that contact with those select individuals may be what is needed! Professionals with group expertise can offer this option.

The facilitator of the group convenes a meeting with those who the dying person has invited and leads a group discussion, keeping the primary focus on the needs and preferences of the person at end of life, as they move through this decision-making model. Although the primary purpose of these groups is to help make decisions concerning the needs of the patient in their medical and physical care needs, the quality of life and contextual features' quadrants open up communication on the social and emotional needs of the person so they too may be expressed. In addition, the group enables the others present to communicate and express the feelings they have also.

Once the group begins and members sense the safety and support, they tend to move quickly to the core issues about which they may have been ruminating and not expressing. Being led by a professional provides the structure and process for ease of communication in a situation that many would have thought not possible. In fact once the group is under way it feels very natural and what is needed for the dying person and others present.

We have noticed a variety of outcomes when these meetings are conducted: reduced pain of a psychological nature tends to occur; resolution of issues; letting go of regrets; reaffirming and valuing existing relations, plus many other personal outcomes. Above all, the group allows for the expression of feelings that so often are not shared. Grieving together and with the person who is leaving is very beneficial for all those involved. Within the group, new relationships may be rekindled and new connections made so that the group setting can support and lift the person emotionally right up until the time of death. We also notice that for the family and friends following the death, the new connections and support networks created earlier help build new relationships among them that did not previously exist. Groups such as these may help the person to "heal" before they die.

Groups may also be constructed which do not include medical or professional personnel; rather, they include family and friends. It is also possible to set up a small group consisting only of family or friends and these can be facilitated to ensure that everyone is offered the chance to say what is needed with a leader making certain that a sense of safety and care is present throughout.

Guided Autobiography Groups

A second focus of our efforts in the area of group work that has direct relevance to these end-of-life issues has been in the context of the guided autobiography, a semistructured, topical, group approach to life review. Typically, the guided autobiography involves a written component, facilitating in-depth personal reflection, and a group experience, reinforcing participation and enhancing recall (de Vries, Birren, & Deutchman, 1995). The self-reflection and private writing allow individuals to organize their thoughts and, in a sense, rehearse what will be shared with others; the opportunity to monitor affectively charged materials that individuals choose to reveal in their groups promotes emotional safety.

A guided autobiography group typically comprises five or six people along with a trained group facilitator. Each person prepares reflections on several major life themes sequentially constructed with the intent to "elicit especially salient memories and form common threads that run through the life that binds the fabric of the life story" (de Vries et al., 1995, p. 166). The themes help participants make sense of their lives and help them identify the unfinished parts of their lives, the regrets, missed opportunities, achievements, and their experience with and anticipation of death.

Reading these prepared thematic statements in the group and receiving the reactions of others helps the participant integrate his or her own story and to experience support and encouragement to finish up those parts of their life that have remained unfinished or incomplete. This frequently leads to desires to contact and speak with certain people; explaining, forgiving, and reconnecting help meet many of the needs that people have within their family and social communities.

Our experience with this process, sketches of which are described below, has allowed us to observe some of the many benefits of participation including the integration of new understandings of the self, others, and the world (Brown-Shaw, Westwood, & de Vries, 1999) as well as the construction and presentation of "models to buffer transitions, to bridge historical times, and to communicate values" (de Vries, Birren, & Deutchman, 1990, p. 6). Life stories provide the personalized context within which issues of life and death, growth and grief, values and beliefs, and choices and decisions perhaps can be best understood.

The leader and other group members assist in offering new perspectives on experiences and affirming the self-worth and value of the individual, their strengths and courage. Individuals gain new insights from the realization of their individuality as well as from commonalities of experiences. Here, the role of the group leader is particularly important in establishing the norms guiding how individuals address the group and treat one another. The group leader should be modeling behaviors and teaching basic communication skills while using proven facilitation and group management skills such as initiating, clarifying, focusing, blocking, limiting, and encouraging consensus. An effective, supportive, safe group permits taking risks in telling one's story and having it heard and witnessed; individuals feel accepted by such a group and acceptance leads to increased communication and belonging, two of the major themes identified by Kuhl (2002) in his powerful study on what people want at the end of life.

Our work with the guided autobiography at life's end has taken place with those nearing the end of their lives—both chronologically and physiologically—and with those dealing with the end of the life of a loved one. Given the extent to which life stories frequently turn on issues of death and loss, these two perspectives are not mutually exclusive; however, in the former case, our work has brought us into contact with veterans of the second World War (Westwood, 1998).

A goal of this health promotion group work was to examine the impact of war experience on the subsequent lives of these men now in their 80s and 90s, promoting personal integration and trauma repair. Death and dying were common themes in the stories reported, both implicitly

and explicitly. These men readily spoke about their age-related concerns with and preparations for death. Moreover, these men spoke of the legacy of war and of having witnessed death, having been beside it and having been a part of it. Many of these discussions took place for the first time in these long lives and many felt unburdened and freed by this opportunity. Similar sorts of outcomes have been noted in some of the groups we have conducted in care facilities for older adults where, given the safe space and opportunity, discussions naturally turned to death preparedness.

In the case of those surviving the death of a loved one, the guided autobiography groups have an appearance superficially similar to grief support groups. The guided, structured, storied nature of this approach, however, renders these two types of groups significantly different. In the sharing and witnessing of a life story, as in the guided autobiography, bereft individuals piece together the story of a life made incomplete by the loss. They are telling their stories and the stories of their deceased loved ones. In such a manner, they are able to articulate, often for the first time, the essence of their grief—who is missing and what is missing. So too are they able to attempt to construct a story that somehow weaves together the now disparate pieces of their lives.

Guided Autobiography with Group Enactment

The many gains made possible by participation in the guided autobiography include increased awareness of life's achievements; however, it is also possible to uncover some of the stumbling blocks which may have restricted individuals from fulfillment in a number of ways (Brown-Shaw et al., 1999). In such cases, a critical event may remain unresolved and incomplete, although now labeled and apparent. Brown-Shaw et al. (1999) refer to this as the diagnostic function of the guided autobiography in that participants express those aspects of the self and story in need of change, including reparation and/or restoration, which call for attention in order to take the individual to another level of self-understanding. Kenyon and Randall (e.g., 2001) refer to this as the potential for "restorying." In such a way, the guided autobiography provides the frame of the story and the context of the event and what is needed is some way in which to retell the story and incorporate a new understanding of the event (see **Figure 19–1**).

The case of Tom illustrates how an enactment taking place within a group context facilitates the resolution of unexpressed issues—in this case, the grief that Tom has been left with all of his life as the result of the early death of his father. An adaptation of that appears in Westwood, Keats, and Wilensky (2003). Tom is a business executive. He is currently married with two young adult children. In his guided autobiography, he spoke of the difficulties that he was having with his wife and children. He attributed these problems to unresolved grief over the loss of his father when he was a 13-year-old boy. He reported feeling "empty" and "emotionally distant" from his family. Through discussion with the group and the group facilitator, Tom anticipated that revisiting and reenacting this time in his own early adolescence would enable him to move emotionally closer to his own young family.

As Tom's primary issue was related to unresolved grief, he wanted to revisit the time of his father's death where he would have an opportunity to tell his father all of the unspoken thoughts and feelings of his adolescent experience. In Tom's situation, his father had languished at home with a terminal illness for a year and a half before he died. Tom was not aware that his father's illness was terminal and was left shocked on the night of his father's death. On this evening, Tom's mother awakened him with news of the seriousness of his father's illness and the announcement of his death. In addition, Tom's mother prohibited him

from attending his father's funeral, leaving Tom with much unfinished business around his father's death. We agreed that the enactment would focus on the scene in Tom's bedroom where his mother awakened him and spoke about his father's death. However, this time, during the enactment, Tom decided that she would take him from his own bed to that of his father's where he could speak to him before he died. This was determined to be the primary scene for Tom's therapeutic enactment.

Once the major scene was established, it was determined that Tom's enactment should be in the evening, similar to his original experience, as this would set the contextual stage for an effective therapeutic experience. Additionally, discussion ensued about the group process, safety and containment, preenactment anxiety, and possible postenactment reactions. Inclusion, control, affection, and trust among members established a highly cohesive group container that could hold a healing space for Tom's enactment.

Tom was encouraged to think about group members who could play roles that would support the enactment. It was noted that on the night of Tom's enactment, everyone was highly engaged and ready for the enactment process to begin. This was evidenced by Tom's openness to the experience, as he began to weep when he stood up within the circle of group members that had formed around him.

In this highly emotional state, Tom began to speak about his experience as an adolescent boy and the impact of his father's illness. Due to Tom's emotional struggle, it was decided to add an important feature into the process. The leader/therapist felt it was important for Tom to describe a special time he recalled with his father. He knew that this moment would serve to support Tom during the process. Tom's emotional state changed to pride as he told us of the time he and his father went camping on the shore of the ocean when the tide suddenly rose and the land around them disappeared. Tom's father took him

Figure 19–1   FIVE PHASES OF THERAPEUTIC ENACTMENT

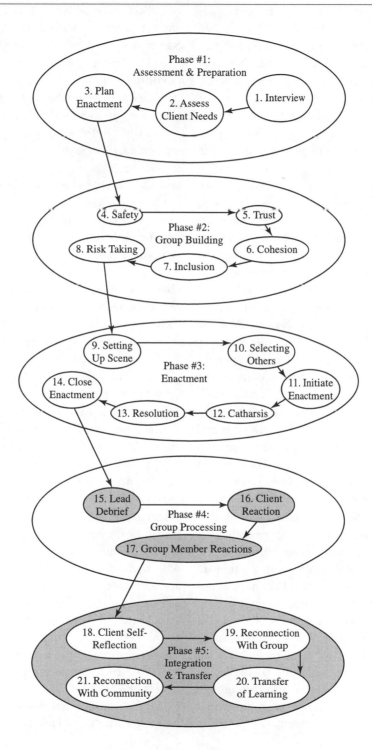

up on his shoulders and walked through the water to bring Tom to safety. To reinforce this important moment of care and protection from Tom's father, the leader thought it was important to reenact this moment in the group. He suggested that Tom reenact the scene by having him be carried across the water by his father. Tom chose a group member to play the role of his father and the enactment began. During the water crossing, intimate memories were rekindled and Tom spoke about them to the group. There was a greater understanding by everyone about the importance of this precious moment, heightening what he had lost or missed because of his father's early death. This short enactment prepared Tom for the scene of grieving to follow.

Once Tom had completed this short enactment with his father, he decided that he needed to call his close friend Jack to help support him in the helplessness and loneliness that would follow. He stated that he needed Jack to hear him speak to his father and needed to lean on Jack's supportive friendship. The leader then proceeded to set the scene related to the night Tom's father died. Group members assisted in quickly constructing a makeshift bedroom with a bed for himself and his brother, along with his parent's bedroom beside it. The leader invited Tom to describe in as much detail as he could, the time, colors, textures, and relevant memories of that night. In this process, we experienced him returning to that moment, as if he was there in the present. This heightened the experiential aspect of the enactment process. The leader encouraged Tom to select a group member that could act as his double—someone who could be him in the event he might not be able to enact sections of the event himself. The double would be able to stand in, so Tom could stand back and see the scene from a distance. Once the scene was set up, the leader assured Tom that he would walk him through the enactment, stopping to check in with him about the pacing and experiential aspects.

As Tom and the leader had prepared, Tom began the scene by being awakened by his mother and told his father was gravely ill and about to die. She walked Tom into his father's bedroom where Tom knelt by his father's bed. At this point, Tom buried his head on his father's chest and expressed his deep grief at not being there with him in his final moments. The leader directed Tom as he spoke about what he missed, what died inside of him when his father passed away, what it had cost him as a young man growing up, what he had wanted, and what he needed from his father in order to parent his own children. Once the scene was complete, Tom was able to stand back and move more into a present-centered reality awakening to what he had just done and the physical and emotional experience of relief and freedom. In stepping back, Tom was able to see more clearly what he received from his father and what his father would have probably said to him as a way of conveying his love and support. The experience of resolution and repair occurred when Tom embraced his present-centered self and permitted himself to grieve his father's death.

When the enactment was completed, Tom returned to sit among the group members. After a brief pause, we asked Tom if he wished to hear the experiences of other members that carried the roles of friend, family members, and double. Tom agreed and each individual spoke first from their perspective as a role player emphasizing any essential and helpful understanding they had, and next how the experience impacted them personally. The leader then gave other group members who witnessed the enactment an opportunity to speak about their own personal experiences of participating as observers. It was noted that, in addition to participating in the enactment as players or witnesses, the group processing experience increased the bonding of members and deepened the experience of safety within the group. Last, processing personal reactions by the leader ensured that the event was completely debriefed before moving on or closing the group.

Upon following up with Tom after the first week and then one month later, we were pleased to hear Tom report that he had found a renewed sense of life and an intimacy with his wife and children that filled that emptiness that he reported in our initial interview.

Summary

The deeply personal nature of life's end is shared by its deeply interpersonal and social nature and further informed by cultural, political, and societal influences (not addressed herein). Dying and death are as much social as they are physiological and biological. The decisions that are made are constructed in the context of important others from medical and social environments with information that is both spoken and not spoken. Grief resulting from the death of a loved one is considered the essence in the understanding of individuals and their intimate relationships.

These social phenomena and others seem particularly well suited to consideration in a group context given their involvement of others. We have considered this context in the foregoing pages, highlighting our work with ethical decision-making groups, the guided autobiography and including reference to group enactment. There exists great potential for such efforts at the end of life. For such potential to be realized, skill and concern are key so as not to add to the burden of those already suffering. In an honest, supportive, and nurturing group environment, however, individuals can effectively communicate about some of the many issues of life's end and continue to grow.

Exercises

EXERCISE 1

Think about a person you know who is at the end of life and review that individual's need for decision making.

EXERCISE 2

Reenact a moment in your life as Tom did in the guided autobiography group.

References

Anderson, R. (1970). *I never sang for my father*. New York: New York American Library.

Ashenburg, K. (2002). *The mourner's dance: What we do when people die*. Toronto, Canada: Macfarlane, Walter & Ross.

Bradley, E. H., Fried, T. R., Kasl, S. V., & Idler, E. (2000). Quality-of-life trajectories in the end of life. *Annual Review of Gerontology and Geriatrics, 20*, 64–96.

Braun, K. L., & Kayashima, R. (1999). Death education in churches and temples: Engaging religious leaders in the development of educational strategies. In B. de Vries (Ed.), *End of life issues: Interdisciplinary and multidimensional perspectives* (pp. 319–335). New York: Springer.

Brown-Shaw, M., Westwood, M., & de Vries, B. (1999). Integrating personal reflection and group-based enactments. *Journal of Aging Studies, 13*, 109–119.

Butler, R. N. (1969). Ageism: Another form of bigotry. *The Gerontologist, 9*, 243–246.

Cicirelli, V. G. (2000). Healthy elders' early decisions for end-of-life living and dying. *Annual Review of Gerontology and Geriatrics, 20*, 163–192.

Deck, E. S., & Folta, J. R. (1989). The friend-griever. In J. K. Doka (Ed.), *Disenfranchised grief: Recognizing hidden sorrow* (pp. 77–89). Lexington, MA: Lexington Books.

de Vries, B. (Ed.). (1999). *End of life issues: Interdisciplinary and multidimensional perspectives*. New York: Springer.

de Vries, B. (2001). Grief: Intimacy's reflection. *Generation, 25*, 75–80.

de Vries, B., Birren, J. E., & Deutchman, D. E. (1990). Adult development through guided autobiography: The family context. *Family Relations, 39*, 3–7.

de Vries, B., Birren, J. E., & Deutchman, D. E. (1995). Method and uses of the guided autobiography. In B. Haight & J. D. Webster (Eds.), *The art and science of reminiscing: Theory, research, methods, and applications* (pp. 165–177). Washington, DC: Taylor & Francis.

de Vries, B., & Blando, J. (2000). Friendship at the end of life. *Annual Review of Gerontology and Geriatrics, 20*, 144–162.

de Vries, B., & Johnson, C. L. (2002). *The death of friends in later life. Advances in life-course research: New frontiers in socialization* (pp. 299–324). New York: JAI Press.

de Vries, B., & Rutherford, J. (2004). Memorializing loved ones on the World Wide Web. *Omega, 49*, 5–26.

Erikson, E. H., Erikson, J. M., & Kivnick, H. Q. (1986). *Vital involvement in old age: The experience of old age in our time*. New York: Norton.

Gottlieb, B. H. (1988). *Marshaling social support: Formats, processes and effects*. Newbury Park, CA: Sage.

Hays J. C., Gold, D. T., Flint, E. P., & Winder, E. P. (1999). Patient preference for place of death: A qualitative approach. In B. de Vries (Ed.), *End of life issues: Interdisciplinary and multidimensional perspectives* (pp. 3–21). New York: Springer.

Heffner, J. E., Fahy, B., & Barbieri, C. (1996). Advance directive education during pulmonary rehabilitation. *Chest*, 109, 373–379.

High, D. M. (1993a). Why are elderly people not using advance directives? *Journal of Aging and Health*, 5, 497–515.

High, D. M. (1993b). Advance directives and the elderly: A study of intervention strategies to increase use. *The Gerontologist*, 33, 342–349.

Hopmeyer, E., & Werk, A. (1994). A comparative study of family bereavement groups. *Death Studies*, 18, 243–256.

Jones, M. (1985). *Secret flowers: Mourning and the adaptation to loss*. London: Women's Press.

Jonsen, A., Siegler, M., & Winslade, W. J. (1992). *Clinical ethics* (3rd ed.). New York: McGraw Hill.

Kastenbaum, R. J. (2004). *Death, society, and human experience*. New York: Allyn & Bacon.

Kenyon, G. M., & Randall, W. L. (2001). Narrative gerontology: An overview. In G. Kenyon, P. Clark, & B. de Vries (Eds.), *Narrative gerontology: Theory, research, and practice* (pp. 3–18). New York: Springer.

Klass, D., & Marwitt, S. (1989). Toward a model of parental grief. *Omega*, 19, 31–50.

Kuhl, D. R. (1999). Exploring spiritual and psychological issues at the end of life. Unpublished doctoral dissertation, University of British Columbia, Vancouver.

Kuhl, D. R. (2002). *What dying people want: Practical wisdom for the end of life*. New York: Public Affairs.

Kuhl, D. R., & Westwood, M. (2000). A narrative approach to integration and healing among the terminally ill. In G. Kenyon, P. Clark, & B. de Vries (Eds.), *Narrative gerontology: Theory, research, and practice* (pp. 311–330). New York: Springer.

Lerner, M. (1970). When, why and where people die. In O. G. Brim, Jr., H. E. Freeman, S. Levine, & N. A. Scotch (Eds.), *The dying patient* (pp. 5–29). New York: Russell Sage Foundation.

LeShan, L. (1982). In M. N. Bowes, E. N. Jackson, J. A. Knight, & L. LeShan (Eds.), *Counseling the dying* (pp. 6–7). New York: Nelson.

Lester, D. (1993). The stigma against dying and suicidal patients: A replication of Richard Kalish's study twenty-five years later. *Omega*, 26, 71–76.

Lieberman, M. A. (1993). Bereavement self-help groups: A review of conceptual and methodological issues. In M. S. Stroebe, W. Stroebe, & R. O. Hansson (Eds.), *Handbook of bereavement: Theory, research, and intervention* (pp. 411–426). New York: Cambridge University Press.

Luptak, M. K., & Boult, C. (1994). A method for increasing elders' use of advance directives. *The Gerontologist*, 34, 409–412.

Magee, J. J. (1988). *A professional's guide to older adults' life review*. Lexington, MA: Lexington Books.

Moss, M., & Moss, S. Z. (1989). The death of a parent. In R. A. Kalish (Ed.), *Midlife loss* (pp. 89–114). Newbury Park, CA: Sage.

Nash, P. (1992). New horizons for widowed persons: A caring program. *Psychology: A Journal of Human Behavior*, 29, 44–47.

Silverman, P. R., & Klass, D. (1996). Introduction: What's the problem? In D. Klass, P. R. Silverman, & S. L. Nickman (Eds.), *Continuing bonds: New understandings of grief*. Washington, DC: Taylor and Francis.

Teno, J., McNiff, K., & Lynn, J. (2000). Measuring quality of medical care for dying persons and their families: Preliminary suggestions for accountability. *Annual Review of Gerontology and Geriatrics*, 20, 97–119.

U.S. Bureau of the Census. (1990). *Census of population and housing: Summary population and housing characteristics*. Washington, DC: U.S. Government Printing Office.

Vachon, M. L., & Stylianos, S. K. (1988). The role of social support in bereavement. *Journal of Social Issues*, 44, 175–190.

Westwood, M. (1998). *Life review program for Canadian veterans*. (Report prepared for Veterans Affairs Canada and the Royal Canadian Legion.) Vancouver, British Columbia.

Westwood, M. J., Keats, P. & Wilensky, P. (2003). Therapeutic enactment: Integrating individual and group counseling models for change. *Journal for Specialists in Group Work*, 28, 122–138.

Yale, R. (1989). Support groups for newly diagnosed Alzheimer's clients. *Clinical Gerontologist*, 8, 86–89.

BIBLIOGRAPHY

Birren, J. E., & Cochran, K. N. (2001). *Telling the stories of life through guided autobiography groups*. Baltimore: Johns Hopkins Press.

Kuhl, D. (2002). *What dying people want: Practical wisdom for the end of life*. New York: Public Affairs.

Part Four

Settings for Group Work

Settings for group work for older people are ubiquitous. In this section of the book, we address traditional settings as well as settings that are less traditional for older people, such as the workplace. Shafer, a business consultant, presents retirement and preretirement preparation in Chapter 20. Then the work in the section moves on to more traditional settings. Black, Kelly, and Rice discuss group work in retirement communities in Chapter 21, a change that for most people requires a great deal of adjustment as they give up their homes of a lifetime. Chapter 22 provides some insight into day care settings and services and presents groups that serve both the patient and the caregiver. Black, Friedlob, and Kelly offer a mélange of groups to conduct in board-and-care homes, and provide numerous resources in Chapter 23. As people grow older and face nursing home living their ability to be active lessens. Amella discusses the research on groups in long-term care in Chapter 24. Lastly, in Chapter 25 we move to the acute care setting, which has changed immensely over the past five years. Edlund and Finch talk about the use of the Internet and telehealth to facilitate patient education and support in the hospital setting and upon discharge from the hospital.

Chapter 20

Retirement Preparation Groups

Patricia Shafer

Key Words

- Construct of retirement
- Best practices
- Patterns of adjustment
- "Good" retirement
- Newly retired
- Special interest groups
- Four modes, seven stages
- Transition map

Learning Objectives

- Understand demographic and cultural aspects of aging
- Establish a time frame for group facilitation
- Reflect on variations in individual adaptations to retirement
- Appreciate unique needs of subgroups
- Understand exercises and tools to enhance transition
- Experience personal inquiry

Introduction

Opinions about the appropriate age for and best approaches to retirement change over time driven by politics, economics, and social convention. The construct of retirement was formalized during the Great Depression of the 1930s, when older employees were moved out of the workforce to make way for younger people. By the close of the 20th century, in a competitive business environment, more people were encouraged, forced, or chose to leave the workforce at earlier ages. Various groups characterized and promoted retirement as an appealing stage of life. New and multifaceted expectations related to retirement arose in an era of average life span extending well into the 70s.

Best practices suggest that formal programs should exist inside organizations to help people gradually phase in to retirement, supported by group practices to prepare for actual retirement. Effective planning helps workers develop a positive attitude toward retirement while they are working and increases satisfaction with the retirement process (Corporate Executive Board, 2004). However, the availability of retirement planning and transition options and tools varies considerably.

A recognized certification process or body of course work does not exist to fully equip professionals to support preretired and newly retired people. It is desirable for retirement counselors— who may be human resource managers, clinical counselors, industrial and social psychologists, psychotherapists, social workers, retirement community managers, consultants, and/or life coaches—to develop an understanding of the spectrum of physical, emotional, and financial changes that occur in retirement. With this knowledge, practitioners can develop engaging instruction, interventions, and coaching protocols to serve preretired and newly retired people.

Goal of Group Practices

The primary goal of group practices is to support newly retired people in an integrated inquiry into the proposition that retirement is a state of mind and an unfolding series of events with many factors in play, not a pre-scripted absolute. This focus of attention enables people driven by work schedules and responsibilities to become motivated by personal desires and equipped to achieve life goals specific to retirement.

This chapter provides an overview for understanding effects of retirement on people's lives, and introduces group exercises to aid and enhance transition. The framework integrates and supplements aspects of five models of retirement preparation used across industry, government, community centers, extension services, counseling offices, and a variety of other settings. The five models are planning, counseling, adult education, human potential, and life planning (Cohen & Anderson, 1999) (see **Table 20–1**).

Group practices should incorporate expertise and tools available from both human resources and financial professionals holding specialized financial planning credentials. Examples are certification for Preretirement Education and Planning, as well as the designation of Certified Retirement Counselor (CRC). In addition, frameworks, curricula, and discussion prompts for preretirement and newly retired groups exist to focus on specific subjects such as coping with loss

(*Everyday Psychologist*, 1999) and replacing such losses with social networks, play, creativity, and lifelong learning (Valliant, 2003).

Efficacy and Benefits

A review of the literature reveals that few longitudinal studies exist on longer-term effects of retirement and certain life-course choices. For group exercises, it is generally believed that the greatest participant benefits are achieved in a period extending from one year before to two years after a career or formal work ends. This is the cohort described as newly retired people— those who are approaching or have recently passed the milestone of retirement. Notably, the traditional definition of *retirement* as an exit from the workforce is increasingly obsolete. A working definition in the early 21st century is "an exit from work following eligibility for pension, Social Security, and/or early retirement benefits."

Erikson (1950) described eight ages in the course of a life, suggesting that mature adulthood is a period for achieving "ego integrity." Group practices to support newly retired people help achieve ego integrity by providing a dimension of structure and discipline to the act of self-reflection by older adults. Group practices help create personal "destinations" that emerge through explored feelings and solidify through planning and action. The process of identifying "destinations" threads together the retirement objectives of making peace with the past, envisioning and accepting a new role in life, overcoming fears of becoming irrelevant, discovering bounds of personal capacity, adjusting to financial realities, and redefining relationships (Rich, Sampson, & Fetherling, 1999).

Broadly, opportunities and challenges for retirement groups involve reformulation of personal identities through: (a) acquisition of a "Third Age" perspective, (b) looking inward for self-discovery, (c) visioning and exploring possibilities, (d) making choices and implementing

Table 20–1   FIVE MODELS OF RETIREMENT PREPARATION AND ADAPTATION

Planning	Counseling	Adult education	Human potential	Life planning
Most popular	Focus: psychological adjustment goals	Retirement seen as developmental stage involving changing life patterns	Underlying theme is retirement as transition, time of renewal	Comprehensive approach used at all ages and stages
Typical in corporations, government— Retirement viewed as economic event, decline	Retirement viewed as time of interpersonal challenge, crisis—concerns of mal-adaptation	Emerged from principles of adult education outline in 1970s	Goal is facilitation of individual goals and enhanced personal flexibility	Philosophy of life as continuum, with most satisfying retirements based on future-focused decisions throughout life
Focus—practical: • Benefits • Finances • Legal • Health care	Programs may be conducted with individuals or in small groups	This model commonly used in colleges and community organizations	Relies on personal strength theory and identification to plan for effective retirement	Holistic approach considers range of factors: finances, relationships, physical and mental health, learning, etc.
Often involves presentations from experts to those anticipating retirement impact—with supporting materials	Focus on anticipating, addressing problems with desired future state orientation	Integrates lectures, group discussion, presentations, interactive work in humanistic, participant-centered approach	Requires skilled group facilitators eliciting highly individualized choices	Planning tools balance potential risks, rewards
Group size—small or large	Counselor's role is to impart successful coping skills		Groups should be no more than 30 in size to accommodate full involvement	
		Comprehensive content centers on enhancing self-esteem and independence		Personalized planning in group setting involving facilitated use of self-learning tools

Adapted from: J. Cohen & C. Anderson, 1999.

goals (Newhouse & Goggin, 2004). This reinforces self-respect in a society that strongly links personal worth with one's work.

Patterns of Adjustment

Extreme cases of overidentification with work may be characterized as "Work Identity Syndrome" and require multistep exercises enabling newly retired people to find meaning outside of work (Edmondson, 1998). Most people spend their adulthood working in structured settings surrounded by other people. A typical workday is regulated, and work occupies 33% of an average day. Thus, those people who strongly identify with work are prone to onset of boredom and questions of self-doubt in retirement: What have I accomplished? What will make my life matter?

In general, the experience of newly retired people is positively or adversely affected by a number of factors—foremost among them are circumstances leading to retirement (voluntary or involuntary), health, wealth and an ability to absorb a reduction in income, and marital status. Racial status may be a factor, too. Retirees who report health and financial challenges tend to be less well educated, are more likely to be minorities, and receive a higher share of income from public sources.

There are neither average nor optimal practices for supporting newly retired people. Effective group practices help individuals to define and pursue a subjective interpretation of "good" retirement that is unique to each individual retiree and his or her circumstances (see **Table 20–2**). Individuals able to transition from past work to a vision of their futures adjust most successfully. Successful adjustments involve group activities that foster individual internalization of change (Bridges, 2003).

Newly retired people may find themselves in one of four modes: (1) Transition to Old Age/ Rest (time for slowing down); (2) New Beginning (freedom to pursue long-awaited goals);

(3) Continuity (just another transition in life); or (4) Imposed Disruption (not fair, frustrating) (Hanson & Wapner, 1994). In addition, the transition to retirement may also involve stages of more or less positive orientation: Honeymoon (immediately following retirement, encompassing a spectrum of feelings from ebullience to loss); Disenchantment (continued sense of loss for months or years, sometimes leading to depression); Reorientation (reevaluation of retirement decision and alternative lifestyle resulting in return to work and or satisfaction); Stability (adaptation) (Atchley, 1976).

There is no predictable flow to the pace or order in which people move through these stages, nor will every individual experience all stages.

Group Size and Participation

One reason that organizations do not provide retirement planning is a belief that personal aspects of retirement make it an individual

Table 20–2 PERSONAL DEFINITION OF RETIREMENT

	Very much %	Somewhat %	Very much/ Somewhat %
Spending more time with family and friends	54	24	78
A chance to relax	48	25	73
A chance to have more fun	48	25	73
Receiving retirement benefits: Social Security or pension	49	23	72
A chance to do things you never had time for	47	25	72
A chance to travel	38	28	67
Doing volunteer or charity work	19	39	57
Slowing down & working fewer hours/part-time	24	32	56
Working for enjoyment, not money	25	27	53
Chance to stop working for pay, completely	23	25	48
Having to do some kind of work to help pay bills	15	28	42
Chance to leave main career to try a different type of work	12	17	28
Feeling less useful or less productive	7	14	20

Adapted from The AARP Working in Retirement Study, 2003.

endeavor best addressed in individual counseling. In actuality, group settings are an appropriate and effective forum for exploring retirement and the transition to retirement. Groups provide an expanded social network and a sense that participants are surrounded with allies, thus countering concerns that retirement leads to social isolation.

Principles of effective group dynamics already discovered, refined, and published on topics such as reminiscence, remotivation, reorientation, and life planning are adaptable to group practices with newly retired populations. A group size of six to eight participants works well in most settings, combining camaraderie and group learning with individualized attention. Even participants with unique physical and emotional circumstances can be successfully served in groups (Noffsinger, 1999). Groups of up to 30 are acceptable if content and exercises are designed to be primarily informational and instructive. Groups intended to be both interactive and reflective should be smaller and more intimate in size (Cohen & Anderson, 1999) (see **Table 20–1**).

Perceptions of Retirement

Retirement is no longer perceived as an official demarcation between working and not working. More than 80% of baby boomers (cohort born between 1946 and 1964) believe that they will stretch out their work lives, moving in and out of the workforce after retirement (AARP, 1998). Current workers aged 50 to 70 aspire to dynamic retirements, with more than half including *working for enjoyment, not money*, in their definition of retirement. Most people envision retirement as a combination of leisure, new experiences, time spent with family and friends, and decisions about how to stay active. Only 20% anticipate feeling less useful or less productive (AARP, 2003). A key decision involves choosing among three paths: (1) stop working completely, (2) continue to work part-time or part-year, or (3) retire for a period of time and then reenter the workforce full- or part-time (Naleppa, 1999). Thus, continuation of work in some capacity and intermittent work reentry are increasingly common.

Despite widespread positive perceptions of retirement, there are adults for whom retirement looms negatively—32% of baby boomers in at least one significant segmentation analysis (AARP, 1998). It is critical that group exercises to support the newly retired encourage hopeful attitudes and address an array of concerns held by adults who feel ill prepared or pessimistic, and may require more support and information. These participants are characterized in two categories: the Strugglers and the Anxious. The profile of the former is median household income significantly below the average baby boomer, a majority being female, with little or no savings for retirement. The latter profile is median household income somewhat below the average, some savings, but low confidence in sufficiency of finances and health care coverage.

Financial topics can raise previously unanticipated issues and have a polarizing effect in groups. Some newly retired people feel wealthier due to lower expenses related to fuel costs, wardrobe, lunches, and so on. Conversely, a newly retired person may be poorer and therefore more stressed as a result of retirement. Notably, American workers tend to overrate their preparation for retirement, particularly savings required for housing, food, and health expenses. The impact on women can be pronounced given that, on average, women earn less than men, women spend more years as unpaid caregivers outside the workforce, and a rising divorce rate means more retiring women are single and supporting themselves financially (*Seattle Post-Intelligencer*, 2002). For group participants with financial concerns writer Ernest Hemingway's admonition that "*retirement* is the ugliest word in the language" may resonate.

Designs for Special Interest Groups

Generally, groups anticipating retirement are quite diverse—with a mix of gender, race, ethnicity, economic strata, and lifestyle. It is also appropriate to organize special interest groups based on criteria that can reflect or help create common bonds. More nuanced group segmentation can add value to respective experiences.

Early Retirees

Some corporate practices have moved to encouraging retirement as early as 52 to 55. The younger a worker is when leaving a job, the higher the probability that such a departure is not truly voluntary. Early retirees are more likely to feel "pushed out to pasture" and unappreciated. Such circumstances can prompt feelings of depression among people who still enjoy working, who believe they can contribute, or who have financial concerns. Transition groups composed of early retirees have much in common with one another.

Women

The story of retirement is no longer just about men. Women working in the 1960s became the first generation of females in large numbers to form long-term careers and enter professional ranks (such as doctors, managers, and educators). The literature is somewhat contradictory regarding whether men and women have different levels of satisfaction in retirement. However, there are indications of fundamental differences between women professionals and nonprofessionals (such as clerical, administrative, and support staff). Women professionals are more likely to feel a sense of loss in retirement while women nonprofessionals may feel relief (Price, 2003). Women who experience more yearlong employment gaps prior to retirement are somewhat more likely to report satisfaction in retirement than women who worked continuously (Cornell, 1998).

Couples

Retirement tends to be a happy time for couples. But the transition to retirement can foster marital strife. Both men and women report more conflict and decline in marital quality, with improvements occurring two years postretirement (Moen, Jungmeen, & Hofmeister, 2001). The greatest conflict occurs when one spouse moves into retirement while the other continues to work, especially when the husband retires and the wife is employed. When husbands and wives retire at about the same time, men are happier in their marriages. Couples that struggled in marriage before retirement are likely to incur more marital tension postretirement. Group design and delivery for newly retired couples should incorporate content on the special issues couples face, as well as skills development in communication and conflict resolution.

Functional Limitations

The vast majority of workers, even those aged 65 and older, are in generally good health without functional limitations. In addition, the trend away from physically demanding jobs should further extend working lives and overall mobility. In health matters, early retirees and those who have worked at physically demanding jobs are statistically more likely to have acute or chronic episodes of poor health, or a limiting physical condition. Additional group activities to meet health needs, alleviating chronic musculoskeletal conditions for example, will complement intellectual and emotional group activities to support newly retired people. Group practices should include advising participants to have a physical examination. Interventions have shown that a health check, counseling, and a written health plan have positive benefits. Exercise prescription schemes should be avoided without appropriate evaluations (National Health Service, 2000).

Prework for Guiding a Group

In preparing to guide a group, the facilitator should determine the ideal number of participants and choose a comfortable and convenient site for running the group. Letters of invitation describing the purpose of the group, the length of time it will be run, and an outline of activities should be sent to eligible participants with an RSVP required to assist the facilitator in planning. The group should then be structured so that participants have had some similar work experiences and share some commonalities besides the pending retirement. An agenda describing the proposed meetings should be distributed during the first meeting of the group with input solicited from the group regarding additional experiences they might enjoy or wish to discuss.

Facilitator Self-Exploration

Facilitators must be sensitive to experiences likely to be encountered by newly retired people. It is desirable for any group facilitator to a have significant work history that permits him or her to picture the realities of retirement. The following self-exploration exercise is relevant for facilitators striving to more fully connect with group participants.

For the facilitator: picture yourself as a newly retired person and write down key thoughts from your personal imaginings.

- Will you be 50? 60? 65? 70?
- What impressions do you have of retirement?
- Are you looking forward to retirement, or not? Why?
- Do you anticipate having any worries—financial, health, or otherwise?
- What is your current level of preparation for retirement?

Participant Self-Assessment

Group practices should include self-assessment tools presented by the facilitator to gauge degrees of participant readiness for retirement and group involve-ment. Tools can be distributed to participants prior to group formation or at the session's opening and before beginning instruction and dialogue. Self-assessments can be revisited on group completion to determine changes in attitude and adaptation, as well as what action steps were completed.

Use of a self-assessment tool creates self-awareness for participants regarding their retirement readiness in practical and emotional terms (see **Table 20–3**). Such tools also help illustrate that retirement is a process involving multiple factors and responses.

Structure and Components of a Transition Process

Retirement involves individuals learning how to live effectively in an ongoing state of retirement. This learning involves looking within to determine what work has meant and what is desired following this important life milestone. Group practices are organized to guide participants through a transition process to retirement. Like other transitions that make sense of life changes, retirement transition generally occurs in three stages: (1) Endings, in which individuals recognize and celebrate opportunities and losses; (2) Neutral Zone, a "time-out" of exploration that can feel new and exciting or unproductive, unconnected, and frightening; and (3) New Beginnings, a launching of new priorities (Bridges, 2003).

An illustration of the key components to help move participants through these three stages is expressed in the Retirement Transition Map (see **Figure 20–1**). These components, covered in numerical order, serve as a framework for discussion, activity, and interactive elements of group practices for newly retired people.

It is possible to provide participants with an understanding of key aspects of retirement and a sense of the process in a tightly organized workshop delivered in one day. Another option, particularly effective when begun up to a year in advance of retirement, is a series of lunches or brown-bag

Table 20–3   RETIREMENT READINESS SELF-ASSESSMENT

Readiness statements	Yes	No	Not Sure	Comments
I have completed a retirement planning process.				
I have a retirement plan.				
My plan addresses many aspects of retirement such as finances, health care, relationships, work, and hobbies.				
I have reviewed my plan with a trained financial adviser.				
I have reviewed my plan with important people in my life including my spouse/partner and children.				
I have identified how long I expect to live and considered how this affects my retirement plan.				
I understand what benefits are available to me, including Social Security, pensions, and retirement accounts.				
I have completed a health check.				
I take care of my health—diet, exercise, and medication.				
I have made arrangements for nursing home or extended health care in the future.				
I have decided whether I will continue to work and how.				
I have taken the time to dream about retirement, including hobbies, interests, and social activities.				
I am optimistic and looking forward to the retirement phase of life.				

This assessment is a tool to aid group participants in reflecting on their level of preparation for retirement. There is no "scoring" necessary. Responses generate thinking and discussion, and aid in action planning. Copyright-Compel, LTD 2004.

meetings facilitated inside an organization by its Human Resources Department and delivered by an internal employee or outside consultant. A fuller and more robust format is designed around the Retirement Transition Map over a minimum of five weeks, with each group session lasting two hours. Participants are encouraged to read, reflect, and journal between sessions. Group work is divided as follows:

- Week 1—understanding the journey: This is a group formation session including facilitator and participant introductions; icebreakers; overview of group goals and procedures; facilitator-provided survey of facts, figures, and fallacies of the retirement experience; and distribution of relevant materials. A useful handout would be a list of retirement-related resources, or a retirement guidebook if one has been created. Supporting exercise: It is important to acknowledge retirement, first, as an ending, and to set a tone of the group sharing the journey toward retirement. Participants individually highlight a list of places they have worked, positions held, and major responsibilities. The information is then transferred onto individual chronological time lines, denoting certain events as emotional peaks and valleys.

Figure 20–1 RETIREMENT TRANSITION MAP

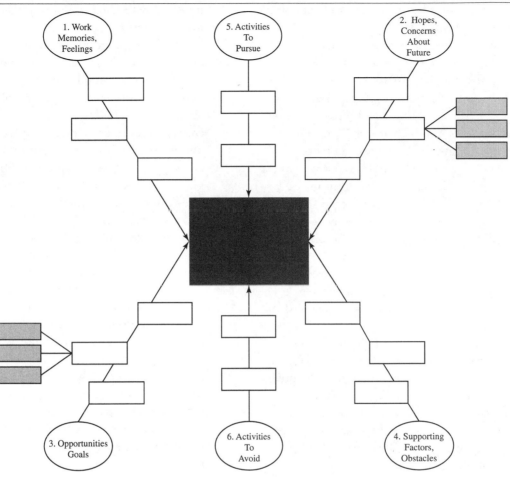

Participants are instructed to continue enhancing the time line on their own between Week 1 and Week 2.

- Week 2—completing the past/reviewing one's career: This session builds on the time line completed in Week 1 by focusing on Items 1 and 2 in the Retirement Transition Map—work memories and feelings, as well as hopes and concerns about the future.

Supporting exercise: Participants review their time lines. They then reflect on questions such as: How did you choose your work? What are defining moments of the time line? What have you most enjoyed? What are the disappointments? What are you most proud of? Are there any unresolved feelings or things left undone? Consequently, what are hopes and concerns about the future? Then, one participant shares his or her work "story" with the group, focusing on what work has meant. Using this as an example, participants share their stories. If the group is small, stories can be shared one-by-one with the whole group. For larger groups, paired shares are sufficient. Each individual transfers key takeaways to boxes on his or her Transition Map.

- Week 3—anticipating the future/accepting a new role: This session combines Transition Map Items 3 and 4—attention to perceived opportunities and goals, as well as factors that could support or prove obstacles to achievement. To generate open thinking, this week can be positioned as "Developing a Hypothesis of the Ideal Retirement" or "Looking into a Crystal Ball." Participants need to be reminded that most people retire without planning or an articulated picture of retirement. Newly retired people should be encouraged to think of themselves as having an open horizon, and therefore, an opportunity to envision—even fantasize—about possibility.

Supporting exercise: Using a board or series of paper sheets covering a wall, participants brainstorm as a group the qualities and characteristics of an ideal retirement. Ideas are proposed and captured as quickly as they come under headings such as Post-Retirement Work; Hobbies/Activities; Relationships; Money/Finances; Health; Learning/Self-Development. Participants choose from the lists and or add individually three to five opportunities or goals for each category. Then, they individually consider supporting factors and obstacles that could affect preferred opportunities and goals. Information is captured on the individual Transition Maps.

- Week 4—choosing preferred alternatives: This session provides a venue for participants to be specific about activities that they would like to pursue and avoid in retirement (Items 5 and 6). It is critical that this session guide participants to prioritize and make choices, limiting themselves to some degree. Logically, activities should link back to opportunities and goals identified in the previous week, but they do not have to. Further completion of the Transition Map continues as a support tool.

Supporting exercise: Any tools that are creative ways to encourage prioritization can be used in this session. For instance, participants can each be given $100 of play money, or a collection of marbles. They must make decisions about which items are worth trading for, and how are they weighted. With $100, for example, is one of the activity choices such a priority that it is worth "investing" $50?

- Week 5—clarifying a personal retirement vision: This session completes the group experience, prompting participants to draw from all that they have learned in order to clarify and summarize personal retirement visions. The purpose is to move from review and visioning to action planning. It is an opportunity to creatively codify concrete steps toward a preferred retirement experience. The session should include a celebratory ritual to achieve closure and launch participants onto their retirement journey.

Supporting exercise: There are numerous ways to conduct a supporting exercise for this session. A left-brained linear approach involves participants creating a forward-looking time line as an extension of the time line completed in Week 1. The time line extension works backward from "End of Life" to ten years, to five years, to one year, to next month. Participants transfer priorities from Week 4, and then create individual steps and milestones toward achieving the goals.

Summary

The transition to retirement will continue to increase in importance as more people retire earlier and live longer. As with other life transitions, retirement is an excellent focus for group work led by human resource managers, clinical counselors, industrial and social psychologists, psychotherapists, social workers, retirement community managers, consultants, and life coaches.

It is logical that there is an established link between preparation for and satisfaction with retirement, but organizations devote limited resources to helping people make the transition. Specific issues, concerns, and aspirations addressed in a safe, comfortable environment can be openly acknowledged and a new life phase anticipated and articulated. Ideally, this facilitated group experience should occur between one year before and two years after official retirement. Newly retired people represent a need and demand to be ably filled by nonprofit and for-profit providers in the public and private sectors.

Exercises

EXERCISE 1

Create a 6-week agenda for running a retirement group.

EXERCISE 2

List the requirements for an effective retirement group facilitator.

EXERCISE 3

Describe how you would apply one tool to a retirement group.

References

AARP. (1998). *Baby boomers envision their retirement: An AARP segmentation analysis—Executive summary*. Washington, DC: AARP.

AARP. (2003). *Staying ahead of the curve 2003: The AARP working in retirement study—Executive summary*. Washington, DC: AARP.

Atchley, R. C. (1976). *The sociology of retirement*. Cambridge, MA: John Wiley & Sons.

Bridges, W. (2003). *Managing transitions: Making the most of change* (2nd ed.). New York: Perseus.

Cohen, J., & Anderson, J. (1999). Life planning: An effective model for retirement planning. Education. *Journal of the International Society for Retirement Planning*, (Summer), 5–10.

Cornell Gerontology Research Institute. (1998). His and her retirement? The role of gender and marriage in the retirement process. *Roybal Issue Brief*. Retrieved June 12, 2004 from *www.applied-gerontology.org*

Corporate Executive Board. (2004, February). Key findings: Pre-retirement programs.

Edmondson, C. M. (1998). *Disconnecting from the workplace: How to balance your life and begin intentional living today*. West Indies: MJP.

Erickson, E. (1950) *Childhood and society*. New York, New York: W. W. Norton & Co. Inc.

Everyday Psychologist. (1999). *The psychology of retirement: How to cope with a major life transition*. Arlington Heights, IL: Business Psychology Research Institute (BPRI) Press.

Hanson, K., & Wapner, S. (1994). Transition to retirement: Gender differences. *International Journal of Aging and Human Development, 39*, 189–208.

Moen, P., Jungmeen, E. K., & Hofmeister, H. (2001). Couples' work/retirement transitions, gender, and marital quality. *Social Psychology Quarterly, 64*(1), 55–71.

Newhouse, M., & Goggin, J. (2004). *Life planning for the 3rd Age*. San Francisco, CA: Civic ventures. *www.civicventures.org*

Naleppa, M. J. (1999). Late adulthood. In E. D. Hutchinson (Ed.), *Dimensions of human behavior: The changing life course* (pp. 257–288). Thousand Oaks, CA: Pine Forge Press.

National Health Service (NHS) Health Development Agency. (2000). *Pre-retirement health checks and plans literature review*. (preparation for identification of pilot site concerned with the provision of pre-retirement advice and services). London.

Noffsinger, E. (1999). Increasing quality of care and access while reducing costs through drop-in group medical appointments. *Group Practice Journal, American Medical Group Association*. (January).

Price, C. (2003). Untitled study of how occupation directly impacts a woman's retirement. Ohio State University. Retrieved June 24, 2004, from *http://researchnews.osu.edu/archive/womret.htm*

Rich, P., Sampson D., & Fetherling, D. (1999). *The healing journey through retirement: Your journal of transition and transformation*. New York: John Wiley & Sons.

Seattle Post Intelligencier. (2002). Many factors make retirement tough for women. (July, 5).

Valliant, G. E. (2003). *Aging well: Surprising guideposts to a happier life from the landmark Harvard study of adult development*. New York: Little, Brown.

Resources

- AARP. (2003). Staying ahead of the curve: The AARP working in retirement study. *http://www.research.org*
- Chapman, E. (1997). *Comfort zones: The comprehensive guide to retirement* (4th ed.

revised by Haynes, M.). Menlo Park, CA: Crisp.
- International Foundation for Retirement Education (InFRE) Certified Retirement Counselor Designees (listed by state). *www.infre.org*
- National Preretirement Education Association. *www.npea.com*
- Zelinski, E. J. (2003). *The joy of not working: A book for the retired, unemployed, and overworked*. Berkeley, CA: Ten Speed Press.

Chapter 21

A Model of Group Work in Retirement Communities

Janet E. Black

James J. Kelly

Susan Rice

Key Words

- Elaborating skills
- Empowerment
- Explicit norms
- Implicit norms
- Nonviolent conflict
- Open-ended groups
- Role modeling
- Self-selection
- Termination

Learning Objectives

- Define the concept of empowerment
- Describe the skills needed by workers in the forming stages of a group
- Describe one example of nonviolent direct communication
- Describe the skills needed by workers in the performing phase of a group
- Identify two ways to assist group members in dealing with termination issues
- Describe some of the positive and negative consequences of open-ended groups
- Describe the process involved in dealing with problem members of groups
- Describe the most important needs of residents living in retirement communities

Introduction

Group work can be an important method of providing supportive services to a retirement community setting. A review of the literature on groups for older persons (Corey, 2004; Kottler, 2001; Toseland, 1995) suggested that the many benefits include reduction of loneliness, isolation, and rejection, conditions often associated with the process of aging in our culture. Groups may also provide increased self-awareness, provide support and socialization opportunities, and help the participants learn new and more successful ways of dealing with issues. Why groups specifically within the retirement community setting? Data from the Census Bureau (2001) show that the oldest-old population has been rapidly increasing in number. In 1960, about 900,000 individuals lived to be 85 or older. In 1990, that number tripled to 3 million, and in the 2000 census, the number had increased again by 1.3 million. By 2050, the Census Bureau's estimates suggest that more than 18 million people over the age of 85 will be living in the United States. Many of these people will be living in retirement communities, which will become an increasingly important setting for working with older adults (U.S. Bureau of the Census, 2001; Folts & Muir, 2002). Those most at risk for future institutionalization include those who have high rates of functional disability, very old average age, and high prevalence of living alone—the same characteristics of most retirement settings, and of those who self-selected the program described in this chapter. While it is true that social support alone cannot prevent institutionalization, most people prefer to "age in place" as long as possible, and social support does slow down the negative emotional consequences that accompany greater physical frailty.

The importance of social supports, particularly for older adults, has been consistently documented in the literature (Hooyman & Kiyak, 1999; Siebert, Mutran, & Reitzes, 1999; Wojciechowski, 2000). Social support gives a person a sense of belonging and acceptance, and social support networks can positively influence one's physical and emotional well-being (Hooyman & Kiyak). Wojciechowski examined the use of and satisfaction with social support networks among older adults living in a retirement community. Findings indicate that both formal and informal support networks were important components in maintaining the residents' well-being. Siebert, Mutran, and Reitzes examined the relationship of friendship and life satisfaction ratings in older adults, and found that the "friend role" is more important in predicting life satisfaction than other variables, including income, marital status, and educational level (p. 530).

This chapter is divided into four parts. Part I describes a specific project and its evolution over time to respond to needs and realities, using students at an urban college campus as group leaders for a series of weekly support groups in a nearby retirement community. This specific project uses group work in two ways—as a methodology for training students to work with groups of older

people, and as a support-group service for people living within a retirement community. Each of these purposes has individual goals and objectives, at the same time as each is an integral part of the whole project. Part II describes the developmental group work issues that emerge, in parallel fashion, in the classroom and in the retirement community. Part III discusses some of the structural issues in coordinating such a program. Part IV briefly summarizes the outcomes of this program, in terms of fulfilling its purposes.

Description of the Project

In a large urban area on the West Coast is a retirement community composed of more than 9000 residents, who desired independent living, but in a sheltered, gated community. The community is 40 years old, and when it first opened, the corporation marketing the community targeted active, new or preretirees in their late 50s or early 60s. They were successful in their targeting, and the units quickly filled up. They were sold as "cooperatives," meaning that residents paid a price for the unit they lived in, and then a monthly maintenance charge for the upkeep of the grounds. Prospective residents were required to have the entire purchase price (which excluded low-income persons) and were required to be capable of "independent living." This history is necessary because it is important to understand the present-day flavor of this community, and points to significant background knowledge that helps to understand the needs of group members within the context of their retirement community setting.

At the present time, the community has "aged," and the average age is 80, rather than 60. Clearly, its residents are a much frailer population than when they moved in and have different needs. Additionally, these residents, who were middle class then, are now retired and so, despite having an adequate place to live, they tend to have much lower incomes. These changes have been largely ignored by the developers of this community, who continue to target healthy, 50ish people who are looking for an active place to retire—golf course, numerous activity clubs, churches, and so on. There is a medical clinic within the community, on a fee-for-service basis, but there continues to be the requirement that all residents must be able to live independently. The reality is that many residents have part- or full-time homemakers and/or caregivers, but there is no official sanctioning or brokerage of these services.

A program of weekly support and discussion groups began when a group of residents approached the nearby state university. They said that they would like to have some interaction with students and residents would welcome some assistance in setting up discussion or support groups, which would be different from the usual activity groups offered in their community. The fulfillment of this request, on their terms, illustrates the belief that empowerment is one of the primary purposes of social work. It is a method by which practitioners can help clients to help themselves in facilitating the interaction between them and their environments for purposes of problem solving (Galinsky & Schopler, 1995; Hepworth, Rooney, & Larsen, 2002; Kurland & Salomon 1996; Theuma, 2001). Empowerment is both a process and an outcome; and it occurs within an environment of interaction in which support, mutual aid, and validation for one's perceptions and experiences are received.

After discussion between the interested residents and key members of the university faculty who possess expertise and interest in working with older adults, a program eventually emerged. It was a partnership between residents and the university's department of social work, with assistance from other areas including the psychology department. The people responsible for the program were residents of the retirement community, including a president, vice president, secretary, and treasurer. A faculty member from the university was the liaison, a role that included teaching a two-semester course in which students would attend class, learn about group work, and then lead (or colead) weekly groups in the community. The faculty member also provided supervision to the students regarding their weekly groups at the retirement community. Students were juniors or seniors, and included majors in psychology, social work, gerontology, nursing, and anthropology. In order to meet an identified need of retirement community members who were in need of support services, but were unable to attend an out-of-home group, or who were not comfortable in a group setting, additional program elements were added. These included weekly in-home visits with homebound residents by students in the program. To provide additional socialization and stimulation opportunities, workshops and potluck dinners involving all members of the support groups and the student leaders were developed. The program serves only a minute segment of this retirement community of 9000—approximately 60 people at any one time. They are a self-selected group, and tend to be frailer, older, and less mobile than the general population. They tend to live either with a spouse or alone, suffer serious health handicaps, and want an opportunity to talk more or less openly about the difficult situations they face.

Students also self-select this program, although a faculty member interviews them before they begin their internship, to explain the program and assess their level of interest and potential. They are required to have an interest in working with older people, and in group work, but are not required to have any specific kinds of experiences. They originally were required to be willing to commit to both semesters of the course and stay with the same group members (and individual home visitor) for the entire year. This has changed over the 25-year history of the program. As budgets have tightened, students have less room in their programs of study for elective credit, and the structure was changed to a one-semester commitment. The focus also changed, to pay attention to the "frailty" of the members, and now includes a life review segment, in which the focus of the individual home visits is to systematically conduct and tape a formal life review, which is later presented to the member. An outgrowth of this program has also been adapted in Northern California and is structured as an intergenerational learning class, at four different sites. This is important, because it demonstrates the importance of flexibility and the ability to be flexible in meeting both university and community needs. On a historical note, there was a time when the program's very existence was threatened and the university and community came together to lobby for the continuance of the program. They were able to demonstrate that there was value to both students and senior residents and that it would be in everyone's interest to find the funding to continue the program. The faculty member working with the students and residents plays an extremely active role in the administration of the overall program, as well as the teaching, and group work supervision aspects of it.

Developmental Group Work Issues—Students and Residents

A variety of models are used to describe stages of group development (Chen & Rybak, 2004; Corey, 2004; Corey & Corey, 2002; Gladding, 1999; Kelly & Berman-Rossi, 1999; Tuckman, 1965), but whatever language is used, a process emerges whereby members of a group change, over time, from an aggregate of people into an interactive, mutually dependent, and mutually influenced unit. Tuckman's classic (1965) alliterative taxonomy of the forming, storming, norming, performing, and adjourning phases of group work enables students to analyze their groups in relation to their stage of development. A more recent taxonomy (Anderson, 1997) presents the TACIT model, an acronym for Trust, Autonomy, Closeness, Independence, and Termination.

This model shows groups developing through the preaffiliation stage (where trust is the major issue), to the power and control stage (where autonomy is the major issue), to the intimacy stage (where closeness is the major issue), to the differentiation stage (where interdependence is the major issue), and finally to the separation stage (where termination is the major issue).

Early on, the point is made to the students in the classroom that they are struggling with the same stages of group development and the same crises that members of the retirement community are dealing with in their group settings. Modeling is used to demonstrate worker tasks, and process analysis using class discussion, case vignettes, and experiential exercises assists students in recognizing the patterns in both sets of groups.

Preaffiliation

In the preaffiliation stage of the classroom unit, students are anxious about the year ahead, about their tasks, and about their future relationships both with each other and with the older group members. Brandler and Roman (1999) describe the initial tasks of the social work practitioner as including "helping to create an atmosphere that allows for safe expression of intimate private feelings. Trust, nurturing, consistency, safety, and low frustration must be provided to facilitate risk taking and promote growth" (p. 16). Group members need to interact with each other to deal with this issue so that they can own the group as they progress. There is much class discussion about how the classroom group will hopefully become a mutual support group, just as they hope the community group will provide support to the residents. Gitterman and Shulman's (1994) classic work on mutual aid and vulnerable groups listed a group of skills needed to create such a support system, including:

1. Directing members' transactions to each other
2. Inviting members to build on each other's contributions
3. Reinforcing mutual support and assistance norms
4. Examining group sanctions
5. Encouraging collective action and activities
6. Clarifying members tasks and role responsibilities
7. Structuring collective decision making

Steinberg (2002) identified mutual aid as "the *raison d'être* of social work with groups" (p. 35). "It seeks to establish a relationship not only between the worker and group members but among members as well in the name of creating limitless sources of help" (p. 37). Basic group work skills that facilitate group interaction—including the leader hearing and encouraging the member-to-member dialogue, supporting group members with encouragement and reinforcement, empathizing and giving feedback—promote the development of a mutually beneficial support system (Chen & Rybak, 2004; Corey, 2004; Kurland & Malekoff, 2002). As students learn that the classroom is also run along this model, they gain familiarity and comfort in the process they take to weekly groups in the retirement community. Delineating this parallel process and these skills very specifically allows the forming process to proceed, as students clearly define their purpose in being together.

It is understood that most students begin group work with many fears (Corey, 2004; Kurland & Salmon, 1998). These include a fear of harm (being harmed by the group, or harming the members), a fear of not knowing what to do, fears about intimacy, and fears about differences between themselves and group members. Initial anxieties are expressed in questions such as, "What will I say to the group members? What if I insult someone? What if someone starts to cry?

What if no one talks? What do the participants really expect of me?"

An additional factor for students to consider is that they are most often placed as coleaders in a group, and so they need to develop a relationship with another student to allow them to work with their client groups. Corey (2004) discussed major advantages and disadvantages of coleadership of groups; particularly relevant are the benefits from the experience and insights of two therapists, and the ability to provide a group combined strengths of a team approach. The most challenging issue for coleadership is for the two leaders to develop a successful working relationship where they can work cooperatively. This issue is dealt with in classroom sessions as well to help students feel some level of comfort with their new leader.

The older members are struggling with the same issues, although they voice their concerns in their own context: "What do I have in common with these people? What if nobody likes me? What if they make fun of my problems? What if I start to cry?" When the students come to this realization, it is enormously relieving to them and is the beginning of the transformation from the preaffiliation stage to the power and control stage. They recognize their own commonality, their own purpose, and the tasks that they will need to deal with together. This recognition also helps them understand what they need to do in the initial stages of group development in the community—namely, to assist the residents to find their own commonality, purpose, and tasks. At every step, the processes occurring in the classroom are examined for their relevance for the community. For example, if the students participate in a programmatic exercise, after it is finished there will be a discussion about how the exercise could be adapted for use by their groups.

Another aspect of the preaffiliation stage has to do with knowing the parameters of the kind of group experience that the leader is providing. Support groups differ from "therapy" groups, and it is important to honor the contract that is set up between members and leader. Rice (2004) cautions workers who are dealing with older populations to avoid delving into problems that elicit stronger emotions than the group is prepared to deal with. On the other hand, the concept of "support" means that members are entitled to nag and complain, and the worker needs to listen, without allowing himself/herself to feel burdened with an unreal responsibility for "doing something" about every grievance that is aired. This balancing between too much and too little relates to accurately assessing how frail members are, and not treating them as frailer than they really are!

Power and Control

One of the factors that makes a support/discussion group different from "normal" social intercourse is that the rules about what is socially appropriate vary. In "real life," if someone says to an older person, "How are you feeling?" they know that the correct answer is "Fine," regardless of the truth. Unless a friend is talking to you on an intimate basis, sharing honest feelings (especially when they are painful or negative) quickly drives away the casual acquaintance. In a group setting, members need to learn that the rules are different, that honesty is appreciated and necessary for intimacy to grow. Honesty leads to conflict, and most people are uncomfortable with conflict. Members need to have the experience of seeing a conflict emerge, be openly dealt with, and resolved rather than denied or avoided. Because many people (students too) have their own issues with conflict, the power and control stage of groups becomes crucial in furthering group development.

In a retirement community, people are anxious to be and to have "good neighbors." They are often reluctant to cross the boundary from acquaintance to friend because of the risk involved that if the friendship does not work out, the "neighborhood" will be strained. As people

become frailer, and more dependent on the good will of neighbors, the risk becomes more unacceptable. As a consequence, residents enter the groups with trepidation related to arguing or fighting, and will try to smooth over any conflicts that occur. Leaders need to become comfortable with their own feelings about conflict, to encourage group members to do the same.

It is useful to teach students a model of nonviolent direct communication, which they then often teach the members of their groups. The model (Lieber, Lantieri, & Roderick, 1998) can be varied and involves seven specific components of directly expressing one's feelings in a way that lets the other person (or people) hear the concern, rather than being threatened by the disagreement. The steps include:

1. I feel (describe your feelings, using words that refer to feelings)
2. When (describe the specific behavior of concern)
3. Because (specify how the offensive behavior affects you)
4. I would prefer (describe what you want)
5. Because (describe how you would feel— be sure to use words that refer to feelings)
6. Then (identify the consequences for the other person "changing")
7. What do you think? (ask for the other person's reaction)

In the classroom, students have the opportunity to practice this new way of communicating. Optimally, this process is facilitated by attempting to create an open, accepting environment where students can feel free to make mistakes and to learn, and to disagree with each other and the instructor when issues come up that make them uncomfortable. For example, the major assignment in the course is a weekly journal, which is kept by each student, which is a description of what they do with their groups, the process that they observe, and their own feelings. Students quickly learn that this is an enormous amount of work and is often emotionally painful. When the assignment is discussed in class, it is really important for the instructor to allow criticism of the assignment, to hear students' concerns, and to be clear about his/her own purposes for changing or not changing in response to student pressures. When done successfully, this is clear role modeling for the student in how to behave with the group when your leadership is questioned. The distinction between being questioned and being threatened is an important one and has to do with the confidence of the leader in his/her strengths. For beginning students or social workers, this is complicated by the fact that they often do not feel much confidence in their roles, and yet they need to act as if they do in order to deal with conflict effectively. Anderson (1997) described this as the central issue of autonomy where the power of people within the group begins to be shared more equally by the leader and the members, and posits that it is necessary for further group development to occur. Gitterman (2002) described the initial stages of groups being focused in the worker's (leader's) authority. This testing process is a normal process and essential so the group can move on with its work and develop a deeper sense of trust.

It is important to be aware that norms of groups are often implicit, rather than explicit. For example, it would be rare that a group leader would tell everyone where to sit, but after a few weeks patterns emerge. If one person is consistently isolated, or conversely, placed at the head of the table, then it might be important to point out the norms that have been developed so that the group can discuss it—and decide if those norms are helping or hindering the development of the group. For example, if a person who is hard-of-hearing is consistently sitting with their "worse ear" toward the group, they lower their chances of fitting into the group.

Intimacy and Differentiation

When a group's members have come to some understanding of who they are, and how they will work, their focus moves to the tasks that they have set for themselves. In a retirement community setting, the members are often struggling with creating adaptive responses to life changes. One perspective of role theory says that alterations must be made in the "preferences, values, role norms, and behaviors that comprise one's social identity." Since for older people life transitions often involve limitations that challenge their old identity, and threaten their sense of well-being, roles need to be modified to be comfortable. Through focusing on life review, discussing similarities in shared experiences and problem solving, members of the group become more competent in dealing with the multiple losses and changes that accompany old age.

The differentiation or performing stage of group development has been characterized as the "work phase" (Shulman, 1999). A number of specific worker skills are delineated that are necessary for the completion of the tasks that the group sets itself. Some of these elaborating skills, which encourage intermember communications include:

1. The skill of containment, in which the worker refrains from jumping in too quickly as members speak
2. The skill of focused listening, which involves listening while keeping in mind the purpose of the group and the here-and-now mood of the group
3. The skill of questioning, in which the member is assisted in his elaboration of the problem, situation, or conflict under discussion
4. The skill of exploring silences, which helps the members understand the nature of silence—whether it is thoughtful, resistant, or helpless.

5. The skill of reaching from the general to the specific, which involves helping members to focus on details so that the result of the group discussion and interaction can be helpful to the group as a whole, as well as each individual member of the group.

All of these skills allow the group to grow together, while giving each other mutual aid, in their support/discussion group format.

Yet another issue that is important for students to explore deals with self-disclosure; how much is the right amount and how much is too much. When used appropriately, the facilitator can be a model for group members and can demonstrate how to disclose and what he or she is willing to risk (Jacobs, Masson, & Harvill, 2002). The dilemmas of when and how to self-disclose include looking at the degree to which the facilitator is also a member of the group and balancing one's own needs against the needs of group members (Maram & Rice, 2002).

Separation

Termination is often the phase of group development that is dealt with least effectively, because it arouses so many issues for group members and group leaders. Many authors (Chen & Rybak, 2004; Corey, 2004; Kottler, 2001) identify the critical skills involved with the termination or ending phase of a group as being of major importance. Birnbaum and Cicchetti (2000) and Toseland and Rivas (2001) suggest that termination needs to begin in the first minutes of the first session—that members need to understand that they are working within some time frame, toward some ultimate purpose.

In the classroom, as the semester begins to draw to a close, students struggle with what they have and have not accomplished, what they will do in the future, and the inevitability of time passing regardless of the circumstances of the moment. They learn that for the retirement group members, they are struggling with the same issues: "Was it worth my time? Did the rewards outweigh the costs?" Just as some students decide that gerontology is not the field they want to pursue, some older residents decide they no longer want to attend a support/discussion group. It is important, as part of termination, to allow people to feel acceptance about their decisions, not to feel like a failure because they did not get what they originally expected to get from the experience. On the other hand, there is often genuine sadness as an experience that gave much joy is ending.

Students often struggle with not wanting to say goodbye. They make promises to continue visiting the members of their group that they will not be able to keep, because it is too difficult to deal with the pain of saying goodbye and dealing with their feelings of abandoning their older members. If they are helped to explore those feelings in class, they are then able to go to the group settings and help their residents explore similar feelings.

For the residents, who have the option of continuing with the group in the next academic year, the dilemma is a bit different—is it worth the trouble of getting emotionally involved with this person if we have to say goodbye? An honest and open confrontation of these issues allows all participants to have a sense of closure that is needed to retain the long-term benefits of the group process.

Most residents and students can relate to the example of thinking about a long-term relationship that ended abruptly—because of death, divorce, or physical lack of proximity—without having the chance to talk about what the relationship meant. What most people do is to downplay the importance of the whole relationship because it is easier than feeling that it wasn't worth enough to deal with the pain of separation. Compare that to a relationship where goodbyes were said and participants had the chance to think together about what worked and what did not work. The loss is still painful, but the memories are more complete and can include the positive ones as well as the hurtful ones. If we want participants to remember and benefit from their group experiences, they need to be able to discuss what it meant to them.

Students are asked to participate in termination exercises, which they usually then adapt for their groups. For example, in one class, each student was asked to write, on a separate index card, something they admired about each person in the class. Each person then received all of the index cards with his or her own name on it and had a tangible piece of evidence as to some of their strengths. One year, there was a student who was doing very poorly in the class, who had difficulty with his groups, and who alienated the other students. The authors felt some apprehension about this exercise, because there was concern about students "getting back" at this individual by being cruel in their statements. However, with clear directions that this exercise was not about what you "liked or didn't like"—but something that you could admire about each person, their unanimous (and separate) feedback was that they admired this student's persistence in the face of so much difficulty. Certainly the recognition that the field of gerontology was not appropriate for this particular student was made easier by knowing that it did not make the student "bad."

Another helpful piece of termination allows members to think, in a nonjudgmental way, about what they would do differently if they had to do it over again, giving people the tools to benefit from every experience they have. At every phase of the group process, members and leaders are encouraged to examine their own process to ensure that they are benefiting from it to the maximum degree possible.

Structural Issues—Students and Residents

One of the distinctive characteristics of this program is that all of the groups are open-ended. For many years of the program, there was a core group of "regulars" who had been with the program since its inception, and stated a preference for long-term commitment to the group. The reality is that the membership is constantly changing. Members get sick for months at a time, so that when they return the group has a different flavor and texture. Members bring visiting friends and relatives for one or two sessions, and juggle their participation in the group with physician appointments and family occasions.

There are both positive and negative consequences of this type of group (Chen & Rybak, 2004; Corey, 2004). Positive features include the added motivation and stimulation provided by members being at different points in the growing process. New members can directly see the benefits of attendance through the enthusiasm of old members. Older members reaffirm their commitment to the group as they take on leadership roles. Open-ended groups are also less threatening than closed groups, as members have the ability (and the right) to distance themselves when discussions get too "heavy." They do not, in practice, use that ability very often, because the group becomes so important to them—but knowing they *could* use it is both a freeing and empowering feeling. Additionally, issues of trust and confidentiality are more easily confronted and discussed, because the group more closely emulates real life, which has arrivals and departures.

There are negative aspects as well, including the problem of repetition of stories (which is sometimes a problem with groups of older people in any circumstances), and a general slowing down of the process of group development because of the addition of new members. The group may have some difficulty maintaining cohesion if the membership fluctuates greatly throughout the semester period. Additionally, the leader must stay attuned to the need to orient newly joined members who have not gone through the initial stages of the groups' "growing pains."

The student-workers need to be aware of these factors and deal with them as they affect group process. Although this is one area where the student learning group optimally does not parallel the community group, in some instances there is at least one student who drops out. Additionally, since the structure of the program has changed to allow for a one-semester commitment, there often is a complete change of leadership at the midpoint of the year. Through an examination of how this affects the learning group, workers are helped to understand the dynamics of open- and closed-ended groups in a dynamic way.

Because the groups are self-selected, there is less control over size than is sometimes desired. For example, one of the groups in our program had 16–18 members attending each meeting, yet the group adamantly opposed a split into two groups. On the other end of the continuum, a group of only six regular members often flounders because of absences, and struggles to have a purposeful discussion with two or three members, and two leaders. Although the faculty liaison can influence the inclusion of new members into specific groups, using that influence needs to be balanced against the desire to keep the groups as empowered as possible. Since the group takes place in a community setting, members often know other members at least by sight or reputation and have clear preferences as to whom they want to get to know better, and whom they would choose to avoid.

Every group has certain "difficult clients." These people can be described as those whose behaviors in the group present problems that are difficult to manage; they are the clients to whom

you are not able to respond in a helpful or effective way (Corey, 2004; Kottler, 2001; Shulman, 1999). Examples of such types of people include monopolizers, the silent group member, the withdrawn member, the restless or agitated group member, and the unmotivated group member. It seems helpful to include this in a discussion of structural factors rather than of developmental factors because it underscores the inevitability of these occurrences. Consequently, the leader is less tempted to simply expel the problem member from the group. An understanding of why people act in certain ways, and knowing that they are often playing out concerns of the group as a whole, can facilitate the leader's intervening in a beneficial way.

For example, why does a monopolizer monopolize? A common assumption is that they want all of the attention; yet the underlying feeling of that person is often that they do not deserve any attention. A discussion that helps people look at their motives for behavior, especially behavior that attracts negative attention, allows every member of the group to learn, and it avoids alienating the person whose behavior provides that learning for each member.

Outcomes

The program has two major purposes: to train students to work with groups of older people, and to be a support group for people within a retirement community. How effective is this program? The first purpose is easier to assess, because students are used to being asked about effectiveness. Student evaluations of this course are consistently high—usually the most positive of all of the courses taught by these authors. Students feel that the time and energy have been worth it, because they have learned, because their choices have become clearer to them, and because they have gotten on-the-job training. The comment that "this is the most useful course I've taken in my whole college career" is fairly common, as we go through the process of termination in the classroom. Most students end this experience with much more certainty about their career choices—they are either sure that they will do group work with seniors, or they are sure they want to work in a different area. We feel that both of these attitudes demonstrate success, as the students now know, with a greater sense of reality, what career they are moving toward. A study of hundreds of students from different cultures by Eyetsemitan (2002) showed that in most individualistic cultures (such as the United States), young people are more willing to work with older people when they perceive older people to have "positive" personal traits (they are caring), "positive" interpersonal traits (they are helpful), and "positive" needs (they need companionship). In comparison, if their stereotypes of older people are negative in these three areas (they are crabby or stubborn, they are arrogant or bossy, and they are demanding), young people are less willing to work with them. The experience of getting to know older adults significantly and dramatically changes the students' idea of who older people are. Students have remained in contact with university faculty as they have become professionals in the field of aging, including directing senior centers and working in hospitals, nursing homes, and other retirement communities.

For seniors in the community, the results are more anecdotal, but are even more unanimously positive. One woman who has been in the group for five years is fond of going up to strangers and saying, "You know, my own son doesn't know me anymore because of this program. I used to be a mouse who never said anything because I had such a low opinion of myself, and now I know I'm a terrific person—that's what I've learned in this group." We have seen a woman deteriorate physically, and regress from walking, to a cane, to a walker, to a wheelchair—and yet she continues to attend group sessions. She attributes her ability to remain in an independent living situation primarily due to the support of the friends that she has made in her group. Perhaps independent living is not always the most desirable outcome—but this woman, in this situation, defines living independently as success. After a long-time member of the men's group died, his widow called and told me that the group had been the most important event of her husband's week for the five years before his death—and that she was grateful, as he had been, for its existence. The potluck dinners, held twice a year, give the residents a reason to care about food. While the potlucks have changed (as residents grow frailer) from home-cooked meals to store-bought, the preparation and presentation remains an important gift that these (primarily) women can give to each other. An interesting study of 63 women examined the meaning of communal meals (Fjellstroom, 2000), and suggested that for women who are living alone, these communal meals recreate meaning and nurture the establishment of friendship networks. These testimonials are what make the group a success. Numerous lives may not be changed dramatically, but individual lives are improved—by individual definitions of what is important. This seems, to us, to be the epitome of social support—to enable people to fulfill their own goals of achievement.

Summary

This chapter described a program within a program, one that allows students to learn about group work with older adults and simultaneously provides continuing supportive group work services to a portion of retired elderly people living in the community. It is important for leaders to understand the phases of group development and how different tasks are required of the leader in each phase. Modeling is demonstrated to be an important part of teaching leadership to students, and empowerment to members. The parallels between the classroom and the community group are described with attention paid to the differences as well. Hopefully, this material can give the impetus to further community programming of support groups.

Exercises

EXERCISE 1

Choose one of the following activities to try out in class or with an informal group of colleagues:

1. Take a package of fortune cookies. Have each participant read one and discuss how it applies to them and how accurate it is.
2. Have the group break into pairs, and in each dyad, find two ways you are alike and two ways you are different from each other. When the group reconvenes, have one spokesperson discuss their findings.

Both of these exercises can be used in the "forming" stage of groups, to help group members forge a common bond. After you have tried it out, choose one exercise and think of how you could adapt, or change the rules, to assist the group members in understanding the "storming" stage of group development.

EXERCISE 2

This exercise is a five-step process to nonviolent communication and consists of the following steps, to use to tell another person something that is upsetting you.

1. Describe the way you feel when something specific occurs that another person does.
2. Describe the consequences for you—what you do with those feelings.
3. Describe what you would prefer the other person to do—in clear, behavioral terms.
4. Describe the rewards (the new consequences) that would occur if the other person did change.
5. Ask for the other person's reaction.

For example: Older woman to adult daughter whom she sees too infrequently (according to her own perception): "When three weeks go by between visits from you, I feel lonely and abandoned. Then I start to feel that I haven't been a good mother, that you really don't care what happens to me. I would really like it if you could manage to visit at least once a week. If you did, I think when we did see each other, it would be more pleasant, because I wouldn't be so angry with you. What do you think about all that?"

Try out this process with another person. Notice your own feelings and your partner's responses. Discuss each of your reactions to conflict, and the differences between handling it nonviolently (as above), and in more confrontational ways.

EXERCISE 3

Think of a relationship in which you never had the opportunity to say goodbye—someone who died unexpectedly, a friend who moved away without your discussing your feelings with each other, a romantic relationship that went sour and was abruptly terminated by either of you. Write that person a letter in which you tell them the positive and negative feelings that you had about them, the best and worst thing that you took away from that relationship, and what you would do differently if you had to do it over again. Does this exercise change the perception you have of this old relationship? How?

References

Anderson, J. (1997). *Social work with groups: A process model.* New York: Longman Press.

Birnbaum, M., & Cicchetti, A. (2000). The power of purposeful sessional endings in each group encounter. *Social Work with Groups,* 23(3), 37–52.

Brandler, S., & Roman, C. (1999). *Group work: Skills and strategies for effective interventions.* New York: Hayworth Press.

Chen, M., & Rybak, C.J. (2004). *Group leadership skills: Interpersonal process in group counseling and therapy.* Belmont, CA: Brooks/Cole-Thompson Learning.

Corey, G. (2004). *Theory and practice of group counseling.* Belmont, CA: Brooks/Cole-Thompson Learning.

Corey, M. S., & Corey, G. (2002). *Groups: Process and practice.* Pacific Grove, CA: Brooks-Cole.

Eyetsemitan, F. (2002). Perceived elderly traits and young people's helping tendencies in the United States, Ireland, Nigeria and Brazil. *Journal of Cross-Cultural Gerontology,* 17(1), 57–69.

Fjellstroom, C. (2000). The meal as a gift—The meaning of cooking among retired women. *Journal of Applied Gerontology,* 19(4), 405–423.

Folts, W. E., & Muir, K. B. (2002). Housing for older adults: New lessons from the past. *Research on Aging,* 24(1), 10–18.

Galinsky, M., & Schopler, J. (1995). Social group work competence: Our strengths and challenges. In R. Kurland & R. Salmon (Eds.), *Group work practice in a troubled society—Problems and opportunities* (pp. 33–43). Binghamton, NY: Hayworth Social Work Press.

Gitterman, A. (2002). Reflections on dealing with group member's testing of my authority: In R. Kurland & A. Malekoff (Eds.), *Stories celebrating group work: It's not always easy to sit on your mouth* (pp. 185–192). Binghamton, NY: Hayworth Social Work Press.

Gitterman, A., & Shulman, L. (Eds.). (1994). *Mutual aid groups, vulnerable populations, and the life cycle.* New York: Columbia University Press.

Gladding, S. T. (1999). *Group work: A counseling specialty.* Edgewood Cliffs, NJ: Merritt.

Hepworth, D. H., Rooney, R. H., & Larson, J. A. (2002). *Direct social work practice: Theory and skills.* Pacific Grove, CA: Brooks/Cole.

Hooyman, N. R., & Kiyak, H. A. (1999). *Social gerontology: A multi-disciplinary perspective.* Needham, MA: Viacom.

Jacobs, E., Masson, R., & Harvill, R. (2002). *Group counseling strategies and skills.* Pacific Grove, CA: Wadsworth Group, Brooks/Cole.

Kelly, T. B., & Berman-Rossi, T. (1999). Advancing states of group development theory: The case of institutionalized older persons. *Social Work with Groups,* 22(2/3), 119–138.

Kottler, J. A. (2001). *Learning group leadership: An experiential approach.* Needham Heights, MA: Allyn and Bacon.

Kurland, R., & Malekoff, A. (2002). *Stories celebrating group work: It's not always easy to sit on your mouth.* Binghamton, NY: Hayworth Social Work Press.

Kurland, R., & Salmon, R. (1998). *Teaching a methods course in social work with groups.* Alexandria, VA: Council on Social Work Education.

Kurland, R., & Salmon, R. (1996). Making joyful noise: Presenting, promoting and portraying group work to and for the profession. In B. L. Stempler & M. Glass (Eds.), *Social group work today and tomorrow: Moving from theory to advanced training and practice* (pp. 22–31). Binghamton, NY: Hayworth Social Work Press.

Lieber, C. M., Lantieri, L., & Roderick, T. (1998). *Conflict resolution in the high school: Skills for classrooms: Skills for life.* Cambridge, MA: Educators for Social Responsibility.

Maram, M., & Rice, S. (2002). To share or not to share: Dilemmas of facilitators who share the problem of group members. *Groupwork,* 13(2), 6–33.

Rice, S. (2004). Group work with the elderly. In P. Ephross & G. Greif (Eds.), *Groupwork with populations at risk.* New York: Oxford University Press.

Shulman, L. (1999). *The skills of helping individuals, families, groups and communities, 4th ed.* Itasca, IL: F.E. Peacock.

Shulman, L. (2002). Learning to talk about taboo subjects: A lifelong professional challenge. In R. Kurland & A. Malekoff (Eds.), *Stories Celebrating Group Work: It's Not Always Easy to Sit on Your Mouth.* (pp. 139–156) Binghamton, NY: Hayworth Social Work Press.

Siebert, D. C., Mutran E. J., & Reitzes, D.C. (1999). Friendship and social support: The importance of role identity to aging adults. *Social Work,* 44(6), 522–534.

Steinberg, D. (2002). The magic of mutual aid. In R. Kurland & A. Malekoff (Eds.), *Stories celebrating group work: It's not always easy to sit on your mouth* (pp. 31–38). Binghamton, NY: Hayworth Social Work Press.

Theuma, C. (2001). Social group work: A journey of discovery. In T. B. Kelly, T. Berman-Rossi & S. Palombo (Eds.), *Group work: Strategies for strengthening resiliency* (pp. 203–214). Binghamton, NY: Hayworth Social Work Press.

Toseland, R.W. (1995). *Group work with the elderly and family caregivers.* New York: Springer.

Toseland, R. W., & Rivas, R. F. (2001). *An introduction to group work practice.* Boston: Allyn & Bacon.

Tuckman, B. W. (1965). Developmental sequence in small groups. *Psychological Bulletin,* 63, 384–399.

United States Bureau of the Census. (2001). *http://www.census.gov/population*

Wojciechowski, T. (2000). *Social support networks among older adult residents of a continuing care retirement community: An exploratory study.* Unpublished thesis, California State University, Long Beach, Department of Social Work.

Resources

Gitterman, A. (2001). Vulnerability, resilience, and social work with groups. In T. B. Kelly, T. Berman-Rossi, & S. Palombo (Eds.), *Group work: Strategies for strengthening resiliency* (pp. 19–33). Binghamton, NY: Hayworth Social Work Press.

Day Care Services

Barbara Haight

Jean Kittredge
Duchesneau

Key Words

- Adult day care
- Adult day health care
- Caregiver
- Community resources
- Inappropriate institutionalization
- Individual plan of care
- Social adult day care
- Support group
- Therapeutic activities

Learning Objectives

- Define *adult day care*
- Differentiate the two models of adult day care
- Identify five elements in an individual plan of care
- Give an example of how a participant's needs can be met through participation in a group experience
- Identify three ways a caregiver's needs are met in the group experience
- Describe two community resources that enhance day care center programs

Introduction

Adult day care centers offer a special place for the daytime care of adults who need professional supervision but who do not need 24-hour institutional care. Many adults are isolated or no longer have access to traditional family members. Centers offer fun, friendship, and acceptance to frail or disabled persons who might otherwise be isolated with their problems. For example, one such center, the Geriatric Adult Day Center in the Bronx, created a holistic family milieu that made people feel safe and at home when visiting there for a day. This center involved clients in their own care and facilitated healing and growth in mind, body, and spirit through the warmth and care engendered there (Sanfilipo & Forker, 2003). Good day care centers can create a safe environment where participants might improve or maintain physical and cognitive skills, receive a nutritious meal, and participate in group experiences. Good day care enhances the self-esteem of the participants and provides caregivers of the frail and disabled with a reliable resource and source of respite. This chapter is about the history of day care centers and the many types of groups that are conducted in them. The focus will be on those programs that primarily serve older adults as the woman portrayed in **Figure 22–1**.

History and Development of Adult Day Care

Day hospitalization programs for the mentally ill date from the 1920s in Europe (Padula, 1983). However, the development of adult day care for the aged had a slow beginning in the United States. The U.S. psychiatric community in the 1940s established programs, similar to those in Europe, for patients at well-known centers: the Menninger Clinic and the Yale Psychiatric Clinic. The day hospital program is still popular today in the mental health community. Dr. Lionel Cosin followed the psychiatric model in developing the first British geriatric day hospital in 1950. It was designed to reduce inpatient hospital stays and used a multidisciplinary approach. In the 1960s, adult day care was introduced to the United States

Figure 22-1 OLD FRIENDS

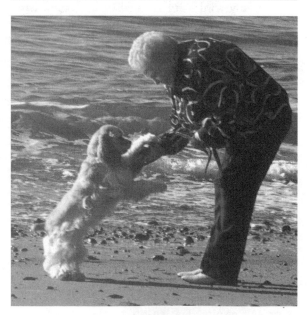

A new friend or an old friend remembered? Interaction with animals allows participants to express affection and share experiences they may have had with an animal of their own.
© Photos.com

when Dr. Cosin established a program based on his British model at Cherry State Hospital in Goldsboro, North Carolina (Padula, 1983).

The Medicare (Title XVIII) and Medicaid (Title XIX) programs of care for the aged and disabled, enacted in the early 1960s, focused on acute medical care. Nursing homes were the only form of insured long-term care, and reimbursement for their services was provided only in conjunction with hospitalization for an acute medical problem. In many cases, this led to inappropriate institutionalization of older people (Blum & Minkler, 1980). Inappropriate institutionalization also had a human cost. It was found that the quality of life for older adults who remained in the community and received care was better than for those who entered long-term care facilities. Pending legislation would allow those who receive homebound services to receive them in an adult day care center. The Medicare Adult Day Services Alternative Act of 2003 would give Medicare beneficiaries who qualify for home health benefits the right to receive them in the most appropriate setting (National Association of Day Services of America [NADSA], 2004).

By 1973, there were fewer than 15 adult day care programs in the United States. That same year, Congress amended Title XX of the Social Security Act and passed Title III of the Older Americans Act. These public policy changes were aimed at assisting older people to achieve or maintain autonomy and to prevent or reduce inappropriate institutionalization through provision of community and home-based care alternatives. A funding source was now available for such services as:

- Adult day care
- Case management
- Counseling
- Foster care
- Homemakers
- Information and referral
- Nutrition

- Recreation
- Transportation

In a 1974 policy change, the DHEW decided to encourage alternatives to institutionalization and agreed to make Medicaid funds available to states for adult day care centers. The number of adult day care programs has grown steadily. In 1978, 300 programs existed. The National Institute on Adult Day Care formed in 1979 renamed itself in 1995 to become the National Adult Day Services Association. By 1989, a national survey identified 1400 adult day centers in 49 states. And in 2000, there were an estimated 4000 adult day care programs throughout the USA (Senior Spectrum, 2001).

Although day care has grown immeasurably in the past 20 years, most U.S. counties do not have enough day care centers. Cox (2003), in an address to the American Society on Aging, said that more than 5000 new centers are needed to meet the nation's requirement in both rural and urban areas. Innovation is especially necessary to meet the rural need where the population is not large enough to support an ongoing day center and where there are not enough professionals to run a center.

Brewer, Stein, and Williams (1997) developed an innovative plan to organize "moving respite care" with only two part-time staff members. Churches in rural communities provided space and home health agencies provided necessary medical care. Two nurses, who started the program, carried the resources from one community to another and provided a half day of care and activities for people with dementia. An evaluation of the program showed it was effective in improving client function and in decreasing caregiver perception of burden.

Adult Day Care Models

As adult day care developed, arriving at a definition of what it does has posed problems for researchers, practitioners, and legislators. Early researchers in the field attempted to characterize programs by using models. These models typically categorized programs as social models or medical models. Social models provided daily socialization, entertainment, protection, shelter, and lunch, whereas medical models provided the aforementioned as well as supervisory nursing, medications, and other medical treatments, such as dressing changes. Regulatory and funding statutes also tried to approach definition by using models. Under Title XIX (Medicaid), participants must need active health care services (medical, nursing, or rehabilitative therapies) and then the cost of day care is reimbursed by Medicaid. Title XX (Social Security Act) and Title III (Older Americans Act) do not have this requirement and will partially reimburse social day care.

Professionals in the field struggle with the model approach. Most agree that programs are a blend of both the social and medical approaches, which allows programs to serve the diversity of needs presented by participants and respond to these needs creatively. These models remain today, but only the medical model is certain to receive reimbursement from Medicare (Bayer, 2004). Day care itself is a bargain. Generally the cost is $57 a day, a small percentage of what it would cost to be in a nursing home. Adult day care centers primarily serve the frail elderly and those with dementia. Medicaid pays for a little more than half of the nation's cost, families pay for 47%, and long-term-care insurance pays for only 1% (Cox, 2003).

Definition

In 1984, the National Institute on Adult Daycare (NIAD), a constituent unit of the National Council on the Aging, Inc., proposed the following definition as part of its national standards for providing adult day care:

> Adult day care is a community-based group program designed to meet the needs of functionally impaired adults through an individual

plan of care. It is a structured, comprehensive program that provides a variety of health, social, and related services in a protected setting during any part of a day, but less than 24-hour care. Individuals who participate in adult day care attend on a planned basis during specified hours. Adult day care assists its participants to remain in the community, thus enabling families and other caregivers to continue caring for an impaired member at home (NIAD, 1984, p. 20).

This definition distinguishes adult day care from other forms of care that may have components of adult day care and that may serve similar populations. It also allows adult day care to address adult populations that are not aged but could benefit from adult day care, such as those with degenerative neurological diseases, victims of head trauma, those with disease-related cognitive impairment, and the terminally ill. Adult day care leaders then created a member organization of adult day care, the National Adult Day Services Association (NADSA), an organization whose mission it is to enhance the success of its 558 members. This member organization also uses the above definition of day care (NADSA, 2003).

Part of a Continuum of Care

There are those who would argue that the more layers the care-delivery system has, the more fragmented the understanding of the various components becomes; services are duplicated and the cost of providing services increases. Others would argue that having a range of options from which to develop an individualistic support system is the preferred goal. Adult day care uniquely answers the complaints of the first argument and provides the benefits of the second.

Because adult day care programs offer a basic core of services, whether they lean toward the social or medical model, they are successful in providing the assessment, services, and support needed to meet their clients' needs. When the older adult and his or her family are faced with needing care and support for the older adult in order to remain at home rather than live in a nursing home, they become champions of the day care concept (Coleman, 1997). A major problem encountered by day care programs is educating the people they could and should serve about the value of their services and about the ability of adult day care to forestall the need for more intensive types of care. When it is time to use other components of the continuum of care, adult day care programs can offer appropriate referral, assurance, and support to their participants and their families as they make care-giving decisions. Day care provides both direct and indirect care to caregivers (Jegermalm, 2002). Adult day care also offers group interaction as shown in **Figure 22–1**.

Figure 22–2   GROUP INTERACTION

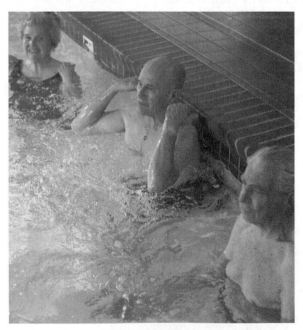

Group interaction builds a sense of community. Physical exercise is important in maintaining strength and mobility. Exercises can be adapted as needed, taking participants' limitations into account.

© Photodisc

The Adult Day Care Setting

Day care programs are developed by organizations endeavoring to meet the special needs of a specific group of people and their caregivers. They usually begin with limited resources for starting a program. Therefore, it is not uncommon to find adult day care programs in diverse settings such as community centers, churches, or other spaces that can be used on a shared basis with other organizations. In one community, the parish nursing association set up small day care units in their respective church basements with funding from the various churches and from grants. Very few programs, at least initially, have the resources for a setting that is specifically designed for the purpose of housing an adult day care program. Even a small day care program is expensive to begin.

Regardless of where the program is housed, the atmosphere of the setting should convey to the participants and their families both warmth and security such as the dining room setting in **Figure 22–3**. Change of any kind, particularly for those who are physically and/or mentally frail, is a barrier to participating in care alternatives. The more comfortable the participants and their families feel about the new environment and the staff who provide the care, the less uncomfortable they will feel about the change in routine. Some day support programs do not necessarily include professional support. Their main objective is to provide social interaction with peers and staff members for those who need it (Ross-Kerr, Warren, Schalm, Smith, & Godkin, 2003).

Ideally, there should be enough space to work in large or small groups. If therapy is provided, separate space should be available to house the required equipment and to meet any privacy needs of the participants. Particularly since privacy became a government-regulated concern through the Health Information Privacy and Portability Act (HIPPA, 2003). There should be a place where a client can go to be alone for a period of rest and quiet. Some people are just not joiners, even though they come to day care. These personality differences among older people need to be considered with allowances made for solitary activities (Dorrite, 2003). Outdoor space is desirable for activities as well as just being outdoors when the weather is pleasant.

Groups: An Integral Part of Program Structure

The essence of working with older adults in the adult day care setting is the group process. The adult day care staff needs a thorough understanding of how to use group techniques to create a therapeutic program that meets participants'

Figure 22–3 AT DINNERTIME

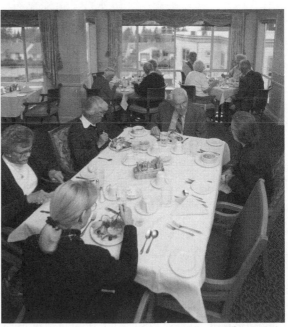

A nutritious meal offers the opportunity for social interaction and reinforces appropriate eating skills. The staff can help participants with physical impairments learn to use adaptive equipment.
© Photodisc

needs. Creating a group-work program for day care begins with meeting the needs of the participants through the individual assessment process. This assessment, performed by a trained professional staff person, should be documented with information about the participants' abilities in the following prioritized areas.

- Physical status, limitations, and goals
- Mental status, limitations, and goals
- Emotional status, limitations, and goals
- Functional status (activities of daily living and instrumental activities of daily living)
- Nutritional status and limitations
- Social history and support system
- Personal strengths and positive aspects of the individual's present life
- Current and past interests
- Participant's personal goals
- Family's or caregiver's expectations

From this assessment, an individualized plan of care can be established to meet each participant's goals and expectations. Because many participants may have similar needs, mutual goals can be accomplished by using the group process. One way to tie participant goals to group formation is to link needs to related activities (see **Table 22–1**).

Table 22–1 is only a beginning. It can be expanded by the needs of a particular center's current participants and the creativity of the staff. While each day may have certain program elements that are routine, such as exercise, other elements should vary to make the program meet the participants' individual needs and wishes. The activities offered need to reflect an adult theme. They need to be meaningful to the participants. Childlike activities have no place in an adult day care program unless children are present. Families and the public will receive the wrong impression of the program's value if they perceive that the activities do not have a therapeutic or recreational purpose for the participants. However, one exception might be the use of soft toys and dolls for people

with dementia as substitutes for attachment figures. The real concern is that older people should never be treated in childish ways nor regarded as children. Reenactment of past times activities and interests remembered from childhood may be appropriate in some circumstances (Knocker, 2002). An example of how groups are formed and the varied needs of participants met through one group activity are illustrated by the following:

> It was the Tuesday before Easter. Vases filled with bright yellow daffodils were on each of the tables in the kitchen area. Hands had been washed and aprons donned by the participants joining this morning's baking session. The staff had premeasured muffin ingredients and made the yeast bread dough, but there was still a lot to do. Mamie and Kay chatted back and forth as they mixed the muffins. While most of the men chose to read the morning newspaper, Clarence had joined the women, eager to make the bread-dough bunnies. Even Marilyn, usually restless and withdrawn, was sitting calmly with the group, watching the progress Mamie and Kay were making with their mixing. There was talk of Easter and Passover traditions and the spring weather that was making the flowers and trees bud out. Clarence decided that the bigger dough bunnies needed small companions and delicately formed the dough into smaller shapes. When the mailman brought the day's mail, he lingered a few moments longer than usual, remarking on the delightful aroma. Even those who had chosen not to be part of the group were enticed to join in when it was time to scrape the bowls.

From the example, it is evident that the baking group on this particular morning allowed the participants to work on many of their individual needs and also to share in a group experience. There were elements of sensory stimulation, physical exercise, emotional support, socialization, and creativity.

In theory, the use of the group process has measurable outcomes. When this technique is

Table 22–1   Participants' Needs and Related Activities

Participants' need	Related activity
Emotional expression	• Art therapy • Peer discussion • Reminiscence group • Singing • Writing
Health promotion	• Group work with therapist • Health education groups • Speakers and demonstrations
Intellectual stimulation	• Crossword puzzles • Current events • Discussion group • Logic/reasoning games • Memory games
Physical exercise (Large-motor movements)	• Armchair exercise • Balloon volleyball • Bowling (adapted) • Dancing • Walking
Physical exercise (Small-motor movements)	• Board and card games • Cooking and baking • Crafts • Setting the table
Sensory stimulation	• Dancing • Gardening • Music • Pet visitation • Sensory stimulation games • Singing
Social stimulation	• Discussion groups • Intergenerational activity • Parties and special events • Remotivation therapy

Source: Based on Webb, 1989.

applied to group work in the day care setting, the measurable outcome is how well the group work helps the individual client reach the goals established in his or her individual plan of care.

It is only fair to point out that in the adult day care setting, participants also should be allowed time to enjoy solo activities, to have quiet time, and to work one-on-one with staff. An example is the participant who expressed an aversion to dogs and cats. When the group was to have pet visitation from the Humane Society, she was allowed to exclude herself from participation in the group experience and even from the area. The staff supported her feelings without pressure or prejudice.

Another example is the gentleman who kept a journal. Each day after the noon meal, he was encouraged to write in his journal. On occasion he wanted to discuss the thoughts he was recording with a staff member. Accommodating individual preferences of a particular client is an important part of meeting the client's total needs.

The physical and mental ability of the participant mix may also determine how much supportive interaction is required from the staff. In forming a group where the participants function at a high physical and/or mental level, the members may be able to participate more in preparing the materials needed for a particular activity. In many adult day care programs, there is a wide range of ability. While each participant should be encouraged to exercise his or her highest degree of ability, having groups that have mixed ability levels works to everyone's advantage. Those who function well feel they are helping, and those less able stretch to do their best.

One of the benefits of working with older adults in the adult day care setting is seeing the renewal of an individual's self-esteem. Many individuals have had recent experiences with loss of ability that have placed their self-worth in jeopardy. When they are able to help others, to feel a sense of community, and to regain or maintain skills, they can go forward with life. Many clients in day care are experiencing dementia. Patients who are physically disabled but mentally alert do not always enjoy being placed with dementia patients. It is necessary to have several levels of programming to be able to serve all populations fully.

There are other factors that influence how group work is applied to the adult day care setting. The size of the population served and the number and capability of the staff determine how and which group techniques are applied. In small social model programs, it may be to everyone's benefit to work as a single group, moving through the day on a structured schedule.

Programs that serve a large number of clients or have a heavy emphasis on medical services may structure their schedules to allow groups to be formed to work on specific goals.

At Redwood Elderlink in Escondido, California, the adult day care program follows the social model structure and each day serves 15 to 20 participants over 60 years of age. It is a nonprofit program that grew out of a full-service retirement community's desire to serve seniors who lived in the community at large. On a given day, the staff may work with participants who have one or more of the following medical conditions:

- Arthritis
- Depression
- Hearing impairment
- Mild to moderate dementia (Alzheimer's type)
- Parkinson's disease
- Stroke
- Visual impairment

The program accommodates participants who are in wheelchairs and/or use walkers or canes. It accepts participants who can feed themselves and who do not require more than one person's assistance to transfer.

The center is open Monday through Friday and offers a full-day and half-day format to clients and their families. The noon meal is included in both formats as an important component of the program content. The activities surrounding the serving and eating of the meal are important in maintaining physical and social skills. The meal offers participants opportunities to learn to use adaptive equipment and engage in social communication, and it fosters a sense of community.

The day is structured so that participants have a variety of opportunities to work on their particular needs through the group process (see **Table 22–2**). Because this program currently serves a small number of people and has a limited staff, the participants work as a single group moving

Table 22–2   Structure of a Day in the Redwood Elderlink Program

Time/Who	Purpose	Activity choice	Equipment/Supplies	Leader
9 a.m./All	Social stimulation Intellectual stimulation Nutrition	Current event Group discussion Morning snack	Newspaper Day/date board Coffee and muffins	Center staff
10 a.m./All	Large-motor stimulation	Exercise Walk	Chairs Beanbag weights Ball and balloon	Exercise therapist
11 a.m./All or 2 groups	Memory stimulation Intellectual stimulation Fine-motor stimulation	Reminiscence group Cooking and baking	Library materials Ingredients and utensils	Center staff/ volunteer
11:45 a.m./All	Prepare for lunch	Toileting and hand wash		

Noon/All	Nutrition	Lunch	Hot meal delivered to
			  center from retirement
			  home
				Center staff

1 p.m. Rest period	Solo activities One-on-one	Quiet time Books and magazines	Background music Reclining chair	Center staff available

2 p.m./All
or 2 groups
	Large-motor
	  stimulation
	Fine-motor stimulation
	Intellectual stimulation
	Social stimulation
	Sensory stimulation
		Craft class
		
		Music/singing
		
		Bingo and bowling
		Pet visitation
			Craft materials
			
			Guest entertainers
			
			Appropriate equipment
				Center staff/
				  volunteer
				Community resource
				  person

3 p.m./All	Nutrition	Afternoon snack	Juice and cookies	Center staff/ volunteer
3:45 p.m./All	Individual reassurance	Prepare for leaving Toileting	Personal belongings	Center staff
4 p.m./All	Participant departure			

through the day on a structured schedule. Each month a calendar is prepared so that participants and their families know what activities are planned and when special entertainment and events are scheduled.

Even with careful preparation, a day may not run smoothly for a variety of reasons, and adjustments are necessary to handle the unforeseen. On one occasion, the weather changed from sunny to dark and blustery due to thunderstorms. The participants became anxious and concerned about how they were going to get home. It took an all-

out effort by the staff to keep them focused on the afternoon activity. The curtains were drawn and bowling was substituted for the scheduled activity so that there was a lot of physical involvement and noise of their own making to drown out the thunderclaps. By the time the participants were ready to leave, the storm was over.

Programs serving a small number of people become close knit. New clients need to be helped to integrate into the existing group. It is not uncommon to find one or two participants for whom the role of welcoming the new participant enhances their own goals.

Similarly, small groups more acutely feel the loss of someone who is no longer able to attend the program. It is important to allow the group members to express their feelings when a loss occurs. If the person has become ill or requires more care, the group may wish to send a card or show support for the family. The death of a participant is the hardest loss, and the staff may wish to have a spiritual counselor speak to the group.

The Unheralded Group: Caregivers

The individual participant is rarely the seeker of services provided by adult day care centers. It is the caregiver who, often reluctantly, seeks the adult day care program as a source of respite from the physical and emotional burden of providing care. Often, day care is a stepping-stone to institutionalization. But the respite obtained from the periodic day care allows caregivers peace of mind and the opportunity to replenish their own psychological resources while keeping their loved ones at home (Gaugler et al., 2003).

Most day care centers offer some form of support and counseling for the caregivers, usually in the form of a group meeting. On a regular basis the group meets with a professional facilitator who is knowledgeable about older adults. Some centers will schedule several such meetings to accommodate the time constraints of the caregivers. Adult children who work may find an early morning or brown-bag lunch meeting fits their work schedules better than an afternoon or evening meeting time. Similarly, spouses may find that it is more convenient to meet closer to the time they transport the participant to the center (see Chapter 18 on support groups).

Another consideration of caregiver group formation is the caregivers' emotional needs. Spouses, particularly men caring for women, may

have concerns different from those of adult children caring for parents. Since the purpose of group work with caregivers is to provide an appropriate setting for them to share experiences, gain insight, and find support for their roles, the makeup of these groups is particularly important (see **Table 22–3**).

The facilitator of meetings with caregivers needs to allow individuals to express their feelings and to seek solutions from members of the group. The facilitator also has to have a carpetbag of resources to answer specific, technical concerns that are frequently expressed. Professionals—psychologists, financial planners, and attorneys—may be needed to bring peace of mind to caregivers with special problems.

Support groups for caregivers are common and important groups for families using day care. The day care center serves as a convenient place to meet with caregivers. The day care staff cares for the person with dementia, and the support meeting can take place at the end of the day, when the caregiver picks up the person with dementia, or at

Table 22–3   CONCERNS EXPRESSED IN CAREGIVER SUPPORT GROUPS

Spouses
- Managing resources
- Loss of conjugal fellowship
- Assuming responsibility for personal care
- Lack of freedom
- Handling behavioral changes

Adult children
- Reversal of the parent-child role
- Juggling career and/or family schedules
- Invasion of privacy
- Guilt about not doing enough
- Financial burden

Other caregivers (relatives or friends)
- Unwanted responsibility
- Lack of proper authority
- Time commitment

the beginning of the day. Cummings (1996), who introduced a psychoeducational support model for care-giving spouses of early-stage Alzheimer's patients, created one example of a support group. However, the only evaluation of the program was by case examples, and case example evaluation is not enough to determine program effectiveness. Gallagher and Hagen (1997) actually evaluated a similar 10-week program and found that scores on patience, tolerance, and understanding increased significantly from pretest to posttest, thereby supporting the efficacy of a psychoeducational program. Another intervention group, a cognitive-behavioral support group for spouses that focused on problem solving and cognitive restructuring, was compared to an information-giving group. The two groups, cognitive-behavioral and information-giving, differed on only two measures, assertion and marital adjustment, but not on measures of psychological distress, leading the researchers to suggest the need to evaluate specific components of the group intervention to determine what does in fact help caregivers (Gendron, Poitras, Dastoor, & Perodeau, 1996). Other researchers concluded that support groups are not for everyone as they found little change in their research with support group interventions (Gage & Kinney, 1995).

Enhancing Programs with Community Resources

Adult day care programs can stretch their staff and financial resources to add program diversity by using community resources. In many communities, adult education programs and community colleges offer instruction on various topics if the adult day care center will agree to be a community classroom. The adult day care participants look forward to visiting instructors who present special activities, and the adult day care program receives exposure as a community resource.

Volunteers who are willing to support the program with their time and talents offer extra support to participants and staff. By using this type of support, staff can plan special activities such as an outing to a ball game or a picnic in a local park.

Youth organizations, such as Scout troops, are looking for experiences with older adults to complete the requirements of merit badges. In some cases, they are seeking an opportunity to talk with older people, but often the Scouts can prepare and present a special program.

As a rule of thumb, most adult day care programs strive to provide dignified experiences for clients at the lowest dollar cost. Through liaisons with groups that also have a desire to serve older adults and the community, all programs are winners.

Summary

Whether the group work in the adult day care setting is formal or informal, it must preserve the dignity and quality of life for everyone. By choice, no one would volunteer to be a participant in such a program, for we all value our independence and autonomy. Programs of adult day care strive to restore and maintain the frail older person at his or her highest level of functioning, in the least restrictive environment, for as long as possible. They also seek to support the caregiver with the physical and emotional burden of caring for a loved one.

Exercises

EXERCISE I

Mr. M. suffered a stroke six months ago, which left him partially paralyzed. He is mentally alert but has difficulty expressing himself. During his rehabilitation, he learned to dress, feed, and toilet himself and to walk with a quad cane. Since he has been at home, he demands that his wife attend to his needs and is losing much of his ability to care for himself.

Mr. M. has been enrolled in the adult day care program because his wife is feeling exhausted and overwhelmed by his behavior.

1. Identify three needs to include in Mr. M.'s plan of care.
2. Suggest three group activities that would help Mr. M. achieve his care goals.
3. Describe how you would support Mrs. M.'s situation.

EXERCISE 2

You are a program aide in an adult day care program. You have noticed that several of the participants have broken and rough fingernails. Your program director has given you permission to lead a nail grooming activity.

1. Briefly outline how you would organize this group activity.
2. Make a list of supplies you will need and their cost.
3. What other health promotion issues related to the hands can be discussed?
4. Name one community resource that might help you.

EXERCISE 3

Music is a favorite group activity among older adults. They love to listen to, sing with, and dance to melodies they remember from various periods in their lives. A volunteer is scheduled to play some oldies from the 1940s. You wish to expand and enhance her visit.

1. Research the popular composers of the 1940s and their best-loved songs.
2. What dance steps were popular in the 1940s?
3. Name two ways music helps achieve participant care goals.

References

Bayer, K. Adult day care: Vol. 2. LT Connections. Retrieved on May 16, 2004, from *http://www.hospicomm.com/adultdaycare.htm*

Blum, S. R., & Minkler, M. (1980). Toward a continuum of caring alternatives: Community based care for the elderly. *Journal of Social Issues, 36*(2), 133–152.

Brewer, B., Stein, M., & Williams, D. (1997, January). Roving rural respite care for the elderly. Presented to the 125th annual meeting of the American Public Health Association.

Coleman, P. (1997). The use of support groups in an adult day health center. *Journal of Gerontological Nursing, 23*(11), 41–3.

Cox, N. Most U.S. counties don't have enough adult day care centers. Today's Seniors Network.com. Retrieved May 16, 2003, from *http://www.todaysseniors network.com/need_for_day_care.htm*

Cummings, S. (1996). Spousal caregivers of early stage Alzheimer's patients: A psychoeducational support group model. *Journal of Gerontological Social Work, 26*(3), 483–498.

Dorrite, M. (2003). Quality of life in VA day treatment center male patients: Association with sociodemographic variables and relationships with hopelessness and depression. *Dissertation Abstracts International, 64,* (4-B).

Gage, M., & Kinney, J. (1995). They aren't for everyone: The impact of support group participation on caregiver's well-being. *Clinical Gerontologist, 16*(2) 21–34.

Gallagher, E., & Hagen, B. (1997). Outcome evaluation of a group education and support program for family caregivers. *Gerontology and Geriatrics Education, 17*(1), 33–50.

Gaugler, J., Jarrott, S., Zarit, S., Stephens, M., Townsend, A., & Greene, R. (2003). Respite for dementia caregivers: The effects of adult day service use on care giving hours and care demands. *International Psychogeriatrics, 15*(1), 37–58.

Gendron, C., Poitras, L., Dastoor, D., & Perodeau, G. (1996). Cognitive-behavioral group intervention for spousal caregivers: Findings and clinical considerations. *Clinical Gerontologist, 17*(1), 3–19.

Jegermalm, M. (2002). Direct and indirect support for careers: Patterns of support for informal caregivers to elderly people in Sweden. *Journal of Gerontological Social Work, 38*(4), 67–84.

Knocker, S. (2002). Play and metaphor in dementia care and dramatherapy. *Journal of Dementia Care, 7*(4), 33–37.

National Adult Day Services Association (NADSA). Medical adult day services alternative act of 2003 (Issue Brief). Retrieved on May, 16, 2004, from *http://www.nadsa.org/Issue%20Briefs/S2655.htm*

National Institute on Adult Daycare. (NCA). (1984). *Standards for adult day care.* Washington, DC: National Council on the Aging.

Padula, H. (1983). *Developing adult day care: An approach to maintaining independence for impaired older persons.* Washington, DC: NCA.

Ross-Kerr, J., Warren, S., Schalm, C., Smith, D., & Godkin, D. (2003). Adult day programs: Who needs them? *Journal of Gerontological Nursing, 29*(12), 11–17.

Sanfilippo, J., & Forker, J. (2003). Creating family: A holistic milieu at a geriatric adult day center. *Holistic Nursing Practice, 17*(1), 19–21.

Senior Spectrum. History of adult day services in the United States. Retrieved on May 16, 2001, from *http://www.seniorspectrum.com/Adb/history.htm*

U.S. Department of Health and Human Services. Health information and portability act. Retrieved in May, 2003, from *http://privacyruleandresearch.nih.gov/*

Webb, L. C. (1989). *Planning and managing adult day care: Pathways to success.* Owing Mills, MD: National Health.

BIBLIOGRAPHY

Abraham, I. L., Onega, L. L., Chalifoux, Z. L., Maes, M. J. (1994). Care environments for patients with Alzheimer's disease. *Nursing Clinics of North America, 29*(1), 157–172.

Adler, G., Kuskowski, M. A., & Mortimer, J. (1995). Respite use in dementia patients. *Clinical Gerontologist, 15*(30), 17–30.

Alzheimer's Association. (1996). *The respite care manual. Chicago, IL: Alzheimer's Association.* (Call No. WM 220 R434 1996.)

Alzheimer's Association. (1995). *Respite care guide: how to find what's right for you.* Chicago, IL: Alzheimer's Association. (Call No. WM 220 R4345 1995.)

Brunk, D. (1996). A rising star: Adult day services find a place in the constellation of services. *Contemporary Long Term Care, 19*(10), 34–46.

Burnside, I. M. (Ed.). (1980). *Psychosocial nursing care of the aged* (2nd ed. pp. 145–159). New York: McGraw-Hill.

Burnside, I. M. (Ed.). (1986). *Working with the elderly: Group process and techniques* (2nd ed.). Boston: Jones & Bartlett.

Cefalu, C.A., Ettinger, W. H., & Espeland, M. A. (1996). Study of the characteristics of the dementia patients and caregivers in dementia-nonspecific adult day care programs. *Journal of the American Geriatrics Society, 44*(6), 654–659.

Currie, A., McAllister-Williams, R. H., & Jacques, A. (1995). A comparison study of day hospital and day centre attenders. *Health Bulletin, 53*(6), 365–372.

Handy, J., & Bellome, J. (1996). Adult day services: The next frontier. *Caring, 15*(12), 24–33.

Henry, M. E., & Capitman, J. (1995). Finding satisfaction in adult day care: Analysis of a national demonstration of dementia care and respite services. *Journal of Applied Gerontology, 14*(3), 302–320.

Flint, A. J. (1995). Effects of respite care on patients with dementia and their caregivers. *International Psychogeriatrics, 7*(4), 505–517.

Gray, J. (1994). Creating an Alzheimer's group respite service. *Spectrum National Association for Senior Living Industries, 8*(4), 21–23.

Greenwood, A. (1996). An idea becomes reality. *Nursing Standard, 10*(29), 26–27.

Kosloski, K., & Montgomery, R. J. (1995). The impact of respite use on nursing home placement. *The Gerontologist, 35*(1), 67–74.

Maahs, S. E. (1995). Pioneering nurse-managed adult day care. *Nursing Spectrum, 5*(19), 8.

Noyes, L. (1996). Making a respite stay comfortable. *Provider, 22*(3), 85–86.

Reifler, B. V. (1995). What I want if I get Alzheimer's disease. *Archives of Family Medicine, 4*, 395–396.

Rudin, D. J. (1994). Caregiver attitude regarding utilization and usefulness of respite services for people with Alzheimer's disease. *Journal of Gerontological Social Work, 23*(1/2), 85–107.

Sayles-Cross, S., & DeLorme, J. (1995, May–June). Worried, worn out and angry: Providing relief for caregivers. *ABNF Journal, 6*(3), 74–77.

Shantz, M. (1995, Winter). Effects of respite care: A literature review. *Perspectives, 19*(4), 11–15.

Stephenson, C., Wilson, S., & Gladman, J. R. (1995). Patient and carer satisfaction in geriatric day hospitals. *Disability and Rehabilitation, 17*(5), 252–255.

Standards and Guidelines for Adult Day Care. (1992). Washington, DC: NCA, 11(3), 14–19.

Wagner, P. (1995, July). Colors of the spectrum: Medical adult day care nursing. *Nursing Spectrum, 5*(14), 16.

Warrington, J., Eagles, J., & Day, M. (1995, March). Care for the elderly mentally ill: Diurnal confusion? *Health Bulletin, 53*(2), 99–104.

Williams, B., & Roberts, F. (1995). Friends in passing: Social interaction at an adult day care center. *International. Journal of Aging & Human Development, 41*(1), 63–78.

Yee, D. L., & Capitman, J. A. (1995). Reaching financial viability in adult day care. *Journal of Long Term Home Health Care, 14*(3), 19–36.

Resources

- Illinois Geriatric Education Center (Producer), (1992). Designing diverse therapeutic environments and programs for persons with Alzheimer's and related dementias [Videocassette]. (No. WT 155 VC. No.236 1992 pt. 2. Available from Illinois Geriatric Education Center, Chicago, IL.)
- National Alzheimer's Association, Annotated Bibliography on Adult Day Programs and Dementia Care. This publication is designed to serve as a reference guide to day center staff, caregivers, and experts in the field of aging. There are two main sections: Section I—Adult Day Programs, Section II—Dementia Care. The bibliography is indexed by subject matter. To order, send $7.95 plus $2.00 for shipping and handling to: National Alzheimer's Association, Attn: Inquiries Processing, 919 N. Michigan Avenue, Suite 1000, Order No. PF 1052, Chicago, IL 60611; phone: 800-272-3900. Also available from NCA, Attn: Rose Russell, Department of Administrative Services, 409 Third Street, Second Floor, Washington, DC 20024; phone: 202-479-6957.
- Newton, G. (2002). Marketing adult day services to business and working caregivers. Winston-Salem, NC.
- Newton, G., & Henry, R. S. (1994). Referral source marketing for adult day programs. Winston-Salem, NC: Bowman Gray School of Medicine of Wake Forest University.
- Norman, J.L., & Horton, E. R. (1996). Adult day care therapeutic activity manual: A continuous quality improvemnt approach. Gaithersburg, MD: Aspen.

Video

- Bowman Gray School of Medicine of Wake Forest University (Producer). (1996). The adult day center entrepreneur: making money for your mission with money-making ventures [1 videocassette, 1 audiotape, and manual]. Winston-Salem, NC.
- Bowman Gray School of Medicine of Wake Forest University, Dementia Care and Respite Services Program (Producer). (1992). Adult day program marketing series [5 videocassettes]. (Call no.: WT 29 VC no. 205 1992). Winston-Salem, NC: c1992.
- Bowman Gray School of Medicine of Wake Forest University (Producer). (1996). Continuous quality improvement! Total quality adult day services! [1 videocassette, 1 audiocassette, and manual]. Winston-Salem, NC.

Chapter 23

Groups in Board-and-Care Homes: Multidisciplinary Approaches

Janet E. Black
Sally A. Friedlob
James J. Kelly

Key Words

- Confidentiality
- Life skills
- Relationships
- Developmental processes/tasks
- Scanning
- Multidisciplinary team

Learning Objectives

- Describe a comprehensive model program for treating older adults at a board-and-care facility.
- Explain the individual professional roles and their relationship to standard roles in a multidisciplinary team approach to treating aged clients in a care home.
- Explain the advantages and disadvantages of a large group in a board-and-care home.
- List five relevant activities that facilitate the developmental tasks of aging and decrease social isolation; also list the rationale for their use.
- Explain the advantages of the community-based model of treatment described in this chapter, and how it provides a continuum of care for clients.

Residents of Board-and-Care Homes

Providing group work services to older adults residing in a board-and-care environment presents a variety of challenges, including careful selection of the type of group work intervention(s) that will most benefit the clients, the group work model, and the delivery of the program itself. Board-and-care homes (also referred to as residential care facilities) are one of several types of community-based, long-term care facilities that provide services to older adults. They provide "more extensive services and protective oversight than other residential settings, such as congregate apartments, but a lower level of services than is offered by nursing homes" (Regulatory measures, 1995, vol. 7).

As is true in other sectors of the aging population, the average resident living in the board-and-care setting is likely to be "older and more disabled than was true a decade ago" (Regulatory measures). Board-and-care homes frequently include a mixed population of physically frail elderly people, cognitively impaired elderly people, and persons with mental health problems. When planning programs for delivery in board-and-care homes, attention needs to be given to the characteristics of the residents themselves, both physical and psychological, to provide a framework for the development of a program of services. Group leaders need a thorough understanding of the developmental processes and maturational stages that individuals experience during their lifetime.

The literature about older adults describes a variety of theories about aging and the various life cycle issues and developmental tasks that are associated with the aging process. While there is some agreement about the various tasks and life cycle issues, it is important to remember that all older adults do not age in the same manner or at the same rate. There are individualized levels and degrees of maturation, development, and life cycle experiences which are influenced by both internal and external factors (Foos, 2003; Moody, 1998). Notably, for each individual, cultural factors must be considered because such factors shape not only clients' expectations and reactions to aging, but also all significant others, including health professionals, with whom the older adult interacts.

In the same way, multiple perspectives must be considered in any discussion of the aging process and age-related deficits. Physical changes may include declining endurance, loss of strength and muscular coordination, increased susceptibility to illness and injury, visual changes, and auditory impairments (see Chapter 12). While the majority of older adults retain their mental functioning, the speed at which information is processed is often slower, and diminution of recent recall is common. Older adults may experience difficulty in integrating sensory input and output, and at times display confusion. According to the first Surgeon General's Report on Mental Health (U.S. Department of Health and Human Services, 1999), almost 20% of people over the age of 55 experience mental disorders that are not part of "normal aging." "The most prevalent mental disorders among older adults include anxiety disorders, which affect an estimated 11.4% of people over age 55. Severe cognitive impairment affects 6.6% of the population over age 65" (Promoting Older Adult Mental Health, 2002, p. 5). Approximately 4.4% of people in this age group are affected by mood disorders, including major depression and other forms of depression (Promoting Older Adult Mental Health). Physiological and psychological changes are interwoven. An older adult who presents with a mental disorder in fact may be undergoing physical changes, such as an auditory impairment, a reaction to a medication, or a reaction to the social environment, such as social isolation or boredom.

Furthermore, maturity for every individual depends on previous sequential developmental phenomena (Erikson, 1950), because during each period of human development there are unique presenting issues and opportunities. Individuals move through a process of adaptation to these issues and opportunities at differing rates, and learn and grow in the process (Erikson, 1950; Moody, 1998). Moody describes old age as a "time when we are likely to come face to face with questions about ultimate meaning" (p. 71). The tasks of defining that meaning and the resulting satisfaction with one's life are critical issues for all older adults.

When stress interrupts development, however, individuals may adapt by regressing or stagnating. For example, for an individual who has lived independently for the majority of his or her life, a move to a board-and-care facility is a highly stressful life event. To cope with the loss of autonomy, self-direction, status, and material possessions, an individual may adapt by blending into the surroundings, thereby inhibiting growth and/or failing to maintain his or her current level of functioning. Conclusively, when working with individuals in a board-and-care setting, one needs a thorough understanding of the developmental processes and related phenomena. Health care professionals can then assist clients in adaptation that encourages growth by providing experiences that foster more successful coping skills and facilitate development tasks. Additionally, professionals can assess the overall physical and mental status of clients in order to coordinate appropriate interventions in a timely manner.

In his classic work, Peck (1968) identified three tasks for aged people, which remain viable for the board-and-care population who are left on the sidelines. These tasks center on the ego in terms of: differentiation rather than work-role preoccupation, body transcendence rather than body preoccupation, and ego transcendence rather than ego preoccupation. Foos and Clark (2003) emphasized the importance of the "person-in-environment-congruence" for individuals, which includes: (1) social congruence with comfort and adaptation levels in social relationships; (2) psychological congruence including a sense of continuity and sense of self-image; and (3) physical congruence, in which the environment needs to allow individuals to maintain some roles and complete everyday tasks. These issues are critically important to the program development for individuals residing in board-and-care homes, as these needs dictate programmatic themes and substance.

The debate over the homogeneity or heterogeneity of persons in board-and-care homes led to a major shift in such facilities' demographics. Previously, young patients with psychosocial disabilities were admitted along with seniors. The current placement practice includes individuals undergoing the normal aging processes and three categories of seniors with an additional variety of special problems. The first of these three categories is clients carrying a diagnosis of persistent schizophrenia who have been confined in hospitals for a major part of their lives. These individuals have coped with stress by regressing to earlier developmental stages. They have deficits in their social and emotional development, cognitive functioning, and perceptual motor development.

They are typically withdrawn, shy, and egocentric, and they have poor posture and poor fine coordination. They have difficulty learning new tasks by trial and error, abstracting a sequence of ideas, and visualizing covert imagery. Long after the schizophrenic symptoms have been in remission, they have retained regressed behaviors acquired during their years of institutionalization.

Individuals with other psychosocial disorders in remission are a second type of client. These clients cannot manage in an independent setting and need the support and structure a board-and-care home offers. They, too, have social and emotional deficits, and often lowered cognitive functioning is involved. Typically, they have difficulty in forming interpersonal relationships and demonstrate poor problem-solving abilities.

Individuals with neurological and medical conditions constitute a third category of client. These clients are found less frequently because board-and-care settings require independence in ambulation, continence, and self-care. Because those with neurological conditions must meet these requirements, the neurological involvement is minimal. Generally, the neurological condition involves upper motor neurons. There may be a lesion located in the brain that was caused by a cerebrovascular accident (stroke) or head injury; or there may be lesions located in the extrapyramidal system that are caused by Parkinson's disease. In either case, deficits in perception, problem solving, personality, behavior, proprioception, sensation, stereognosis, hearing, sight, coordination, and voluntary or involuntary motion may be present.

While age is the common denominator, the board-and-care population confirms the findings presented in the literature which assert that the maturational process is individual. Despite the individual problems and deficits, aging is the one homogeneous factor shared by all board-and-care clients, and thus they are all dealing with similar life stage issues. After carefully considering all the forgoing issues of clients residing in board-and-care facilities, we are impressed by the need for interventions that facilitate growth and adaptation. We believe group treatment is particularly beneficial in view of the 11 pervasive therapeutic factors which Yalom (1995) in his cornerstone book on group psychotherapy identifies and discusses in depth. These are: instillation of hope, universality, imparting information, altruism, the corrective recapitulation of the primary family group, development of socializing techniques, imitative behavior, interpersonal learning, group cohesiveness, catharsis, and existential factors. By reason of our combined years of clinical experience, we assert that these curative factors are present not only in traditional group psychotherapy, but also in a range of groups led by practicioners of the various fields of human services, such as occupational therapy, movement therapy, music therapy, and art therapy, which are psychotherapeutic, therapeutic, and task oriented. (See also Chapter 16.)

The ability to assimilate life markers encountered in old age and to put them into a meaningful context, given the entirety of one's life, contributes to successfully carrying out the developmental tasks of aging and successful adaptation in aging. Significantly, a major cognitive characteristic of the geriatric life stage is the ability to retrieve past memories with clarity and detail. Herein lies an important asset that can be the foundation for building structure and function in successful adaptation. While the focus of this chapter is not reminiscence, as a group intervention it is important to state that the phenomenon of reminiscence is an essential element in the continuing development of the older adult (see Chapters 14 and 15). Reminiscence is instrumental to growth in social and emotional development (Birren & Schaie, 2001; Corey & Corey, 2002). The ability to retrieve and share past memories can be utilized as an effective means of

intervention in board-and-care homes because it is the one element that cuts across all special problems of individuals in these homes (Butler, Lewis, & Sunderland, 1998).

Regardless of their impairment, all individuals respond to familiar activities that draw upon previously learned tasks and experiences. Familiar activities employ well-known motor schemes and facilitate abstract imagery and conception of end results. Activities utilizing established learning skills increase self-confidence and self-esteem. Therefore, they promote pleasurable experiences that encourage trust. A major benefit of employing a range of group interventions for all clients is the marked opportunity to bring about an environment that facilitates the tasks of aging which have been impacted by the institutional board-and-care environment. Strategic group interventions have an impact on the naturally occurring process of life review, important for putting into perspective one's successes as well as one's unresolved conflicts during the later stages of life (Corey & Corey, 2002; McInnis-Dittrich, 2002; Molinari, 1994). Movement, visualization, cooking, art, music, task planning, and activities of daily living, for example, provide opportunities not only for life review but also for growth and adaptation in all areas of human development—physical, sensory, perceptual, cognitive, social, and emotional. These phenomena, according to Willard and Spackman (Crepeau, Cohn, & Schell, 2003), are intricately interwoven, and issues, stresses, or gains that take place in one area often bring changes in another.

The Advantage of the Multidisciplinary Team

Many professional groups have practiced multidisciplinary teamwork and collaboration for many years, but only recently has the concept received attention in the professional literature. Berg-Werer and Schneider (1998) define interdisciplinary collaboration as "an interpersonal process through which members of different disciplines contribute to a common product or goal" (p. 698). Bronstein (2003) identifies five core components of interdisciplinary collaboration: interdependence, newly created professional activities, flexibility, collective ownership of goals, and reflection on process. The multidisciplinary team approach to planning and implementing a rehabilitation program has a distinct advantage in the board-and-care setting. During a two- to four-hour session, a team can employ a variety of activities and specific practice applications so that growth in one area influences growth in another area. Furthermore, a variety of modalities facilitates the clients' motivation, attention span, and tolerance for sitting and for group interaction. In our experience, the use of a multidisciplinary team approach to group activities in a board-and-care home might include a social worker, occupational therapist, movement therapist, art therapist, and various skill building activities in one or multiple group sessions.

Each team member can provide experience in his or her area of expertise. Ideally, the team members complement each other so that the blending of resources facilitates effective, methodical treatment planning. The movement therapist, for example, can initiate the session by providing a group experience that stimulates pleasure centers in the body. This pleasure stimulation is critical because clients who have been sedentary and have had little sensory stimulation often fail to experience pleasurable body sensations, a lack that decreases risk-taking behaviors in perception, cognition, and socioemotional growth. Thus, movement facilitates experiences that increase trust, decrease anxiety, and encourage growth in integrating sensory and motor abilities. The occupational therapist can then introduce an activity that requires increased attention span, orientation, concentration, and tolerance to sitting. The occupational therapist also can promote maintenance of cognition stim-

ulated during movement and can facilitate an increase in functional levels by utilizing familiar, simple, problem-solving tasks, that can be readily recalled and mastered. The social worker and the nurse can expand on the treatment process by assisting clients in integrating their group experience through verbalization.

A major advantage to a multidisciplinary team approach is that a large number of clients can be treated in a group setting. Although the current literature emphasizes small-group treatment, a large group can be treated effectively with a team approach. Such an approach can ensure the inclusion of all clients in each session which is vital in working with this type of client. Thus, team members can serve as cotherapists who provide mutual support and assistance in facilitating and processing a session. An additional advantage to utilizing a multidisciplinary team approach is that each team member can provide training for students in his or her respective field, and the participation of students provides several advantages. They bring enthusiasm, youth, and stimulation to board-and-care clients. They offer an opportunity to encourage clients to impart advice drawn from past experiences and assist in student training, which closes the generation gap and promotes mutual growth, especially in self-confidence and self-esteem. By sharing knowledge and wisdom with the younger generation, clients experience a sense of what some have called "generativity"— "one cares for what one has generated in this existence; each stage of life, once given, is woven into the fates of all" (Moody, 1998, p. 451). This is important for clients who are cast in a dependency role and can experience the reversal of that role in sharing with others.

Furthermore, during group activities students can be paired with clients requiring individual attention outside of the group process. Thus, in a large group, one-on-one treatment can be provided. Another benefit in utilizing students is that students learn early in their training about resources offered by other disciplines, as well as about ways to work with other disciplines to provide more effective client treatment. (See Chapters 6, 26, 27, 28, 29, and 30, which elaborate on teaching students.) Still another advantage of the team approach is that other services can be provided during group activities. For example, as previously discussed, medical as well as psychosocial needs are important to address; doctors and nurses can assess patients individually for such concerns during a session. Medical students can also be included in the group process, along with social work and occupational therapy students. In addition, young doctors must be oriented early in their training to be sensitive to these clients' total needs. This training still is often not included in the medical model nor in the nursing model.

Volunteers can be another effective resource for the team. They can include individuals who would benefit equally from group process to meet their emotional and social needs. For example, community members such as senior citizens or young psychiatric clients who have been isolated can be extremely helpful. In addition to being sensitive and empathetic to clients, these individuals can meet their own needs to be altruistic and to give and receive nurturance. Because volunteers need guidance and structure, however, the team must take care to plan for sufficient volunteer guidance. (See Chapter 10 about collaborating with volunteers.)

Development of Interpersonal Relationships

To initiate a program at a board-and-care facility utilizing a multidisciplinary team approach, three essential interpersonal relationships must be carefully developed. These are the relationships among members of the multidisciplinary team itself, between team members and the board-and-care personnel, and between team members and the clients.

Relationships within the Multidisciplinary Team

Working with older adults can be an extremely rewarding experience, but can also be very draining and discouraging at times. Unique characteristics of older people that particularly impact group work with this population include physical and sensory limitations, variable attention spans, interference from external factors (i.e., medication side effects, scheduling conflicts with other medical or psychological needs of the client), and the need for a slower and more deliberate pace in the group process (Corey & Corey, 2002; McInnis-Dittrich, 2002; Toseland, 1995; Toseland & Rivas, 2001). Corey and Corey (2002) sum up group work with older adults to be more directive, less confrontive, more supportive, and more an ongoing function of teaching members ways of expressing themselves and listening to others. Coleadership in group activities and the use of a multidisciplinary team to provide the group experiences are, in our experience, realistic and very satisfying solutions. Coleadership also seems most appropriate in these settings as it efficiently reaches large numbers of individuals and can effectively provide services that meet psychosocial needs as well as deal with developmental and age-related tasks and issues. Issues in coleadership of a group have been given a great deal of attention in group work literature and are discussed further in Chapter 9.

Multidisciplinary team members (staff) must be experienced professionals with a strong background in group leadership and cotherapy. Coleaders need to communicate on multiple levels. Concurrent with dual communications and client group processing, they must guide and supervise students, volunteers, and board-and-care personnel. The demands of the position include sharp attention to detail, including constant scanning of each individual; sensitivity to the environment at all times; and continual dynamic processing of the various interactions. Judgments about setting up interactions, intervening, facilitating, and integrating material as it develops are minute-by-minute processes. These qualifications are absolutely necessary if leaders are to undertake, without disaster, a large group of 20 to 30 clients in a board-and-care facility.

Team members need to be flexible, open to new ideas, and willing to explore their own feelings and defenses. Although each person contributes knowledge unique to his or her profession, each must be open to sharing responsibilities. Often, skills overlap professional boundaries. Territoriality can be destructive to group cohesion. It can have a negative impact on clients, who are generally sensitive to staff process issues, by producing anxiety and conflicting attitudes toward supportive figures. On the other hand, conflicts cannot be overlooked; denial does not preclude conflict, and feelings will emerge covertly or overtly. Either way, denial is deleterious to the prime work of the team, namely, client adaptation.

Conflicts can be discussed during regularly scheduled staff meetings. Differences of opinion, however, also can be dealt with during a treatment session. Toseland and Rivas (2001) have found in their work with groups that this method sets an effective model for clients, but reminds the person working with groups to carefully evaluate and decide which situations can be appropriately dealt with in the group itself without damaging consequences. When this technique is used, the staff members pull their chairs into the middle of the group with the clients around them and discuss issues face to face until there is closure. Staff then return their chairs to the outer circle with the clients and continue with treatment. The authors have found this approach to be effective in group work with older adults. It affords opportunities to: (1) build trust toward staff, because they are open; (2) recognize that staff are human, with human flaws and feelings, rather than condescending, inexperienced young people who think

they are in control; (3) avoid staff resentment, which might build through a session when feelings were not discussed and which would affect client treatment; (4) prevent splits between staff and clients; and (5) model methods for clients to express feelings.

The final opportunity is worth expanding. Many clients are resentful and angry toward family members, board-and-care personnel, and other clients even though involvement, such as that shown in **Figure 23–1**, contributes to well-being. They may resent team members who they feel are controlling their lives by requiring group participation. Many have been taught that anger is not a polite feeling to express; because they fear rejection if anger is expressed, they repress their feelings. Unexpressed anger perpetuates depression and physiological illness and can lead to decompensation. By dealing with conflict openly, staff model communication skills and demonstrate that they have neither died nor become ill, nor have they been offended by another's anger. They also demonstrate the possibility of growth and increased warmth in a relationship in which taboo subjects can be discussed. Again, this method can be utilized only in an atmosphere where highly skilled leaders have established a close working relationship.

When working in larger groups, many dynamics are coming into play and the team members and coleaders must be aware of interactions and side conversations or behaviors that are taking place. Therefore, they must seat themselves so that they can watch each other and pick up cues from facial expressions, body gestures, and eye contact. Body language can help them employ the skills and the confirming judgments previously discussed.

Team Relationship with Board-and-Care Personnel

The relationship between the multidisciplinary team and the board-and-care personnel needs to be carefully cultivated. While board-and-care operators are receptive to improving the quality of their programs and thereby maintaining their certification status, they may be threatened by the overwhelming power they have assigned to a professional team. Often, they fear they will be under scrutiny by the team, who will find fault with their programs or levels of care and recommend that their certification be suspended. This apprehension can be advantageous in assisting clients. Mere team presence encourages board-and-care operators to maintain and upgrade services provided for clients, utilize client monies ethically, and interact with clients respectfully. On the other hand, the presence of team members can evoke resentment and resistance. Personnel may experience disruption in their regular routines and may displace their frustrations onto clients, thereby hindering the team's primary purpose.

Therefore, before initiating a client-centered group, the coleaders must establish rapport with the board-and-care operators and personnel. Purposeful inclusion of personnel in treatment sessions, with verbal or written credit for their participation, is essential. Courtesies, such as assisting personnel with cleanup, also are important. In general, the team needs to be sensitive to the needs of the personnel. Existing creative programs and positive client involvement must be acknowledged. Nevertheless, personnel may view the team as condescending in usurping leadership roles. Some of the personnel may have been highly involved with clients over many years and may feel the so-called experts are negating their efforts.

In addition, personnel must deal with what they view as the insurmountable and draining issues of caring for older adults and perhaps mentally ill clients on a 24-hour basis. Therefore, personnel may feel resentful toward team members entering the home one session per week with a full entourage of staff offering "ideal" advice. Of course, the personnel may feel gratitude, relief, hope, and stimulation by having additional support and assistance. The team, however, must be aware of the total perspective. Everyone needs the esteem derived from receiving credit for a job well done. In several recent studies of board-and-care operators (Eckert, Cox, & Morgan, 1999; Mares, Young, McGuire, & Rosenheck, 2002) caregivers describe personal gratification from their work, and demonstrate strong motivation in the face of low reimbursement, difficult clients, and less-than-supportive community environments. These attributes need to be acknowledged and encouragement given to continue this challenging work. As previously discussed, the results of recognition are reflected in client attitudes and care. Mutual exchange of ideas should be given mutual professional respect. Finally, the therapeutic relevance of maintaining this special relationship needs to be imparted to students who can hinder the process if this training is omitted.

Figure 23-1 Social Interaction

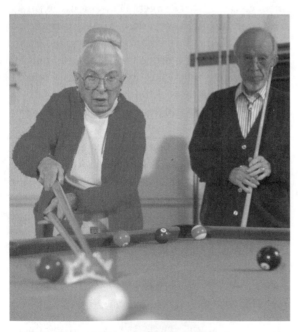

Ongoing social interactions are important.
© Photodisc

Relationships Between Team and Clients

The importance of the relationship between the team members and the clients should be underscored. A well-functioning team with respect for one another does not pass unnoticed by clients. As discussed in earlier chapters, the process of aging and the addition of a mental illness or debilitating physical illness present many challenges for the multidisciplinary team members, the board-and-care operators and staff, and, most importantly, the clients themselves. Individuals choosing to provide services to this population in a community-based board-and-care home need to be aware of the multiple issues involved and be able to demonstrate flexibility, creativity, and an ability to work within multiple systems of care and constituency groups. An important factor in providing groups in residential settings is that the group members live in the same environment and have ongoing contact with one another before and after the group sessions or activities (Shulman, 1999). These ongoing relationships impact the group process and are also affected by the group experience and activities themselves. Careful attention must be directed to observed issues between clients that surface during group sessions, and these concerns need to be dealt with in the group setting itself if appropriate, or during individual time with the client(s) involved. Additionally, board-and-care staff may be able to share important information with the team members regarding residents' behavior before and after group sessions, thus becoming an important member of the multidisciplinary team approach to resolving issues.

Another important factor to consider in the relationship between the team members and the clients is that most groups in board-and-care homes are open ended, and groups will experience loss of members as well as introduction of new members into the group milieu. Because of the changing nature of the group members, the group likely requires more structure and has less continuity, and special attention needs to be paid to processing the loss of group members and welcoming new members. Significantly, loss of group members may be synonymous with death. Yalom (1980), in the classic *Existential Psychotherapy*, states that life and death are interdependent; they exist simultaneously, not consecutively; death whirs continuously beneath the membrane of life and exerts a vast influence upon experience and conduct. All human beings develop defenses against a focus on death. The aged continually must face the death of friends and companions and their own immortality. Shulman (1999) discusses the importance of working not only with the clients in the group, but the group as the client as well; this is an important concept for group work in this type of setting. Additionally, health care professionals may experience what Yalom called "death anxiety" when the topic of death arises. Team members must be prepared in staff postgroup debriefings to discuss such countertransference so as to move the client group process forward.

A Model Program

Initiating the Program and Entering the Board-and-Care Home

In some instances, individuals who are providing the group activities described above or other programs in a board-and-care home are employees of the facility itself, or a parent company, which owns and operates multiple facilities, either statewide or within a local geographic area. In these cases, the team is a part of the board-and-care home staff themselves, and entry into the facility and relationships with caregivers have built-in legitimacy and purpose. More often, the program in these facilities is delivered by an outside entity (an individual or a multidisciplinary team) that is based at another institution with a focus on community intervention strategies. In these cases, entry into the board-and-care home is more challenging, and may take many months of negotiation and discussion. One might consider these individuals "consultants" to the facility, bringing in a special service or program that was not previously available. Kaiser (1997) lists five structural elements of the consultation process which would be necessary: (1) contract development describing the services to be provided; (2) plan of services, to include assessment of the needs and nature of the site; (3) contact with the caregiver and clients; (4) reporting of activities, and (5) evaluation of the services.

While there is abundant literature on consultation services, there is little written that specifically addresses the special circumstances of consulting and providing program elements to a community-based facility serving older adults and/or psychiatrically impaired individuals. The basic consultation skills presented by Munson (2002), would seem to apply to these special circumstances. Consultants need to demonstrate exceptional interpersonal skills, a stable personality, conceptual sophistication, and, most importantly, a good sense of timing.

In the model presented in this chapter, entry into the board-and-care facility was not a problem as the collaborative partnership model within a geographic community facilitated entry. In January 1975, the psychiatry service in a large medical center reorganized from a medical model to a community psychiatry model. Each inpatient ward became a mental health center serving clients living in a particular geographical catchment area in the community. Each center was to provide inpatient crisis treatment, establish a multipurpose satellite center for outpatient treatment, establish working relationships with and provide education about mental health for community members, and assist clients in utilizing the community's resources. One philosophical belief in initiating such a program was that the rapport established among the medical center, the community, and the clients on a more personal level would ultimately have a greater benefit for clients with mental health disabilities than traditional medical models. Staff could better assist clients in making a transition from the hospital to the community by providing services that helped clients remain in the community for longer periods of time with shorter rehospitalization periods. They could encourage clients to seek help before hospitalization became a necessity.

Introduction of the Program

In the spring of 1977, the authors were actively involved in program development with the research team at the community satellite center. The satellite was housed in a progressive community church, which allowed use of its facilities as part of the church's commitment to community action programs. The postdoctoral social worker, Jim Kelly, was involved in expanding his clinical skills and also in serving as a consulting expert in the field of gerontology. The occupational therapist, Sally Friedlob, was codeveloper and clinical coordinator for a life-skills training and research program designed to assist clients with psychosocial disabilities in reintegrating into the community. She was also instrumental in developing evening resource programs at the satellite center. Older adults were a target population that the mental health center had not reached. To meet the needs of the aged population, the two team members decided to initiate an evening program once a week at the satellite center. They proposed the plan to a third team member, Jan Black. She was the social work service community program supervisor. She was included because the medical center's Social Work Department had a successful postdischarge follow-up program in place, and she had ongoing relationships with numerous board-and-care facilities.

Because the authors and the community social work service had laid extensive groundwork, the board-and-care operators were receptive to the idea. The satellite center was chosen for the group work for specific reasons: (1) to involve the aged clients in a community experience, thereby decreasing feelings of isolation and feelings that they were society's castoffs; (2) to utilize the satellite center for a variety of community programs and to obtain community acceptance and participation; (3) to connect the older adults with the existing state geriatric program housed within the church; (4) to involve some of the clients in a possible grandparent program with preschool children; (5) to increase motivation and functional capacity by providing the stimulation of a new environment; (6) to increase reality orientation by holding the group in a special room at the same time each week; and (7) to provide stimulation by enabling clients to experience a weekly ride in an automobile.

In the first two attempts to initiate the program at the satellite center, the clients failed to attend. Therefore, for the third session the authors decided to take the program to the facility. They found that failure to attend was due to poor communication between day and evening personnel, lack of personnel coverage, low personnel interest, transportation problems, and financial problems. The physical needs of many of the clients dictated that meeting in the board-and-care setting would be logistically preferable. In addition, a large number of clients could receive desperately needed services. Although half of the clients were not qualified for direct services at the medical center, the authors believed that they were justified in treating the entire population because the community psychiatry model encourages exchanges in services and programs among a variety of agencies.

The population was mixed and included outpatients with chronic psychosocial disabilities, former state mental hospital residents, and older adults from the community who needed the structure provided by a facility. Upon seeing familiar clients who had actively participated in a resocialization program 18 months earlier, the occupational therapist was appalled by their appearances. They had regressed in social skills, they displayed retarded motor activity, they were emaciated and showed little affect, and their grooming and clothing were poorly kept. More of the board-and-care population were withdrawn and appeared depressed.

After interviewing clients, the authors found that few knew the names of people with whom they were living. During mealtimes, clients rarely spoke to each other. Most sat isolated all day; some drank coffee and smoked cigarettes, watching television occasionally. Most slept much of the day and evening. Three full meals were served daily and clients were given an evening snack. Although the rooms were bare, the facility was kept clean and neat. The authors concluded that a major contributing factor to the apparent depression of the clients was the lack of nurturance, interpersonal connections, and stimulation. The authors also concluded that their earlier impressions about the relevance of group interventions were well grounded. A program was designed to include a range of strategically placed group interventions.

Creative Staffing and Administrative Issues

The authors decided to implement the program one evening per week for a three-hour period (6 p.m. to 9 p.m.) after the dinner hour, because this time frame avoided interfering with the responsibilities of the board-and-care personnel. The authors functioned as cotherapists and included in their team a highly experienced registered movement therapist, occupational therapy students, social work students, nursing students, and medical students. The students rotated through the program; the number of weeks of participation depended on their schedules. Older adults from the community volunteered to assist in programming.

A unique part of the program was that a group of young outpatients served as volunteers. These young adults, who had completed an intensive inpatient life-skills training program (Friedlob, 1982), had been discharged to their own apartments or to cooperative housing. They had increased their social skills during the training, but they required community follow-up in order to maintain treatment gains. Most were overly concerned with their own well-being—an egocentrism that inhibited their awareness of others and affected their social skills. The young adults met with the multidisciplinary team for dinner before the board-and-care evening program, going out for dinner or rotating dinners at the outpatients' apartments. Everyone contributed money toward groceries, did the shopping, and assisted in cooking the meal. The group used the dinner hour to plan the board-and-care session and to purchase ingredients for the session's cooking activities. Another unusual aspect was that some of the young adults living in the board-and-care home formed relationships with their peers and participated in the volunteer program. These outpatients formed friendships that they continued throughout the week. Some of the young adults formed relationships with older adults at the board-and-care home and worked individually with them during a session. These social interactions and the young people's sense of altruism decreased their self-conscious behaviors and their psychiatric symptoms by allowing them to be less concerned about their own psychological well-being and social adequacy.

The cotherapists served as role models, providing leadership in program development, clinical expertise, client and student education and supervision, liaison with the medical center's research team and administrative personnel, and liaison with the university faculty. The cotherapists also were responsible for coordinating programmatic needs with the board-and-care administration. Arrangements for space, refreshments, and equipment (such as pianos) were made. The team continually strove for a combined effort in setting goals, planning implementation, and communicating about health care and staffing issues. The team was able to manage the varied needs of 20 to 30 board-and-care clients for the reasons previously discussed (see the previous section, "Advantage of the Multidisciplinary Team").

Implementing this program was beneficial to the medical center, the taxpayers, and to the board-and-care facility. The board-and-care home received free services from skilled professionals who would have been far too expensive for it to employ. Furthermore, the activity program contributed to the status of the home in maintaining its certification. The taxpayers saved money in that the cost per day of hospitalizing a client is more than that of maintaining a client in the community. The medical center paid only small stipends to students and no salary to volunteers. The occupational therapist was able to treat a large number of outpatients during the weekly sessions. The postdoctoral social worker and the movement therapists were paid a flat consultant fee by the psychiatry service, which saved tax money.

Although money was tight, supplies essential for board-and-care residents to maintain the functional level required to remain in board-and-care, for example, cooking equipment, cooking ingredients, and project materials, qualified as occupational therapy life skills treatment interventions. As such, funds and materials were provided by the Occupational Therapy Department, and as well, by the DAV (Disabled American Veterans).

Program Goals

The ultimate goal of the program was to enhance clients' adjustive resources and therein facilitate growth and adaptation. Group experiences were aimed at providing opportunities for: reality orientation, sensory stimulation, socalization, friendship networks, and community integration.

Capitalizing on retained strengths (physical, sensory, perceptual, cognitive, social, and emotional)

- Retraining in lost skill areas
- Building confidence in retained skill areas
- Supporting independence (by allowing decision making and encouraging autonomy in carrying out tasks when feasible).
- Increasing self-esteem (through opportunities listed above)

Program Structure

A routine program structure is important in assisting older adults with retention of recent memories and reality orientation. When these individuals know exactly what to expect, their sense of physical security and their self-confidence to risk participation are increased. Furthermore, motivation can be encouraged if the routine provides a pleasurable experience. For the aged, pleasure can be derived simply by purposeful activity that has been mastered by repeated familiar rehearsals and/or experiences. Routine need not lead to boredom. Creativity can be explored within a structured program. The information summarized in **Table 23–1** is an outline of the basic plan used in this program, the rationale for the sequencing of events, and examples of related creative activities that were incorporated into the familiar routines.

LARGE GROUP INVOLVEMENT

Burnside (1976) stated that students often get carried away and feel that group work is like cooking potatoes—one more will not matter very much. Yalom (1995) stated that unless clients are carefully selected, the majority of the patients assigned to group therapy will terminate treatment discouraged and without benefits. In managing a large, unselected group, the authors found quite the contrary. The leaders of this group, how-

ever, were highly skilled and experienced, and they had the advantage of adequate support systems. A number of guidelines for managing a large group have already been discussed, but a few additional comments are necessary. First, clients must never be treated like just another potato. In undertaking the program, the leaders carefully considered the physical and emotional needs of each client. Furthermore, the coleaders were responsible for ensuring that each client was actively acknowledged and included in each session.

The primary technique found to be relevant for this size group was scanning. The coleaders observed each individual successively clockwise and then counterclockwise throughout the session. At any given moment, cotherapists were aware of the physical location, facial expressions, verbalizations, and so on, of a particular client. Periodically, while one coleader or allied staff member directed an activity, the other co-leaders scanned the group, picking up behaviors that required intervention. For example, one client's left leg began quivering while he was standing with the group doing an exercise. A cotherapist used eye contact and subtle hand signals to direct a student to assist the client, who was able to complete the activity from his chair. To help with scanning and other activities, higher-functioning clients and team members can be seated next to those who need assistance. Staff can be redirected as necessary. Staff members should be positioned so that they can clearly see each other. Following are three other strategies for large-group management.

Small Groups. With adequate staffing, the large group can be broken into smaller groups. One method utilized in the program was to assemble the entire group for a given activity in order to explain it, and then to break into smaller groups. Upon task completion, group members rejoined to share their small-group experiences briefly. Leadership for each small group was carefully assessed, given the assets and limitations of

Table 23–1   Outline of Basic Program Plan, Rationale for Sequence, and Associated Activities

Regularly structured program	Rationale for programmatic sequencing	Example of creative activities
Opening greetings	Orient to a purposeful beginning. Orient to new individuals. Reinforce memory of familiar persons. Convey feelings of individual importance by remembering client's name. A name or nickname is extremely important for self-identification. Names have many meanings and implications. "This is who I am."	Through movement: Say your name and everyone will say your name and copy your movement. Game: New staff and students will go around the room and try to remember everyone's name and movement (with creative cueing when students stumble; it is important to remember everyone). Clients sometimes feel good if they can stump a student briefly.
Getting clients who have not attended because they are isolated in their rooms, outside, or sleeping	Everyone needs to feel that he or she is important enough to be remembered. Everyone likes to feel included in the group process rather than left on the fringes. Clients need to be included early in the session to reinforce participation and orientation to date, time, and place.	Other clients assisted in getting each other once relationship had been formed. Younger clients who played guitars serenaded older clients in group. Familiar jokes and storytelling before joining the group can be instituted to motivate clients.
Movement therapy	Developmentally, movement emerges from other abilities. Movement is the plane on which primal learning must take place, and it is the cognitive level that must be integrated before higher thought processes can evolve (Levy, 1974). Movement therapy creates a warm atmosphere and pleasurable physical experiences. Movement therapy decreases anxiety to prepare the group for forthcoming activities. Movement therapy increases interaction and trust among individuals through shared experiences without having to verbalize cognitively integrated experiences (at the early stage).	Movement geared to expressing aspects of a particular holiday. Movement that grows out of a client's spontaneous action or reaction.

Regularly structured program	Rationale for programmatic sequencing	Example of creative activities
Music therapy period: music (harmonica, percussion, brass) and movement	Music was often used in conjunction with movement. Music stimulates affect, mood, and expression of feelings and is a catalyst for linking the present with the past and future. Music was generally a natural outgrowth of movement. Clients frequently broke out in song after moving or wanted to perform for others; for example, one man brought his harmonica to play; another a guitar. Singing familiar songs from a book printed in large type stimulated vision, hearing, and following a familiar sequence and helped task conceptualization. Promoted increased trust and camaraderie among individuals.	Individuals in movement spontaneously pantomiming piano playing from time to time sat at the piano and played familiar songs while the group moved. Percussion instruments were included in a sing-along. Instruments were spontaneously created from familiar objects such as wax paper and combs.
Task-planning group	Clients are now ready to sit for a longer period, with increased attention span and receptivity to ideas. Familiar tasks involving decision making increase self-esteem and the feeling of autonomy. Tasks require negotiation, compromise, expression of feelings, and sharing of ideas. High-level thought processes are now ready to evolve.	Planning next week's treat or special program. Planning a group project and carrying it out; for example, making simple learning toys for the children at Head Start (using familiar pictures from magazines for flash card words). Planning homework activities, such as taking a walk with a friend. Planning utilization of the community's resources.
Life skills activity: cooking	By this time, clients need a break that reinforces participation. Response is positive to oral gratification. Cooking, which involves familiar, simple problem solving and follow through, reinforces higher-level thought processes and can be an extremely pleasurable and beneficial venture.	

(continued)

Table 23-1 Outline of Basic Program Plan, Rationale for Sequence, and Associated Activities (continued)

Regularly structured program	Rationale for programmatic sequencing	Example of creative activities
Verbal psychodynamic group	Part of closure requires integration of evening's experience through verbalization. Clients need to convey unexpressed thoughts and feelings. Clients have been stimulated and need to calm down before retiring.	Formal group psychotherapy, and psychotherapy as a component of human service groups, initiated by social worker.
Formal goodbye	Orient clients to time. A formal goodnight hug or hand-shake for each person reinforces personal worth and friendship. Provides reassurance of closure for those worried that they will not see the staff again. Provides hope that "We will meet again" (during the early stage).	Goodbye songs such as "Goodnight Irene" and the "Goodbye, Farewell" song from *The Sound of Music* can be sung at the door.

team members. The small-group leader had to be able to give directions clearly and to handle group issues. An occupational therapy student, for example, was able to manage an art group that stimulated remote recall and then discussed content and process issues. A volunteer outpatient was able to lead a small group successfully in a cooking activity, such as baking a stir-and-frost cake, while a student served as an assistant. This strategy increased the level of participation and the self-esteem for the volunteer.

Dyads or Pairs. These proved to be another constructive means of working with a large group. Clients who worked in pairs created new friendships that carried over to daily routines. One pair, for example, began to take the bus to the satellite center twice per week, where they interacted in a therapeutic social club and participated in the senior citizens' lunch program. Dyads were utilized in task activities, such as

making a Christmas decoration. They were used to personalize a group activity. For example, the leader directed the group members to turn to a neighbor and discuss what he or she thought about the current topic. In addition, dyads were used in training clients to ask for help, and sometimes a buddy system was instituted for the forthcoming week. Another advantage of the dyad is a staff member, volunteer, or another client can be assigned to pair up with clients who are withdrawn or on the fringe of the group. Subsequently, such clients ease into the group and become less alienated.

Individual Treatment. Clients were treated individually while the group was concurrently convening, because clients frequently had individual problems and needs. As they formed trusting relationships with team members, they expressed pent-up feelings that they had repressed due to fear or isolation. For example, one aged woman had been placed in the facility by the county after she had been hospitalized for a broken hip because she needed supervised aftercare. She was worried about her house, belongings, and garden. She was so concerned that she rarely left her room and rarely attempted to exercise her hip as directed, to increase strength. She needed someone to listen and to empathize with her. A medical student was assigned to work with her for 30 to 35 minutes a week. The session was not only of benefit to the woman, but benefited the student. In expanding his medical training; he learned that the needs of an aged patient may far exceed the physical treatment required to heal a broken hip. He found that healing was also facilitated by attitude and motivation. These needs might not be apparent to a medical team without a holistic approach to treatment. Frequently, clients relied on team members to divulge negative feelings toward the board-and-care personnel. This is a delicate subject and will be discussed in more detail (see the section on "Problems, Obstacles, and Management" later in this chapter).

Group Interventions

Movement Therapy

Beginning in the 1940s and running through the 1960s dance and movement therapy was a developing field and gained recognition as a significant mind-body healing process. In the early 1970s, movement-oriented activity emerged as an adjunctive form of treatment in psychiatric rehabilitation. Dance/movement therapy is the psychotherapeutic use of movement as a process that furthers the emotional, cognitive, social, and physical integration of the individual (American Dance Therapy Association, 2004). For this program, movement therapy sessions were structured to provide a secure environment in which clients could increase what Foos and Clark (2003) call "person-in-environment congruence." Movement

therapy also was meant to increase mobility and decrease physical deterioration which impacted cognitive functioning. Predictable activities instilled reassurance in clients who felt unsteady and insecure about their kinetic capabilities. For clients who were experiencing a diminution of strengths, these sessions increased self-confidence and a positive self-image. Movement became a metaphor for personal and social equilibrium. Designated times for large-group activities, dyads, and individual expression were built into the program. The large group offered skills in coping with interactions similar to those needed to cope with a large group of people on a day-to-day basis.

Interactions that required less intimacy were facilitated to: (1) provide clients overwhelmed by large-group interactions with time-outs; (2) promote privacy, which is often excluded from the board-and-care experience; (3) provide an opportunity for each individual to explore and express his or her own creativity; and (4) provide time to work out individual issues. For example, clients were directed to find a familiar way to move their arms. Navigating large muscle movements with a group was self-satisfying, on the one hand, and on the other, beginning with a large group in this way was comforting for clients who had difficulty tolerating intimacy. Over time, the large group became more personal. For example, clients were directed to form a circle, turn, and give the person in front of them a back rub.

Small-group activities, such as finding a familiar way to balance together, encouraged not only trust and warmth, but also autonomy that emerged from dependency. Dyads promoted an increased opportunity for intimacy and interpersonal skills. An activity such as mirroring with another individual (one person pretends to be looking into a mirror; the other is the mirror image and copies the looker) promoted an exchange of eye contact, facial gestures, postures, and feelings, and led to one-to-one verbal exchanges following the activity. Individual activities also encouraged a sense of mastery and accomplishment. Some individual movement was integrated with the large-group activity. For example, during movement charades, a client showed off his or her expertise and abilities by pantomiming an activity he or she enjoyed while everyone guessed what was being enacted. Each performance ended with group applause. The movement sessions began and ended with a large-group activity. The final activity was to stand in a circle holding hands, find balance together, and finally let go in order to find one's own balance. This reinforced a sense of relatedness to others and to self, and promoted trust in others and in self. The basic group structure served to orient group members to time and also to the life cycle—that is, there was a definite beginning, middle, and end during each session.

Movement therapy directives stimulated familiar body motions and encouraged discussions about each client's achievements, which reduced the imposed impersonal institutional experience, and increased clients' sense of identity. For example, when directed to "Find a way you like to move your arms and we'll follow you," one woman began to do the crawl stroke. She then related to the group that she had been an avid swimmer when she was a young girl growing up in Sweden. Her memories stimulated and encouraged a very shy Mexican man, who rarely initiated conversation, to act out the crawl stroke and share that he too had enjoyed swimming in his youth.

Familiar movements that were coupled with familiar music encouraged individuals to talk about instruments they had liked to play. These instruments were provided during succeeding sessions and incorporated into the weekly routine. One man played the harmonica; three played the piano; one, the organ; and two, the guitar. These individuals were encouraged to take turns providing the background music during the movement

sessions. Musical instruments contributed to the self-esteem, stature, and dignity, not only of those who played the instruments, but also of the mobile participants. For example, the organ music stirred up associations about music accompanying ice skaters. The "Skaters' Waltz" was played while people pretended to ice skate. The activity further stimulated a variety of related memorable life event markers that the group examined. Such associations sometimes awakened life's disappointments. One man who, in childhood, had been groomed to dance with a major ballet company shared a life event that changed the direction of his career goals and dreams. He expressed unvoiced feelings and obtained support and an alternate perspective about his disappointment from the group. Movement also promoted sensory input through tactile, visual, and auditory stimulation.

Music Therapy

The poet Longfellow declared music is the "universal language of mankind" (Kipfer & Chapman, 2001). McInnis-Dittrich (2002) discussed the healing properties of music, and how music is an effective tool in group work with older adults. The National Association for Music Therapy (AMTA) (1999) substantiates these facts: "Music is a form of sensory stimulation, which provokes responses due to the familiarity, predictability, and feelings of security associated with it." Crowe (1999), past president of the AMTA, asserts that music therapy can make the difference between withdrawal and awareness, between isolation and interaction, between chronic pain and comfort— between demoralization and dignity. Clients were extremely responsive to music. A regularly scheduled group developed as an outgrowth of the movement therapy group. Music increased motivation, pleasure, mental alertness, and animation. Furthermore, music proved to be an excellent agent for promoting developmental tasks. Period music, in particular, brought out a variety of moods and often stimulated moods correlated with past events, encouraging clients to share feelings verbally with the group. Melodies and songs evoked associations with life events that highlighted periods of self-direction. The natural progression of music sessions led to activity and discussion that promoted engagement and a sense of identity. For example, one man who was delusional stopped his grandiose talk and began to tell a story about an experience he had had at a USO (United Service Organizations) dance and demonstrated several fancy steps he knew, including the fox trot and the rumba. For an individual to spontaneously break out in solo, with group members intently listening and then applauding enthusiastically, was not unusual during a music session. In following sessions, people might call out a favorite singer or piano player, clapping and demanding an encore performance. A man shared with great pride that as a young man he had studied voice at Juilliard, and for the first time in many years, sang in front of a group, and the crowd sprang to their feet and cheered.

After hearing a folk song, another man recalled chopping wood with his father and then recalled his role on the family farm in Missouri. His anecdotes encouraged others to share meaningful stories. Such tales helped restore personal dignity. Music's universal appeal also closed the generation gap. For instance, one regressed young man, who was a talented musician and a rocker at heart, was pleased to play standard tunes and slower contemporary songs on the piano for the group. In return, the older clients expressed gratitude through applause and sing-alongs, which facilitated his engagement and social-appropriate interactions. Clients who had been angry at the younger man because of his "noisy music" began to accept him and relate to him. In addition, they were willing to give special time for him to play rock music on the guitar, and he was willing to adapt some of his favorite pieces to meet their needs. Music therapy offered continuity by pro-

viding a do-re-me link to the past, a here-and-now present, and a direction toward the future. For these reasons, music spontaneously rippled into other activities to assist in integrating the experience. For example, at the end of an evening's session, the group convened at the door while the staff serenaded the clients with a good-bye song, and the clients responded through song and perhaps a farewell tune.

Art Therapy

The earliest expressed emotion through artwork appears on the walls of cave dwellers. At the beginning of the 20th century, psychiatrists such as Carl Jung became interested in art and its relationship to illness. However, art therapy as a distinct human service profession emerged in the 1930s.

Art therapy utilizes art media, images, the creative art process, and patient/client responses to the created art productions as reflections of an individual's development, abilities, personality, interests, concerns, and conflicts. Art therapy practice is based on knowledge of human developmental and psychological theories which are implemented in the full spectrum of models of assessment and treatment including educational, psychodynamic, cognitive, transpersonal, and other therapeutic means of reconciling emotional conflicts, fostering self-awareness, developing social skills, managing behavior, solving problems, reducing anxiety, aiding reality orientation, and increasing self-esteem (The American Art Therapy Association, 2003).

Art was not a regularly scheduled part of the program, but it was periodically employed as a highly effective agent of the developmental process. Initially, group members would declare, "I can't draw." Staff emphasized that artistic ability was not the purpose of the activity. Art was a means to an end; namely, it was used to facilitate large-group and/or small-group discussion. For example, one directive was to: (1) fold the paper in three sections; (2) in the first section, choose a color that creates a feeling you had about a historical event that happened during your lifetime; (3) in the second section, write what the event is and write a word that describes how you felt at the time; (4) in the third section, write a word that describes how you feel as you think about it now. Sometimes the colors were not included in the discussion but were used solely to facilitate associations. Other times, the use of color was tied into the discussion. Directing clients to draw symbolic figures or markings was incorporated in a similar way. The cotherapists facilitated the discussions and encouraged young staff members to learn from clients. For example, one could learn a great deal about historical events firsthand. The result was that clients who often felt abandoned by society felt included and useful. During art sessions, clients frequently discovered that they had many things in common with each other. Three clients were surprised to learn that they had all grown up in the same town in Ohio. These discoveries encouraged alliances and interactions outside the sessions.

Occupational Therapy: The Developmental Task Group

Occupational therapy with its strong foundation in both physical medicine and psychosocial rehabilitation is the solid marriage of the arts and the sciences, including occupational science. Occupational therapy (OT) emerged from the Mental Hygiene Movement that promoted humane treatment for mental patients in the early 1800s and the first occupational therapy association was established in 1817. (See Chapter 27 for more on occupational therapy.) The field blossomed after World War I and again after World War II. The Arts and Crafts Movement became an essential intervention for shell-shocked and injured soldiers. The 1940s Immigrant Settlement Movement, which asserted that occupation is a major contributing factor in the health of the individual, sealed occupational therapy's importance in the medical and human services fields. Occupation as applied to occupational therapy may be, but is not necessarily, related to vocation. Rather occupation is defined as purposeful activity. This definition is based on the premise that advanced cognition sets humans apart from other animals, and therefore humans have an innate need to engage in activity. Wilcox (1993) stated that purposeful activity is a "central aspect of the human experience." In other words, humans are occupational beings whose existence is filled with numerous occupations. "Occupation is motivated by humans' need to explore and master themselves and their world" (Kielhofner & Burke, 1985). Purposeful activity—or occupation—encompasses skill, competence, initiation, social acceptance, and satisfaction. It affects each individual's physical, emotional, and spiritual well-being.

A major goal of the occupational therapist is to assist clients in securing functional "skills for the job of living" (Hinojosa, 2004). Moreover, it follows that OT is a natural fit in community-based multidisciplinary public health settings that prepare clients to live independently in the community (Scaffa, 2001). Clark, Azen, Zemke, Jackson, Carlson, & Mandel (1997), in the largest randomized, controlled trial of OT practices to date, the "Well Elderly Study," compared 361 culturally diverse seniors who were divided into three groups. One received OT activity interventions, another social activities, and the third no intervention. Among other results, the study concluded that social activity alone appeared to be no more effective than no treatment at all when compared with social activity employing OT theoretical principles.

The developmental task group has been employed as a treatment method since the 1960s. The task group provides a unique approach to preventative medicine and was a prime intervention utilized with the board-and-care residents.

The advantage of employing the developmental task group was that it not only promoted autonomy in performing simple problem-solving and decision-making skills, but it also encouraged using these skills with others. Typically, in a task group, the end result is secondary to the developmental process. In their overview of group models, Howe and Schwartzberg (2001) spotlight Fidler and Fiedler (1969) who wrote:

> Task accomplishment is not the purpose of the therapy group but, hopefully, the means by which the purpose is realized. It is seen as the catalytic agent which elicits behavior and interaction, brings into focus both functional capabilities and limitations, facilitates collaboration in working through problems, and provides a concrete reality faction against which to measure learning and achievement.

In working with older adults, however, the authors found that the end result was equally important. Clients needed to be able to conceptualize an end result, experience mastery in task completion, and believe they could still make a contribution. To meet these needs, familiar tasks that drew on past memories, abilities, motor activities, and assets were presented. For example, one task was to plan, set up, and participate in an old-fashioned barbecue. The developmental task group was designed to facilitate skills in each phase of the activity process. Cole (1998) described these phases as: Phase 1—Planning, which begins after a brief introduction by the facilitator and usually starts with brainstorming; Phase 2—Doing, that is carrying out the plan soon after completion; Phase 3—Evaluation, which includes reflection of behavior and its consequences, feelings of members about the group, and evaluation of task accomplishment.

The board-and-care developmental task group combined both directive and facilitative approaches. In the directive method, the leader defines a group, selects activities, and structures the group in ways that she knows to be therapeutically appropriate for a specific group of patients (Cole, 1998). While the task emerged from client requests, the coleaders defined the barbecue as a task and a structured seven-step problem-solving method was introduced and implemented. Once the structure was laid out, the coleaders functioned as advisory/resource persons. Without assuming responsibility for the group, the coleaders facilitated group process and made learning possible. The development task group provided a means for:

- Engaging clients in purposeful and fulfilling activity
- Increasing independence by encouraging clients to contribute ideas drawn from past experiences
- Providing gratification and success
- Fulfilling narcissistic needs for self-actualization while providing an opportunity for sharing in a cooperative venture
- Promoting communication skills, social interaction, and generalizing experiences to the community
- Providing repeated opportunities to perceive cause-and-effect relationships
- Providing parallel play-work situations that encourage modeling and imitation
- Providing opportunities for problem solving, carry through, and observable results
- Increasing sitting tolerance and attention span
- Increasing risk-taking behavior by increasing physical and psychological security
- Increasing self-confidence and self-esteem
- Providing opportunities for evaluation, change, and growth

A COMMUNITY-ORIENTED DEVELOPMENTAL TASK GROUP

One afternoon a week a group of elderly veterans residing in the board-and-care participated in occupational therapy sessions. Initially, these veterans were resistant to the concept of occupational therapy because, as one client put it, "I made enough wallets when I was in the VA hospital." However, the resistance was soon overcome by the group's purpose: to make learning toys for the children in the nearby Head Start preschool. The group structure was similar to the developmental task group as previously explained. The occupational therapist served as the liaison between the Head Start administrator and the client group. In between planning sessions, the clients constructed the learning toys. For example, one vocabulary and language toy involved woodworking and decoupage. The group process was an essential component of the task group. For instance, one client who led the puppet-making activity had been a private in the Army. Another veteran who had been a lieutenant scoffed at the notion of taking direction from such an enlisted man. While aging may include changes in status, this poignant vignette highlights the loss of stature the institutionalized client experiences secondary to a traumatic separation from the mainstream of life. The professional facilitated the group process by validating the client's feelings and helping him gain a different perspective about the experience. Subsequently, he was able to give others a leadership opportunity, and preserve his self-image by serving as an advisor. In response, other group members became more tolerant of his interpersonal style.

The developmental task group also assisted in filling such voids through purposeful activity/occupation, which instilled a sense of accomplishment and contribution. The task group project culminated in the clients presenting the toys to and planning and preparing a party for the children at the children's Head Start school. The social work postdoctoral fellow, along with the OT, accompanied the group to the school and co-led the group process. He also co-led the posttask evaluation session, the following week.

Occupational Therapy: Life-Skills Training

Cooking Activities. Brown (1982) found that training in life skills should closely correlate with skills required in a particular living environment. This correlation reinforces retention of learned skills and encourages utilization and autonomy in skill application. Although board-and-care facilities do not allow clients in the kitchen (county health laws prohibit clients from handling foods in the kitchen), simple cooking activities using developed task group methods were planned and carried out in the dining area. The authors found that issues relating to foods were extremely meaningful. Food invokes a variety of personal feelings and associations. To enhance the many therapeutic aspects incurred by a cooking activity, an art therapy approach was utilized after one cooking session. The art paper was divided into thirds. In the first section, clients were directed to remember a particular meal shared with their families by diagramming where each person sat. Foods served at that meal were drawn in the second section. Colors, markings, and/or drawings depicting feelings during that particular meal were placed in the last section, encouraging life review. Clients talked about their own values, habits, and feelings and then compared these. For example, many found that their parents did not allow discussions during mealtime. For others, mealtime was the only time family members gathered to share stories, jokes, and daily happenings and to plan family events. The discussion assisted clients in integrating feelings about current mealtimes. Clients also compared food preferences, mourned current losses involving consumption of favorite foods, and planned the preparation of foods, such as old-fashioned ice cream sundaes.

Activities such as the above, coupled with pleasurable cooking experiences, promoted social interaction during eating and the generalization of socialization during daily meals. Upon arriving during one dinner hour, the authors were gratified to find clients chatting, sharing, and calling each other by name. In addition, the authors found a way around the county health laws in order to assist one middle-age client. The client was able to assist kitchen staff for minimal pay after the doctor wrote in the chart that assisting in the kitchen was essential in the client's rehabilitation. Thereafter, this client's role, image, self-esteem, and ability to take on responsibility and social skills improved.

Other Life Skills Activities. The evaluation of a number of clients showed individual life-skills needs (Brown & Munford, 1983). Training in communication, health care, hygiene, budgeting, community resources, and time management skills was initiated when necessary. For example, one man with a progressive neurological condition was beginning to have difficulty dressing himself. His motor activity was retarded, and he displayed tremors upon voluntary motion. Inability to care for himself would lead to either rehospitalization or transfer to a nursing home facility. The occupational therapy student was assigned to work individually with him for part of each session. The patient's goal was to maintain his level of independent functioning for as long as possible.

Life-skills training was sometimes employed in the group setting. For example, during one developmental task group, the members filled out a weekly schedule balancing each day with work, rest, and play. They chose homework assignments, such as taking a walk to the market for a snack with a buddy. The group members reviewed task accomplishments, difficulties, and areas for growth during the following week's session.

Other Therapeutic Modalities

Children

Wallach, Kelley, and Abrahams (1979) pointed out that institutionalized elderly people are deprived of the psychosocial stimulation provided by family interactions, because the frequency of visits by families who are available tends to decrease as the stress, guilt, and resentment toward the patient's dependency develops with lengthening institutionalization. In their study, patients reported increased social interaction, reduced daytime sleeping, increased mobility, and decreased voluntary confinement after consistently interacting with high school students. Throlow and Watson (1974) provided one of the earliest rationales for an intergenerational model when they studied sixth graders who participated in 45-minute sessions twice a week with a geropsychiatric population. After 11 weeks, the aged people demonstrated significantly greater improvements than did the control group in the areas of self-awareness and self-esteem. Corey and Corey (2002) and Moody (1998) described the use of intergenerational programming with older adults and children/adolescents that had a significant positive impact on an issue that causes much distress among both age groups—loneliness and social isolation.

Occasionally, team members and board-and-care personnel brought children to participate with clients. Clients became animated, laughing and smiling with the children. Children facilitated the loosening of defenses and encouraged displays of warmth. For example, one client's cultural background had customs about appropriate touching; thus, he rarely touched others and never hugged them. The client was able to respond positively to a child's touch. An 89-year-old man had difficulty communicating with others because of his poor vision and hearing. He actively engaged a small child throughout a movement session. He cooed and waved at her and played peek-a-boo. Children also stimulated clients' childhood associations, which were reviewed and processed during verbal sessions.

Pet-Facilitated Group Therapy

Pets also provide meaningful experiences for aging and chronically ill people (Barba, 1995; Raina, Walter-Toews, Bonnett, Woodward, & Abernathy, 1999; Willis, 1997). There is a large body of literature on the positive effects on health of elders who have pets. One older woman who was confined to a wheelchair was able to hide a cat in her room (some health laws prohibit live-in pets). Although she was depressed about living in the care home, the maneuvering and secrecy involved in feeding and maintaining the cat were thrilling. She had difficulty relating with the other clients, so the cat became her one reliable living contact. She held it on her lap and petted and hugged it. When she began to trust team members who worked with her individually, she shared her mischievous undertaking with them. As other clients found out about the cat, they became cohorts and helped her with management, leading to her increased socialization and ultimately to her group participation. Pets, like children, stimulated childhood associations and other life event markers related to animals.

Problems, Obstacles, and Management

Although the programs described in this chapter were well planned, well coordinated, and adequately staffed, problems were encountered. Obstacles were expected because the authors were well aware that any program has its drawbacks. Problems were managed with team planning and strategies. One major problem in maintaining the program was surviving the changing conditions. Because the home had three owners within a three-year period, relationships had to be established with each new administration; furthermore, the staff changed monthly and sometimes weekly. Often, the new evening personnel had not been oriented to the program and were overwhelmed when the team appeared with a full crew and program plan. Some of the new personnel were offended when team members requested that they maintain routines, such as serving coffee after the task group. Some served the coffee before the authors could explain the rationale and disrupted the program.

At first, the authors attempted to remedy this situation by calling the staff on the afternoon of the group. Communication between the day and evening personnel was poor, however. Therefore, the team decided one of them would orient the personnel on arrival while the other would initiate the program. Then personnel were included in the refreshment period and other festive events such as holiday parties. Personnel were encouraged to join the group at will. The team was conscientious about postgroup clean-up, especially in the dining room where uniformed personnel had already completed their evening work by setting up the dining room for the following morning. Sometimes the team judiciously decided to reset the tables.

Providing alcoholic beverages on special occasions is another concern. In our society, alcohol is a significant object; the ability to consume alcohol is a mark of maturity. General rules and restrictions imposed on the aged living in an institution, especially rules and restrictions about alcohol, promote low self-esteem and self-confidence about their ability to maintain their autonomy. At the Michael Reese Institute in Chicago, the geriatric program encourages the inpatients and staff to dress formally for dinner one night a week, and wine is served with dinner. As a result, self-image and hope for the future were observed to increase during the session. The authors also found a similar outcome when one beer was provided during barbecues and special holiday events. There are several precautions that need to be taken to prevent deleterious effects, however. Some board-and-care clients may be alcoholics, some may be on medications that cannot be ingested with alcohol, or some may have a low tolerance for alcoholic beverages. Therefore, knowing the medical history of each client is important.

Clients frequently wanted to place the authors in an omnipotent role. This was both a blessing and a curse and often evoked conflicting feelings. Clients experiencing a loss in dignity improved their future outlook because of the power they invested in the team to help them with their plight. Although the team was instrumental in alleviating some of the problems, the team had to be tactful in order to prevent possible punitive actions to clients by the board-and-care staff and possible termination of the program. Clients confided in the team, and sometimes team members felt torn about their alliances. For example, when the woman who was hiding a cat in her room confided in the team, the team had to decide whether the cat might create a health problem and had to determine other possible consequences of failing to report the animal to the owner. In the end, the authors decided that the benefits the woman derived from having the cat outweighed the possible problems and decided to overlook the situation.

Other issues were not as easy to overlook. For example, several clients accused personnel of misappropriating their funds. The team decided that the best way to deal with the situation was to report the issue to the medical center's community social work service, which was responsible for quality assurance in board-and-care settings. When the community social worker probed the situation, the operator called for a team conference and demonstrated that the clients were confused and had fabricated stories.

Confidentiality

The issue of confidentiality with clients is an important one. Whether clients were correct in their perception about a situation was not always as important as the thoughts and feelings they were able to express confidentially. Common themes were loss of dignity, low self-esteem, help-lessness, and lack of control. Some of their attitudes and behaviors were found to be defenses against their anger and underlying hurt. The single most important quality in helping clients cope is empathy. Empathy skills include listening, helping the client to express his or her feelings, and conveying feedback that the client has been understood (Hepworth, Rooney, & Larsen, 2002). Confidentiality must expressly be discussed when utilizing volunteers and most likely requires them to complete signed agreements.

Staff Debriefings

An important component of not only a multidisciplinary team group approach, but also of coleadership for all group interventions, is that the role of each coleader and assistant leader must be examined prior to instituting a program and then reviewed periodically throughout the program. For example, for a given group one coleader took the lead in presenting a topic or facilitating a process. At the same time, the other coleader scanned the group and provided group-ready guidance for a member who was disengaged from the group or on the fringe of the group. Group debriefings clarified roles and individual client/group needs. Cotherapists as a part of the same group, like clients, sometimes had different perceptions about a group experience. Staff pre- and postgroup sessions facilitated a more productive group process. Additionally, staff could address program obstacles as they arose. A case can be made for the inclusion of volunteers in debriefing meetings. In the program highlighted in this chapter, volunteers were included in a segment of the staff meetings, as they were an essential part of the team and the intervention strategies. This not only contributed to the well-being of the board-and-care clients, but also to the self-esteem of the young outpatient volunteers. Again, confidentiality was always a primary focus.

Summary

Group work activities are an excellent treatment modality for residents in a board-and-care setting, particularly those activities that provide opportunities for individuals to develop a sense of self, to decrease social isolation, and to feel empowered by participating in their own treatment process. Individuals with a wide range of problems and deficits can be included in such a treatment program. A major advantage of the therapeutic technique of group work is that it can take many forms such as movement, cooking, art, music, and activities of daily living. These activities provide opportunities for growth and adaptation in all areas of human development.

In undertaking a program at a board-and-care facility, employing a multidisciplinary team is preferable. This approach can be beneficial in that a large number of clients can be treated in a group setting by utilizing skilled coleaders directing a variety of assistant leaders. The large group can be divided into small groups, dyads, and individual group treatment. A team member can provide experiences in his or her area of expertise to complement and enhance experiences provided by other team members. Ideally, team members need to be flexible in sharing responsibilities, because territoriality can be destructive to group cohesion. There are three interpersonal relationships that must be carefully cultivated: between the multidisciplinary team members, between the team members and the board-and-care personnel, and between the team members and the clients. In addition, a multidisciplinary team is cost effective in that a variety of services can be provided to a large outpatient group. Creative staffing can assist in this process. There is a substantial cost benefit in maintaining clients in the community in comparison with the cost of hospitalization. We as clinicians are focused on quality-of-life issues; to be able to ensure support in improving quality of life, we must, however, be accountable to administration.

The quality of life for the patients in the program described in this chapter was enhanced primarily in terms of social-skills gains. Clients who had initially appeared withdrawn, emaciated, and unkempt showed improved grooming, became animated and involved in activities, and formed relationships with others. Clients acknowledged each other by first name or last name for endearment. Conversations at mealtimes became spontaneous, one-on-one friendships formed, clients independently initiated trips to the satellite center by bus, and drinking in local taverns decreased. Two major changes were noticeable: clients developed interpersonal relationships that continued without staff facilitation, and when the physical environment began to deteriorate in terms of upkeep, food, and finances, the interpersonal relationships and morale remained high.

Another important issue was the model of program development and delivery that was used in this example. The concept of a geographical catchment area approach means that all of the potential service providers in a particular area are coordinated, and services are provided across agency and institutional boundaries. The current fragmentation of service delivery systems to both older adults and individuals with persistent mental illness treats individuals and symptoms, but loses sight of the whole person and their connection with their community. Historically, the medical model and institutional care have been the more commonly identified resources for those individuals needing structure and assistance in their living environment.

The literature clearly demonstrates that an adequately funded and integrated system of care works, and that, in fact, chronically and severely mentally ill persons experience both higher levels of functioning and quality of life (Lamb, 1998; Lamb & Bachrach, 2001; Segal & Riley, 2003; Smith, Hull, Hedayat-Harris, Ryder, & Berger, 1999). The authors of this chapter clearly advocate for this coordinated system of care approach to serve older adults and severely and persistently mentally ill individuals that can benefit from the supervision and specialized program of a board and care environment.

The 1999 landmark Supreme Court decision in *Olmstead v. L.C.*, 527 U.S. 582, "Affirmed the right of individuals with disabilities to live in the community rather than in institutions whenever possible." In an effort to implement the Olmstead decision, the President has issued an executive order which requires coordination among numerous agencies that administer programs affecting access to the community for people with disabilities (The President's New Freedom Commission on Mental Health, Final Report, 2003). This precedent-setting legal decision and subsequent mandate for coordination of care and development of appropriate community resources to serve individuals with a mental health condition is applauded by the authors, and provides a hopeful outlook for the future of coordinated service delivery systems.

Exercises

EXERCISE 1

Part 1: Work with one other classmate or a small group of your classmates. Lay out a box of crayons and unlined paper. Each person is to take a piece of paper and fold it in thirds. Then, each recall a historical event in his or her lifetime. Each is to imagine where he or she was at the time, people with whom he or she was involved, and related objects and events. Each person is to imagine how he or she felt at the time, to choose a color to represent his or her feelings at the time, and to express the events and feelings on the first third of the paper. Artistic ability is not required. Participants may wish simply to put a color or two or a symbolic figure on paper. Next, in the middle section of the paper, each writes a feeling word that describes his or her feeling at the time of the event. Finally, in the third section of the paper, each writes a word that describes his or her feelings about the event as it is thought about now.

Part 2: Each person identifies a song(s) she or he associates with her or his event.

1. Allow time for each person to share his or her events.
2. After each person shares, other group members are to imagine how that person felt in one or two feeling words. The members each have a turn to tell the speaker their two words. The speaker responds by validating or invalidating the words.
3. Allow time for spontaneous interaction by members—for example, two members may have common themes.
4. Process past and present feelings and attempt to put the events into perspective.

EXERCISE 2

Work with a group of classmates. Make a circle. Each person is to think of an activity he or she has enjoyed performing. One person is to pantomime the activity while the rest of the group guesses what the person is doing.

EXERCISE 3

Work with a group of classmates to plan refreshments for the next class meeting using the following systematic problem-solving method. The resources you need for this exercise are a chalkboard and chalk or newsprint, tape, and a marker. Start by selecting a leader who is to verbally outline and guide the group through each of the directives below, to call upon group members, and to write the suggestions, and so forth on the board.

1. State the problem to be solved (e.g., provide refreshments for the next class session)
2. Brainstorm as many ideas as you can without judging whether or not an idea

is good or bad. Sometimes a bad or silly idea turns out to be valuable, and a good idea turns out to be impractical.

3. Go through each idea, one by one, and list the advantages and disadvantages of each. For example, a fine cabernet sauvignon might be welcome after all the homework in this class, but it may not be allowed in the classroom; it may even be seen as promoting drinking on campus, which the school's administration may be attempting to reduce.

4. Now, choose which of the many ideas that have been presented are feasible to use.

5. Decide the what, who, when, and where of each selected idea. Outline the resources you need (e.g., transportation to the grocery store) and the people with whom you may need to consult.

6. Set a date and carry out the plan.

7. Next class, while you enjoy your refreshments, discuss the outcome of your plans: What went well? What would you improve upon for the next time? How did you feel about your participation in the group?

Exercise 4

Make a circle with your classmates to form a group. Recall the 11 therapeutic factors identified by Yalom and listed earlier in the chapter. Then, choose one or more of the previous exercises that you completed and discuss which curative factors were present during the exercise and how they impacted your experiences.

References

American Association of Retired Persons. (1997). Ensuring a responsive long term care system: New challenges for a new century. *Perspectives in Health and Aging, 12*(1), 106.

American Art Therapy Association. (2003). What is art therapy? Retrieved May 31, 2004, from *http://www.arttherapy.org/aboutarttherapy/about.htm*

American Association of Dance Therapy. (2004). What is dance/movement therapy? Retrieved May 31, 2004 from *http://www.adta.org/*

American Music Therapy Association. (1999). *http://www.musictherapy.org/quotes.html*

Barba, B. E. (1995). The positive influence of animals: Animal-assisted therapy in acute care. *Clinical Nursing Specialist, 9*, 199–202.

Berg-Weger, M., & Schneider, F. D. (1998). Interdisciplinary collaboration in social work education. *Journal of Social Work Education, 34*, 97–107.

Birren, J. K., & Schaie, K. W. (Eds.). (2001). *Handbook of the psychology of aging*. San Diego, CA: Academic Press.

Bronstein, L. R. (2003). A model for interdisciplinary collaboration. *Social Work, 48*(3), 297–306.

Brown, M. A. (1982). Maintenance and generalization issues in skills training with chronic schizophrenics. In J. P. Curran & P. M. Monti (Eds.), *Social skills training* (pp. 1–47). New York: Guilford Press.

Brown, M. A., & Mumford, A. (1983). Life skills training for chronic schizophrenics. *Journal of Nervous and Mental Diseases, 171*(8), 466–470.

Burnside, I. M. (1976). Overview of group work with the aged. *Journal of Gerontological Nursing, 2*(6), 14–17.

Butler, R., Lewis, M. I., & Sunderland, T. (1998). *Aging and mental health* (6th ed.). Boston: Allyn & Bacon.

Cole, M. B. (1998). *Group dynamics in occupational therapy: The theoretical basis and practice application of group treatment*. Slack, Inc: Thorofare, New Jersey.

Corey, M. S., & Corey, G. (2002). *Groups, process and practice*. Pacific Grove, CA: Brooks/Cole.

Crepeau, E. B., Cohn, E. S., & Schell, B.A. (Eds.). (2003). *Willard & Spackman's Occupational Therapy* (10th ed.). Philadelphia, PA: Lippincott Williams & Wilkins.

Crowe, B. (1999). Quotes about music therapy. American Music Therapy Association. Retrieved May 31,2004, from *http://www.musictherapy.org/quotes.html*

Eckert, J. K., Cox, D., & Morgan, L. A. (1999). The meaning of family-like caring among operators of small board and care homes. *Journal of Aging Studies, 13*(3), 333–348.

Erikson, E. (1950). *Childhood and society*. New York: Norton.

Fidler, G. S., & Fiedler, J. W. (1969). Occupational therapy. New York: Macmillan.

Foos, P. W., & Clark, M. C. (2003). *Human aging*. Boston: Allyn & Bacon.

Friedlob, S. X. (1982). The development of a life skills training program for chronic schizophrenic patients: Three case studies. Unpublished papers.

Hepworth, D. H., Rooney, R. H., & Larsen, J. A. (2002). *Direct social work practice: Theory and skills.* Pacific Grove, CA: Brooks/Cole—Thompson Learning.

Hinojosa, J. (2004). New York University, Steinhardt School of Education, Department of Occupational Therapy. Retrieved May 31, 2004, from *http://www.nyu.edu/education/steinhardt/db/departments/11*

Howe, M. C., & Schwartzberg, S. L. (Eds.). (2001). *A functional approach to group work in occupational therapy.* New York: Lippincott Williams & Wilkins.

Kaiser, T. L. (1997). *Supervisory relationships: Exploring the human element.* Pacific Grove, CA: Brooks/Cole.

Kipfer, B. A., & Chapman, R. L. (2001). *Roget's International Thesaurus* (6th ed.). New York: Harper & Row.

Kielhofner, G., & Burke, J. P. (1985). Components and determinants of human occupation. In Williams and Wilkins (Eds.), *A model of human occupation: Theory and application* (pp. 12–36). Philadelphia: F. A. Davis.

Lamb, H. R. (1998). Deinstitutionalization at the beginning of the new millennium. *Harvard Review of Psychiatry, 6*(1), 1–10.

Lamb, H. R., & Bachrach, L. L. (2001). Some perspectives on deinstitutionalization. *Psychiatric Services, 52*(8), 1039–1045.

Linhorst, D., Hamilton, M., Young, E., & Eckert, A. (2002). Opportunities and barriers to empowering people with severe mental illness through participation in treatment planning. *Social Work, 47*(4), 425–434.

McInnis-Dittrich, K. (2002). *Social work with elders: A biopsychosocial approach to assessment and treatment.* Boston: Allyn & Bacon.

Mares, A. S., Young, A. S, McGuire, J. F., & Rosenheck, R. A. (2002). Residential environment and quality of life among seriously mentally ill residents of board and care homes. *Community Mental Health Journal, 38*(6), 447–469.

Molinari, V. (1994). Current approaches to psychotherapy with elderly adults. *Directions in Mental Health Counseling, 4*(3), 3–13.

Moody, H. R. (1998). *Aging: Concepts and controversies.* California: Pine Forge Press.

Munson, C. (2002). *Clinical social work supervision.* Binghamton, New York: Haworth Press.

Olmstead v. L.C., 527 US. 581, (1999).

Peck, R.C. (1968). Psychological developments in the second half of life. In B. L. Neugarten (Ed.), *Middle aging and aging* (pp. 88–92). University of Chicago Press.

The President's New Freedom Commission on Mental Health: Final Report. (2002). Retrieved April 21, 2004, from *www.whitehouse.gov/infocus/newfreedom/chapter4/2004*

Raina, P., Walter-Toews, D., Bonnett, B., Woodward, C., & Abernathy, T. (1999). Influence of companion animals on the physical and psychological health of older people: An analysis of a one year longitudinal study. *Journal of the American Geriatrics Society, 47,* 323–329.

Regulatory measures, licensure found to improve quality in board and care homes. (25 September 1995). *Brown University Long-Term Care Letter, 7*(18), 1042–1386.

Segal, S. P., & Riley, S. (2003). Caring for persons with serious mental illness: Policy and practice suggestions. *Social Work in Mental Health, 1*(3), 1–17.

Scaffa, M. (2001). *Occupational therapy in community-based practice settings.* Philadelphia: F. A. Davis.

Shulman, L. (1999). *The skills of helping individuals, families, groups and communities.* IL: F. E. Peacock

Smith, T. E., Hull, J. W., Hedayat-Harris, A., Ryder, G., & Berger, J. (1999). Development of a vertically integrated program of services for persons with schizophrenia. *Psychiatric Services, 509*(7), 931–935.

Throlow, J., & Watson, C. S. (1974). Remotivation for geriatric patients utilizing elementary school students. *American Journal of Occupational Therapy, 28,* 469–473.

Toseland, R. W., & Rivas, R. F. (2001). *An introduction to group work practice* (4th ed.). Boston: Allyn & Bacon.

Toseland, R. W. (1995). *Group work with the elderly and family caregivers.* New York: Springer.

U.S. Department of Health and Human Services. (1999). Mental health: A Report of the Surgeon General. Rockville, MD.

U.S. Department of Health and Human Services. (2002). Promoting older adult health: Aging network partnerships to address medication, alcohol and mental health problems. Washington, DC: U.S. Substance Abuse and Mental Health Services Administration.

Wallach, H. F., Kelley, F., & Abrahams, J. P. (1979). Psychosocial rehabilitation for chronic geriatric patients: An intergenerational approach. *The Gerontologist, 19*(5).

Wilcock, A. (1993). A theory of the human need for occupation. *Occupational Science, 1*(1), 17–24.

Willis, D. A. (1997). Animal therapy. *Rehabilitation Nursing, 22*(2), 78–81.

Yalom, I. D. (1980). *Existential psychotherapy.* New York: Basic Books.

Yalom, I. D. (1995). *The theory and practice of group psychotherapy* (4th ed.). New York: Basic Books.

Resources

- Butler, R, Grossman, L. K., & Oberluk, M. R. (1999). *Life in older America.* New York: Century Foundation Press.
- Clark, F., Azen, S. P., Zemke, R., Jackson, J., Carlson, M., & Mandel. D. (1997). Occupational therapy for independent living older adults: A randomized controlled trial. *Journal of American Medical Association*, 278, 1321–1326.
- Ryan, D., & Doubleday, E. (1995). Groupwork: A lifeline for isolated elderly. *Social Work with Groups*, 18(2–3), 65–78.
- Schneider, R. L., Kropf, N. P., & Kisor, A. J. (Eds.). (2000). *Gerontological social work: Knowledge, service settings and special populations.* Belmont, CA: Wadsworth Press.
- Sheikh, J., & Yalom, I. D. (1996). *Treating the elderly.* San Francisco: Jossey-Bass.

Acknowledgments

The authors would like to thank Jane Manning, registered dance therapist, for her clinical contributions to this project. Suzanne Silverstein, MA, ATR, is greatly appreciated for her art therapy consultation. George Saslow, MD, served as an educator, role model, and group work consultant. Murray Brown, MD; Richard Chung, MD; Fran Kelly, OTR; Norma Donigan, MSW; Betsy Alkire; and Judith Coleman Maurella provided the necessary support to survive the system.

Group Work in Long-Term Care Facilities

Elaine J. Amella

Key Words

- Continuity theory
- Eden Alternative
- Family groups
- Long-term care continuum
- Nursing assistant groups
- Online groups
- Preadmission and orientation groups
- Resident and family councils
- Skilled nursing facility
- Support groups
- Tobacco cessation groups
- 12-step groups
- Therapeutic groups

Learning Objectives

- Define the continuum of long-term care
- Apply Atchley's continuity theory to the long-term care group process
- Recognize the need for innovative groups that meet staff, resident, and family needs in long-term care facilities
- Discuss the range of therapeutic and support groups that can function within long-term care facilities

- Identify how groups can assist residents and families to maintain control over the quality of their lives

Residential facilities for older adults offer broader options than once existed. Today, larger numbers of older adults may choose to live along a continuum from retirement communities to traditional nursing homes. In 2004 (Centers for Medicare and Medicaid Services), it was reported that 1.4 million adults live in skilled nursing facilities (SNFs) and it is estimated that another 1 million live in assisted-living facilities (ALFs) and residential care facilities (RCFs) (California Advocates for Nursing Home Reform, 2004). The type of service required by the individual determines the place of residence.

The U.S. Census Bureau (2004) divides agencies into: (1) nursing care facilities providing inpatient nursing and rehabilitative services; (2) community care facilities for the elderly providing residential and personal care services including board-and-care homes (see Chapter 23); (3) homes for the elderly providing a range of services that do not include nursing care; and (4) continuing care retirement communities (CCRCs) that include ALFs providing nursing care as well as retirement and traditional CCRCs. Medical-model day care centers (see Chapter 22) that offer therapeutic services are usually included in the long-term care continuum. Within all of these facilities, there is an opportunity for individuals, their families, and caregivers to come together in groups to facilitate the transition to a new environment, to organize and govern their affairs, to offer socialization, and to receive therapeutic services. This chapter will outline groups that serve older adults and others along the continuum of long-term care. For purposes of this chapter, older adults living in a long-term care facility will be termed residents.

Theoretical Perspective: Continuity

The move to a CCRC, where the individual usually resides in a free-standing unit or apartment, might be much less disruptive than a move to a SNF, where 24-hour nursing care is required, yet both moves signal a change of reduced independence and a loss of the familiar. The couple moving into their own CCRC apartment has to prioritize their belongings, choosing among possessions acquired over a lifetime. The individual admitted to a nursing home after a serious hospitalization must leave behind everything that cannot fit into a few dresser drawers and a small closet. Additionally, all require a mechanism to adjust to this life passage, derive some sense of control, begin to establish a new social network, and perhaps become involved in therapeutic interactions. Groups can facilitate these adaptational processes wherever they are through a methodology of mutual aid. For example, a church could set up a transitional group for the elders of the church community and invite speakers representative of a variety of long-term care sites. The seniors would learn about each site and a facilitator could encourage discussion that would help each individual find the right place for him or her and facilitate a move.

Atchley (1999) provided continuity theory as a model to help the health care provider examine needs of older adults in light of ever-changing issues and the individual's own growth. Continuity theory identified the "primary goal of adult development as adaptive change, not homeostatic equilibrium" (p. 6). Atchley sees continuity as a feedback system where the *life structure* influences *decision making*, *actions*, and *results*; any one of these four constructs can double-back and influence future adaptation. Within the life structure construct are three other concepts of: (1) *mental patterns* such as personality, self, worldview, personal goals, and life strategies; (2) *life patterns* such as living arrangements, relationships, activities, and health practices; and (3) *health*.

If aging is seen as a time of continued development, the potential for psychological and social growth continues. Through the psychological transcendence of aging, personal attributes such as creativity and ingenuity are required and valued. Social roles change and the self-centered perspective of younger years moves to a more nurturing role, such as caregiver. This adaptation of social roles as well as exploration of new life perspectives may be fostered through group work for families, caregivers, and residents. If health care professionals consider elements of this model when constructing the best context for older persons to thrive physically, psychologically, and socially, then they are taking a holistic approach to addressing resident needs. Atchley's life structure construct is used in this chapter to provide structure for the three sections under which group work is considered: mental patterns, life patterns, and health.

Mental Patterns

Support Groups

Support groups for residents, families, and caregivers emerge as key elements of the mental pattern concept. Over the years, support groups evolved as a readily recognizable way of seeking help among persons dealing with similar problems and change. Support groups in the long-term care continuum vary from traditional 12-step programs such as Alcoholics Anonymous or Overeaters Anonymous for persons living in CCRCs to support groups for stroke survivors in a SNF. However, residents and families are not the only ones to benefit from groups. In a novel support group, Burack and Chichin (2001) developed a support group for nursing assistants caring for nursing home residents at the end of life. Based on earlier research where three educational sessions were given to the nursing assistants in a large, urban nursing home, the support group addressed the emotional needs of the aides who were often faced with losing a resident with whom they had worked for extended periods of time. In many cases the aides became a surrogate family for the dying resident and the sense of attachment was extremely strong. In a text outlining their complete program, the aims of the group research were: (1) to explore the aides' feelings, experiences, and needs in caring for the dying especially when the resident chose not to have life-sustaining treatment; and (2) to determine the efficacy of the group (Chichin, Burback, Olson, & Likourezos, 2000).

Using the usual support group methodology, a loosely guided discussion occurred between members of each participant group of four to eight aides (total $n = 35$) and the group leader who was one of the investigators, thus a knowledgeable resource. The aides reported informal support from peers and nurses on their unit when they experienced a resident death, but most stated that staff were left to cope on their own without the institutional support so often found in hospice or critical-care hospital areas. The aides often felt frustrated that they were instructed in how to meet resident or family's needs during the dying process, but no one paid attention to their needs. During the support group sessions, aides reminisced about particular residents, large and small acts of caring, the reciprocal nature of their relationships with residents, interactions with families, and those families' decisions about end-of-life care, as well as their difficulty with postmortem care of someone with whom they were close. On a scale of 1 to 5, with 5 being the most positive rating, these 35 aides rated the group on 10 items regarding the group process and their recommendations to others; with a range of 3.9–5.0, their mean response was 4.5 demonstrating the need for further work on support groups for formal caregivers in long-term care.

FAMILY SUPPORT GROUPS

Family support groups in long-term care often cluster around several issues—reduction in isolation, the ability to share ideas, affirmation of the care giving role, sharing of strategies to cope and solve problems (Barusch & Peak, 1997). Additionally, some facilities have specialized support groups for families of residents with specific problems such as Alzheimer's disease where information sharing may be a key function. Contrary to the myth, families and friends continue to be involved with nursing home residents and wish to remain informed (Campbell & Linc, 1996). Groups are a way for those goals to be met through open communication and information sharing.

Peak (2000) developed and evaluated an eight-week group that had as its goal, support of socio-emotional needs as well as education, therapy, growth, and socialization (p. 56). Enrolling both new resident and incumbent families ($n = 19$), this project combined elements of the traditional support group and an orientation group. Running three times over 15 months, a curriculum of six topics was developed that assisted families with recognition of the resident's need, developed strategies to deal with both the family's own needs and those of the resident, heightened awareness of their own responses, and provided an opportunity to share experiences and expertise.

An interesting component of the project was the addition of a social work student who independently visited residents and developed specific activities that contributed positively towards visiting and passed these on to families in the support group. In postintervention questioning, families rated as most positive: information sharing regarding Medicare and Medicaid rules, information about dementia and medication, and appropriate activities for a visit. Despite self-rated decline in their resident's health during the months the group was held, members reported less guilt associated with nursing home placement, found visiting easier after group participation, and reported a greater understanding of their loved one's situation. Thus, this small study showed that the family support group continues to have benefits for families even during the resident's progressive decline. With innovative additions, such as social work or recreational therapy assistance for determining ways to interact with residents, the positive interaction between family and resident can be preserved or augmented.

RESIDENT SUPPORT GROUPS

These groups take many forms depending on level of functioning, cognition, specialized needs, and interests. While the most familiar types of support groups may be disease related such as dementia or stroke groups, in keeping with Atchley's (1999) model, continuation of former groups can be established within a long-term care community. Mosher-Ashley and Rabon (2001) compared differences between older and younger persons (n = 160) attending Alcoholics Anonymous (AA) meetings using measures of emotional support, depression, loneliness, and life satisfaction. Dividing the participants into three groups for analysis, the oldest group (65+) was found to have the lowest depressive symptoms and the greatest life satisfaction, which the investigators attributed to many years of sobriety—a positive accomplishment. When long-term sober alcoholics (n = 17) were asked to explain why they

still participated in AA meetings after 10 to 36 years of sobriety, an analysis of responses using a constant comparative method showed four primary themes that mirrored the AA mission: social, spiritual, service, and support (Osborne, 2003). The investigators described the diverse participants as "people of remembrance" and as such choose to keep in touch with their past while adapting to change, reinforcing the continuity model. Adding further support to the ongoing need for sobriety support groups in older age is a study by Vaillant (2003) who followed two groups of males (n = 194), college students and inner-city adolescents who met DSM-III criteria for alcohol abuse from 1940 to the present. At age 70, chronic alcohol dependence was rare with only 12% of the college students and 10.5% of the adolescents still abusing alcohol. For those abstaining, the best predictor of sobriety was continued AA attendance. Twelve-step groups may have a real place within long-term care facilities as many residents may be in recovery and find that participation in groups such as AA offers a chance for continued socialization, affirmation of shared values, and positive self-esteem.

While a number of therapeutic groups are offered in long-term care facilities, the critical differential between them and leisure activities is the overall objective. For example, if a music program is planned as a form of reminiscence therapy to meet the needs of preselected residents or if it is a sing-along with all invited, the goals are very different; the former is therapeutic, the latter is an activity. Rehabilitation professionals in the areas of recreation, art, music, movement, and drama therapy have expertise in the assessment of resident needs based on an evidence-based model; they will determine short- and long-term goals and then devise a plan of care with measurable objectives that may include therapeutic group work as part of their interventions. Therapeutic groups require skilled professionals with expertise in the modality, as they will need to adapt the group process and the context of the group to meet the needs of participants as sessions evolve (Carter, Andel, & Robb, 2003). Minimization of these modalities into simple activities that para- or nonprofessional staff can accomplish undermines the therapeutic goals.

One of the most common therapeutic modalities used in long-term care is music therapy, as it has repeatedly been shown to be effective as a positive influence on depression and in changing behavior in persons with Alzheimer's disease. **Figure 24–1** shows a group combining music therapy with exercise. For example, within an adult day care center among persons with moderate cognitive impairments, a therapeutic music group reduced agitation as measured by the Cohen-Mansfield Agitation Inventory (Jennings & Vance, 2002). However, in a critical review of studies that proposed to examine the influence of music therapy sessions on persons with dementia, Lou (2001) recommends the longitudinal biopsychosocial effects of music on this population be investigated rather than short-term outcomes. This valid critique must be tempered with the knowledge that dementia is a progressive disease, and if residents are studied for longer periods, it may be harder for investigators to tease out the effects of longer exposure to the intervention and affects of brain deterioration.

Eden Alternative

A recent paradigm that has received much attention in long-term care is the Eden Alternative—a model developed out of funding from the New York State Department of Health in the early 1990s. Thomas (1996), who received the original grant and has since trademarked the model, posited that life for residents of nursing homes was marked by loneliness, helplessness, and boredom. He went on to re-create a homelike environment through the use of environmental adaptations—plants, animals, and children; staff education; and empowerment of direct care-giving staff and residents. Many facilities adopted the Eden

Alternative while evidence of its effectiveness was viewed skeptically by some as outcomes were noted in studies that used subjective measures (Hinman & Heyl, 2002; Ruckdeschel & Van Haitsma, 2001). One study (Coleman et al., 2002) showed no improvement in resident outcomes and a slight improvement in staff retention, while several (Barba, Tesh, & Courts, 2002; Bergenman-Evans, 2004) reported positive data on resident outcomes. One of the principles of the model is that there is a minimization of group activities and a spontaneous environment is promoted (Thomas). As such, the Eden Alternative deemphasizes the use of groups for either therapeutic or support purposes and proposes that these groups should spring from the wishes of residents—an idea that lacks authenticity, especially in the face of years of research that supports group work as a meaningful modality to promote change and adaptation. While most would agree that a homelike environment is better than a sterile institution, further research is needed before valid methods such as professionally organized and led group work are dismissed in long-term care facilities.

Life Patterns

Residents' Councils and Family Councils

Two groups that fall into life patterns include those that deal with the resident's and family's adjustment to and control over their lives and socialization. Two of the longest-standing groups within long-term care facilities are the residents' council and the family council; often having mutual goals, they will be considered together. The federal government actually requires those agencies receiving Medicare and Medicaid funding to support these activities: "The facility must provide a resident or family group, if one exists, with private space" (Code of Federal Regulations, 2003). Most states require resident and family councils and have regulations governing those members of the agency, usually administrative, who will be responsible to the councils and accountable for enacting recommendations. New York State, for example, requires each facility to provide the space for a "family and friends council" to meet. Staff and visitors must be allowed to attend. Legislation also requires designation of a person who will provide assistance to the group and respond to written requests from the group (Friends and Relatives of the Institutionalized Aged, 2003).

The goal of both residents and family councils is usually to provide a means for both groups to influence the management of the long-term care facility in a democratic forum (Safford, 1994). These councils are often a conduit for information from the stakeholders to administration and back, but may also serve as a way to organize the life of the facility through social events and celebrations. The organization of the councils may be strictly or loosely run; however, the leadership is usually elected from among the interested parties and usually holds office for a specified period of time.

Having an organizational structure that allows for accountability as well as a way of recording information to ensure that grievances raised are addressed compels the usual committee structure of chair, vice or cochair, and secretary. Because fund-raising is usually not an expectation of these committees, having a treasurer may be optional. To ensure representation for residents who may be away from the facility or have health problems, it is often useful to have alternates chosen for leadership positions. Many times these councils follow parliamentary procedure as outlined in texts such as *Robert's Rules of Order* (Robert, Evans, Honemann, & Balch, 2000). A health care group leader, often a social worker or recreation therapist, may need to coach both residents and families in appropriate ways to report problems using the chain of command as well as dealing with routine business. It may be advantageous to include someone from the ombudsman office as a yearly visitor to these

groups so members can be informed of ways to report serious problems. The National Long-term Care Ombudsman Resource Center Web site provides a listing of all state ombudsman programs. See http://www.ltcombudsman.org/static_pages/ombudsmen.cfm. A listing of national advocacy groups that can assist families and residents in the governance of facilities is found in **Table 24–1**. Many of these organizations have either an e-mail list or chat rooms where families or residents can find information and support—offering a virtual group of the 21st century!

Preadmission and Orientation Groups

These groups are sometimes differentiated from formal support groups as they usually have set goals and a rather fixed agenda. Often managed by marketing staff, these groups familiarize new residents and families with the facility and its routines and answer any questions. New social contacts can be fostered while residents and their families adapt to change in another network. Policies can be explained so that anxiety is lessened and expectations are made clear. It is recommended that the orientation group meet at least twice at the convenience of the families, so residents who are adjusting to the facility have time to formulate questions and are able to begin integration (Safford, 1994). If key persons within the organization can be present for introductions and questions, the residents and families become aware of the entire community and the commitment of the facility to improving the quality of life of all residents.

Health

Although health promotion has been a critical goal in community and primary care, the management of acute and chronic disease was formerly the goal of most long-term care facilities that offered services to the frail older adult. With the

Table 24-1 Virtual Groups Sponsored by Advocacy Organizations*

Caregiver.com		http://www.caregivers.com
Children of Aging Parents (CAPS)	(800) 227-7294	http://www.CAPS4caregivers.org
ElderCare Online		http://www.ec-online.net
Family Caregiver Alliance	(800) 445-8106	http://www.caregiver.org
Friends and Relatives of Institutionalized Aged (focus is on New York state but is an excellent resource and long-standing advocacy group)	(212) 732-5667	http://www.fria.org/contact_us.html
National Family Caregivers Association	(800) 896-3650	http://www.nfcacares.org
Well Spouse Foundation	(800) 838-0879	http://www.wellspouse.org

* All Web addresses verified 6/17/04.

continuum of long-term care expanding, health promotion and self-care management of chronic illnesses become more important as older adults become more active participants in their own health care. Health groups have become a new paradigm for long-term care facilities.

Tobacco Cessation

Tobacco cessation provides an excellent model of a health-related intervention that is amenable to group work. In a recent study commissioned by the Center for Social Gerontology (2001), a focus group of white and African-American older adults described lifelong tobacco use habits that started, for most, around age 10—this translated to a range of 50 to 70 "pack years" of smoking for most of these individuals. While their rationale for starting tobacco use was the usually sited factors—peer pressure and desire to improve self-image—a few from this cohort were actually encouraged in tobacco use by their physicians to help "calm their nerves" or lose weight. Although those who were in contact with other persons and children gave reducing second-hand smoke exposure as a reason to curtail or quit smoking, the primary reason these older adults wished to quit was for their own health. Barriers to quitting smoking included: fear of gaining weight, lack of will power, lack of awareness of helpful resources, and disbelief that tobacco cessation products really worked. Facilitators of smoking cessation were

Figure 24-1 Promoting Health Through Exercise

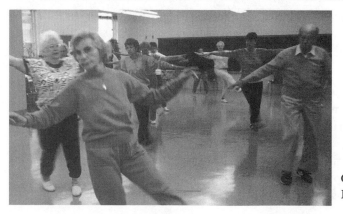

Courtesy of Bill Branson/National Cancer Institute.

willingness to change and a desire to feel and become more healthy, and knowing someone who had died from a tobacco-related illness—an unarguable reality in this age group. Armed with data from this study and information from the Smoking Cessation, Quality of Life and Older Persons Web site as well as techniques for group work outlined in the American Lung Association's "Quit Smoking" Web pages (2004), a group leader could initiate a successful age-appropriate tobacco cessation group in a CCRC or ALF.

Change of lifelong behaviors that fail to promote health may not be as difficult to achieve among long-term residents as many stereotypes suggest: you can teach an old dog new tricks! Using Atchley's model or one of the change models that are being successfully used in health care settings, such as the Transtheoretical Stages of Change (Prochaska, 2003; Prochaska, Velicer, Prochaska, & Johnson, 2004), which has been used for smoking cessation, decreasing weight in persons with diabetes, and decreasing risky behaviors, the group leader could initiate a very positive gathering of older adults who wish to take on this challenge. As the cohort of older adults who will enter long-term care facilities in the near future begins to change from passive receivers of health care to advocates for self-management of health, health groups could become as popular a method of group work for health professionals as caregiver support groups are today. In fact, health groups composed of caregivers themselves might actively take on health goals rather than just referring participants to other agencies for managing these issues.

Summary

Using Atchley's continuity theory to address lifelong change, group work within long-term care facilities is moving proactively to address change in the later stages of life. Whether groups deal with mental patterns, life patterns, or health, the professional leader is challenged to involve participants in decision making, developing plans, and evaluating results so that change will promote the highest quality of life. New paradigms should be considered in group work, such as health groups for residents and caregivers, continuation of former groups such as 12-step programs, groups for formal caregivers, and referral to virtual online groups. In a time of decreasing resources, it is important for group leaders to ensure that the groups they lead are evidence based and are achieving the desired outcomes, as well as to advocate for continued group work as essential to the fiber of long-term care communities.

Exercises

EXERCISE 1

Contact 12-step programs in your area to see if any currently have groups within CCRCs or ALFs and whether they would consider starting a group in one of these facilities.

EXERCISE 2

Join an online discussion group in one of the virtual support groups given in **Table 24–1** to determine how the topics discussed may be different from and similar to group discussions within facilities. Note common themes.

EXERCISE 3

Using one of the therapeutic methods discussed in other chapters (e.g., guided autobiography in Chapter 15), consider how the group process might change across settings from CCRC to SNF.

EXERCISE 4

Attend a residents' council or family council meeting in a long-term care facility and attempt to determine if outcomes achieved through this group methodology were more effective than those achieved through individual efforts.

EXERCISE 5

Become familiar with the legislation in your state regarding the requirements for these groups and their administrative accountability to the councils.

References

American Lung Association. (2004). Quit smoking. Retrieved July 17, 2004, from *http://www.lungusa.org/site/pp.asp?c=dvLUK900E&b =33484*

Atchley, R. (1999). *Continuity and adaptation in aging: Creating positive experiences*. Baltimore: Johns Hopkins Press.

Barba, B. E., Tesh, A. S. & Courts, N. F. (2002). Promoting thriving in nursing homes: the Eden Alternative. *Journal of Gerontological Nursing, 28*(3), 7–13.

Barusch, A. S., & Peak, T. (1997). Support groups for older men: Building on strengths and facilitating relationships. In J. Kosberg & L. Kaye (Eds.), *Elderly men: Special problems and professional challenges* (pp. 262–278). New York: Springer.

Bergman-Evans, B. (2004). Beyond the basics: Effects of the Eden alternative model on quality of life issues. *Journal of Gerontological Nursing, 30*(6), 27–34.

Burack, O. R., & Chichin, E. R. (2001). A support group for nursing assistants. *Geriatric Nursing, 22*(6), 299–307.

California Advocates for Nursing Home Reform. (2004). What you need to know about residential care facilities. Retrieved July 17, 2004, from *http://www.canhr.org/RCFE/RCFEfactsheets/rcfe_needtoknow_fs.htm*

Campbell, J. M., & Linc, L. G. (1996). Support groups for visitors of residents in nursing homes. *Journal of Gerontological Nursing, 22*(2), 30–35, 54–55.

Carter, M. J., Andel, G. E., & Robb, G. M. (2003). *Therapeutic recreation: A practical approach*. Prospect Heights, IL: Waveland Press.

Centers for Medicare and Medicaid. (2004, March 31). MDS Active Resident Count Report. Retrieved July 17, 2004, from *http://www.cms.hhs.gov/states/mdsreports/rescnt.asp?date=6*

Center for Social Gerontology, University of Michigan (2001). Tobacco cessation program research: Focus group research report. Retrieved July, 17, 2004, from *http://www.tcsg.org/tobacco/BPCSG-Report_01.pdf*

Chichin, E. R., Burback, O. R., Olson, E., & Likourezos, A. (2000). *End-of-life ethics and the nursing assistant*. New York: Springer.

Code of Federal Regulations. (2003). Title 12, Volume 1 CITE: 42CFR483.15, 512-513.

Coleman, M. T., Looney, S., O'Brien, J., Ziegler, C., Pastorino, C. A., & Turner, C. (2002). The Eden alternative: Findings after one year of implementation. *Journals of Gerontology Series A-Biological Sciences & Medical Sciences, 57A*(7), M422–427.

Friends and Relatives of the Institutionalized Aged. (2003). Family organizations. Retrieved July 17, 2004, from *http://www.fria.org/consumers_family.html*

Hinman, M. R., & Heyl, D. M. (2002). Influence of the Eden alternative on the functional status of nursing home residents. *Physical & Occupational Therapy in Geriatrics, 20*(2), 1–20.

Jennings, B., & Vance, D. (2002). The short-term effects of music therapy on different types of agitation in adults with Alzheimer's. *Activities, Adaptation & Aging, 26*(4), 27–33.

Lou, M. (2001). The use of music to decrease agitated behaviour of the demented elderly: The state of the science. *Scandinavian Journal of Caring Sciences, 15*(2), 165–173.

Mosher-Ashley, P., & Rabon, C. E. (2001). A comparison of older and younger adults attending Alcoholics Anonymous. *Clinical Gerontologist, 24*(1-2), 27–38.

Osborne, E. (2003). Why do people with long-term sobriety continue to participate in Alcoholics Anonymous? *Dissertation Abstracts International, 62*(2A). (95015–95050).

Peak, T. (2000). Families and the nursing home environment: Adaptation in a group context. *Journal of Gerontological Social Work, 33*(1), 51–66.

Prochaska, J. O. (2003). Staging: A revolution in helping people change. *Managed Care, 12*(9 Suppl.), 6–9.

Prochaska, J. O., Velicer, W. F., Prochaska, J. M., & Johnson, J. L. (2004). Size, consistency, and stability of stage effects for smoking cessation. *Addictive Behaviors, 29*(1), 207–213.

Robert, H. M., Evans, W. J., Honemann, D. H., & Balch, T. J. (2000). *Robert's Rules of Order* (10th ed.). Cambridge, MA: Perseus.

Ruckdeschel, K., & Van Haitsma, K. (2001). The impacts of live-in animals and plants on nursing home residents: A pilot longitudinal investigation. *Alzheimer's Care Quarterly, 2*(4), 17–27.

Safford, F. (1994). Group work in long-term care. In I. Burnside & M. G. Schmidt (Eds.), *Working with older adults: Group process and techniques* (3rd ed. pp. 227–239). Boston: Jones & Bartlett.

Title 42-Public Health, Chapter IV-CMS. Requirements for states and long term care facilities. Subpart B - Requirements for Long Term Care Facilities: Sec. 483.15 Quality of life c.3. U.S. Government Printing Office.

Thomas, W. H. (1996). *Life worth living*. Acton, MA: Vander Wyk & Burnham.

U.S. Census Bureau. (2004). 2002 NAICS Definitions: 623 Nursing and Residential CareFacilities. Retrieved July 17, 2004, from *http://www.census.gov/epcd/naics02/def/NDEF623.HTM*

Vaillant, G. (2003). A 60-year follow-up of alcoholic men. *Addiction,* 98(8), 1043–1051.

Chapter 25

Groups for Older Persons in Acute Care Settings

Barbara J. Edlund
Nancy J. Finch

Key Words

- Information
- Psychoeducation
- Support
- Caregiver
- Partnerships
- Telehealth
- Self-help
- Web-based

Learning Objectives

- Discuss the role of groups in the acute care setting, identifying at least four types of groups appropriate for older persons in acute care settings
- Describe two considerations for groups of older persons in the following areas: size of group, length of group meeting, frequency of meetings
- Discuss common considerations in conducting groups of older persons
- List four important qualities of the nurse who leads groups of older persons
- Note at least two inclusion criteria and two exclusion criteria for groups of older persons in acute care settings

Currently, older adults are hospitalized more frequently and suffer more chronic diseases than any other age group (Cotter & Strumpf, 2002). Hospitalizations in the acute care environment are primarily for scheduled surgeries and the management of complications from a chronic illness diagnosis. Group settings, for the purposes of education and support, have long been used to assist patients in managing emotional stress and adjusting to chronic illnesses. Consequently, the concept of using "self-help groups" to support and meet the needs of a congruent group of patients is not a new one (Shepherd et al., 1999). Over the last decade, however, the traditional format of groups in the acute care setting has waned because of the shortened length of stays and the more severe acuity level of patients. Nurses, believing that group work is an effective treatment modality for older adults, struggle with maintaining groups in a rapidly changing health care environment.

In light of these changes, there is a need to review the traditional format of groups for older adults in the acute care setting and modify as well as develop nontraditional alternatives for this therapeutic modality. This chapter discusses the role of groups in the acute care setting, the movement from more traditional to nontraditional group offerings and the benefits of maintaining this therapeutic modality in the overall care of the hospitalized older adult.

Overview

Articles and books about groups for older persons cover a wide range of topics: types of groups, advantages, outcomes, and recommendations. Therapeutic groups emerged in the early 1900s as a means of addressing psychological problems (Klemm et al., 2003) and include groups focused on education, self-help, psychoeducation, and support groups for both patients and caregivers (Peak, Toseland, & Banks, 1995). Therapeutic groups are now common as individuals, caregivers, and families organize themselves to solve their own problems.

Over the last several decades, more has been written about groups for older adults in the acute care setting. There are advantages to groups: time economy, older persons are less afraid in groups, other group members rather than a powerful group leader can provide support, loneliness can be decreased by feeling acceptance from the group members, and members can identify with others. Groups offer social support providing participants with a sense of security, an opportunity to share experiences and concerns, and increased worthiness and belonging. This sense of belonging and security often enables older adults to respond better in groups than as individuals. Groups can decrease the negative effects of institutionalization because they are viewed as safe settings for patients to model or try new behaviors.

In a study of elderly veterans and their caregivers, researchers found that those veterans receiving care and whose wives participated in a support group had lower health care costs in both the inpatient and outpatient settings. This resulted in total cost savings for the care recipient (Peak, Toseland, & Banks, 1995) by decreasing complications and readmissions to the acute care setting.

The benefits of including a therapeutic group in the recovery of a hospitalized older adult are well documented. The changing health care environment with shorter hospital stays, however, has necessitated that nurses, in many instances modify the traditional group format to include more nontraditional offerings to better meet patient needs. The inpatient unit still remains the point of contact for informing the patient and family of the existence and benefits of participating in a therapeutic group specific to the health problem of the individual. In the past, the patient may have attended several sessions before being discharged, now a patient often begins the group work after discharge in the outpatient clinic setting.

More recently, advances in technology have made it possible to offer nontraditional forms of support to meet patient needs. For example, online (e.g., Internet, computer mediated) cancer support groups provide information, personal and professional support, shared experience, and patient advocacy (Madara & White, 1997). In this instance, the nurse introduces the patient to this form of support while still in the hospital. Booklets with instructions can be given to patients interested in participating in this method of support after discharge. In addition, a demonstration by the nurse on the clinical unit on how to access Web sites for information can be included (Bowles & Dansky, 2002).

Telehealth with the use of videophone technology provides another option for patient and caregiver education and support. Through this method, a nurse in the inpatient or outpatient setting communicates via interactive videophone with homebound patients to provide information and assist patients and families to manage symptoms and cope with the disease and its treatment (Dimmick, Mustaleski, Burgiss, & Welsh, 2000). The benefits of these innovative nontraditional methods of offering group support are that of avoiding some of the pitfalls of traditional support groups such as inconvenient times, distance from the hospital or outpatient clinic, transportation, and child care concerns (Finfgeld, 2000; Oravec, 2000). Ultimately, the patient benefits from having choices to participate in either a traditional or nontraditional support group option or a combination of both.

Types of Groups for Acute Care Settings

There are a number of types of groups in which older adults may participate in the acute care setting. The following sections describe these groups and their defining characteristics.

Educational Groups

The goal of an educational group is to provide information. The nurse leader is able to educate more individuals more efficiently using a group format. The members become co-teachers in the group as they share information and experiences (Webster & Austin, 1999). Hospitals often employ a specific nurse designated to coordinate patient education. The coordinator partners with staff nurses to provide needed information and resources for patients. The goal of teaching facilitates patient self-management.

Psychoeducational Groups

The goal of a psychoeducational group is to develop coping skills through learning about the disease and its treatment. This group is similar to the educational group in imparting information, however, a skilled nurse leader assists patients with improving problem-focused coping skills for successful community living. Group meetings are frequently characterized by a focus on the concerns of individual members who take turns receiving assistance from the group (McCallion & Toseland, 1995). Psychoeducational groups are characterized by an expectation of a high level of self-disclosure, and for this reason such groups may be closed to new members once the group has started (Sundeen, 2001). This is done to encourage the development of intimacy and feelings of safety and comfort as members share personal successes and difficulties coping with a particular health problem. However, the issue of whether a group of this type is closed or open to new members is subject to discussion.

Self-Help Groups

The goal of a self-help group is for lay members to share common experiences, work together to gain control over their lives, express empathy and support for one another, and use their strengths to gain control over their lives (Murray, 1996). These types of groups can deal with a variety of personal, social, and medical problems. This type of support group is led by a member elected by the group or is self-appointed by virtue of being the one who brought the group together. Self-help groups may occur in an outpatient setting as patients come for treatment or in follow-up appointments after discharge from the hospital (Lieberman, 1988).

Support Groups

The goal of a support group is to help members cope with the stresses associated with living with a particular disease and to sustain and enhance their coping abilities. Members participate at their own pace. Members give and take as they interact with other members. A lay group member leads this type of group. Psychological closeness is encouraged by the knowledge that members share similar concerns that are often not well understood by others. The group serves as a resource for social contacts and an informal network for social support (Stuart & Laraia, 2001). Support groups assist individuals to cope with a particular health problem. They differ from psychoeducational groups in that the latter assist individuals experiencing problems in coping with the illness situation and are led by a skilled professional. A number of writers classify support groups as a type of psychoeducational group because teaching, self-disclosure, and skill building also occur. The reader should not get bogged down in the various definitions of groups but recognize what is needed in a particular situation and who can best facilitate the group to meet the needs of patients and their families. Support groups exist for caregivers of a patient as well as for the patients themselves.

CAREGIVER SUPPORT GROUPS

The goal of a caregiver support group is to help caregivers cope with the stresses of caregiving and to sustain and enhance their coping abilities. During sessions, members are encouraged to listen empathetically, support each other, give and receive advice about effective coping strategies, share ways to manage physical problems, and provide each other with hope (McCallion & Toseland, 1996). Caregiver support groups can reduce caregiver stress, decrease depression, and mobilize support systems among the family and community (Wright, Bennet, & Gramling, 1998). In addition, telephone interventions have assisted family caregivers to develop problem-solving techniques (Davis, 1998; Grant, Elliott, Giger, & Bartolucci, 2001).

Telehealth

The goal of telehealth support groups is to provide information and support to participants simultaneously at two or more different locations. A variety of mechanisms of telecommunications such as telephones, computers, videophones, interactive videos, and teleconferencing are used (Dimmick, Mustaleski, Burgiss, & Welsh, 2000). "The strength and promise of telehealth lies in providing increased access to health care services by augmenting existing services, not replacing them" (American Nurses Association, 2004).

WEB-BASED GROUPS

The goal of online (e.g., Internet, computer mediated) support groups is to provide information, personal and professional support, shared experiences, and patient advocacy (Klemm et al., 2003). Online support offers 24-hour access, anonymity, and information. This method avoids the visual distraction of age, gender, and social status while allowing patient and caregiver to access information in the comfort and privacy of the home (Madara & White, 1997).

The disadvantages of telehealth and Web-based groups are that some older adults may be afraid of the technology and are overwhelmed by what they have to learn. The initial cost of equipment for the hospital or clinic as well as the patient may be too high. While older adults may have computers in their homes, they may not have the needed program to access the group being offered. Some videophones run off the TV screen, but participants in this format can only see the group leader and not the other members of the group. This is done to maintain confidentiality. For those older adults who prefer the familiarity of the group setting and immediate social support, telehealth and Web-based support groups do not meet this need. However, for those older adults who are homebound and familiar with computer technology or are not afraid to learn, these nontraditional approaches are a lifeline linking patients and their caregivers to others with similar problems and needs (Finkelstein, Speedie, Lundgren, Demiris, & Ideker, 2001).

Patient Population Groups in the Acute Care Setting

Cancer, heart disease, and stroke are among the leading causes of morbidity and mortality among older adults. Groups in the acute care setting have for some time assisted both older patients and their families to deal with the physical and psychosocial concerns related to these major health problems. Examples of specific patient groups for older adults in the acute care setting are discussed in the following sections.

Groups for Cardiac Patients

Groups for cardiac patients are well documented in the literature. Clearly, patients benefit from education about their conditions from structured group support. For example, cardiac rehabilitation is a structured process that begins with a cardiac event and continues throughout life. Cardiac rehabilitation is available to individuals who have coronary artery disease and who have experienced a coronary event. Emphasis is placed on making lifestyle changes to prevent further disease and complications.

Cardiac support groups have been used as an intervention to cope with depression following a myocardial infarction (MI). Psychological distress, such as anxiety, anger, fear of death, loss of control, and problems with interpersonal relationships, has been described in patients following an MI (Warren & Whall, 2001; Carney et al., 1997). Frasure-Smith and colleagues (1995) found that major depression was related to a seven- to eight-fold increase in mortality 18 months following an MI. Warren and Whall (2001) describe a support group intervention developed to help MI survivors cope with depression. Although the outcomes were not systematically measured, anecdotally, both patients and family members verbalized feelings of distress, found support, and reported feeling less alone.

A nurse-facilitated support group for cardiac rehabilitation clients was conducted over a 20-week period (Eakes, Mayo, & Whicker, 1997). This support group pilot program gave participants a forum in which to both give and receive support as they undertook dramatic lifestyle changes. The high level of compliance evidenced by the rate of attendance at the weekly sessions was considered an indication of the value members placed on the support group.

Sudden cardiac death (SCD) is a major health problem in the United States. Life for such patients after an implantable cardioverter defibrillator (ICD) includes many difficulties in adaptation. Patients identified physical concerns about the sensation of being shocked, medications, difficulty sleeping, as well as psychological concerns about fear, changes in mental functioning, changes in lifestyle, loss of control, driving, and spousal overprotectiveness (Doolittle & Suave, 1995; Sneed & Finch, 1992). Patients with an ICD may have severe anxiety about the fear of future shocks and depression after experiencing ICD shocks (Bourke, Turkington, Thomas, McComb, & Tynan, 1997; Hegel, Griegel, Black, Goulden, & Ozahowski, 1997).

Support groups for ICD implantation are beneficial in reducing stress and enhancing adjustment and are recommended for family-focused interventions (Dougherty, 1997). Qualitative reports from patients and their spouses after support group intervention indicated positive adjustment to the device, improved ability to cope, and increased satisfaction with life (Badger & Morris, 1989; Molchany & Peterson, 1994; Sneed, Finch, & Michel, 1997). Lastly, the support group offers help in coping with the possibility of death through the therapeutic friendships established in the group.

In peer-support groups, activities are built on peer support. The groups are led by persons who have had experience with the same diagnoses, but professionals may be involved as well. Johansson (1998) describes peer-support groups for individuals with heart disease. For example, an exercise physiologist may conduct classes related to structured physical activity or professional lectures given by nurses or dietitians on nutrition may address the benefits of healthy eating. Nevertheless, all of the groups can be considered peer support because the mutual aid component is strong (Shepard et al., 1999).

Participation in a support group after a cardiac event was reported by Hildingh and Fridlund (2003). Patients who participated in a special program of support through group activities and education had increased their physical activities and eventually stopped smoking. Because of the positive outcomes, the researchers recommended the use of peer-support groups as a support strategy in long-term rehabilitation after a cardiac event.

Groups for Cancer Patients

Groups for cancer patients and their families have existed for almost 30 years and were first reported in the 1970s (Klemm et al., 2003). These groups have been diagnosis specific or have dealt with general treatment issues and are coping with cancer.

Participation in a support group may foster hope, offer emotional support and confidence, and allay psychological problems and physical concerns (Liberman, 1988). Among patients with cancer, participation in self-help groups may provide new coping strategies and result in a lower depression rate and a decrease in anxiety and mental exhaustion (Chelser & Chesney, 1995; Cope, 1995; Gray, Fitch, Davis, & Phillips, 1997).

More recently, cancer patients have utilized the Internet as a means of support and the number of Internet cancer support groups has risen dramatically (Madara & White, 1997). Several studies have reported on the benefit of videophones in the self-management of elderly persons with cancer and other chronic diseases (Rooney, Studenshi, & Roman, 1997). This form of telehealth has been associated with an improvement in quality of life for patients (Dimmick, Mustaleski, Burgiss, & Welsh, 2000).

Groups for Patients in Rehabilitation

Stroke is the third leading cause of death in the United States. It is the principal cause of severe, long-term disability (American Heart Association, 2004). Stroke patients now go home before they have reached their rehabilitation potential. Many of these individuals need assistance with activities of daily living, household management, and transportation. Greater responsibility has fallen on family caregivers to provide this help and support services. Approximately 80% of stroke survivors rely on family caregivers to continue rehabilitation through home-based programs (Family Caregiving Statistics, 2004).

Although the caregiving experience can have many positive aspects, it can also have negative physical and psychological consequences. Caregivers report problems with depression, sleeplessness, back pain, headaches, stomach disorders, and, more frequently, loneliness and isolation (Chenier, 1997; Ostwald, 1997). A study by Bakas and colleagues (2002) found that caregivers of stroke survivors expressed needs and concerns in five major areas: information, emotions and behaviors, physical care, instrumental care, and personal responses to caregiving. Web-based support groups and nurse specialists available online to answer questions and provide information for caregiver's of stroke survivors are cited as very helpful to long-term rehabilitation (Steiner & Pierce, 2002).

Tran and colleagues (2002) used videophone technology to offer instructional and emotional support to homebound caregivers of stroke patients. This method demonstrated a cost-effective approach to providing support for caregivers and allows them to achieve the best long-term outcomes for the stroke patient in the home (Gresham, Duncan, & Stason, 1995).

Developing a New Group: An Example

Background

Approval of implantable cardioverter defibrillators (ICD) by the Food and Drug Administration occurred in 1985. The early literature following implantation focused on the medical complications of this life-saving device. Little was known, however, about how individuals adjusted to living with the device and what interventions were helpful in assisting patients and their families with this adjustment. Two advanced practice nurses, one expert in cardiology and the other a nurse faculty researcher with cardiac expertise, discussed the need to learn more about the adjustment and needs of individuals with an ICD. They used a focus group methodology to determine if there was a need for a therapeutic group for this patient population.

Focus groups were useful techniques to investigate specific needs of this patient population. Focus groups allowed the nurses to get close to the participants' understanding of their needs and to learn about their experiences and perspectives. The results of several focus groups held with patients and their families documented the need for a therapeutic group and led to the development of an ICD support group (Sneed & Finch, 1992). In the focus groups, patients expressed fear, anxiety, loss of control, and loss of independence as a result of living with the device. In addition, they expressed the fear of being shocked (which did occur early in the technology of this implantable device but now is less of a concern because of technological advances), fear of death, loss of self-esteem, pain, problems sleeping, depression, and worry because few health care workers knew about the device. Further, patients indicated they were not able to drive because of the danger of being shocked with the implanted device. This posed problems and was a great inconvenience. Spouses also had similar issues but, in addition, worried about role changes within the family and how family members would react. They also expressed the need to be very protective of their spouse, some expressed being too overprotective. This valuable information from patients and families provided the impetus for developing a patient and family ICD support group.

Planning the Group

With the need clearly documented, the advanced practice nurses developed a survey to assess interest, commitment to attend, preferable times and day of the week, and number of sessions per month. Patients in the hospital received the survey and were asked to complete it. The survey was also mailed to former patients who were presently being followed in the outpatient clinic. Inclusion criteria for group participation included patients with an ICD and their family members and caregivers.

The information from the survey was helpful in planning the day and time of the support group. The ICD clinic was held every Monday in the Outpatient Department. The decision was made to hold the support group an hour before the start of clinic and to hold the support group twice a month to reach as many patients and their families as possible. The advanced practice nurses then reviewed the literature on group process and met with a psychiatric liaison nurse to review group process and structuring a group. They discussed the role of a group facilitator and the benefits of a coleader. They became familiar with Yalom's curative factors in group work. These include altruism, cohesiveness, learning, guidance, catharsis, identification, insight, hope, and existential factors (Yalom, 1983). These factors promote the participants' development of more adaptive patterns of behavior (see Chapter 4).

They reviewed the ground rules for conducting a group as well as the length of sessions, room accommodations (especially for those patients in wheelchairs), access to parking, and food for the support group sessions. The nurses explored how to manage conflict in the group, deal with a disruptive member, and how to handle emotions. The psychiatric liaison nurse was extremely helpful and knowledgeable about conducting groups. While the advanced practice nurses knew about group process, they had never conducted a support group for patients and their families.

Planning with a coleader from the beginning was very helpful. Ideally, one facilitator should have experience with group process and group dynamics and the other be an expert in caring for that population. In acute care settings today, it may be difficult to utilize nursing staff as facilitators because of the high acuity of patients. Also, many nursing units are experiencing retention issues and high turnover rates due to the shortage of nurses. Shared leadership for conducting groups or a rotating team approach may be more feasible today given heavy workloads and the nature of the acute care setting.

The advanced practice nurses also reviewed the qualities of a good leader working with older adults in a group. These included caring about older people, respecting older people, and possessing an ability and desire to learn from older people. Furthermore, leading a group of older adults in the acute care setting requires an understanding of the biological aspects of aging. Further, it requires patience, sensitivity, and a commitment to the important work of the group. In addition, communication with the other members of the health care team was important so that they were informed of the group's purpose and supported its efforts.

Groups for older adults have some unique aspects. The nurse leaders recognized that group members may need assistance or transportation getting to a group. The nurse leaders also realized group members were dealing with multiple health problems and that it was important to help members keep their expectations realistic. The leaders also knew that group members could become ill, deteriorate, or die, and the remaining members would need to deal with this. In addition, shorter well-planned sessions benefit the frail elderly who may tire easily. Further, group leaders may have to use a small portable microphone to be heard in the group setting as well as plan for some assistive devices to aid those members with hearing deficits.

Conducting the Group

The first meeting of the support group was held on the first Monday of the month, an hour before the clinic appointments began in a conference room. The session conducted by the advanced practice nurse with expertise in cardiology lasted for one hour. The nurse coleader was present as well. Five patients and their caregivers attended. Introductions were made at the beginning of the session. Patients indicated how long they had the device. In addition, they discussed their issues or concerns and any signs or symptoms they were experiencing. A number of the patients told of their experience receiving a shock and how many times this had occurred. The group continued to meet twice a month on the first and third Mondays of the month with an average attendance of four to six patients and their caregivers in the conference room in the clinic. Light refreshments were served at group meetings.

As the group membership grew (10–20 patients and caregivers), the meeting was moved from the conference room to a large waiting room in the clinic. Also, patients soon took a more active role in the leadership of the group. Initially, the patients took turns sharing the leadership role with the nurse. Eventually two patients shared the leadership role so that by the end of the first year of the support group, the support group was totally patient led. Patients handled the conflicts within the groups themselves and rarely was the nurse leader required to intervene. The nurses sought informal feedback from the patients and caregivers as to how the group was going and whether it was meeting their needs. The responses were overwhelmingly positive. As the group continued to meet, many patients came only once and told their story. This experience validated for them that others were like them and that they would be "okay" too. Over time, refreshments were omitted at the suggestion of the groups and only coffee was served.

Early in the third year of the group, the need emerged to have separate groups for patients and caregivers for some period of time during the one hour meeting. Clearly caregivers had some different issues than the family member for whom they were providing care. To address this need the first half of the meeting included all in attendance. During the second half of the hour caregivers and patients split into smaller groups. One of the advanced practice nurses attended each of the groups.

As technology and the needs of patients changed, the group sessions were held only once a month. The monthly meetings alternated between a social format and an educational format with guest speakers. The attendance at the meetings varied with more patients and caregivers attending the educational monthly meeting. At the annual December meeting, a Christmas luncheon sponsored by the pacemaker vendors was provided for the support group. At this meeting a cardiologist always spoke and then answered any questions of the group. Usually, there were 30–45 people in attendance at this holiday luncheon.

Patients and caregivers suggested topics for educational meetings, and the nurse facilitator planned the speakers and facilitated these meetings. A variety of speakers were involved in the educational meetings. They included: a cardiologist describing new technologies and current issues, research nurses discussing current studies and their findings, a pharmacist addressing new drugs on the market, a dietician reviewing diet concerns and foods high in sodium content, a psychiatric liaison nurse teaching relaxation techniques, a pastor dealing with spiritual issues and the matter of advanced directives, and an exercise physiologist talking about the importance of maintaining weight, strength, and flexibility. Group participants also received a demonstration in Tai Chi and several pursued this independently of the group.

The atmosphere for the educational sessions was informal. Verbal comments by group members were strictly voluntary. Confidentiality was ensured so that patients and family members could be open in their discussions. The nurse leader summarized the major topics of the session, mentioned the upcoming agenda, and sought input from the group as to any final thoughts or comments. Sometimes the group members spent a few minutes talking privately to the group facilitators or to the other recipients after the sessions ended.

Evaluating the Group

A variety of approaches were used to evaluate the outcomes of this support group. Initially, feedback was obtained informally from both patients and caregivers. They were asked about the helpfulness of the group in terms of support and the usefulness of information provided. Tools that can be used to measure behavior changes include pregroup and postgroup measures and long-range measures to determine more lasting effects. Factors such as pain, depression, level of anxiety, hopefulness, coping skills, problem-solving strategies, and activities of daily living can be measured with standardized instruments.

Questionnaires and surveys were used to obtain feedback about the ICD group as the years went on. Evaluation of the group content in terms of goals and objectives, guest speakers, and ongoing needs and desires from the group members were determined. Ongoing feedback was necessary and important for future planning so that sessions would appeal to the needs of the group. Groups that have been meeting for a long period of time tend to become social sharing sessions as well as educational forums. Evaluation is an extremely important component of the group process, and results of the questionnaires are useful to guide future groups. The ICD support group discussed in this example continues to meet today and is in its 14th year. This is evidence of the important role support groups have in assisting patients and families to manage their health. Interestingly, this ICD support group is launching a support forum on the Internet. (See Exercise 4 at the end of the chapter for the Web site.)

Maintaining Groups

Marketing existing groups in acute care has become an issue primarily due to shorter hospitalizations. Patients are admitted to short stay units for various surgical procedures and are discharged within 24 hours. During this episode of care, patients and their caregivers are often overloaded with information about self-care. They cannot begin to assimilate the amount of information until after discharge. Studies have shown that patient knowledge and coping issues are highest during the first three months after discharge from acute care (Doughtery, Pyper, & Benoliel, 2004). These are the critical time periods that patients can benefit greatly from groups.

It is essential for the nursing staff to communicate information about the group to other specialty units and clinics where the patients are seen in follow-up. The group leader also needs to communicate to the physicians and social workers within the acute care setting about the group. Information about the group can be included in the take-home teaching packet. Phone calls after discharge can be used to communicate and remind patients about existing groups. Using flyers and posters in the nursing units and outpatient clinics is another marketing method. Publishing information in local newspapers and hospital newsletters are ways to get the word out. Posting information on Web sites and chat rooms specific to the patient's diagnoses has become a popular venue.

Summary

In this chapter, a variety of issues regarding groups for older persons in acute care settings are addressed. The types of groups that can be conducted are described and examples given for traditional and nontraditional approaches. Initial planning for such groups is reviewed, as well as problem situations, education and training, and special considerations for conducting groups for older adults. Evaluation of groups and marketing ongoing groups also are addressed. Throughout the chapter, patience, flexibility, and an understanding of aging are noted as essential qualities for group leaders. The groups for older persons that have been described may not work in every acute care setting. However the value and benefits of support groups for patients and caregivers are well documented and still regarded as an important component of patient and family care. With the advent of technology, nontraditional approaches for providing support offer additional ways of providing patients and families with information and support. The challenge for nurses is to assess patient and family needs and suggest the best ways in which to provide the information and support needed for self-care.

Exercises

EXERCISE 1

Develop a specific plan for assessing the need for an inpatient group seeking input from patients, families, and nursing staff.

EXERCISE 2

Interview the nurse leader of a current caregiver support group about the experiences of starting the group.

EXERCISE 3

Attend a peer-led support group and a profession-ally led support group. Contrast and compare these two groups.

References

American Heart Association. (2004). *Heart disease and stroke statistics* (2004 update). Retrieved March 16, 2004, from *http://www.americanheart.org/presenter*

American Nurses Association (2004). Retrieved July 1, 2004, from *http://www.ana.org/readroom/tele2.htm*

Badger, J. M., & Morris, P. L. (1989). Observations of a sup-port group for automatic implantable cardioverter defibrillator recipients and their spouses. *Heart Lung,* 18(3), 238–243.

Bakas, T., Austin, J. K., Okonkwo, K. F., Lewis, R. R., & Chadwick, L. (2002). Needs, concerns, strategies, and advice of stroke caregivers the first 6 months after discharge. *Journal of Neuroscience Nursing,* 34(5), 242–251.

Bourke, J. P., Turkington, D., Thomas, G., McComb, J. M., & Tynam, M. (1997). Florid psychopathology in patients receiving shocks from implanted car-dioverter-defibrillators. *Heart,* 78, 581–583.

Bowles, K. H., & Dansky, K. H. (2002). Teaching self-man-agement of diabetes via telehomecare. *Home Health-care Nurse,* 20(1), 36–42.

Carney, R., Tevelde, A., Freedland, K., Sarni, J., Simeone, C., & Clark, K. (1997). Major depressive disorders in coronary artery disease. *American Journal of Cardiology,* 60, 1273–1275.

Chenier, M. C. (1997). Review and analysis of caregiver bur-den and nursing home placement. *Geriatric Nursing,* 18(3), 121–126.

Cope, D. (1995). Functions of a breast cancer support group as perceived by the participants: An ethnographic study. *Cancer Nursing,* 18(6), 472–478.

Cotter, V., & Strumpf, N. (2002). *Advanced practice nursing with older adults.* New York: McGraw-Hill.

Davis, L. D. (1998). Telephone-based interventions with family caregivers: A feasibility study. *Journal of Fam-ily Nursing,* 4(3), 255–270.

Dimmick, S. L., Mustaleski, C. Burgiss, S. G., & Welsh, T. (2000). A case study of benefits and potential savings in rural home telemedicine. *Home Healthcare Nurse,* 18(2), 124–135.

Doolittle, N. D., & Suave, M. J. (1995). Impact of aborted sudden cardiac death on survivors and their spouses: The phenomenon of different reference points. *Ameri-can Journal of Critical Care,* 4(5), 389–396.

Dougherty, C. M. (1997). Family-focused interventions for survivors of sudden cardiac arrest. *Journal of Cardio-vascular Nursing,* 12(1), 45–58.

Dougherty, C. M., Pyper, G. P., & Benoliel, J. Q. (2004). Domains of concern of intimate partners of sudden cardiac arrest survivors after ICS implantation. *Jour-nal of Cardiovascular Nursing,* 19(1), 21–31.

Eakes, G. G., Mayo, C., & Whicker, S. (1997). *Rehabilitation Nursing,* 22(4), 173–176.

Family Caregiving Statistics. (2002). In National Family Caregivers Association. Retrieved July, 1, 2004, from *http://www.nfcacares.org/NFC2002_stats.html*

Finfgeld, D. L. (2000). Therapeutic groups online: The good, the bad, and the unknown. *Issues Mental Health Nursing,* 21, 241–255.

Finkelstein, S. M., Speedie, S. M., Lundgren, J. M., Demiris, G., & Ideker, M. (2001). TeleHomeCare: Virtual visits from the patient's home. *Home Health Care Management & Practice,* 13(3), 219–226.

Frasure-Smith, N., Lesperance, F., & Talajic, M. (1995). Depression and 18-month prognosis. *Circulation,* 91(4), 999–1005.

Grant, J. S., Elliott, T. R., Giger, J. N., & Bartolucci, A. A. (2001). Social problem-solving telephone partner-ships with family caregivers of persons with stroke. *International Journal of Rehabilitation Research,* 24(3), 181–189.

Gresham, G. E., Duncan, P. W., & Stason, W. B. (1995). *Post-stroke rehabilitation.* Clinical Practice Guidelines, Public Health Service, pub 95-0662.

Hegel, M. T., Griegel, L. E., Black, C., Goulden, L., & Oza-howski, T. (1997). Anxiety and depression in patients receiving implanted cardioverter defibrilla-tors: A longitudinal investigation. *International Jour-nal of Psychiatry Medicine,* 27(1), 57–69.

Hildingh, C., & Fridlund, B. (2003). Participation in peer support groups after a cardiac event: A 12-month fol-low up. *Rehabilitation Nursing,* 28(4), 123–128.

Johansson, P. (1998). Model of long-term rehabilitation of patients with heart and lung disease. *Socialmedicinsk Tidskrift,* 8, 427–432.

Klemm, P., Bunnell, D., Cullen, M., Sonfji, R., Gibbons, P., & Holecek, A. (2003). Online cancer support groups: A review of the research literature. *Computers, Infor-matics, & Nursing,* 21(3), 136–142.

Lieberman, M. A. (1988). The role of self-help groups in helping patients and families cope with cancer. *CA: A Cancer Journal for Clinicians,* 38, 162–168.

Madara, F., & White, B. J. (1997). On-line mutual support: The experience of a self-help clearinghouse. Informa-tion referral: *Journal of the Alliance of Information Referral Systems,* 19, 91–107.

McCallion, P., & Toseland, W. (1995). Support group interventions with caregivers of frail older adults. *Social Work with Groups,* 18(1), 11–25.

Molchany, C. A., & Peterson, K. A. (1994). The psychological effects of support group intervention on AICD recipients and their significant others. *Progress in Cardiovascular Nursing,* 9(2), 23–29.

Murray, P. (1996). Recovery as an adjunct to treatment in an era of managed care. *Psychiatric Service,* 47, 1378.

Oravec, J. A. (2000). On-line medical information and service delivery: Implications for health education. *Journal of Health Education,* 31(2), 105–110.

Ostwald, S. K. (1997). Caregiver exhaustion: Caring for the hidden patients. *Advanced Practice Nursing Quarterly,* 3(2), 29–35.

Peak, T., Toseland, R., & Banks, W. (1995). The impact of a spouse caregiver support group on care recipient health care costs. *Journal Aging and Health,* 7(3), 427–499.

Rooney, R. M., Studenski, S. A., & Roman, L. L. (1997). A model for nurse case-managed home care using televideo. *Journal of the American Gerontological Society,* 45(12), 1523–1528.

Shepherd, M. D., Schoenberg, M., Slavich, S., Wituk, S., Warren, M., & Meissen, G. (1999). Continuum of professional involvement in self-help groups. *Journal of Community Psychology,* 27, 39–53.

Sneed, N. V., & Finch, N. (1992). Experiences of patients and significant others with automatic implantable cardioverter defibrillators after discharge from the hospital. *Progress in Cardiovascular Nursing,* 7(3), 20–24.

Sneed, N. V., Finch, N. J., & Michel, Y. (1997). The effect of a program of psychosocial nursing support on the early adjustment of patients and families with new ICD's. *Progress in Cardiovascular Nursing,* 12(2), 4–14.

Steiner, V., & Pierce, L. L. (2002). Building a web of support for caregivers of persons with stroke. *Topics of Stroke Rehabilitation,* 9(3), 102–111.

Stuart, G., & Laraia, M. (2001). *Principles and practice of psychiatric nursing.* St. Louis, MO: Mosby.

Sundeen, S. (2001). Psychiatric rehabilitation. In S. Stuart & A. Laraia, (Eds.), *Principles and practice of psychiatric nursing.* St. Louis, MO: Mosby.

Tran, B. Q., Buckley, K. M., & Prandoni, C. M. (2002). Selection and use of telehealth technology in support of homebound caregivers of stroke patients. *Caring,* 21(3), 16–21.

U.S. Department of Health and Human Services. *Clinical Practice Guidelines,* 6 (AHCPR Publication No. 95-0662). Rockville, MD.

Vesmarovich, S., Walker, T., Hauber, R. P., Temkin, A., & Burns, R. (1999). Innovations in practice. Use of telerehabilitation to manage pressure ulcers in persons with spinal cord injuries. *Advances in Wound Care,* 12(5), 264–269.

Warren, J. R., & Whall, A. L. (2001). Development of an intervention to cope with depression following myocardial infarction: A nurse-facilitated cardiac support group. *Journal of Gerontological Nursing,* May, 24–25.

Webster, C., & Austin, W. (1999). Health related hardiness and the effect of a psychoeducational group on client symptoms. *Journal of Psychiatric Mental Health Nursing,* (6)3.

Woods, N. F., & Earp, J. L. (1978). Women with cured breast cancer: A study of mastectomy patients in North Carolina. *Nursing Research,* 17, 279–285.

Wright, L. K., Bennet, G., & Gramling, L. (1998). Telecommunication interventions for caregivers of elders with dementia. *Advances in Nursing Sciences,* 20(3), 76–88.

Yalom, I. D. (1983). *Inpatient group therapy.* New York: Basic Books.

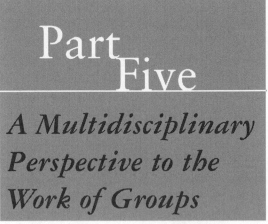

Part Five

A Multidisciplinary Perspective to the Work of Groups

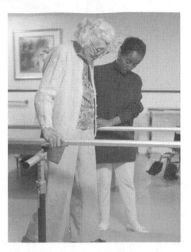

Part 5 provides a multidisciplinary perspective to the work of groups. Traditionally, the nurse and the social worker have used groups as interventions. In Chapter 26, Haight discusses the history of group work by nurses and highlights the groups that nurses have traditionally led. Mitcham, Burik, and Wicks, in Chapter 27, describe an occupational therapist's use of groups. They provide a fresh perspective and a new understanding of the work done by occupational therapists. To complement the chapter on occupational therapy, in Chapter 28 Wise and Brotherton share their insights on groups in physical therapy. They complement the written word with clear pictures of therapeutic exercises conducted in groups. In Chapter 29 we return to the longer-established tradition where Gibson and Kunz present a social work perspective.

Chapter 26

A Nursing Perspective

Barbara K. Haight
Irene Burnside

Key Words

- Conversation deprivation
- Reality orientation
- Reminiscence
- Sensory retraining
- Somatic preoccupation
- Verbosity

Learning Objectives

- Describe the historical growth of group work by nurses with aged clients
- List seven group modalities for the aged in which nurses have excelled
- List six other terms that may be used for reminiscence
- Describe four therapeutic values of reminiscence
- Analyze specific adaptations made by nurses in group therapy with the aged
- Synthesize nurses' unique contributions to group work with the aged

Burnside's introduction to group work in the late 1960s presented difficulties. When she decided to conduct groups with aged nursing home residents, she found that she was not welcomed by the nursing home. She was told that nurses did not do group work—that only social workers and psychologists did. To enable Burnside to work with groups, a local physician wrote orders for group work on the charts of those patients Burnside had chosen for group work.

Burnside felt a great need for supervision in that initial group experience because her prior group work had been with young adult schizophrenics. At the time, she had no background working with older adults in groups. However, she could not find a preceptor knowledgeable about older adults. She was advised to seek out a psychiatrist at a large urban medical center who had published about the aged. She told him the director of the hospital had referred her to him. When she stated her request, he replied, "You've got to be kidding," and refused to help her. The learning process that she subsequently used is best known as "flying by the seat of one's pants." Because she did not recommend that process for others, she wrote her first group book in the early 1980s. The first group she conducted moved her so much that she tried to capture that two-year experience by writing descriptive articles (Burnside, 1969a, 1970a, 1970b, 1971). What she learned in that pragmatic experience aided her greatly in teaching students and in running future groups. Fortunately, times have changed: both gerontological and psychiatric nurses are now sought as leaders of groups. We have Burnside to thank for our acceptance, a pioneer who influenced many nurses. This nurse still remembers a workshop delivered by Burnside, in which she ran a demonstration group of dementia patients whom she had never met before. At the end of the group session, she presented each group member with a brand new $5 bill as token payment for their time spent participating in the group. Each dementia patient examined the bill closely. The men took worn wallets out of their hip pockets, while the women opened their purses, and all carefully and proudly put their earned money away.

Acts such as these made Burnside a legend as an author, group facilitator, and speaker. She widely influenced numerous future gerontological nurses to work in groups with older people.

Overview

This overview serves as a short history of nurses' involvement in group work. Nurses began doing group work in the 1950s, but the name of one of the first group-leader nurses remains unknown. Truly a pioneer and an effective leader, she was the unidentified nurse coleader described in the classic work by Linden (1953). Then in 1968, Terrazas, a nurse, coauthored an article with Yalom on group therapy for psychotic elders in a state hospital in California. Following this introduction, Burnside wrote the second article on group work in 1969. In addition to these early articles, the first nurse-authored book to contain substantive material on group work with elders by nurses appeared in 1973 (Burnside, 1973). This book affected process and content in older adult groups. Morrison (1973) described her master's-level work in group therapy for older women who used health clinics more than normal. Blake (1973) described her leadership of a group for the

aged in a large public institution. She based her work with demented individuals on ego psychology, and Holtzen (1973) worked with a group in a similar setting and reported themes of depersonalization, isolation, hopelessness, and lack of trust in her observations. Other chapters by nurses about groups included Stange (1973), who creatively explored use of props, sensory stimulation, and social graces with aged women on the back ward of a state hospital; and Holland (1973), who co-led a group of stroke patients in a chronic disease rehabilitation hospital with a coleader who was a social worker. The nurse– author said her leadership style varied from that of her partner. She described her approach as activity centered in contrast to the verbal style used by the social worker.

Everson and Mealey (1978) wrote the most complete and best article for nurse instructors wishing to teach nursing students to be group leaders with older adults. This article continues to be highly recommended for nurses supervising students doing group work, as is the article by Tappen and Touhy (1983). Smith (1980) described her leadership problems when running groups for chronically ill, institutionalized psychiatric patients. Although Smith did not focus specifically on older people, her information is applicable for nurses planning to begin groups with older people. Smith pointed out that "on first making a decision that a therapy group should be established, one automatically sets up a chain reaction of decision making. The initial decision involves choosing group members" (p. 1301).

These statements sound deceptively easy, but new nurse group leaders should not be misled. If cooperation is not forthcoming from the agency officials where the group is to take place, the start can be difficult. Smith also points out that one needs the expertise and assistance of those with knowledge about group work. Another essential point for a nurse group leader is that the leader must strive to achieve balance in the amount of control she or he exercises as a leader because "a group leader must give the direction where necessary, but must remember that a certain amount of freedom gives the group its potential to grow" (Smith, 1980, p. 1303). The leader must also give freedom to students so that all may grow in the experience. At the start, students need to allow themselves floundering time while they practice their leadership roles. (See Chapter 10 on leadership.)

Nickoley-Colquitt (1981) examined the effectiveness of preventive group interventions for older clients. She noted that during the past decade, group approaches emphasizing health promotion have emerged and prevention is one part of health promotion. Nickoley-Colquitt reviewed 18 group interventions involving the family members of an aged population. In spite of great diversity in the groups examined, all the groups had one focus in common: to provide health-promotion interventions for older adults who were experiencing stressful changes. As health promoters, nurses are particularly well qualified to conduct group work with frail or cognitively impaired older adults. This is because of their orientation to wellness (rather than illness) and prevention (rather than disease processes and diagnosis).

Groups for frail older adults often begin slowly, with exceedingly high anxiety in the members. Reducing anxiety, pain, and discomfort so that the members will remain in the group is the first task of the leader in the initial meetings. Nurse–authors Janosik and Phipps (1982, p. 252) note that "There is an erroneous impression among some health workers that group work is inappropriate for the elderly because they have little capacity for change or because their quality of life cannot be sustained during the sunset years." The slow beginning of nurses in conducting group work with older clients is probably related more to the ageist attitudes of the day than to adjusting to the recently acquired role of group leader. Burnside observed that at times nurses as leaders were not taken very seriously, and this was probably because nurses had been viewed in old traditional roles, such as the carriers of bedpans, dispensers of pills, and writers of charts. Today, fortunately, most have a more modern view of nursing.

Janosik and Phipps (1982) wrote about problematic behaviors occurring in group work with older adults. Their long list of problematic behaviors—callousness, compartmentalization, somatic preoccupation, verbosity, denial, confabulation, regression, selfishness, and repetitiousness—presents a negative view but should be a challenge to any present-day leader! The negative nature of the listed behaviors could discourage the neophyte leader, particularly as these authors gave no list of positive behaviors that might enhance the group experience. Leaders need to understand that the behaviors of staff, leaders, or members may contribute to the emergence or continuance of such problematic behaviors in the group. Our own approaches and interactions may be responsible for difficult behaviors we see in elders.

Many older people do not want to be in a nursing home. They may use regression and selfishness as coping strategies because of their anger at being there. Burnside believes verbosity is closely related to conversation deprivation and continues because the leader does not insightfully redirect the conversation in the group. Many older adults have no one to listen to them; but a group experience provides many listeners and multiple sounding boards. Some group members' somatic preoccupations and concern about bodily symptoms may well be attributed to the leader's neglecting to provide nurturance and care to the members, or, as Burnside states, somatic preoccupation may be directly related to the initial anxiety of the group members. These problem behaviors decrease considerably during the life of the group as the leader listens and empathizes. However, when group leaders are nurses, older adults feel free to discuss their physical complaints, thereby prompting some of the somatic preoccupation to continue.

Nursing Groups Today

In the past, nurses have actively led the following groups: reality orientation, validation therapy, reminiscence, health promotion, and sensory retraining, music, and support groups. (Some of these groups were mentioned in Chapter 3 or have entire chapters devoted to them in this book.) To this list, nurses have added a multitude of new and innovative groups. Both old and new groups will be presented in the following paragraphs.

Reality Orientation

A nurse helped to pioneer reality orientation (RO) groups when they began in Tuscaloosa, Alabama, in the 1960s (Taulbee & Folsom, 1966). Scarbrough, also a nurse, continued to further refine the area of reality orientation classes (Drummond, Kirkoff, & Scarbrough, 1979). Spector, Orrell, Davies, and Woods (2000) reviewed the literature on the effectiveness of RO for managing dementia and suggested a positive effect on cognition and behavior. Thus, opinions on the usefulness of RO remain mixed. Reality orientation is such a straightforward group intervention; nursing assistants as well as nurses can easily conduct it. To teach nursing assistants, Haight created a self-learning module for the nursing assistants in a Veterans Administration hospital. This hospital had a system of earning points toward promotion and pay raises, so there was an incentive for even the night shift to participate in the learning module. The process and content of the self-learning module was evaluated with a test at the end of the module. Many of the assistants who completed the module went on to conduct RO groups. Having the assistants conduct these groups resulted in two positive outcomes: pride and increased job satisfaction for the assistants, and a

more intense reality orientation environment because all personnel participated in the milieu of RO, a requirement for a successful program. In many ways, RO is passé compared to new modalities, but RO serves many purposes within institutions and should not be abandoned.

Validation Therapy

Validation therapy was started by a social worker but widely adopted by nurses, particularly in Europe where many nurses and nurse assistants receive mandatory training in validation therapy before starting work in a nursing home. Scandland and Emershaw (1993) compared validation therapy to RO, and found no differences between pretest and posttest for either intervention. But Day (1997), reviewing the validation therapy literature, suggests validation therapy offers another option for care, and like RO, we should not abandon it. But we should not adopt validation therapy too hastily as Briggs (2004) recently reported that there was insufficient evidence to support conclusions that validation therapy was effective for people with dementia or cognitive impairment.

Reminiscence Groups

Nurses have a long history of running reminiscence groups. Ebersole (1976) may have been the first to write about it when she shared her work in a chapter in Burnside's book. Cook (1998) conducted a reminiscence group in a nursing home and found that the reminiscence group improved life satisfaction significantly. Other nurses are involved in either reminiscence groups or life review, such as McDougal, Blixen, and Lee-Jen (1997) who published a landmark study in which they described the success of psychiatric nurses in billing for a life review when they visited depressed homebound older people. Ashida (2000) looked at the effect of reminiscence music therapy sessions on changes in depression in people with dementia and found significant decreases in depression after five days of reminiscence-focused music therapy. She was able to combine two modalities for excellent outcomes. Puentes (2000) also tested reminiscence as a teaching tool for the enhancement of nursing skills in communication. Nurses are very diverse in their application of reminiscence as an intervention and as such have contributed a great deal to the field of reminiscence. The multidisciplinary study of reminiscence is fully discussed in Chapter 14.

Reminiscence is also helpful in getting older people to mobilize psychological resources and to master their emotional burdens. Four common modes of group work nurses often incorporate into a reminiscence group can be seen in **Figure 26–1**; they are reality orientation, remotivation, music, resocialization, sensory stimulation, art, and poetry. **Figure 26–2** shows how a variety of modalities can be incorporated into a group.

Health-Related Groups

In addition to the above three categories of groups, nurses also pioneered health-related groups (Heller, 1970; Holland, 1973; Holtzen, 1973; Murphy, 1969). Health-related groups were perhaps a natural for a nurse to lead because

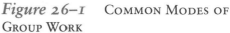

Figure 26–1   COMMON MODES OF GROUP WORK

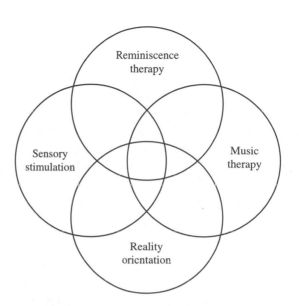

of the nurse's interest in holistic health, in prevention, and in alleviation of distress and pain. For example, Ferszt, Heineman, Ferszt, and Romano (1998) created a grief group that was transformative. Members expressed their feelings through art therapy activities. Through this group, women overcame their grief, learned to see

Figure 26–2

Small group completing a task together.

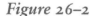

themselves in new roles, and gained support for these roles, while challenging old stereotypes about themselves.

Another common type of group, support groups, has helped nurses recover from chemical dependency. The mutual goals of these support groups are recovery and improvement of self-image. As members, nurses have the opportunity to talk to peers about the problems related to their jobs that led to chemical dependency (Miller, 1997). The conversation and mutual support lead to recovery and better health.

Sensory Retraining Groups

Scott and Crowhurst (1975), two Canadian nurses, conducted sensory retraining programs to put patients in touch with their environment and one another. Heidell (1972) also wrote about this group modality. The program combines activities that are designed to reawaken or maintain all of the senses: sight, sound, taste, smell, and touch.

One of Burnside's early articles (1969b) was about the use of sensory stimulation with older adults in a nursing home. That group experience taught her the value of props, the importance of food and beverages, and the use of touch within a group. Interestingly, what was once sensory retraining is now called Snoezelen, a multisensory experience using high-tech equipment and a more intense environment to deliver sensory stimulation. Nurses as well as occupational therapists have an interest in promulgating this intervention as demonstrated by the great increase in the numbers of publications on Snoezelen and multisensory stimulation in the 1990s (Chitsey, Haight, & Jones, 2002). Schofield (1996) sees value in the intervention as a way to reduce chronic pain. Schofield and Davis (1998) report that some patients experienced a decrease in pain and improvement in overall well-being after participating in Snoezelen groups and sessions.

Music Therapy Groups

Hennessey (1976a, 1976b, 1978) was especially gifted in her use of music therapy groups; Hennessey combined her professional and personal talents in a unique fashion. She was both a nurse group leader and a concert violinist. She aptly described the meld of her music and nursing:

> In the past my life was split in two parts; I kept them carefully separated. I wore different clothes, worked with different people, and used different skills. Few of my musician friends were aware that I was a nurse, and my hospital associates did not know that my violin was a major part of my existence. When I discovered a way to combine work as a health professional and as a musician, it was as though I became a professionally whole person. The dichotomy that had been defined by the nursing world began to disappear, and with the feelings of wholeness, the effectiveness of my work with groups increased.

There are not many who are both nurses and concert violinists able to follow in her footsteps. That does not mean nurses have abandoned music as an intervention but nurses' music groups are mostly music appreciation groups where the group listens to the music of others. McCaffrey and Locsin (2002) suggest music listening as a noninvasive intervention that helps to create a healing environment. In Snoezelen groups, music is played in the background to add to the stimulation of the senses.

Other Nurse-Led Groups

Nurses are often called upon to lead support groups for families. Davidson, Tang, and Titler (2003) created an evidenced-based protocol for family bereavement support after the death of a nursing home resident. The purpose of the protocol was to provide guidelines for family grief support. Former friends are often a vital part of the older adult's social support network. Part of the nurse's role is to help older people maintain their social support systems (Lilly, Richards, & Buckwalter, 2003). Ostwald, Hepburn, and Burns (2003) described a training project for family caregivers. Family caregivers had to learn skills tailored to their family care giving needs. They did so through a workshop, where they often found social support from other members sharing the same experiences. Psychotherapeutic groups run by nurses are fully addressed in Chapter 18. Topical groups differ from all others: for example, using pets as therapy is a new approach to leading a therapeutic group (Hooker, Freeman, & Stewart, 2002). Increasing an older person's physical activity in the company of others is another popular way to help people enjoy their peers while getting stronger. A most innovative and futuristic group is one using the Internet for discussion (Mahoney, 2003). Mahoney used the Internet to discuss vigilance with caregivers. Though the purpose of her project was to get help for her research, the idea of being a part of some whole can contribute to the support of isolated caregivers. As we look to the future, many of our therapeutic groups may take place in chat rooms, with or without a qualified leader.

Special Aspects to Consider

Group Modality Selection

The selection of the appropriate group modality is crucial to the success of the group. It may be necessary to adapt the process of a particular group to conform to older people's needs and abilities. Because nursing deals with persons in transition, it might be well to assess group members using that dimension.

The common adaptations needed in group work with older people should be based on the following:

1. Mutual determination by leader and members of group goals and objectives

2. Assessment of losses, including:
    - Physical (most especially members' hearing, vision, and mobility)
    - Social (especially the death of a spouse and peers and pets)
    - Financial losses (home, income, personal belongings)
    - Status (loss of job, respect), which may result in lowered self-esteem
3. Attention to nutritional needs and fluid intake
4. Attention to sensory losses
5. Skill and expertise of the leader
6. Psychosocial needs of the older person
7. Time and energy of the group leader
8. Resources available:
    - Financial
    - Locations/space for group meetings

The nurse needs to be skilled in the assessment of each person to select the right combination of members and modality. (See Chapter 8 on membership selection.)

Refreshments

Poston and Levine (1980) wrote a provocative article about their group therapy. The members came to a community-oriented psychiatric clinic for help with their depressive conditions. The leader's first attempt at "a conversational group treatment with these patients was unsuccessful." Apparently, that group never developed a sense of cohesion, and splinter groups formed. The patients said they felt worse than before the group experience "because they got upset listening to other patients' problems" (p. 159). Based on what they learned from the failure of the first group, Poston and Levine tried a second method of group treatment. A coffee lounge was prepared to "provide more direct gratification for these patients' needs" (p. 159), and refreshments were part of the group meeting.

The willingness of nurses to be nurturing (even with nonnarcissistic patients) is one way that group work by nurses often differs from that of other disciplines. Because most nurses are nurturing persons, they tend to use nurturing techniques, such as serving food, in their group work with the aged. The literature notes group leaders of other disciplines also doing this. Poston and Levine (1980) describe nurturing behaviors, as do Black, Friedlob, Ruenstein, and Kelly, who in Chapter 23 give an in-depth description of the use of fluids and food in groups.

The forms of refreshments served in groups vary from beverages to special types of snacks, pastries or cookies—and even popcorn! At first it might seem that these are party-only groups. Upon closer observation, a variety of rationales emerge for why nurses might successfully incorporate refreshments into their group work:

- Refreshments provide nurturing for those most in need—narcissistic patients, poorly nourished and/or dehydrated individuals, lonely or alienated members, sensorial deprived individuals.
- Food and drink also provide an easy method for improving social graces.
- The serving of food allows the leader to assess appetite, coordination during eating, likes and dislikes in food, and eating and drinking habits.
- Refreshments can create an element of surprise for those who complain of ennui.
- The nourishment itself (for example, popcorn) can be the theme for reality orientation and reminiscence groups.
- The nourishment can provide an educational theme for a meeting (for example, examining, discussing, and then eating papayas, mangoes, or pineapples).
- If the leader prepares the nourishment, it can provide a poignant moment (for example, a group member cried when Burnside baked an angel food cake for her birthday

and for the meeting: "It's been 18 years since I have tasted angel food cake. It was at my granddaughter's birthday party.").

The nourishment can serve as an instructional aid to a student leader. Questions to be asked about serving food include:

- What do you serve diabetic members of the group?
- How full do you fill the cups/glasses?
- When and why do you use finger foods?
- How do you intervene when a member colors the peeled banana green with the felt-tipped pen used to write the nametags?
- Who will finance the cost of the nourishments?
- What is the best type of glass or cup to use for your group?
- Specifically how will you use the nourishment to improve activities-of-daily-living (ADL) skills or social graces?
- Will you serve the refreshments?
- Will you share the nourishment with the members?
- When in the meeting will you offer the nourishment—before, midway, or after?
- Who will clean up the mess that might occur?

One student in Lubbock, Texas, conducted a reminiscence group at a local nursing home and wrote: "To avoid the institutional look, I used tablecloths, ceramic coffee mugs, brightly colored napkins, and patterned paper plates for all of our meetings. At each session at least one member of our group, man or woman, would comment on how attractive the table looked.

Transference

Transference is a psychological term for transferring feelings we may have about a particular person to a member of the group who resembles that person. The average older person will often reenact the family group in the group life; transference may occur, for example, one member to the other, "You sound just like my brother used to," or older member to young leader, "You remind me of my granddaughter; she talks like that." A nurse with a psychiatric background will be quick to recognize transferences within the group. However, Burnside said it was always startling when the transferences did occur in a group; they tended to catch her off guard. One needs to be sensitive to the occurrence and also to analyze if we are experiencing transformation ourselves and treating group members like grandparents or other relatives.

Nursing students should have an experiential group experience to learn the basics of group process. For example, reminiscence groups of students should be a requirement before they themselves lead a reminiscence group. If they are fortunate, they will have had group work as a part of their educational process.

Education

Following is an example of one nursing curriculum that includes group work. There are seldom separate courses at the undergraduate level, unless some time is given to groups in the psychiatric nursing curriculum. However, some form of group exposure, such as working with health education groups, often takes place in the clinical setting. Nurses are taught that patient teaching is an essential component of their professional role, and essential to promote behavior change (Saarmann, Daugherty, & Riegel, 2000). Patient education projects may take place in community health classes. For example, students in clinical placements in a low-income community high-rise for older people taught health education programs such as "caring for your diabetes" to the residents of the high-rise. They not only had to prepare the teaching program, they had to decide where the group would meet, organize the room, gather refreshments, and make notices to attract people to the program. During the class, they had to lead the group and answer questions. Thus they had a small group-learning experience.

The graduate-level curriculum for clinical nurse specialists at the Medical University of South Carolina included a formal group course. The course covered theory and guidelines for forming groups. The students themselves formed groups and critiqued themselves as they went through the process of forming (getting together), storming (arguing differences), norming (agreeing on rules), performing (actually running the group, and disbanding (terminating the group). Often these student groups were composed of students from several nursing majors and, when beginning the group, they were not well acquainted with one another. However, after the groups were formed, names adopted, and logos created, the group became cohesive. This cohesiveness generated competition among the groups for the best project or presentation, which in turn fed the cohesiveness of the groups.

The students analyzed the group behavior throughout the semester, thus learning about group behavior from hands-on experience. Students also attended one or two community groups that were meeting and wrote about the group process, leadership, the types of members, group behavior, and so forth. They diagrammed the group, looking for the direction of the conversation, the unofficial leader, the scapegoat, and the monopolizer, if any. One of the most unruly and interesting groups the students visited was the faculty at the monthly faculty meeting.

In addition to this formal group course, gerontology students had a group assignment in their clinical course. To do this work students read Burnside's original group text, using the clinical instructor for reference and supervision. Reading the book was an assignment to complete before the clinical actually started so that the contents of the book could be discussed at conference on the first clinical day. The rotation for long-term care was 15 weeks and in that 15 weeks, the student had to write a group plan, select members, hold six group meetings and then evaluate the process of the group. Students often made the same mistakes year after year, the biggest being thinking they had a lot of time to get started when they didn't. Most made the mistake of starting too late because they spent inordinate amounts of time on their plan for the group.

Another mistake students made was to select group members by intuition rather than knowledge. One student, for example, started a current events group and ended up with four alert, interested newspaper readers and two people with dementia. A simple assessment with the Mini Mental State Exam (MMSE) would have averted this mistake. Another student wanted to run a sensory stimulation group for those with dementia. At least two of her group members were in early dementia and felt insulted to be members of this group. They told her and quit. Other students ran gardening groups and discovered that although the patients were able-bodied, they expected the students to do the heavy work. Exercise groups and walking groups were popular until the students realized there was no time for communication and had to remedy the situation by resting halfway and having a meeting. One student bought her group matching baseball caps with a logo. It was always a delight to see this group of disabled people take off with their walkers and their caps.

The most successful group was a beauty group of end-stage Alzheimer's patients. All of the students were excited by the response in this group and wanted to take part, so their leader was not at a loss for help. One week they did shampoos and sets, and another week makeup. The most fascinating day was manicure day. Watching some of these women, who did not care for themselves nor communicate with others and often exhibited behavioral problems, put on their nail polish and

carefully wait for their nails to dry was indeed eye opening. This group showed us different ways to communicate that were so successful. The advantage of student groups is that only a student would think of doing such a group and have such a good time doing it.

At the end of each clinical day the group of students gathered for clinical conference and supervision. Some were devastated by their clinical experience and learned a great deal from their mistakes. They were not graded on the success of their group, but rather on the completeness of their own group evaluation, which they were required to do as one of their final papers. The instructor visited and evaluated the group at least once, and each student did a peer evaluation of another group. The teacher asked each student to analyze the evaluations, to synthesize the information, and draw conclusions regarding the success or demise of their group. By that last presentation day, students had formed a cohesive clinical group and were not afraid to criticize themselves and outline a different plan for next time.

The students were not worried about past mistakes; they learned from them. Many had the confidence to go out and create groups again. They came back to school while in their first work situation and reported that they were running groups and because of this skill had impressed their superiors. As Daley (2001) said, "Clinical nursing practice facilitates both personal and professional development and allows students to practice their profession in a safe environment."

Nurses and social workers are often critical of the other discipline's ability to do group work with older adults. Collaboration with other disciplines can be taught to students while teaching them about groups. In Project Effect, a grant-funded program at the University of Central Florida, graduate students in nursing, social work, psychology, and counseling worked as a nucleus to provide direct services to families. The team defined collaboration as a team-oriented process to reach common goals that could not be achieved alone. The students rated the project as being very valuable to them and will probably continue similar work when they are out in the professional world (Gropper & Shepard-Tew, 2000). Throughout this book we emphasize the importance of working with other disciplines. With all the group work that needs to be done, squabbling over turf seems unnecessary.

Summary

Butler, Lewis, and Sunderland (1991, p. 421) stated "Nurses probably conduct more groups with older persons than do other professionals." This chapter discussed seven common nurse-led groups: reality orientation, remotivation, reminiscence, health-related, sensory retraining, music, and support groups. The increase in publications, theses, and chapters written by nurses in the past 20 years denotes the interest of nurses in group work with older people. Evaluations of group work are often highly subjective; nurses need to change that subjective analysis and move to a research posture. Responsible clinicians who are able to objectively judge the effectiveness of the group experience for members must do evaluations of group work.

The overall goal for group work is to make the later years of life the very best that they can be instead of the worst. King (1982, p. 25) reminds us "No therapeutic modality can fulfill the wants, hopes, and needs of all clients." Yet there is no doubt that groups can change the quality of lives, including those of the leaders! Regardless of what we write or expound, the true teachers are the aged group members. Burnside believed they join our groups out of their great generosity and kindness, to please and help us, and she found that a humbling experience.

Exercises

EXERCISE 1

Read five nurse-written articles about group work with older people. Are there commonalities in the techniques described by each of the authors? List two commonalities and discuss each.

EXERCISE 2

Choose Chapter 27, 28, or 29. Compare and contrast the perspective of that writer with the nurse's perspective presented in this chapter.

EXERCISE 3

Interview a nurse who has conducted group work with older adults. What was her or his motivation to lead such a group?

EXERCISE 4

Select from the reference list of this chapter two nurse-written articles that discuss the theory and practice of group work.

1. Critically read the selected articles.
2. List three concepts regarding groups that appear in the articles.
3. Write one intervention that a group leader might use for each of the three common concepts you identify. Defend your intervention.

References

Ashida, S. (2000). The effect of reminiscence music therapy sessions on changes in depressive symptoms in elderly persons with dementia. *Journal of Music Therapy, 37,* 170–182.

Blake, D. (1973). Group work with the institutionalized elderly. In I. M. Burnside (Ed.), *Psychosocial nursing care of the aged* (1st ed., pp. 153–160). New York: McGraw-Hill.

Briggs, N. (2004). *Validation therapy for dementia.* The Cochrane Library, 2.

Burnside, I. M. (1969a). Group work among the aged. *Nursing Outlook, 17*(6), 68–72.

Burnside, I. M. (1969b). Sensory stimulation: An adjunct to group work with the disabled aged. *Mental Hygiene, 53*(3), 381–388.

Burnside, I. M. (1970a). Group work with the aged: Selected literature. *The Gerontologist,* 10(3), 241–246.

Burnside, I. M. (1970b). Loss: A constant theme in group work with the aged. *Hospital Community Psychiatry,* 21(6), 173–177.

Burnside, I. M. (1971). Long-term group work with hospitalized aged. *The Gerontologist,* 2(3), 213–218.

Burnside, I. M. (1973). *Psychosocial nursing care of the aged.* New York: McGraw-Hill.

Butler, R. N., Lewis, M. I., & Sunderland T. (1991). *Aging and mental health: Positive psychosocial and biomedical approaches* (4th ed.). New York: Merrill.

Chitsey, A., Haight, B., & Jones, J. (2002). Snoezelen: A multisensory environmental intervention. *Journal of Gerontological Nursing,* 28(3), 41–49.

Cook, E. A. (1998). *Effects of reminiscence on life satisfaction of elderly female nursing home residents.* Unpublished doctoral dissertation, School of Nursing, The University of Texas at Austin.

Daley, B. (2001). Learning in clinical practice. *Holistic Nursing Practice,* 16(1) 43–54.

Davidson, K., Tang, J., & Titler, M. (2003). Evidence-based protocol: Family bereavement support before and after the death of a nursing home resident. *Journal of Gerontological Nursing,* 29(1), 10–28.

Day, C. R, (1997). Validation therapy: A review of the literature. *Journal of Gerontological Nursing,* 23(4), 29–34.

Drummond L., Kirkoff L., & Scarbrough, D. (1978). A practical guide to reality orientation: A treatment approach for confusion and disorientation. *The Gerontologist,* 18(6), 568–573.

Drummond L., Kirkoff L., & Scarbrough, D. (1979). *Leading reality orientation classes: Basic and advanced.* Arlington Heights, IL: Intercraft.

Ebersole, P. (1976). Reminiscing and group psychotherapy with the aged. In I. M. Burnside (Ed.), *Nursing and the aged* (1st ed., pp. 214–230). New York: McGraw-Hill.

Everson, S. J., & Mealey, A. R. (1978). Baccalaureate nursing students as leaders in geriatric groups. *Journal of Nursing Education,* 17(7), 17–26.

Ferszt, G., Heineman, L., Ferszt, E., & Romano, S. (1998). Transformation through grieving: Art and the bereaved. *Holistic Nursing Practice,* 13, 68–73.

Gropper, R., & Shepard-Tew, D. (2000). Project EFFECT: A case study of collaboration and cooperation. *Nursing Outlook,* 48, 276–80.

Heidell, B. (1972, June). Sensory training puts patients "in touch." *Modern Nursing Home,* 28, 40.

Heller, V. (1970). Handicapped patients talk together. *American Journal of Nursing,* 70(2), 332–335.

Hennessey, M. (1976a). Group work with economically independent aged. In I. M. Burnside (Ed.), *Nursing and the aged* (1st ed., pp. 231–244). New York: McGraw-Hill.

Hennessey, M. (1976b). Music and group work with the aged. In I. M. Burnside (Ed.), *Nursing and the aged* (1st ed., pp. 255–269). New York: McGraw-Hill.

Hennessey, M. (1978). Music and music therapy groups. In I. M. Burnside (Ed.), *Working with the elderly: Group process and techniques* (1st ed., pp. 255–274). North Scituate, MA: Duxbury Press.

Holland, D. L. (1973). Co-leadership with a group of stroke patients. In I. M. Burnside (Ed.), *Psychosocial nursing care of the aged* (1st ed., pp. 187–201). New York: McGraw-Hill.

Holtzen, V. (1973). Short-term group work in a rehabilitation hospital. In I. M. Burnside (Ed.), *Psychosocial nursing care of the aged* (1st ed., pp. 161–173). New York: McGraw-Hill.

Hooker, S., Freeman, L., & Stewart, P. (2002). Pet therapy research: A historical review. *Holistic Nursing Practice,* 16(5), 17–23.

Janosik, E., & Phipps, L. (1982). *Life cycle group work in nursing.* Monterey, CA: Wadsworth.

King, K. (1982). Reminiscing psychotherapy with aging people. *Journal of Psychiatric Nursing and Mental Health Services,* 20(2), 21–25.

Lilly, M., Richards, B., & Buckwalter, K. (2003). Friends and social support in dementia caregiving. *Journal of Gerontological Nursing,* 29(1), 29–36.

Linden, M. (1953). Group psychotherapy with institutionalized senile women: Study in gerontologic human relations. *International Journal of Group Psychotherapy,* 3, 150–170.

Mahoney, D. (2003). Vigilance: Evolution and definition for caregivers of family members with Alzheimer's disease. *Journal of Gerontological Nursing,* 29(8), 24–30.

McCaffrey, R., & Locsin, R. (2002). Music listening as a nursing intervention: A symphony of practice. *Holistic Nursing Practice,* 16(3), 69–77.

McDougal, G., Blixen, C., & Lee-Jen, S. (1997). The process and outcomes of life review psychotherapy with depressed homebound older adults. *Nursing Research,* 46, 277–283.

Miller, P. (1997). Support systems of nurses recovering from chemical dependency: A pilot study. *Holistic Nursing Practice,* 11(4), 56–70.

Morrison, J. M. (1973). Group therapy for high utilizers of clinic facilities. In I. M. Burnside (Ed.), *Psychosocial nursing care of the aged* (pp. 142–150). New York: McGraw-Hill.

Murphy, L. N. (1969). A health discussion group for the elderly. In *ANA Clinical Conferences*. Atlanta, GA: Appleton-Century-Crofts.

Nickoley, S. (1978). Promoting functional level of health and perception of control in elderly women in the community through supportive group intervention. Unpublished master's thesis. NY: University of Rochester.

Nickoley-Colquitt, S. (1981). Preventive group interventions for elderly clients: Are they effective? *Family Community Health: Journal of Health Promotion Maintenance*, 3(4): 66–85.

Ostwald, S., Hepburn, K., & Burns, T. (2003). Training family caregivers of patients with dementia: A structured workshop approach. *Journal of Gerontological Nursing*, 29(3), 37–44.

Poston, B., & Levine, M. (1980). A modified group treatment for elderly narcissistic patients. *International Journal of Group Psychotherapy*, 30(2), 153–167.

Puentes, W. (2000). Using social reminiscence to teach therapeutic communication skills. *Geriatric Nursing*, 21, 315–318.

Saarman, L., Daugherty, J., & Riegel, B. (2000). Patient teaching to promote behavior change. *Nursing Outlook*, 48, 281–7.

Scanland, S. G., & Emershaw, L. E. (1993). Reality orientation and validation therapy: Dementia, depression, and functional status. *Journal of Gerontological Nursing*, 19(6), 7–11.

Schofield, P. (1996). Snoezelen: Its potential for people with chronic pain. *Complementary Therapies in Nursing and Midwifery*, 2(1), 9–12.

Schofield, P., & Davis, B. (1998). Sensory deprivation and chronic pain: A review of the literature. *Disability Rehabilitation*, 20, 357–366.

Scott, D., & Crowhurst, J. (1975). Reawakening senses in the elderly. *Canadian Nurse*, 71(10), 21–22.

Smith, L. L. (1980). Find your leadership style in groups. *American Journal of Nursing*, 80(7), 1301–1303.

Spector, A. Orrell, M., Davies, S., & Woods, R. T. (2000). Reality orientation for dementia: A review of the evidence of effectiveness. *The Cochrane Library*, 1.

Stange, A. (1973). Around the kitchen table: Group work on a back ward. In I. M. Burnside (Ed.), *Psychosocial nursing care of the aged* (1st ed., pp. 174–186). New York: McGraw-Hill.

Tappan, R., & Touhy T. (1983). Group leader—Are you a controller? *Journal of Gerontological Nursing*, 9(1), 34.

Taulbee, L, & Folsom, J. (1966). Reality orientation for geriatric patients. *Hospital Community Psychiatry*, 17(5), 133–135.

Yalom, I. D., & Terrazas, F. (1968). Group therapy for psychotic elderly patients. *American Journal of Nursing*, 68(8), 1691–1694.

Resources

FILM

- Interacting with Older People [56 minutes, black-and-white, 16 mm]. A two-part training film primarily for nurses. Discusses psychosocial needs of older adults and suggests techniques to use in interacting with them. Wayne State University A-V Center, 680 Putnam, Detroit, MI 48202.

An Occupational Therapy Perspective

Maralynne D. Mitcham

Jerry K. Burik

Alison M. Wicks

Key Words

- Environment
- Meaning
- Occupation
- Occupational challenges
- Occupational choices
- Occupational perspective
- Occupational opportunities
- Occupational strategies
- Participation
- Person

Learning Objectives

- Define the construct of occupation
- Recognize the historical contribution of occupation to health and well-being, and the emergence of the profession of occupational therapy
- Appreciate humans as occupational beings
- Contrast occupational issues in older adulthood to those in earlier phases of the life course
- Recognize the perspectives that occupational therapists bring to working with groups of elders
- Discuss occupational considerations for designing and promoting occupation-based groups for elders

To contribute to the multidisciplinary section of this text, we begin our chapter with an overview of the construct of occupation, how it played a historical role in promoting health and well-being and led to the emergence of the profession of occupational therapy. Although all of us in the health professions share a common heritage, we wish to share a perspective that helps answer the question, "Who put the occupation into occupational therapy?" We continue using an occupational perspective to explore occupational participation throughout the life course, giving attention to the occupational issues in older adulthood and the occupational strategies that ensue. In the latter part of the chapter we present Pierce's (2003) framework for designing occupational experiences and discuss how to apply the framework in the design of group occupations for elders. We conclude by describing "The Well Elderly Study," which empirically demonstrates the effectiveness of occupational therapy in promoting participation in group occupations for well elders. We hope our chapter not only furthers understanding of occupation and occupational therapy, but also promotes collaboration with our colleagues in other health professions who work with elders.

Introducing Occupation

> *Man through the use of his hands, as they are energized by mind and will, can influence the state of his health.*
>
> —*Mary Reilly*

Occupational therapists believe that humans are hardwired for occupation. As a species, humans have a natural tendency to engage their time and energy in occupations that are personally meaningful, socially satisfying, and culturally relevant. Our profession asserts that, throughout the life course, humans make sense of their worlds through the subjective experience of engaging in occupation, and it is this subjective experience that differentiates occupation from general classes of commonly understood activity (Pierce, 2001a). Furthermore, we propose that occupation itself is a health determinant. The ability to engage in a wide variety of occupations is, for the most part, health promoting. Our minds, bodies, and spirits are challenged to respond to stimuli in the human and nonhuman environments and to create responses that enable us to orchestrate lives that have meaning. In contrast, lack of occupation has a deleterious effect on our health. Consider, for example, the rapid physical and mental deterioration of a prisoner held in solitary confinement and you see that occupational deprivation is the greatest punishment a society can impose on its offenders (Whiteford, 2000).

Why the term occupation? Occupo, the Latin root of the word occupation, means "to take possession, grasp, seize, enjoy, or get a start on." Within the profession of occupational therapy, we interpret that definition to mean taking possession of our time and energy, grasping that which holds our interest, seizing an opportunity for new learning, enjoying what we do, and getting a start

on a new way of living—especially after developmental delay, deprivation, trauma, and stress. Occupation enables people idiosyncratically to shape their lives and create patterns of living that are a good fit for the environments in which they live, the spaces they occupy, and the sociopolitical and cultural contexts in which they interact. Occupation is all about the business of living, everyday living, and occupational therapists use occupation as means and end in their practice.

Early Associations of Occupation with Health and Well-Being

In its broadest sense, the origins of occupational therapy can be traced back to the beginnings of time. Using occupation to restore health and well-being is well recorded and historians have provided us with rich descriptions of how people throughout the world have lived their lives and how they have adapted to change over the centuries. Even early mythological figures such as Aesculapius, the god of healing, responded in times of illness and crisis by quieting deliriums with such occupations as songs, farce, and music, while the early Greeks soothed their troubled psyches with poetry and discourse. MacDonald (1976), herself an occupational therapist, suggests that the first occupational therapists were physicians. For example, Hippocrates, the father of medicine, emphasized the body–mind link in all interventions and recommended occupations such as wrestling, riding, and strong exercise. The Romans participated in occupational exercises such as sailing and hunting to maintain their health and well-being. Celsus, a Roman physician, prescribed reading aloud for a weak stomach, and described "several kinds of madness and their cures," recommending the use of occupation "suitable to the temper of each." As time unfolded in subsequent centuries, physicians promoted occupations that related to how workers earned their living, thereby directing intervention to match current lifestyle demands (MacDonald, p. 4).

When the Renaissance spawned new growth in medicine and science, increased interest in philosophy and psychology expanded to include industrial physiology, which addressed topics such as rhythm, posture, and energy expenditure. Occupation was then used for toughening up and recreation, and by the end of the 1700s physicians began classifying occupational exercises as active and passive, differentiating between the quiet rhythms of sewing and playing the piano with the more energetic pursuits of bell ringing and chopping wood. With the advent of the Industrial Revolution, attention was redirected to exploring occupations for maintaining health in a society where fewer members would engage in manual work. Increased interest in psychological medicine grew as society saw the potential for humans to be replaced by machines. The arrival of electricity in the mid-1800s and its use as a form of bodily treatment outstripped previous interest in occupational and mental forms of exercise, and this focus on the physical body is still with us as a society today (MacDonald, 1976).

Meanwhile interest in psychological medicine turned its attention to treatment of those incarcerated with mental illness and the deprivation that resulted from the deleterious effects of inactivity. Cruel treatments, restraint, torture, and punishment characterized life in the lunatic asylums. Key reformers felt that moral rather than physical restraint and mental hygiene were more effective forms of intervention. Consequently, new and more active daily routines were established for patients who began to engage in occupations that were wholesome and might enable them to return to life outside the asylum. Although separate from the mainstream of society and still without the benefit of modern pharmaceutical interventions, occupation was used to reshape behavior and to manage madness. Patients engaged in a daily round of labor and leisure, and improvements were noted in their demeanor, appearance, and overall health. The asylum became a self-contained community with patients engaged in occupations on its farm, or in its mechanical shop, laundry, and kitchen (MacDonald, 1976).

As the 19th century came to an end and the 20th century began, many new movements and social reforms were under way throughout the Western world to improve the health of those who were in any way disadvantaged. For example, the pioneering work of Jane Addams at the Hull House Settlement in Chicago provided an opportunity to study the meaning of occupation for new immigrants whose lives were clearly impoverished by circumstance and culture. Settlement work in cities spread across the United States, modeling itself on the Arts and Crafts Movement of the early 1900s. Well-educated women, who became involved in helping those less fortunate, gained confidence and continued working toward other reforms that ultimately led to women's suffrage in the United States (Quiroga, 1995).

Emergence of Occupational Therapy as a Health Profession

The devastating effects of the First World War made it clear that recuperative occupations were needed to integrate severely wounded soldiers back into civilian life. It was at this point that reconstruction aides emerged to work with soldiers who were invalids in what became known as curative workshops. The first reconstruction aides were recruited from nurses and craft teachers who dedicated themselves to restoring the shattered lives of those who had fought for their country. Whether at home or abroad, soldiers developed new interests and skills to prepare them to cope with and adapt to living with their impairments (Quiroga, 1995).

In the United States, the National Society for the Promotion of Occupational Therapy was formed in Clifton Springs, New York in 1917, and its objectives were to advance occupation as a therapeutic measure, to study the effect of occupation on human beings, and to scientifically dispense this new knowledge. The founders came from social work, medicine, psychiatry, nursing, architecture, and teaching and had strong connections in hospitals, schools, and social organizations. Programs for educating occupational therapists were soon developed and leading physicians established departments and programs of occupation in their hospitals. The active involvement of patients in their recovery moved to a new level of understanding as occupation again showed itself to counter the boredom and inactivity associated with long periods of hospitalization. By the time the Second World War came along, occupational therapists, along with their colleagues in physical therapy, nursing, and medicine, were prepared to ensure the successful rehabilitation of returning soldiers. Following that war, occupational therapists focused their practice on bedside occupations to support people experiencing long periods of hospitalization. The profession of occupational therapy developed along comparable lines in other countries in the Western world and such histories are well documented (Quiroga, 1995).

During the second half of the 20th century, the profession of occupational therapy adapted to advances in health care delivery. With results from research, improvements in medication, and innovations in technology bringing about better outcomes, the profession of occupational therapy became more reductionistic in its outlook and more aligned with the medical model, emulating the scientific approaches of other health professions. For a while the profession lost its focus on occupation, but in recent years that focus has returned with renewed vigor (Whiteford, Townsend, & Hocking, 2000). A call to put the occupation back into occupational therapy has resulted in a broadening of service delivery to include educational and community contexts. Today, no matter in which country you look, you will find occupational therapists working in traditional, acute care, and rehabilitation settings as well as community settings such as home health, long-term care, retirement communities, day care centers, school systems, and industry.

Looking at Humans as Occupational Beings

> *The aspects of things that are most important for us are hidden because of their simplicity and familiarity.*
>
> —*Ludwig Wittgenstein*

Underpinning the practice of occupational therapy is the belief that humans are occupational beings who learn about themselves and their world by participating in purposeful and personally meaningful occupations. Occupational therapists believe that people's occupations—that is, the things they do—are influenced not only by personal values and meaning but also by the physical, sociocultural, and political environments in which people do things. In their classic work, Fidler and Fidler (1978) assert that it is through doing, that the nascent human becomes humanized:

> The ability to adapt, to cope with problems of everyday living, and fulfill age-specific life roles requires a rich reservoir of experiences acquired from direct engagement with both human and nonhuman objects in one's environment. *Doing* is the process of investigating, trying out, gaining experience, responding, creating, and controlling. It is through such action, with feedback from both nonhuman and human objects, that an individual comes to know the potential and limitations of self and the environment and achieves a sense of competence and intrinsic worth (p. 306).

New understandings about humans as occupational beings are emerging as the discipline of occupational science unfolds; for example,

Wilcock examined human occupation from an evolutionary perspective. She developed an occupational theory of human nature in which she proposed that humans, as occupational beings, have an *innate need to use time in a purposeful way* to enable them to accomplish the following crucial components of their lives: (1) provide for immediate bodily needs of sustenance, self care, and shelter; (2) develop skills, social structures, and technology aimed at safety and superiority over predators and the environment; and (3) exercise and develop personal capacities enabling the organism to be maintained and to flourish (Wilcock, 1993, 1995, 1998, 2001).

Others have undertaken research that further contributes to our understanding of humans as occupational beings. Bateson, an anthropologist, believes that "The capacity to do something useful for yourself or others is the key to personhood" (1996, p. 11). Developing personhood through doing is a concept extended in works by Christiansen (1999, 2000) who asserts that "occupations are key not just to being a person, but to being a *particular* person, and thus creating and maintaining an identity" (1999, p. 547).

Perhaps one of the most important outcomes of the study of humans as occupational beings is the recognition and importance of the dynamic interaction across the life course among people, their environments, and the diverse occupations in which they engage. The Person-Environment-Occupation Model, developed by Law et al. (1996), helps occupational therapists understand the dynamic nature of occupational performance. As shown by the overlapping circles in **Figure 27–1**, occupational performance is at the center of the interaction existing between the person, environment, and the engagement in occupation. The capabilities of the person, the press of the environment, and the nature of the occupation all influence the quality of occupational performance throughout the life course.

Occupation Across the Human Life Course

The relationship between person, environment, and occupation changes over time in response to the various opportunities and challenges that shape each stage of a person's life course. The primary occupation for children is play, which is self-focused to satisfy personal needs. Through play children develop physical and cognitive skills as they explore the world and themselves. Children's occupational experiences depend on where and with whom they live, and thus shape their subsequent identities. As individuals undergo the inevitable transition from childhood to adolescence, they experience numerous personal, physical, and social changes, which have a significant impact on them occupationally. Adolescence is a time of tremendous upheaval. Identity issues and dramatic bodily changes greatly influence

Figure 27–1 THE PERSON-ENVIRONMENT OCCUPATIONAL MODEL: A TRANSACTIVE APPROACH TO OCCUPATIONAL PERFORMANCE

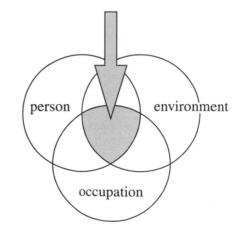

From Law et al. (1996). Used with permission.

occupational performance. Developing a new-found sense of independence is a vital part of preparation for adulthood. Control over occupational choice increases and opportunities to test new boundaries proliferate. Engaging in group occupations with peers is paramount for social development and preparation for the adult world and its attendant responsibilities (Wicks, 2003).

In adulthood, individuals take on new occupations, such as employee, partner, or parent, and some of the occupations in which they previously participated may take on new purpose and meaning. In comparison to occupations early in the life course, adult occupations carry significant economic responsibilities and involve other people, such as caring for children or managing employees; they are more complex and require a greater commitment of time and effort. There are often explicit policies and implicit social expectations associated with adult occupations. These, coupled with adults' personal expectations and motivations for doing, influence occupational performance (Wicks, 2003).

With the demographic shift of the population in the Western world and the baby boomers poised to take flight into retirement, this is an opportune time to put the occupational theory of human nature, which links time use, purpose, and health, to the test with elders. What do people do and not do as they age? Where, how, and with whom do they spend their time? What gives them pleasure? What gives meaning to their lives? These questions form the basis for developing an occupational perspective on aging and are important considerations when designing occupational therapy programs for elders.

One powerful effect of occupation is its organizing ability during times of transition. Think how often we ask a new retiree, "What are you going to do next?" Or "What are you doing with your time these days?" Or we ask a grieving widow, "How are you going to stay busy? How are you going to do everything on your own?"

And the answer to these questions is that, for the most part, people begin new phases of their lives by re-orchestrating what they do: they develop new habits and routines or modify old ones, they revisit former interests or develop new ones, they move to new environments or adapt the ones in which they live. However, if positive or adaptive responses are not forthcoming over time, then people become occupationally dysfunctional and move into a downward spiral that progresses from a cycle of ineffectiveness to incompetence and, ultimately, helplessness.

Elders continue to engage in purposeful and meaningful occupation, but may be required to make occupational adaptations due to physical changes related to aging, changes in relationships following the death of a spouse, or social policy such as retiring from paid employment. In response to such physical, emotional, and social influences, and as long as life continues, people expand their repertoire of occupations by developing new occupations and abandoning others. Cumulative experience in occupations grows over time and people's occupational life course will evolve, adapt, or be transformed into new patterns as interactions between the person, environment, and occupation change.

Research shows that although the majority of elders successfully make the occupational adaptations that accompany aging and continue to lead productive and occupationally meaningful lives, some may have difficulty adapting. Frailty, loneliness, or physical and mental impairments may diminish the number and diversity of their occupations (Baltes & Baltes, 1993; Ranzijn & Grbich, 2001; Ranzijn, Harford, & Andrew, 2002). In the MacArthur Foundation study of successful aging, Rowe and Kahn (1998) propose a three-part paradigm for aging well: avoiding disease, maintaining high cognitive and physical function, and engagement in life. The concept of engagement in life is not only consistent with an occupational perspective of health and well-being but also with the World Health Organization's definition of health and its International Classification of Functioning, Disability, and Health, which promotes a more inclusive and societal approach to looking at disability and health (Wilcock, 1998; World Health Organization, 2001).

As people live longer, their needs for meaningful occupation only increase. Results of time-use studies with elders show tremendous variability in how people spend their time with key differences between men and women as traditional roles for our current generation of elders might suggest. For example, women spend more time in occupations related to homemaking while men spend more time in occupations related to home maintenance. Although many elders engage in a broad repertoire of occupations, time spent in passive and solitary occupations increases with age but not necessarily to the detriment of its value or meaning (Stanley, 1995).

When Wicks (2003) explored the life course of elderly Australian women from an occupational and a feminist perspective, she found four common features to the occupational strategies that the women developed over time. Although the strategies were uniquely situated to meet individual occupational needs, collectively their primary purpose was to create opportunities for meaningful occupation. These occupational strategies were developed at an early stage and refined over time, and there was a clear relationship between the quality and quantity of occupational strategies and level of participation in meaningful occupations. Finally, the effectiveness and refinement of occupational strategies influenced the women's satisfaction with their occupational life course. Three major examples of the occupational strategies developed by the women over time, which positively influenced health, well-being, and satisfaction with the life course, include: (1) creating independence by maintaining a separate identity, pursuing personal leisure interests, or creating personal space; (2) enriching occupational experiences by becoming immersed in available occupations, creating alternative occupations, improvising, and by being willing to try new occupations; and (3) adopting enlightened self-interest, a strategy designed to satisfy personal occupational needs as well as meet the needs of significant others (Wicks & Whiteford, 2004). Awareness and understanding that people develop such occupational strategies across the life course are vital when designing programs to promote occupations for groups of elders.

Designing Occupational Experiences

It is not what a person does, but how involved in the activity a person becomes.

—*Mihalyi Csikszentmihalyi*

One of the cutting-edge approaches to designing occupational experiences comes from Pierce (2001b). She proposes that occupation will only have therapeutic power if it includes three key elements: appeal, intactness, and accuracy. The relationships among these three key elements and their component parts are shown in **Figure 27–2**. First, *appeal* refers to the subjective experience that occupations have for people; second, *intactness* requires that the contextual conditions for engaging in the occupation are appropriate and not contrived; and third, *accuracy* demands that occupational therapists collaborate with people to set up chosen occupations in ways that make sense and meet their goals (Pierce, 2001b, 2003).

Increasing the appeal of an occupation depends on the way in which the components of productivity, pleasure, and restoration each contribute to the subjective dimensions of occupation. Pierce (2003) proposes that all occupations have varying degrees of productivity, pleasure, and restoration inherently embedded within them, and how each of these elements is valued varies with the individual.

Figure 27–2 BUILDING THERAPEUTIC
POWER

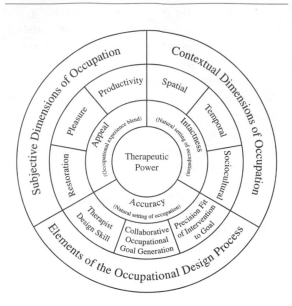

Appeal + Intactness + Accuracy = Therapeutic Power

From Pierce, D. E. (2003). Used with permission.

Rather than having to choose between a sense of productivity or pleasure or restoration, one can structure participation in occupations that combine these elements in highly idiosyncratic ways.

Because our current generation of elders grew up in a time when the Protestant work ethic prevailed, a sense of productivity is a highly desirable state to ensure that one feels useful and valuable to society. In Western cultures, pleasure often seems the very antithesis of productivity, enjoyed only after the work is done. Yet giving and receiving pleasure is a highly personal and often overlooked health-promoting concept as it evokes many different types of human responses: intellectual, emotional, sensual, tactile, physical, and spiritual. Healthy pleasures are life affirming and strongly linked to immune system functioning. In cultures other than Western, pleasure is a central feature of the life well lived (Ornstein & Sobel, 1989;

Pearsall, 1996). Restoration is a frequently overlooked but vital component of the subjective experience of occupation. Much like pleasure, restoration is antithetical to the values of the Protestant work ethic—yet, without sufficient restoration our lives become frantic, frenzied, and frenetic. Encouraging and creating opportunities to nurture resting and quiet-focused occupations are health promoting, especially when they create a newfound sense of energy, improved mood, and increased feelings of well-being (Pierce, 2001a).

Maintaining the intactness of an occupation requires attention to the three contextual dimensions in which occupations take place if a sense of authenticity is to prevail: where, when, and how occupations take place vary tremendously among individuals. According to Pierce (2003), the spatial dimension of occupation relates to the human body and the spaces it occupies. As humans, we respond to different spaces primarily through our senses, with vision and touch finely honed. The ways in which we perceive our bodies in any given space strongly influence our feelings of comfort. Spaces also carry with them meaning. They are not just containers we drop into when we want to do something; consequently spaces and places add further to the authenticity of the occupational experience. The temporal dimension of occupation relates to timing, when and how often we choose to engage in occupation, and the flow of time within an occupation. We are shaped by our circadian rhythms and we each have our own rhythm of doing things. Individual differences usually produce quite strong preferences for different daily, weekly, monthly, seasonal, and annual habits and routines.

The sociocultural dimension of occupation relates to how we like to engage in occupation and the way in which we participate is strongly influenced by our heritage and culture. Social engagement in occupation can move from being completely solitary to highly interactive, from small groups to large groups, from private to public, and the mix and balance are highly individualized. Our cultural background greatly influences the aspects of occupation that we treasure and hold dear (Pierce, 2001b).

Increasing the accuracy of targeted occupations requires sharpening the focus of all the elements of the occupational design process. Occupational therapists need strong design skills so they can collaborate with their clients in establishing occupational goals (what is it that you want to do that has meaning to you?). They must ensure that engaging in selected occupations will make sense and be perceived as authentic and relevant to their clients' lives. Failure to do so will result in insufficient therapeutic power to achieve the desired outcomes (Pierce, 2003).

Promoting Participation in Occupations for Groups of Elders

Pierce's design framework gives us a starting point for looking at the occupational needs and interests of elders when they participate in groups. Acknowledging the importance of the subjective dimension of occupation and withholding our interpretation of what an occupational experience means to another is vital for designing occupationally based groups for elders, for meaning is always in the eye of the beholder. Often health professionals working with elders organize groups and they expect elders to want to participate. They anticipate favorable outcomes, and then are disappointed when neither group is enjoyable for the participants nor do the elders fully participate. We propose that promoting participation in occupations for groups of elders requires further attention at the design stage to three important variables: context, choice, challenge.

Context is a major contributor to environmental press and may help or hinder participation in occupations for groups of elders. In terms of physical contexts, venues for group occupations of elders need to be authentic, attractive, and accessible. A variety of venues, indoor and outdoor, and availability of daytime or evening programs all enhance the range of available group occupations for elders. In contrast, the sociocultural context may enliven or hamper the way in which groups of elders participate in occupations. Often, institutional policies dictate where, when, and how clients spend their waking hours, resulting in a custodial rather than a therapeutic environment (Taft & Nehrke, 1990).

Consider Miguel's recent admission to a nursing home, which strictly regulates the availability of group occupations. Before his devastating stroke, Miguel regularly got up early to drink coffee with his friends at the barbershop. Although it is not feasible for Miguel to get out to a barbershop for his morning coffee, small accommodations to the morning routine could allow Miguel access to an alternative venue in which to drink coffee with a group of men. Creatively framing where, when, and how groups of elders are able to participate in occupations inexorably influences the authenticity and meaning embedded within the group experience.

Choice is one of the most powerful strategies for promoting participation in groups for elders. Elders need opportunity to have a voice in their choice of occupations. Elders will choose to participate in group occupations in accordance with the pleasure they bring them, and the value they provide in fostering feelings of productivity and restoration. Choice is strongly influenced by sociocultural norms, linked to race, status, class, gender, and age (Kondo, 2004).

Consider Saj, a Samoan man at a senior citizens center, who adamantly refused to make scones with the cooking group, yet when asked what he liked to eat, immediately offered to cook a pot of chop suey, his national dish, for the group. Alternatively, consider the resultant sense of control, increased morale, and the positive effect when residents in long-term care facilities are offered a number of choices in their dining preferences (Duncan-Myers & Huebner, 2000).

Occupational choice affirms our occupational identities, shows the world who we are, and strengthens the appeal of engaging in group occupations.

Challenge is an equally powerful element in promoting participation of elders in group occupations if they are to experience what Csikszentmihalyi (1993) calls flow, the feeling of being totally absorbed in the moment. Flow only occurs when the level of challenge matches a person's skills. If the challenge is greater than the skill level, then anxiety and stress prevail, but if the skill requirements are set too low, boredom and apathy set in. Consider the following scenario. Why won't Stella and Mary join the bingo group today at the assisted living facility? Are they disinterested? Why are they resisting? Further discussion reveals that they find playing bingo insufficiently challenging and would rather co-opt another couple of residents playing bridge. Occupational challenges, when "just right," provide a compelling reason for elders to participate in groups.

The WISH Team

To illustrate further how the variables of context, choice, and challenge are used in designing occupations for groups of elders, we describe an example from local practice, in which Mitcham and her occupational therapy students used a group-based approach to design and implement a health promotion and education program for elderly residents at Brighton Place, a low-income housing complex. Funding for the program initially came from a Healthy South Carolinian Initiatives grant at the Medical University of South Carolina (Haight, 1998) and is currently sustained by federal support from the Health Resources and Services Administration (Mitcham, 2002). The program and its evolution are based on work by Clark et al. (1997), Clark et al. (1996), Jackson (1996), and Mandel, Jackson, Zemke, Nelson,

and Clark (1999). A strong community–campus partnership, a hallmark of the program, developed between residents and occupational therapy students, and together they named the program the WISH Team, to represent the components of Well-being, Independence, Safety, and Health.

CONTEXT

Situated in a suburban part of town, close to a large shopping mall, Brighton Place is comprised of 10 detached, single-story buildings, each with 10 one-bedroom apartments and a separate community building that houses the site manager's office, laundry facilities, restrooms, residents' mail boxes, large community room, and small kitchen. The majority of residents are women who live alone but still drive their own cars, and there is a fairly even distribution of African-American and Caucasian residents. The context fosters independence, promotes autonomy, and encourages participation in programs offered by external groups, such as the university.

CHOICE

Central to the ongoing success of the WISH Team is the resident-centered approach and collaborative process of qualitative needs assessment that takes place twice a year. A group discussion is held and residents identify the issues most important to them in the areas of well-being, independence, safety, and health. Residents then choose the order in which they would like to deal with the issues, the frequency with which they'd like to meet, and the day and time. Based on the results of the discussion, occupational therapy students are guided to plan and implement a series of occupation-based health promotion and education sessions that respond to the topics of choice. For example, safety continues to be a popular choice of topic. Women who live alone are concerned about their personal safety, safety in their home, and safety out in the community; consequently, several sessions have focused on these topics.

Sessions are held in the large community room, which is well equipped with small tables and chairs. Active publicity for the sessions includes communicating with the site manager and president of the residents' association, posting flyers in central locations and distributing them to each resident's apartment, and making personal phone calls to remind key participants to encourage others to attend. At the start of the project, sessions were offered on a weekly basis but now have settled into a monthly routine with eight to twelve residents attending each time. Each session lasts approximately one hour and has taken on a familiar shape and rhythm based on residents' choice: arrival, sign in, and greeting; warm-up exercises with music to energize mind and body; presentation of main topic; active participation in small groups to apply concepts from the main topic; summary and take-home message; and closure with refreshments, social interaction, and checking of blood pressure—another choice expressed by the residents. Balancing the familiarity of the shape of the session with the added stimulation of new knowledge from the main topic ensures that residents feel comfortable yet sufficiently challenged.

CHALLENGE

No matter the topic at hand, each session is designed to help participants analyze their own patterns of occupation, and to increase understanding of how participating in occupation exerts an influence on their rhythm of living and current lifestyle. Providing the "just right" challenge requires a multimedia approach to accommodate varying levels of literacy, education, cognition, and typical impairments associated with aging. For example, students have learned principles of graphic design so that written materials for the take-home message are visually appealing, adapted to a suitable reading level, and nonthreatening in their presentation. Customizing the level of challenge for a mixed-ability group of residents is made eas-

ier by having two or three students at each session to provide sufficient and individual attention to upgrade or downgrade participation in the small group activities that follow the presentation of the main topic. Interaction in small groups also provides opportunities for the more able residents to help those less able, and to share experiences validating what they know about promoting their own health. Ongoing and informal evaluation shows that residents have increased their knowledge of topics related to well-being, independence, safety, and health, and want to continue the monthly meeting of the WISH Team.

Validating the Power of Occupation

> When one is older, it is important to have meaning in your life, and the opportunity to do meaningful things.
>
> —Basil Hetzel

Although the WISH Team is a local example of promoting participation in occupations for groups of elders, we bring our chapter to a close by describing a landmark study in the United States that empirically supports the power of group occupations to promote health and well-being for elders. "The Well Elderly Study," a randomized controlled trial, demonstrates that preventive occupational therapy mitigates against the health risks associated with aging. In it, 361 men and women over the age of 60 from a variety of ethnic backgrounds who lived independently in two government-subsidized apartment complexes were randomly assigned to one of three groups for nine months: an occupational therapy group, a social activity control group, and a non-treatment control group. Those who received occupational therapy participated for two hours each week for nine months in group-based intervention, plus they received an additional hour each month of individual intervention.

Occupational therapists provided the intervention using a variety of delivery methods including didactic presentations, peer exchange, personal exploration, and direct experience to help participants incorporate positive changes into their existing and idiosyncratic lifestyles. The group sessions focused on the importance of occupation to overall health and well-being, and how changes and adaptations to one's routine and pattern of occupation promote: (1) increases in personal, home, and community safety; (2) improvements to specific health behaviors such as using principles of joint protection and energy conservation; and (3) gains in engaging in personally meaningful occupations that are congruent with individual attributes, values, goals, and circumstances (Clark et al., 1997).

The effectiveness of the intervention was measured at baseline, after nine months, and again six months later with a battery of standardized and well-known measurements as follows: the RAND Health Status Survey Short Form–36, Functional Status Questionnaire, Life Satisfaction Index 2, Center for Epidemiology Studies Depression Scale, and the Medical Outcomes Study Health Perception Scale. Overall, participants who received occupational therapy experienced more gains and fewer losses on the variables measured than did participants in the social activity and nontreatment control groups. Statistically significant ($P < .05$) gains were made in the areas of quality interaction on the Functional Status Questionnaire, and on the physical functioning, role functioning, vitality, social functioning, role emotional, and general mental health subscales of the RAND Health Status Survey Short Form–36. These gains were sustained six months after receiving occupational therapy, thereby embedding health-promoting changes into participants' daily routines and life roles (Clark et al., 2001).

One of the most important outcomes of the study was the cost-effectiveness of the intervention, approximately $548 for each participant. As examined by Hay et al. (2002), costs for postintervention health care were significantly lower for the occupational therapy group ($967) when compared to the social activity ($1726) and the nontreatment ($3334) control groups, or to a combination of the control groups ($2593). These cost savings are important because overall medical expenditures increase with age even for healthy elders. The significance of "The Well Elderly Study" for the profession of occupational therapy is that it has generated increased interest in working with well elders outside of the medical model and provides a prime example of the power of using occupation to promote health and well-being.

Summary

The way to improve quality of life is not through thinking but through doing.

—Anonymous

Occupation is all about the things people do throughout their lives that have meaning, purpose, and value to them. Throughout time, occupation has had a major influence on health and well-being, and, ultimately, occupation emerged as the domain of practice for occupational therapists. When occupational therapists focus on humans as occupational beings, they direct their practice to use occupation as means and end. The most important contribution occupational therapists make to working with groups of elders is the ability to accurately design authentic experiences that are relevant for everyday living. Occupational therapists enable elders to participate in meaningful occupations by optimizing the contexts in which they participate, maximizing the available choices, and tailoring the challenges to enhance successful occupational performance, thereby promoting health and well-being. Using preventive occupational therapy to help elders develop strategies to organize and orchestrate their lives in idiosyncratic ways and to satisfy their innate needs for purposeful use of time has been validated empirically by "The Well Elderly Study" and shown to be a cost-effective mechanism for intervention.

Exercises

Exercise 1

Look at your own life and identify at least three occupations you believe contribute to your health and well-being. When did you begin these occupations? Through how much of your life course have these occupations been important to you? What would you do if you could not participate in these occupations?

Exercise 2

Look at **Figure** 27–1. Select a specific occupation for a specific person (elder) in a specific environment. List three attributes of the occupation, the person, and the environment. Consider their interaction and think about ways to enhance occupational performance.

Exercise 3

Look at **Figure** 27–2 and think about the three key elements that enhance therapeutic power. List three strategies that you could use to enhance the appeal, intactness, and accuracy of an occupation for a group of elders living in a retirement community.

Exercise 4

Consider three more variables when designing group-based occupations for elders: context, choice, and challenge. For each variable, list three strategies you might employ when designing an occupation-based group for elders living in an assisted living facility.

References

Baltes, P., & Baltes, M. (1993). *Successful aging. Perspectives from the behavioral sciences*. Cambridge: University of Cambridge Press.

Bateson, M. (1996). Enfolded activity and the concept of occupation. In R. Zemke & F. Clark (Eds.), *Occupational science: The evolving discipline*. Philadelphia: F. A. Davis.

Christiansen, C. (1999). Defining lives: Occupation as identity: An essay on competence, coherence, and the creation of meaning. *American Journal of Occupational Therapy, 53*(6), 547–558.

Christiansen, C. (2000). Identity, personal projects and happiness: Self construction in everyday action. *Journal of Occupational Science, 7*(3), 98–107.

Clark, F., Azen, S. P., Carlson, M., Mandel, D., La Bree, L., Hay, J., et al. (2001). Embedding health-promoting changes into the daily lives of independent-living older adults: Long-term follow-up of occupational therapy intervention. *Journal of Gerontology, 56B*(1), 60–63.

Clark, F., Azen, S. P., Zemke, R., Jackson, J., Carlson, M., Mandel, D., et al. (1997). Occupational therapy for independent-living older adults. *Journal of the American Medical Association, 278*(16), 1321–1326.

Clark, F., Carlson, M., Zemke, R., Frank, G., Patterson, K., Ennevor, B. L., et al. (1996). Life domains and adaptive strategies of a group of low-income well older adults. *American Journal of Occupational Therapy, 50,* 99–108.

Csikszentmihalyi, M. (1993). Activity and happiness: Towards a science of occupation. *Journal of Occupational Science, 1*(1), 38–42.

Duncan-Myers, A. M., & Huebner, R. A. (2000). Relationship between choice and quality of life among residents in long-term care facilities. *American Journal of Occupational Therapy, 5*(5), 504–508.

Fidler, G., & Fidler, J. (1978). Doing and becoming: Purposeful action and self-actualization. *American Journal of Occupational Therapy, 32,* 305–310.

Haight, B. K. (1998). Healthy aging project: Promoting and managing health in subsidized housing. The Healthy South Carolina Initiatives, Medical University of South Carolina.

Hay, J., La Bree, L., Luo, R., Clark, F., Carlson, M., Mandel, D., et al. (2002). Cost-effectiveness of preventive occupational therapy for independent-living older adults. *Journal of the American Geriatric Society, 50,* 1381–1388.

Jackson, J. (1996). Living a meaningful existence in old age. In R. Zemke & F. Clark (Eds.), *Occupational science: The evolving discipline* (pp. 339–361). Philadelphia: F. A. Davis.

Kondo, T. (2004). Cultural tensions in occupational therapy practice: Considerations from a Japanese vantage point. *American Journal of Occupational Therapy, 58*(2), 174–184.

Law, M., Cooper, B., Strong, S., Stewart, D., Rigby, P., & Letts, L. (1996). The person-environment-occupation model: A transactive approach to occupational performance. *Canadian Journal of Occupational Therapy, 63,* 9–23.

MacDonald, E. M. (1976). *Occupational therapy in rehabilitation.* Baltimore: Williams & Wilkins.

Mandel, D. R., Jackson, J. M., Zemke, R., Nelson, L., & Clark, F. A. (1999). *Lifestyle redesign. Implementing the well elderly study.* Bethesda, MD: American Occupational Therapy Association.

Mitcham, M. D. (2002). *Community connections: Partners for service and learning.* (D37HP00876). Health Resources and Services Administration.

Ornstein, R., & Sobel, D. (1989). *Healthy pleasures.* Reading, MA: Perseus Books.

Pearsall, P. (1996). *The pleasure prescription. To love, to work, to play—life in the balance.* Alameda, CA: Hunter House.

Pierce, D. E. (2001a). Untangling occupation and activity. *American Journal of Occupational Therapy, 55*(2), 138–146.

Pierce, D. E. (2001b). Occupation by design: Dimensions, therapeutic power, and creative process. *American Journal of Occupational Therapy, 55*(3), 249–259.

Pierce, D. E. (2003). *Occupation by design: Building therapeutic power.* Philadelphia: F. A. Davis.

Quiroga, V. A. M. (1995). *Occupational therapy: The first 30 years 1900–1930.* Bethesda, MD: American Occupational Therapy Association.

Ranzijn, R., & Grbich, C. (2001). Qualitative aspects of productive ageing. *Australasian Journal of Ageing, 20*(2), 62–66.

Ranzijn, R., Harford, J., & Andrew, G. (2002). Ageing and the economy: Costs and benefits. *Australasian Journal of Ageing, 21*(3), 145–151.

Rowe, J. W., & Kahn, R. (1998). *Successful aging.* New York: Random House.

Stanley, M. (1995). An investigation into the relationships between engagement in valued occupations and life satisfaction for elderly South Australians. *Journal of Occupational Science, 2*(3), 100–114.

Taft, L. B., & Nehrke, M. F. (1990). Reminiscence, life review, and ego integrity in nursing home residents. *International Journal of Aging and Human Development, 30,* 189–196.

Whiteford, G. (2000). Occupational deprivation: Global challenge in the new millennium. *British Journal of Occupational Therapy, 63*(5), 200–204.

Whiteford, G., Townsend, E., & Hocking, C. (2000). Reflections on a renaissance of occupation. *Canadian Journal of Occupational Therapy, 67*(1), 61–69.

Wicks, A. (2003). Understanding occupational potential across the life course. Life stories of older women. Unpublished doctoral dissertation, Charles Stuart University, Australia.

Wicks, A., & Whiteford, G. (in press). Gender and occupational participation. In G. Whiteford & V. Wright-St. Clair, *Occupation and practice in context.* Marrickville, Australia: Elsevier.

Wilcock, A. (1993). A theory of the human need for occupation. *Journal of Occupational Science: Australia, 1*(1), 17–24.

Wilcock, A. (1995). The occupational brain: A theory of human nature. *Journal of Occupational Science: Australia, 2*(1), 68–73.

Wilcock, A. (1998). *An occupational perspective of health.* Thorofare, NJ: SLACK.

Wilcock, A. A. (2001). *Occupation for health* (Vol. 1). London: College of Occupational Therapists.

World Health Organization. (2001). *International classification of functioning, disability and health: ICF.* Geneva: Author.

BIBLIOGRAPHY

Christiansen, C. H., & Baum, C. M. (Eds.). (1997). *Occupational therapy: Enabling function and well-being* (2nd ed.). Thorofare, NJ: SLACK.

Christiansen, C. H., & Townsend, E. A. (Eds.). (2004). *Introduction to occupation: The art and science of living.* Upper Saddle River, NJ: Prentice Hall.

Crepeau, E. B., Cohn, E. S., & Boyt Schell, B. A. (2003). *Willard & Spackman's occupational therapy* (10th ed.). Philadelphia: Lippincott Williams & Wilkins.

Hasselkus, B. R. (2002). *The meaning of everyday occupation.* Thorofare, NJ: SLACK.

Hinojosa, J., & Blount, M. L. (Eds.). (2004). *The texture of life: Purposeful activities in occupational therapy* (2nd ed.). Bethesda, MD: American Occupational Therapy Association.

Kielhofner, G. (2004). *Conceptual foundations of occupational therapy.* Philadelphia: F. A. Davis.

Kramer, P., Hinojosa, J., & Royeen, C. B. (Eds.). (2003). *Perspectives on human occupation: Participation in life.* Philadelphia: Lippincott Williams &Wilkins.

Townsend, E. (Ed.). (2001). *Enabling occupation: An occupational therapy perspective* (2nd ed.). Ottawa, Canada: CAOT Publications ACE.

Zemke, R., & Clark, F. (Eds.). (1996). *Occupational science: The evolving discipline.* Philadelphia: F. A. Davis.

A Physical Therapy Perspective: Group Exercise and Education for the Older Adult

Holly H. Wise

Sandra S. Brotherton

Key Words

- Chronic conditions
- Functional limitation
- Group exercise and education
- Health promotion
- Impairments
- Injury prevention
- Intervention
- Older adults
- Physical therapy
- Rehabilitation

Learning Objectives

- Understand the role of the physical therapist in promotion, maintenance, and restoration of optimal physical function and movement
- Describe the benefits of physical therapy group exercise and education in the treatment of impairments associated with conditions commonly found in older adults
- Explain the importance of a needs assessment in the design and implementation of a physical therapy group intervention
- Discuss essential participant, instructor, and facility considerations in the design

and implementation of a physical therapy group intervention
- Identify the components of a physical therapy group exercise and education program
- Discuss implementation strategies designed to enhance the delivery of physical therapy group programs
- Explain how formative and summative assessments can be used to evaluate outcome effectiveness and to guide in the planning of future group interactions

Physical therapy is a primary health care profession with an established theoretical and scientific base and widespread clinical applications in the promotion, maintenance, and restoration of optimal physical function and movement (American Physical Therapy Association [APTA], 2003). Although the use of certain physical therapy techniques for illness and injuries goes back to ancient times, the modern physical therapy profession developed during the 1900s in support of military servicemen in World War I. Physical therapists also played an important role during the poliomyelitis epidemics of the mid-1900s by helping people with polio minimize or overcome the paralyzing effects of the virus (Scott, 2002).

Because physical therapists work with people of all ages, it is critical that they understand a vast array of problems that can affect movement, function, and health throughout the life span. All physical therapists have completed coursework in the medical, biological, physical, and psychological sciences and, at a minimum, graduate from a program of college education. Physical therapist educational programs offer degrees that range from the baccalaureate degree to the clinical doctorate in physical therapy. Some physical therapists seek advanced certification in a clinical specialty, such as orthopedic, neurologic, cardiopulmonary, pediatric, geriatric, or sports physical therapy, and others become certified in electrophysiological testing and measurement. In some countries, the professional education of physical therapists prepares them to be autonomous practitioners (Scott, 2002).

Physical therapists are experts in the management of patients and clients with impairments resulting from musculoskeletal, neuromuscular, cardiopulmonary, and integumentary (skin) problems. **Table 28–1** identifies examples of impairments and conditions that may affect an individual's ability to move and function optimally in their daily lives. Physical therapy services are provided by, or under the direction and supervision of, a physical therapist and include examination, evaluation, diagnosis, prognosis and planning, intervention, and reexamination of the outcomes. The cornerstones of physical therapy interventions are the coordination of an individual's plan of care, patient/client instruction to ensure active participation in health care, and direct interventions in the form of therapeutic exercise and functional training. Often, an important component of a physical therapist's program is directed at preventing injury and loss of movement (APTA, 2003).

Physical therapy practice settings vary in relation to whether the desired outcomes are focused on professional education, treatment or rehabilitation, health promotion, or prevention. Thus, physical therapists work in educational and research centers, outpatient clinics, homes, hospitals, nursing homes, senior citizen centers, fitness centers, and in a variety of other community settings (Scott, 2002). Within these settings, patients and clients access physical therapy services either through a referral from their physician or by self-referral. If the diagnostic process reveals findings that are not within the scope of the physical therapist's knowledge, experience, or expertise, the physical therapist will refer the patient or client to another appropriate practitioner. **Table 28–2** displays exercises that can be performed in a community setting.

Physical Therapy for the Older Adult

Normal age-related bodily changes are often misunderstood by seniors and unnecessarily limit daily activities. A physical therapist, working with the older adult, understands the anatomical and physiological changes that occur with normal aging and can be an important source of information. The physical therapist evaluates the older adult and develops a specially designed therapeutic exercise program that may prevent lifelong disability and/or restore the highest possible level of functioning. Another example of such a program is given in **Table 28–3**.

Screening programs, tests and measurements, evaluations, exercises, therapeutic modalities, and educational interventions allow physical therapists to:

- Increase, restore, or maintain range of motion, physical strength, flexibility, coordination, balance, and endurance.
- Recommend adaptations to make the home accessible and safe.
- Teach positioning, transfers, and walking skills that promote maximum function and independence.
- Increase overall fitness through exercise programs.

- Prevent further decline in functional abilities through education, energy conservation techniques, joint protection, and use of assistive devices to promote independence.
- Improve sensation and joint proprioception.
- Reduce pain (APTA, 2003).

Review of the Literature on Group Physical Therapy for the Older Adult

The following review of the scientific basis for group physical therapy interventions is based on the broad categories of interventions designed to improve balance and reduce or prevent falls, minimize the functional limitations associated with chronic conditions, and promote health and wellness.

Balance and Falls

Numerous studies have been conducted to examine the benefits of various forms of group exercise on balance with older adults. The practice of tai chi chuan has been found to improve balance in community-dwelling elders (Hain, Fuller, Weil, & Kotasias, 1999; Hong, Li, & Skelton, 2000;

Komagata & Newton, 2003) and delay the onset of first falls (Wolf, Barnhardt, Ellison, & Coogler, 1997). Participation in a computerized balance training group also resulted in significantly improved postural stability (Wolf, Barnhardt, Ellison, & Coogler). In addition, improved performance on a test of balance was noted for elderly individuals after engaging in either group aquatic or land-based lower-body exercises (Douris et al., 2003). Fall-prone elderly men who participated in a 12-week group program consisting of strength, endurance, and mobility activities had a lower 3-month fall rate than a control group (Rubenstein et al., 2003). Lastly, group participants in a 12-month program of weight-bearing exercises had fewer falls and performed significantly better on reaction time and 6-minute walk tests than a control group (Lord et al., 2003).

Functional Limitations with Chronic Conditions

Physical therapists combine group exercise and education to improve the health of individuals and reduce the functional limitations that can occur with a variety of chronic diseases. Several

Table 28-1 IMPAIRMENT CATEGORIES AND EXAMPLE CONDITIONS THAT MAY AFFECT MOVEMENT AND FUNCTION

Impairment categories (APTA, 2003)	Example conditions
Musculoskeletal • Posture • Muscle performance • Joint mobility and range of motion • Motor performance • Gait, locomotion, and balance	Amputation Bony/soft-tissue surgery Fractures Inflammation Joint arthroplasty Osteoarthritis Osteoporosis Rheumatoid arthritis Spinal disorders Stress/fecal incontinence

continued

Table 28–1   IMPAIRMENT CATEGORIES AND EXAMPLE CONDITIONS THAT MAY AFFECT MOVEMENT AND FUNCTION (CONTINUED)

Impairment categories (APTA, 2003)	Example conditions
Neuromuscular	
• Neuromotor development	Alzheimer's
• Motor function/sensory integrity	Coordination/balance disorders
– Nonprogressive disorders	Dementia
– Progressive disorders	Hemiplegia
– Acute/chronic polyneuropathies	Multiple sclerosis
• Peripheral nerve integrity	Parkinson's
• Motor function, peripheral nerve and sensory integrity with nonprogressive disorders of the spinal cord	Peripheral nerve injury
	Spinal cord disorders
	Traumatic brain injury
• Arousal, range of motion, and motor control with coma, near coma, or vegetative state	
Cardiovascular/Pulmonary	
• Aerobic capacity/endurance	Cardiac and pulmonary disease
– Deconditioning	Deconditioning
– Cardiovascular pump dysfunction	(cancer, diabetes, etc.)
• Ventilation, respiration/gas exchanged and aerobic capacity/endurance	Hypertension
	Lymphatic system disorders
– Airway clearance dysfunction	Obesity
– Ventilatory pump dysfunction	
– Respiratory failure	
• Circulation and anthropometric dimensions	
Integumentary (Skin)	
• Integumentary integrity	Amputation
– Superficial skin involvement	Bacterial meningitis
– Partial-thickness skin involvement/scar formation	Burns
– Full-thickness skin involvement/scar formation	Cellulitis
	Diabetes mellitus
	Keloid scar
• Skin involvement extending into fascia, muscle, bone, and scar formation	Malnutrition

Table 28–2 SAMPLE ACTIVITIES AND EXERCISES FOR GROUP PHYSICAL THERAPY CLASS FOR COMMUNITY-DWELLING OLDER ADULTS

Class title	Participants	Educational topics	Sample activities & exercises	Outcome measures
Better Balance	Older adults who have experienced > 1 fall in last 6 months	Fall risk factors Proper posture Benefits of exercise Environmental hazards/ adaptations	**Active range of motion exercises** Cervical flexion, rotation, lateral flexion; scapular adduction; trunk extension; hip extension and knee extension; and ankle dorsiflexion **Stretching exercises** Standing corner stretch for pectoralis major Standing stretch for ankle plantar flexors Sitting stretch for hip and knee flexors Supine hamstring stretch (**Figure 28–1**) **Strengthening exercises** Chin tucks Scapular adduction using Thera-band/tubing in sitting or standing (**Figure 28–2**) Wall slides for quadriceps Step up on stair to strengthen hip extensors **Mat exercises: With/without weights** Side-lying hip abduction (**Figure 28–3**) Supine straight leg raises with opposite leg positioned in hip/knee flexion Supine pelvic tilts with both hips/knees flexed and feet on the supporting surface **Balance activities** Standing: Single leg stance (**Figure 28–4**) 　　　　Half-circle "sway" All fours: Balance on hands/knees lifting one leg/arm at a time	Postural assessment Goniometric measurements for ROM MMT FIM Balance-assessment tools 　TUG 　POMA 　BBS

Table 28–3   SAMPLE ACTIVITIES AND EXERCISES FOR GROUP PHYSICAL THERAPY CLASS FOR
OLDER ADULTS IN INSTITUTIONAL SETTINGS

Class title	Participants	Educational topics	Sample activities & exercises (sitting with or without mat)	Outcome measures
On the Move	Nonambulatory frail, older adults in institutional settings	Exercise importance Activities of daily living	**Seated activities (in circle):** Ball activities: Passing, throwing, catching, bouncing, and kicking Parachute (sheet) activities: Lifting it up, tossing an object placed on the sheet up in the air, or rotating the sheet around the circle **Active range of motion exercises** Cervical flexion, rotation, lateral flexion; scapular adduction; trunk extension; knee extension; and ankle dorsiflexion **Stretching exercises** Sitting stretch for hip and knee flexors Supine hamstring stretch (**Figure 28–1**) **Strengthening Exercises** Chin tucks Scapular adduction using Thera-band/ tubing in sitting or standing (**Figure 28–2**) **Mat exercise** With/without weights Side-lying hip abduction (**Figure 28–3**) Supine straight leg with opposite leg positioned in hip/knee flexion Supine pelvic tilts with both hips/knees flexed and feet on the supporting surface	Postural assessment Goniometric measurements for ROM MMT FIM

studies reported benefits obtained from group activities for older adults with chronic musculoskeletal conditions. Older adults with arthritis improved scores on measures of physical performance and mental health after participation in educational classes and standing and sitting dynamic exercise (Gunther, Taylor, Karuza, & Calkins, 2003). Hidding et al. (1993) reported on a randomized, controlled trial that studied the effects of adding supervised group physical therapy to unsupervised individualized home therapy on 144 individuals with a diagnosis of ankylosing spondylitis. Weekly group physical therapy proved superior to individualized home therapy for certain measures of trunk mobility and fitness and had an important effect on global health reported by the participants. In addition, total medical costs decreased 44% for participants in group therapy as compared to 35% for home therapy (Bakker, Hidding, van der Linden, & van Doorslaer, 1994).

Group education and exercise have also been successfully used with individuals with a diagnosis of urinary incontinence or fibromyalgia. Women with urinary incontinence participated in group education and pelvic floor muscle exercise and reported improved scores on all outcome measures (pad tests, incontinence impact questionnaires, visual analogue scales, symptom severity index score) compared to baseline and had better self-rated symptom scores than women who received

Figure 28–1

Supine hamstring stretch.

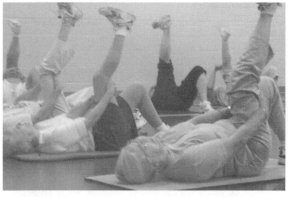

Figure 28–2

Tube row: scapular adduction.

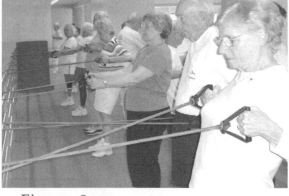

Figure 28–3

Side-lying hip abduction exercise.

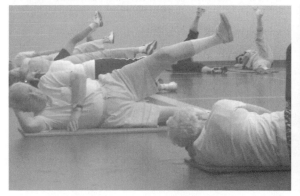

Figure 28–4

Standing single leg balance activity.

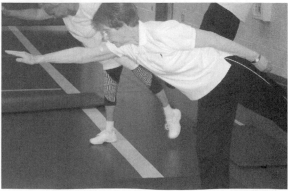

individual treatment for urinary incontinence (Demain, Smith, Hiller, & Dziedzic, 2001). Educational group meetings provided for individuals with fibromyalgia and their spouses or significant others resulted in improved symptoms and quality of life (Bennett et al., 1996; Schacter, Busch, Peloso, & Sheppard, 2003). These group meetings offered participants instruction in stress-reduction techniques, exercises to increase fitness and flexibility, and suggestions to improve exercise adherence.

Additional studies have documented the beneficial outcomes with group physical therapy interventions for individuals with impairments related to chronic neuromuscular conditions. Eng et al. (2003) evaluated the physical and psychosocial effects of an 8-week community-based functional exercise program on a group of individuals with chronic stroke and found that the exercise program improved mobility, functional capacity, balance, and performance of activities. For individuals with Parkinsonism, group training did not improve the gait patterns of the participants but beneficial effects on psychosocial discomfort were reported (Pedersen, Oberg, Insulander, & Vretman, 1990). A qualitative study of the effects of group dynamic water exercise on persons with late effects of polio reported physical and psychosocial benefits for the participants. In addition, the group process appeared to be of great importance not only as a social phenomenon but also as a learning resource (Willen & Scherman, 2002).

Promotion of Health and Wellness

Physical activity programs have also been successfully implemented with groups for the promotion of health and wellness of the older adult (O'Hagan, Smith, & Pileggi, 1994; Lazowski et al., 1999; Brown et al., 2000; King et al., 2002; Timonen, Rantanen, Timonen, & Sulkava, 2002; Taylor et al., 2003; Grant, Todd, Aitchison, Kelly, & Stoddart, 2004). A study of physically frail, institutionalized seniors who took part in the Functional Fitness for Long-Term Care Program, significantly improved their mobility, balance, flexibility, and hip and knee strength compared to a group of elders who performed range of motion exercises only (Lazowski et al., 1999). Similarly, frail elders who participated in low-intensity supervised exercises made significant gains in function, balance, strength, flexibility, and gait speed compared to the control group who performed flexibility exercises only (Brown et al., 2000). Residents of personal care (assisted-living) homes improved their performance on a test of balance following a seated group exercise program that simulated functional activities (Taylor et al., 2003). Significant improvements in function, as measured by the sit to stand test, were found in a group of nursing home residents who participated in group exercises led by a physical therapist when compared to a matched group without the input of a physical therapist (O'Hagan et al., 1994). A program of lower-extremity strengthening exercise was found to improve mood as well as isometric muscle strength in a group of frail older women recuperating from an acute illness (Timonen et al., 2002). A functional exercise program for older, overweight women was found to reduce body mass and blood pressure, improve functional activities (timed walk, weight lifting, and stair climbing), and enhance life satisfaction (Grant et al., 2004). Older adults with mobility impairments significantly improved their physical performance following a program of exercises performed at a senior center, but were not able to sustain the improvements when transitioned to home exercises (King et al., 2002).

Guidelines for Physical Therapy Group Exercise and Education

Physical therapy group exercise and educational classes provide an effective, efficient alternative to individual interventions for older adults. Group interventions may be a part of the rehabilitation program for an individual with impairment(s) associated with a specific diagnosis such as stroke. These interventions may allow participants to spend more time receiving physical therapy compared to those receiving individual treatment only (De Weerdt et al., 2001). Older individuals, who no longer qualify for continued physical therapy for treatment, may be interested in a program of supervised exercise to maximize recovery. In addition, community-dwelling seniors may be attracted to classes designed to promote wellness and prevention of impairments and functional losses associated with aging or disease. Frail elders in institutionalized settings may not have a diagnosis that would qualify them for physical therapy treatment; nevertheless, they would benefit from a program of physical activity to prevent deconditioning and improve function. Group programs appeal to many older adults because of the socialization and support offered through peer interaction.

Assessment of Need

The first step in the establishment of group exercise and education is to assess the need for the activity (Gallichio, Berthold, & Kubik, 2000). Exercise and educational needs may be determined from older adults, activity directors at facilities that provide services to seniors, and health care practitioners. From these individuals, information about current exercise participation, health habits, educational interests, hobbies, and activities can be obtained and used in the development and progression of group classes.

Design and Format

PARTICIPANT CONSIDERATIONS

Goals of the group are more likely to be accomplished if participant membership is determined by diagnosis and/or common functional status. Individuals with specific medical diagnoses such as arthritis, total joint replacement, stroke, and urinary incontinence may be interested in exercise and educational classes designed specifically to address problems associated with the diagnosis. Older adults without a specific diagnosis may be placed in a group based on their functional ability. For example, participants in a program that includes walking or exercises performed in a standing position must all have good standing balance to benefit from the activities. Seated exercise may be more appropriate for frail, deconditioned older adults, who require greater supervision and assistance.

Prior to implementation of the exercise and educational group, written consent and medical release forms should be developed for the older adults to sign (Gallichio, Berthold, & Kubik, 2000; Lewis & Campanelli, 1990). The consent form should outline components of the program including benefits and risks associated with participation in the group intervention. The consent form usually includes a statement that acknowledges voluntary involvement in the group. Participation may be discontinued at any time. A medical release form, once signed by the participant's physician, authorizes the older adults to take part in the group intervention and provides an opportunity for the practitioner to supply important medical information such as diagnosis or activity limitations. Both forms serve to limit the liability of the instructor and/or facility for any adverse event that may occur during the group activity.

The recommended number of participants in a group varies based on the functional and cognitive abilities of the members and the amount of assistance and supervision required. Thus, groups that consist primarily of independent, community-dwelling seniors may be larger than groups comprised mostly of frail, deconditioned elders. Groups of healthy, community-dwelling seniors may have a participant to instructor ratio of 12:1 (J. B. Tomsic, personal communication, May 4,

2004), but optimal participant to instructor ratio for a physical therapy group of frail seniors has been reported to be 4:1 (Nishimoto & Schunk, 1989). It has been suggested that more than an ideal number of members could be enrolled because illness and conflicting appointments affect participation of one fourth to one half of individuals on any given day (Nishimoto & Schunk). Recent information on exercise and educational group interventions suggest that a minimum of two instructors be available, one to lead the class and the remaining instructor(s) to circulate among the participants to assure safety and monitor for proper technique (Gallichio, Berthold, & Kubik, 2000).

Instructor Considerations

Instructors must have knowledge of and interest in leading exercise and educational groups for older adults. Essential qualifications include training in the following areas: exercise and aging, signs of over-exertion, basic first aid, cardiopulmonary resuscitation, and group dynamics (Lewis & Campanelli, 1990). Although not considered an essential qualification, it is desirable for group leaders to be certified as exercise specialists by the American College of Sports Medicine or the National Strength and Conditioning Association (Lewis & Campanelli). The most essential interpersonal skill for leaders is the ability to relate meaningfully to seniors (Lewis & Campanelli). Exercise and health education leaders should also be organized, firm, empathetic, patient, and skilled in providing a mixture of fun and purposeful activities (Lewis & Campanelli).

Facility Considerations

A comfortable, safe, appropriate physical environment can enhance the effectiveness of the group intervention. The physical space should have convenient parking, doorways that accommodate wheelchairs, and bathrooms that are wheelchair accessible and conveniently located. Chairs should be sturdy and comfortable and have armrests to facilitate client transfer from standing to sitting and back to standing. If portions of the exercise program are performed on the floor, the floor covering should be composed of comfortable, firm material such as a short-pile carpet. Handrails should be accessible to provide support for challenging exercises that are performed in the standing position. Handrails can also be used to facilitate transfers from the floor to standing and may serve as a stable attachment for exercise tubing or bands. If audiovisual equipment for educational programming and a sound system for music are used, electrical outlets must be readily available in the classroom. Electrical cords should be out of the walking path or should be taped to the floor to prevent tripping. A room with a thermostat is essential to provide a comfortable temperature for the participants.

The impact of age-related changes in vision and hearing on the ability of the older adult to function in the environment must be considered when assessing lighting, noise, acoustics, and color scheme of the physical space. Bright overhead lighting that can be dimmed during educational sessions or for relaxation exercises is optimal. Blinds or curtains are needed for windows to reduce glare on sunny days. The space should be reasonably quiet without competing noise from heating and air-conditioning units, fans, televisions, or individuals who are talking. Music may be desired as research has shown that some older adults have increased participation in group interventions when exercises are accompanied by rhythmic music (Mathews, Clair, & Kosloski, 2001). However, it is important that the volume and type of music do not interfere with a participant's ability to hear the instructor (J. B. Tomsic, personal communication, May 4, 2004). Appropriate floor covering may help reduce noise and should not distract participants visually.

Components of the Program

Activities and educational programming should be determined in collaboration with participants (Rinne & Toropainen, 1998). Objectives need to be established to guide program development, and outcomes should be evaluated at the end of the session. Participants can be asked to select educational topics of interest from a list developed by the instructor. Most exercise programs for older adults consist of warm-up, stretching, strengthening, balance and coordination, cardiovascular conditioning, and cooldown activities. Simple equipment such as resistive bands and cuff weights for strengthening, balls for balance and coordination activities, and canes and towels for stretching can be incorporated into the exercise program.

Implementation

In order to achieve health benefits from the program, the group intervention should last for a minimum of 8–12 weeks, and participants should meet at least twice a week on alternate days to allow for recovery between sessions (J. B. Tomsic, personal communication, May 4, 2004). If there is an educational component to the class, an hour and a half is recommended for the session. One hour is sufficient for exercise classes without an educational component. For older adults, the best time for a class to meet is in the morning after 9 o'clock.

If participants are meeting for the first time, the session should begin with introductions. The instructors should start by introducing themselves and talking about their professional qualifications. Time should then be allowed for the participants to meet and greet each other. Introductions may be accomplished in a traditional manner by having the participant state his or her name and share some additional information such as where he or she lives. A group roster with names, addresses, and pictures may be desirable to promote interaction among group members. When a new participant joins an established group, the instructor should orient the newcomer to group procedures and introduce the individual to the other participants. It is recommended that the newcomer be in close proximity to the instructor for the first few sessions to learn the exercise routine correctly.

After introductions, an educational topic for the session may be presented. Instructors should establish a warm, comfortable atmosphere for the classes by personalizing the information through the use of questions for the audience about topics such as exercise or whether they have ever been to a physical therapist for treatment. Use of props and visual aids (skeletons or slides) helps the information "come to life for participants." Instructors should encourage questions from the audience but should try to keep members from rambling at length about a personal issue. Due to time constraints, specific concerns of individuals may be addressed after class. Follow-up telephone calls between educational group sessions may help to answer questions and provide encouragement (Schacter, Busch, Peloso, and Sheppard, 2003).

Exercise sessions typically consist of warm-up, workout, and cooldown components and can be performed to music. The warm-up may include deep breathing, reinforcement of proper posture, and range of motion exercises for the cervical region, upper extremities, trunk, and lower extremities. The workout comprises strengthening exercises using resistive exercise bands and cuff weights, balance and coordination activities either standing or while sitting on a ball, and aerobic activities such as dancing or walking. The cooldown component consists of gentle movements, deep breathing, and relaxation exercises. Standing exercises or activities using a ball may need to be modified for frail, deconditioned participants to allow them to perform the exercise while sitting in a chair. Consistent language, demonstration, and feedback facilitate participant motivation and proper exercise performance. Group members should be taught how to monitor their pulse during exercise and asked by the instructors to call their heart rate out loud periodically to ensure a safe intensity of exercise. Participants who have continual difficulty monitoring their exercise heart rate and perceived exertion may benefit from using electronic monitoring devices to ensure that target levels of physical activity are attained (Schacter, Busch, Peloso, & Sheppard, 2003). Finally, it is important to introduce changes to a program incrementally to allow participants to adjust to a new routine, equipment, and instructors.

Evaluation

Initial, formative, and summative assessments should be conducted for group physical therapy classes. For those individuals who are participating in group interventions as part of their rehabilitation plan, a physical therapist examination and evaluation must be performed and appropriate tests and measures administered to assess impairments, to determine a diagnosis and prognosis, and to develop goals and a plan of care. Examples of tests and measures commonly used by physical therapists when working with the older adult include:

- Postural assessment
- Goniometric measurements for range of motion (ROM)
- Manual muscle testing (MMT) for strength
- Self-care and activities of daily living (ADLs) measures such as the Adult Functional Independence Measure (FIM) (Uniform Data Set for Medical Rehabilitation, 1993)
- Balance and gait measures such as:
  - Timed Up and Go (TUG) (Podsiadlo & Richardson, 1991)
  - Performance Oriented Mobility Assessment (POMA) (Tinetti, 1986)
  - Berg Balance Scale (BBS) (Berg, Wood-Dauphinee, Williams, & Gayton, 1989)

The patient or client is re-evaluated periodically to assess progress towards established goals. Formal written questionnaires can be administered before and after the intervention to determine whether or not the established objectives were met.

The physical therapist may choose to use formal and/or informal evaluation throughout interventions provided for nonrehabilitation groups. As previously mentioned, formal assessment may occur before and after the class, but feedback can also be sought informally during the program by asking the older adults what they thought about specific aspects of the educational or exercise session. Through observation, instructors can also assess the older adult's knowledge of prevention, proper technique for stretching, use of proper posture, and ability to monitor heart rate.

Summary

Successful physical therapy group exercise and educational classes provide an alternative to individual interventions for older adults. Collaboration with the older adults to determine educational and exercise needs is important for an effective intervention. Careful consideration should be given to participant characteristics, instructor qualifications, the physical environment, and components of a program prior to implementation. Initial, formative, and summative assessments are used to measure benefits of the intervention.

Exercises

EXERCISE I

Contact a local senior center and assess their need for group exercise and educational classes.

EXERCISE 2

Design a group exercise and educational program for older adults that can be accomplished in a seated position.

EXERCISE 3

Develop an outcomes measure that would evaluate the effectiveness of group exercise and educational classes.

References

American Physical Therapy Association. (2003). *Guide to Physical Therapist Practice* (2nd ed.). Alexandria, VA.

Bakker, C., Hidding, A., van der Linden, S., & van Doorslaer, E. (1994). Cost effectiveness of group physical therapy compared to individualized therapy for ankylosing spondylitis. A randomized controlled trial. *The Journal of Rheumatology,* 21(2), 264–268.

Bennett, R. M., Burchkhardt, C. S., Clark, S. R., O'Reilly, C. A., Wiens, A. N., & Campbell, S. M. (1996). Group treatment of fibromyalgia: A 6 month outpatient program. *Journal of Rheumatology,* 23(3), 521–528.

Berg, K. O., Wood-Dauphinee, S. L., Williams, J. T., & Gayton, D. (1989). Measuring balance in the elderly: Preliminary development of an instrument. *Physiotherapy Canada,* 41, 304–311.

Brown, M., Sinacore, D. R., Ehsani, A. A., Binder, E. F., Holloszy, J. O., Kohrt, W. M. (2000). Low intensity exercise as a modifier of physical frailty in older adults. *Archives of Physical Medicine and Rehabilitation,* 81, 960–965.

Demain, S., Smith, J. F., Hiller, L., & Dziedzic, K. (2001). Comparison of group and individual physiotherapy for female urinary incontinence in primary care. *Physiotherapy,* 87, 235–42.

De Weerdt, W., Nuyen, G., Feys, H., Vangronsveld, P., Van de Winckel, A., Nieuwboer, A. (2001). Group physiotherapy improves time use by patients with stroke in rehabilitation. *Australian Journal of Physiotherapy,* 47(1), 53–61.

Douris, P., Southard, V., Varga, C., Schauss, W., Gennaro, C., & Reiss, A. (2003). The effect of land and aquatic exercise on balance scores in older adults. *Journal of Geriatric Physical Therapy,* 26(1), 3–6.

Eng, J. J., Chu, K. S., Kim, C. M., Dawson, A. S., Carswell, A., & Hepburn, K. E. (2003). A community-based group exercise program for persons with chronic stroke. *Medicine & Science in Sports & Exercise,* 35(6), 1271–1278.

Gallichio, J., Berthold, S., & Kubik, K. (2000). Bridging the gap: Fitness through the ages. *Physical Therapy Magazine,* 8(1), 54–58.

Grant, S., Todd, K., Aitchison, T. C., Kelly, P., & Stoddart, D. (2004). The effects of a 12-week group exercise programme on physiological and psychological variables and function in overweight women. *Public Health,* 118(1), 31–42.

Gunther, J. S., Taylor, M. J., Karuza, J., & Calkins, E. (2003). Physical therapist-based group exercise/education program to improve functional health in older health maintenance organization members with arthritis. *Journal of Geriatric Physical Therapy,* 26(1), 12–17.

Hain, T., Fuller, L., Weil, L., & Kotasias, J. (1999) The effects of t'ai chi on balance *Archives of Otolaryngology-Head and Neck Surgery,* 125, 1191–1195.

Hidding, A., van der Linden, S., Boers, M., Gielen, X., de Witte, L., Kester, A., Kijkmans, B., & Moolenburgh, D. (1993). Is group physical therapy superior to individualized therapy in ankylosing spondylitis? A randomized controlled trial. *Arthritis Care & Research,* 6(3), 117–125.

Hong, Y., Li, J. X., & Skelton, D. (2000). Balance control, flexibility, and cardiorespiratory fitness among older tai chi practitioners. *British Journal of Sports Medicine,* 34, 29–34.

King, M. B., Whipple, R. H., Gruman, C. A., Judge, J. O., Schmidt, J. A., & Wolfson, L. I. (2002). The performance enhancement project: Improving physical performance in older persons. *Archives of Physical Medicine and Rehabilitation,* 83, 1060–1069.

Komagata, S., & Newton, R. (2003). The effectiveness of tai chi on improving balance in older adults: An evidence-based review. *Journal of Geriatric Physical Therapy,* 26(2), 3–16.

Lazowski, D. A., Ecclestone, N. A., Myers, A. M., Paterson, D. H., Tudor-Locke, C., Fitzgerald, C. (1999). A randomized outcome evaluation of group exercise programs in long-term care institutions. *Journals of Gerontology Series A- Biological Sciences and Medical Sciences,* 54(12), M621–M628.

Lewis, C. B., & Campanelli, L. C. (1990). *Health Promotion and Exercise for Older Adults: An Instructor's Guide.* Rockland, MD: Aspen.

Lord, S. R., Castell, S., Corcoran, J., Dayhew, J., Matters, B., Shan, A., & Williams, P. (2003). The effect of group exercise on physical functioning and falls in frail older people living in retirement villages: A randomized, controlled trial. *Journal of the American Geriatrics Society,* 51, 1685–1692.

Mathews, R. M., Clair, A. A., & Kosloski, K. (2001). Keeping the beat: Use of rhythmic music during exercise activities for the elderly with dementia. *American Journal of Alzheimer's Disease & Other Dementias,* 16(6), 377–380.

Nishimoto, T., & Schunk, C. (1989). Group therapy: An alternative treatment approach. *Clinical Management,* 7(4), 16–18.

O'Hagan, C. M., Smith, D. M., & Pileggi, K. L. (1994). Exercise classes in rest homes: Effects on physical function. *New Zealand Medical Journal,* 107, 39–40.

Pedersen, S. W., Oberg, B., Insulander, A., & Vretman, M. Group training in parkinsonism: Quantitative measurements of treatment. *Scandinavian Journal of Rehabilitation Medicine,* 22(4), 207–211.

Podsiadlo, D., & Richardson, S. (1991). The timed "up and go": A test of basic functional mobility for frail elderly persons. *Journal of the American Geriatrics Society,* 39, 142–148.

Rinne J., & Toropainen, E. (1998). How to lead a group— Practical principles and experiences of conducting a promotional group in health-related physical activity. *Patient Education and Counseling,* 33(Suppl. 1), S69–S76.

Rubenstein, L. Z., Josephson, K. R., Trueblood, P. R., Loy, S., Harker, J. O., Pietruszka, F. M., & Robbins, A. S. (2000). Effects of a group exercise program on strength, mobility, and falls among fall-prone elderly men. *Journals of Gerontology Series A-Biological Sciences and Medical Sciences,* 55, M317–M321.

Schacter, C. L., Busch, A. J., Peloso, P. M., & Sheppard, M. S. (2003). Effects of short versus long bouts of aerobic exercise in sedentary women with fibromyalgia: A randomized controlled trial. *Physical Therapy,* 83(4), 340–358.

Scott, R. W. (2002). *Foundations of Physical Therapy.* New York: McGraw-Hill.

Taylor, L. F., Whittington, F., Hollingsworth, C., Ball, M., King, S. V., & Diwan, S. (2003). A comparison of functional outcomes following a physical activity intervention for frail older adults in personal care homes. *Journal of Geriatric Physical Therapy,* 26(1), 7–11.

Timonen, L., Rantanen, T., Timonen, T. E., & Sulkava, R. (2002). Effects of a group-based exercise program on the mood state of frail older women after discharge from hospital. *International Journal of Geriatric Psychiatry,* 17, 1106–1111.

Tinetti, M. E. (1986). Performance-oriented assessment of mobility problems in elderly patients. *Journal of the American Geriatrics Society,* 34, 119–126.

Uniform Data Set for Medical Rehabilitation. (1993). *The Functional Independence Measure.* Buffalo, NY: State University of New York.

Willen, C., & Scherman, M. H. (2002). Group training in a pool causes ripples on the water: Experiences by persons with late effects of polio. *Journal of Rehabilitation Medicine,* 34, 191–197.

Wolf, S. L., Barnhardt, H. X., Ellison, G. L., & Coogler, C. E. (1997). The effect of tai chi quan and computerized balance training on postural stability in older subjects. *Physical Therapy,* 77, 371–381.

Resources

- American Physical Therapy Association. Available at *www.apta.org*
- The Geriatric Section, American Physical Therapy Association. Available at *www.geriatricspt.org*
- Lorig, K., & Fries, J. F. (1990). *The arthritis helpbook: A tested self-management program for coping with your arthritis* (3rd ed.). Reading, MA: Addison-Wesley.
- Newman, L. A. (1995). *Maintaining function in older adults.* Boston, MA: Butterworth-Heinemann.
- The Arthritis Foundation. Available at *http://www.arthritis.org/*
- The World Confederation of Physical Therapy. Available at *http://www.wcpt.org/policies/index.php*
- World Health Organization. (2001). *ICF: International classification of functioning, disability and health.* Geneva, Switzerland: Author.

Chapter 29

A Social Work Perspective

Faith Gibson

John Kunz

Mary Gwynne
Schmidt

Key Words

- Advocacy
- Cooperation
- Confidentiality
- Directivity
- Empowerment
- Host agency
- Least contest
- Multidisciplinary team
- Values and purpose

Learning Objectives

- Describe circumstances in the early and more recent history of social group work that have led social workers to believe they have a duty to advocate for their clients
- Discuss how the values and purposes of social work have contributed to an approach especially suited for work with older persons and their families
- Tell why it is important for social workers in nursing facilities to work closely with nursing staff when planning groups
- List three issues the group social worker should take into account when intervening in response to group members' complaints about their families or the setting in which they are living
- Describe two typical instances in which the nurse's responsibility for safety and the social worker's concern for self-determination have contributed to tensions

Social group work differs from group work led by other health professionals not in its knowledge base, which is shared, but in the values and purposes of social work that guide it. Sometimes these differences alienate social workers from their natural allies, and group services to older people suffer as a consequence. This divergence in practice can occur even when basic values overlap between professions. (See Chapter 31 for further exploration of these similarities and differences.)

After reviewing the circumstances that have given social work its character, this chapter explores misunderstandings that sometimes occur between professionals in host agencies and describes steps the social worker can take to avoid them. The chapter also discusses some of the practical concerns that arise from the juxtaposition of social work values and the desires of older people. Finally, a case study of a small group of physically frail residents illustrates some of the major obstacles and opportunities associated with undertaking group work practice with elderly nursing home residents.

Historical Background

Some social workers feel awkward when first starting to work with older adults, as do many other professionals. A review of four social work textbooks used at a Midwestern accredited undergraduate social work program found that there were no specific sections that focused on group work with older adults (Chen & Rybak, 2004; Corey & Corey, 2002; Corey, Corey, Callanan, & Russell, 2004; Zastrow, 1997). In fact the words *older adult*, *elderly*, or *senior* were not found in the index of any of these books. Only one listed and included a paragraph on life review (Chen & Ryback) that referred to a technique that is used with the seniors. The lack of focus on group work with older adults puts social workers employed in settings which serve older people at a great disadvantage.

Fortunately during the past few years the National Association of Social Workers (NASW) began to advocate for additional competencies in social work education (NASW, 2004). The Institute for Geriatric Social Work, affiliated with Boston University, was formed to further educate social workers on improved practice with older adults (Institute for Geriatric Social Work, 2004). Many clinical social workers in long-term care settings have also benefited from the educational publications developed by the Psychologists in Long-Term Care group (2004).

Gerontological social work now presents the fastest growing sector within the social work profession (Dobrof, 2002). Group work opportunities abound in many different practice settings including hospitals, nursing homes, and other types of residential facilities, adult day services, and community agencies. This chapter briefly describes the historical development of group work within the social work profession from the earliest period of the settlement movement and youth club provision, through the generalist phase to the contemporary position of generalist practitioners and advanced group work specialists. The chapter then concentrates predominantly on group work practice in nursing homes where the employment of social workers is now mandatory but recognizes that many other practice opportunities also exist. With over half of all the members of NASW now self-employed, private practice of group work provides increasing employment opportunities, despite the complexities of securing funding, for generalist social workers and group work specialists alike (Kadushin & Harkness, 2000). The clash of professional perspectives, so damaging to care recipients, is addressed and practical suggestions offered about how social workers might broaden their vision and increase their skills for constructive, cooperative interprofessional practice.

The social work approach to small groups acquired its character in three phases: first, as part of an undifferentiated group work movement; next, as a method within social work; and finally, as a cluster of skills, knowledge, and competencies disseminated throughout the profession. A fourth phase is now emerging in which generalists are undertaking advanced study at masters and doctoral levels to emerge as group work specialists, consultants, teachers, and researchers. As group work developed from a specialty in the second phase to part of the general repertoire in the third, the range of persons it dealt with and the nature of its interventions broadened.

In the first phase, group work began as classes and clubs in settlement houses and youth-serving organizations (Lasch-Quinn, 1993). This work led to optimism about human's drive to health and the growth-generating power of the group. It also caused the group to be viewed as a medium for socialization.

Engaged in teaching new ways to new Americans, the settlement houses dealt with normal people and therefore looked to growth and learning rather than remediation. This created some reluctance later to move into group therapy, which was seen as undemocratic and elitist.

Many of the persons coming to the settlement houses worked in factories, lived in tenements, and were deprived of many of the protections and advantages automatically extended to the middle class. Settlement-house workers advocated for the poor and encouraged them to campaign for themselves. This past is evident in social work's continuing strain of reformism. Social workers are taught the duty of advocacy and the strength of the group to help its members act on their own behalf.

The settlement house offered young people opportunities to make new friends, but beneath this was a more serious purpose—socialization. The intent was to teach people how things were done in America so that they might succeed in their new land. The youth organizations and church groups also had an educative, socially responsible character-building thrust. The first phase took place in the last quarter of the 1800s and the early years of the 1900s, when young families were emmigrating from Europe and young Americans were losing some of the traditional supports they had experienced in rural communities.

The second phase of social work's history began when the government began giving relief in the Great Depression, and social workers broadened their function beyond investigating the poor. In this second phase, social group work moved into the mainstream of social work proper and became one of its three major methods, along with casework and community organization.

The second phase ended when the American Association of Group Workers joined other social work organizations to form the NASW in 1955. Group work was professionalized and then moved into social work as a methodological specialization.

When Gertrude Wilson (1976, pp. 31–32), one of the leaders of the second phase, looked back over half a century of social group work, she recalled that the leadership of the American Association of Group Workers had consisted chiefly of social workers, although only a few years earlier the group work section of the National Conference of Social Work had drawn members from adult education, physical education, agricultural extension programs, and the Children's Bureau. Thus, a narrowing had occurred, as social group work became not a profession in its own right but a method within social work. Ten years after its introduction at Case Western Reserve in 1927, group work was being taught in ten schools of social work. Students had to choose among casework, group work, and community organization; specialization reigned.

In the meantime, two things had happened to group work. First, under the influence of such persons as Fritz Redl, who worked with severely disturbed boys, group work had moved beyond the original growth and task groups to include remediation (Doel & Sawdon, 1999). Second, social work purposes had come to determine its direction.

The third phase saw the end of group work as a separate specialty and the merging of its skills and theory into generalist practice. This was typified by the expectation of the Council on Social Work Education (CSWE) that all students in accredited social work programs would undertake some group work courses, and for many a related group work practice experience during their practicum. For very few would this practice experience be undertaken in a specific group agency (Council on Social Work Education, 2004).

In 1961, four organizations concerned with older adults convened a seminar on "Social Group Work with Older People." In the foreword to the proceedings, Randall stated that it was appropriate that social casework came first in the series of seminars but right after that group work should follow, because group workers had been the first to make some of the adaptations in method required by older people (National Association Social Workers, 1980).

In the same year, William Schwartz (1979), a group worker, theorist, and teacher, had pointed out that social work's new roles in institutional and therapeutic settings indicated that the unit of service should be determined by client need, not by agency or practitioner specialization. In Berman-Rossi's comprehensive collection of his writings (1994), she describes Schwartz's national and international influence on social work, and within it, group work education and practice.

Today Schwartz's vision is largely realized. The generalist is taught to work with individuals, families, groups, or communities as the occasion demands. Group interventions have become part of the training of every social worker. Ideas concerning the need for clarity of objectives, identifying common ground between people, mobilizing mutual aid, mediation between client and system, and the responsibility of the social worker to lend a vision about what is possible are accepted as mainstream ideas in group work practice (Association for the Advancement of Social Work with Groups, 2004).

A fourth phase is emerging in response to changing opportunities and increasing demands. There are both more demands for group work and more sources of reimbursement for social services, including working with small groups in a variety of service settings with people of varied ages and diverse needs. With the rise of private practice and with membership of interdisciplinary teams, more social workers are leading therapy groups. With the growth of mutual support groups, more social workers are organizing and facilitating self-help groups. With social services mandated in nursing facilities, more are working with resident and family groups in settings providing long-term care. Finally, more are engaging in case management, whether as traditional social workers or as relatively distant coordinators and cost con-trollers. In these days of managed care, and in the face of demographic population changes and strident—albeit legitimate—demands for accountability in spending public funds, contemporary social workers, including group workers, struggle hard to remain effective in meeting the needs of vulnerable people (Gitterman & Shulman, 2004; Gitterman, 2002).

In response to this changing climate, differences in education and professional preparation have evolved. Undergraduates are still being trained as generalists, but, in addition to a generalist grounding, graduate students are becoming more specialized. Students electing to work with individuals and families take courses that equip them to lead groups; those seeking careers in social administration and management usually also undertake some training in group process in order to lead work groups.

Social group work has emerged from its 100 year history with values similar to those of the other helping professions—essentially a belief in the uniqueness and worth of the individual and in each person's right to self-determination and respect. In the case of social work, these values are undergirded by a set of assumptions growing out of the profession's past in the youth organization and settlement house, with its optimistic view of human nature and its commitment to fight injustice. The optimism about human nature may have been somewhat tempered by three recent decades of work in protective services. Nevertheless, enough of these underpinning assumptions remain to make social workers critical staff members or guests in host agencies.

Social Work Values and the Older Adult

Social work's values and range fit it for work with older adults. The range refers both to clientele and types of intervention. Social workers' education equips them to serve this heterogeneous population: they can facilitate groups for the well aged, provide support for organizations of older persons engaged on their own behalf, and lead patient and family groups for residents of institutions and those attending adult day care services.

Older persons experiencing losses tend to have multiple needs. The generalist social worker is prepared to work with the individual, family, group, institution, or community and therefore can move—as the earlier group worker could not—from leading a relatives' group to following up the members' concerns about establishing eligibility or securing special resources (Ryan & Crawford, 2002). This capacity is useful when a nurse or physician wants to organize a group around an illness and needs a coleader who will share responsibility for other kinds of follow-up.

Although members of all helping professions operate with an awareness of the client's social systems, it is safe to say that no other profession is so explicitly required by its mission to relate to them and to operate within the parameters of awareness of the psychosocial problems with which diverse people struggle. This perspective is helpful when dealing with a population that includes persons who are disabled, dependent, or institutionalized.

Older persons often present with situational or context-related depression or troubled role transitions. Emphasis on self-determination and client strengths and resiliency combats learned helplessness—the apathetic, passive, depressed kinds of behavior that often ensue when aging persons discover that they have lost control over many aspects of their lives (Phillips & Cohen, 2000). Social workers are taught to engage the healthy residue in the personalities of even severely cognitively or physically disabled older people and their caregivers. Social workers are also taught to contribute to the mobilizing or creation of constructive and responsive environmental conditions and support systems (Fast & Chapin, 2000; Kivnick & Murray, 2001; Ronch & Goldfield,

2003). These writers emphasize a multifaceted positive approach to coping and seek to assist people "whose troubles aren't all in their heads" (Berlin, 2002).

This approach towards mobilizing the potential of individuals and individuals in groups is not new, as illustrated in one of the early accounts of group work with older people. In their book about the Hodson Center in New York during World War II, Kubie and Landau (1953) related how the professional social worker arrived at this prototypical old people's center and quickly developed modes of democratic leadership among these seemingly passive persons, who previously had allowed themselves to be bossed by two or three aggressive members.

The focus on socialization as a process is relevant both for persons moving into a life stage for which there are few guidelines, although some outstanding individual role models exist, and also for aging individuals who are moving into group living. Irving Rosow (1974) wrote movingly about the poor schooling society gives people in preparation for old age. Young people are told clearly what is expected of them, but the old are left to stumble into old-age roles, learning only through criticism and rejection.

Rosow (1974) pointed out that younger authority figures engender a sense of role reversal that stimulates geriatric "difficultness" as a "desperate rearguard action to retain vestiges of dignity, control, and independence that are steadily slipping" (p. 140). Certainly this is true in long-term care settings, where administrators and nurses tend to be middle-aged or younger. Many institutions for older people whose populations are by definition frail and vulnerable, offer few inspiring role models from whom members might learn how to be self-respecting older persons.

Rosow (1974) said that the support of the peer group ordinarily maintains the morale of persons moving as cohorts into new situations, but it is hard for older adults to identify with occupants of a devalued status (pp. 141–143). He proposed apartheid of the old—insulated enclaves of their own where they might make their own rules and find status and comfort (pp. 155–170). Retirement communities have grown in popularity, but not every older person wishes to live in age-segregated communities. What Rosow's formulation does contribute to everyday life is an awareness of the strong need for older persons, especially those moving into sheltered care, to participate in small groups, particularly small groups that can provide not only induction for the newcomers into the system but also opportunities for peer leadership. The social work group offers this kind of help because it fosters opportunities to exercise choice, mutual aid, and concerted action. (See Chapter 21 for a case example.)

The Guest Connection

If social work values and principles equip the practitioner for service to older people, they can also contribute to misunderstandings and conflict with other professions. The more needful the client, the more likely the social worker is to be serving that person in a host agency—that is, in a hospital, a mental health facility, or a nursing home, settings where social work is not the dominant profession. The more vulnerable the clients, the more likely they and their families are to be harmed if they sense disharmony among members of the treatment team.

Interprofessional collaboration is needed in the community also, but the prototypical situation, illustrating the full potential for a clash of values, is found in the nursing home. In all special settings for older people, there are different degrees of disability and correspondingly different levels of care and control. The higher these are, the more important is team communication and cohesiveness.

The social worker may find that it is relatively simple to organize a poetry, music, or reminiscence group for the residents of a board-and-care home or congregate living facility for older people. (See Chapters 21 and 23.) It may be necessary only to check the monthly schedule, get clearance from the administrator, and pay attention to members' interests and competing events. In the same home's nursing unit, arrangements will be more complex.

The social worker who attempts to organize a patient group without consulting the director of nursing is likely to arrive to find that group members are napping, being bathed, are at the beauty parlor or seeing their physician. Equipment may have been tidied away, a troop of Brownie Scouts scheduled for a sing-along, and a competing activity slated for the meeting room.

Before viewing this as sabotage, the social worker would be well advised to look at the logistics of the setting and the condition of the patients. The work schedules of nursing personnel swing around a five-day week and there may be absences and substitutions. The charge nurse on duty when the group held its first meeting may not be there on the date of the second. Nurses' assistants may function on a tight schedule around a predictable patient routine driven by physical care priorities. Other events are likely to be overlooked or forgotten, especially if they do not occur on a daily basis. (Chapter 23 illustrates many of these problems.)

Patients in nursing homes tend to be very old, very frail, or both. Therefore, a group member may be in bed with the side rails up not because someone wanted to keep her out of the group meeting but because she manifested mild confusion and seemed unwell.

Before beginning a group, full consultation with staff is essential. Not only the director of nursing and the administrator but others, including the nursing aides, should have an opportunity to share views, suggest patients, and when feasible, participate in leadership itself. Some group members will go out with relatives just when your meeting is scheduled and others will remain in bed or be at the podiatrist, but these things will be less likely to happen if staff is included in group planning. Chapters 7, 8, 9, 10, 11, and 12 address many of these issues and all emphasize the necessity for careful planning and conscientious consultation with colleagues.

The moral is threefold: in these settings, every other activity is secondary to nursing care, the staff is often stretched thin, and nursing personnel must cope with accountabilities of their own. These factors lead to conflicts, even when the values held by the two professions are either the same or very similar.

Interaction with Other Disciplines

The Social Work Code of Ethics contains six sections that identify values and principles. (See Tables 31–1 and 31–2 in Chapter 31 which list values for social work and nursing.) Two underlying values are universally recognized; related to them are two duties that influence the attitudes that social workers bring to interprofessional collaboration (National Association of Social Workers, 1999). The two values are: (1) respect for the inherent dignity and worth of people, and (2) recognition of the central importance of human relationships. Related duties include confidentiality, autonomy, and advocacy.

Social workers do not have a monopoly of virtue. Other disciplines also believe in the uniqueness and inherent dignity of the individual and in client self-determination; others also respect confidentiality and view themselves as patient advocates. Countervailing this is professional caution. Physicians think they might be sued for practically anything, and nurses have been taught that they are responsible for the physical safety of every patient. They also sense the social worker's view that she or he is the only one in the setting who really cares.

The safety/freedom tension between nurses and social workers should be eased by federal nursing home reform amendments and state regulations that emphasize as patients' rights a greater sharing of responsibility with the resident and family

(U.S. Social Security Act, 1987). A major irritant in the past has been what social workers viewed as the excess restriction of patients by overly cautious nurses. Nevertheless, it has been nurses who provided much of the leadership in the movement toward restraint-free care that has culminated in the new laws.

RESPECT FOR DIGNITY AND WORTH OF PERSONS

The need to respect individual dignity and worth is spelled out for nurses also (McCormack, 2003; Northern, 1998). Because they deal with persons in situations conducive to regression—around the provision of physical care, such as feeding, toileting, putting to bed—nurses are likely to respond to the patient's need for a comforting parental figure. The same patient may present a more coping self to the social worker because much of the business they do together involves decision making and negotiation by the resident and therefore elicits a more mature level of behavior. Nurse and social worker are reacting to different patient expectations and perceptions arising out of the different needs and demarcated responsibilities of service. Their responses will also be influenced by the different way each has been socialized into their profession. If nurses responded as social workers do, the patient might perceive their behavior as distancing and cold.

The social worker is likely to be jarred by the nursing aid who addresses an aged patient as she might a small child ("Still dry, Rosie?"). Excellent nursing practice frowns on this too. Nurses are continually searching for new and better ways to measure nursing quality and therefore improve best practices in nursing home care (Rantz & Connolly, 2004).

RESPECT FOR CLIENT SELF-DETERMINATION

The nurse is also aware of the patient's need for autonomy, and now more than ever the geriatric nurse must be ethically fit to work both independently and as part of collaborative and multidisciplinary teams (Lund, 1998). The social worker is likely to view the nurse as needlessly restrictive, and the nurse to see the social worker as heedless of risks to patient safety. The experienced social worker does not thoughtlessly dismiss safety issues, help a patient out of a wheelchair inappropriately, or promise an outing without consulting a nurse. The patient who requests a cookie may be diabetic. Social workers practicing in health care contexts must be informed about health concerns and their management.

The nurse's education emphasizes responsibility for patient safety. The very family that protests about restrictions may be the first to complain if that patient falls. Moreover, family members will address their complaints to the nurse even though it may have been the social worker who precipitated a change in restraining care arrangements when the patient in the group requested it. As long as the physician and laity are ready to blame the nurse, they must let the nurse set the limits.

The social worker can deal with some of these tensions by helping families to come to terms with their own feelings about placement so that they can act responsibly and determine how much risk taking they are willing to support for their mentally or physically frail relative. Concerning the well-being of any individual patient, the negotiation of agreements about acceptable risk and shared responsibilities should be agreed in care-planning meetings, case conferences, and ideally in family conferences (Ejaz, Noelker, & Schurr, 2002). Relatives' groups co-led by nursing and social work staff members are also appropriate forums in which general principles of risk management can be explored (Toseland, 1995).

CONFIDENTIALITY

Today's nurse is well aware of the right to privacy, both through professional education and through patients' bills of rights. With the new HIPAA regulations, required because of the inherent dangers in sending patient information across the Internet, confidentiality is mandated (Health Insurance Portability and Accountability Act, 1996). (See Chapter 31 for a fuller discussion of the HIPAA requirements.) Confidentiality falters when accountability comes in. The nurse is not supposed to withhold information from the physician, and in the case of the aged patient with dementia, she or he may accept a paying relative's right to know. When the social worker has an obligation to report (as in court-related or guardianship cases), the worker usually deals with confidentiality by indicating its limits to the client, but there are persons who are unlikely to grasp such explanations.

Within the group, confidentiality needs to be an agreed ground rule, and its violation may conflict with another desirable norm, openness. One advantage of coleadership with a member of the nursing staff is that it makes visible the fact of sharing. In the same way, if a patient group wishes to discuss some aspect of service with administration, supporting them rather than taking over this task permits group members to decide for themselves how far they are willing to go.

ADVOCACY

Social workers are taught that they have a duty to advocate for those members of society who are vulnerable, powerless, and oppressed. As born-again activists (Cohen & Mullender, 1999) they often campaign for patients' councils, less medication, and more freedom even when it entails an element of risk. Group workers in particular come from a historical tradition committed to egalitarianism in personal relationships and democratic styles of leadership, even if their actual practice falls short of the ideal. This elicits some unpopularity, especially when the young reformer approaches the task with overtones of moral elitism. What needs to be remembered is that every person working with older people has an obligation to prevent abuse and exploitation (Gutierrez, Parsons, & Cox, 1998). If the social worker is not bent on going it alone, the ethical commitments of the other staff will secure allies in the effort (Cox, 2002).

Three issues should be considered: the definition of the protagonists, the principle of *least contest*, and the interdependence of the individual and his social system.

First, definitions differ. For example, the social worker whose patients are dozing through group sessions may view medication as a chemical straitjacket employed by physicians for the convenience of nurses, especially if the worker was born too late to see the state of psychotic patients before psychotropic medications became available. The physician may counter the criticism by viewing the social worker as a troublemaking upstart. In addition, the administrator may see what the social worker defines as advocacy as disloyalty to the home. Definitions influence interaction.

Second, the principle of least contest suggests beginning with inquiries and quiet negotiation before making negative assumptions about motivation. The physician may be unaware that he or she is medicating the patient into drowsiness and may be willing to reassess the medication in light of a changing situation. The principle of least contest is built on the premise that it is easier to escalate protest than to temper it after defensiveness has been aroused.

Finally, it is rarely in the client's interest to denigrate his or her social system. It is the function or task of the group worker to mediate between persons and their social systems. This is true whether it is an individual and his or her family or a group of residents and the nursing or other staff in the facility in which they live. In attempting to make institutions and persons responsive to client needs, social workers must take care not to harm the client in the process of "rescue." Old persons cannot leave certain systems, such as the family, even if technically they are extruded by their placement and by the family's withdrawal. The individuals continue to see themselves in the context of the family and quite often are seen in that relationship by others. This is why most efforts to serve one at the cost of the other fail. The separation and alienation remain a running sore.

In the same way, the client and the long-term care setting need each other. Therefore, it is not an act of disloyalty to make a setting aware that it is failing its residents. Even the for-profit facility receives its legitimization because it delivers a service to the sick and the very old. If the setting provides good service to patients and their families, it will fulfill its social mission and be confirmed in its profit-earning one. If it falls far below standards, it will jeopardize both. To attack the home without first attempting to change it through ordinary channels is to misserve the clients. The oldest, frailest, and most vulnerable suffer transplantation with difficulty and generally are better served by improvement of conditions where they are. This fulfills the purpose of social work, which aims to promote or restore a mutually beneficial interaction between individuals and society in order to improve the quality of life for both.

A Model for Providing Multidisciplinary Practice

The Mental Health Outreach Program (MHON), formerly based in Duluth, Minnesota, and Superior, Wisconsin, began addressing mental health issues in long-term care in 1992 (Kunz & Larson-Utities, 1998). It started with a pilot program entitled Project CARE. This initial program combined the efforts of one long-term care facility, a psychiatric clinic, and a mental health treatment facility. The results were so successful that it eventually expanded into a partnership with over 20 long-term care facilities. The MHON staff included a psychiatrist, psychologists, several clinical social workers, a nurse, education director, and administrative and support staff.

The model focused on:

1. Treating older adults in their long-term care settings rather than a doctor's office or hospital setting

2. Education of staff at all levels about older adults' mental health using the *Mental Health and Older Adults* video training series (Kunz, 1997). Training topics included older adult development, grief and loss experienced by older adults, therapeutic reminiscence, communicating with moderately and severely affected older adults with dementia, and medications and their side effects. These videos were also used for educating family members.

3. Monthly team meetings were held that included all of the MHON staff plus the facility nursing director, social works, activity professionals, occupational and physical therapists, spiritual care providers, direct care staff, and at times family members. These focused on the ongoing assessment and treatment of the clients, changes in facility milieu, education and coaching of all staff involved, and brainstorming creative solutions for each individual.

The clinical social workers undertook the bulk of the day-to-day individual, group, couples, and family therapy within the facility. The knowledge base and empowerment of this multidisciplinary team approach was of a great value to the social workers. They could, in turn, consult and empower the group and other work done by activity professionals and other facility staff. They used the educational tools developed and gave "on-the-spot" educational inputs to help staff and families adjust their approaches and better understand the clients' needs. This approach contrasted hugely to the more conventional approach of a clinical social worker going into a facility and trying to do all this varied work alone.

Values and Pragmatic Issues in Group Interventions

Older people are very diverse. They include, for example, retired executives and working men, psychiatric patients grown old, people with disparate physical and cognitive disabilities, the chronically or more recently depressed, elderly priests and nuns, women and men, poor and middle-class blacks, rural elders, Hispanics and Latinos who may speak limited English, and downtown skid-row residents. Together they present age, cultural, ethnic, language, and cohort differences that test social work and invite thoughtful attention and differential responses (Anderson & Hill-Collins, 2001; Cox & Parsons, 2000; Spencer, Lewis, & Gutierrez, 2000). (See Chapter also Chapter 32.)

Self-Determination and Reluctant Participation: A Case Example

Gerontological social workers sometimes criticize acute care settings for failing to make a serious commitment to talking therapies for older adults, but social workers are caught in a dilemma of their own. How much should they press aged persons in residential care to participate in the small groups they offer? Even in an age of patients' rights, there is a power differential between professional and resident that most social workers would be reluctant to invoke (Williams, 2002). (Chapter 31 discusses similar issues concerning residents who resist joining groups.) The problem is that those perceived by the professional to be most in need of group services are often the least willing to try them. This dilemma is illustrated by Alice C.

Among the 25 patients in the nursing wing of a large home for older people, there were cognitively alert patients who had cocooned themselves away from contact with other residents who had dementia; not an uncommon problem in many residential facilities. (See Chapters 11 and 12.) Some of the nursing wing residents had special friends who visited from the adjoining boarding unit or they had managed to sustain long established contacts from their local community. A few, however, seemed both lonely and self-absorbed. The social worker believed they needed more stimulation and companionship than the nursing home currently provided. Miss C.'s transfer from the boarding unit to the nursing wing via the hospital brought this into focus.

When Miss C., 92, returned from the hospital having broken her hip, she was restless and unhappy, caught between a desire to go back to the independence of her room in the boarding home and the fears that made her reluctant to give up the safety of the nursing unit. She accused the nurses of wanting to keep her a patient and at the same time always found a reason for not walking when they came to assist her. The social worker could not deal with this problem in a casework relationship because Miss C. had displaced on the social worker much of her anger at the administrator, a woman of similar age, although ordinarily she got along well with both members of staff. The social worker's observation and assessment led her to the opinion that Miss C. might find support from her peers more acceptable.

She approached Miss C. and four other very alert patients who were in poor health. They agreed to try a meeting. One man had multiple sclerosis and another, Parkinson's disease. An 85-year-old woman who had adjusted well to her transfer to the nursing wing was also invited. A fifth candidate agreed to join the group and then withdrew because of a plan to go off-grounds with a relative.

On the day of the meeting, the patient with Parkinson's disease "forgot" and was moving rapidly toward his room when the social worker persuaded him to give it a try. The others gathered with less protest. In welcoming everyone to the meeting, the social worker again repeated that the purpose of the meeting was to give them, as persons with keen intellects, an opportunity to lend one another some company and support. She reiterated her hope that they would decide to meet on a weekly basis. All were polite but cautiously noncommittal, except for the gentle 85-year-old, the one least in need of the program; she remarked that it might be nice to meet regularly in this way.

The social worker waited for others to speak, occasionally howling in items to an essentially silent group. Finally she commented that Dr. M., the patient with the multiple sclerosis, had recently tried acupuncture. The group's interest immediately quickened. All eyes were upon him, Dr. M. smilingly described his experience while the others plied him with questions. For a little while they were truly a group, but they never agreed to meet again.

The following week, Dr. M. was "too tired"; the patient with Parkinson's disease stumped resolutely to his room with a "not today"; and Miss C. was not speaking to the social worker. Only the outgoing 85-year-old was willing—and she could hardly constitute a group by herself. It seemed that Miss C. could not tolerate any contact at all that might threaten her brittle defenses. Later, when she had resolved her ambivalence about remaining in the nursing wing, she readmitted the social worker to her good graces, quite amazed that she could ever have imagined that Miss C. might have been angry. For the two men, isolation seemed a means of conserving their failing energies.

In this instance, the social worker suggested she had had several indispensable ingredients: the separate goodwill of all the members except Miss C., who was temporarily at odds with her; the support of the administrator and the nursing staff, who shared the same concern; and, as potential members, a small group of persons who had much in common.

These persons had had little energy to invest in new relationship, and yet for a moment Dr. M. had shone and his smiling peers had urged him on. Her major unanswered question was how much pressure to exert. During the remainder of her association with the home, she continued to look in vain for a group solution to the problem of how best to meet the needs of the isolated alert patient.

In the same home, two other groups fared somewhat better. The social worker continued to lead an ongoing music group because it was an activity that the alert and less alert residents could enjoy together. (See Chapter 16 on music and other creative arts activities.) After several years, it collapsed under her unwillingness to continue when the nursing aides plucked out the more passive members and the members who had dementia and put them to bed. The original earlier morning meeting time had had to be shifted, and the new time chosen by the nurses was unwelcome to their assistants because it interfered with their opportunity to "finish up."

A reminiscence group designed to provide not only stimulation for the most disoriented members but also education for a social work student continued until her field placement ended. (Chapter 14 discusses reminiscence group work in detail.) Attendance at the music group had required only encouragement and a reminder. The reminiscence group had the support of the paraprofessional staff and the eager willingness of the participants who enjoyed recalling personal memories and welcomed the closer relationships with staff that mutual recall prompted.

Two factors are important in securing initial participation: a good relationship with the social worker and a low level of threat. Even when the social worker is brought in only to lead groups, he or she would be well advised to spend time first getting acquainted with the clients, the setting, and the staff.

At a downtown nutrition site, an extremely marginalized group of seniors attended a current events group, a humanities group, and a men's group designed for heavy drinkers. In each instance, students led the group and the members appreciated contact with younger people. The humanities group provided stimulus for reminiscence of a very structured sort. A male student who quickly saw that the Alcoholics Anonymous formula was not appropriate for these clients ran the men's group. He chose instead to support the flicker of companionship and the limited here-and-now sharing that occurred. His success mirrors that of other student-led groups reported by Soltys, Reda, and Letson (2002). It is worth noting that attendees at these three groups represented a fraction of all the persons who used the center. It was a small pool fed by a big sea. At no time was the need for group activities, as might be judged by the professional, a determinant of participation; older people rightly chose for themselves whether or not to participate.

When attendance is compulsory, nonparticipation takes special forms. Lesser, Lazarus, Frankel, & Havasy (1981) and his associates described the restless, disjunctive behavior of older psychotics in traditional group therapy. Most members were silent; some displayed pseudoconfusion; others addressed irrelevant questions to the physician coleader. When, however, reminiscence was substituted, the same patients became alert and receptive, making it apparent that the disturbed behavior was a method of dealing with the threat the group posed. Similar problems can still occur if group workers try to impose rather than work towards achieving agreement over goals and program, ends and means. The achievement of mutuality remains one of, if not the key objective of social workers who attempt to undertake group work with older people.

Respect for the Individual and the Too-Bland Group

Attention has been drawn to the rejection implicit in offering older people only recreational and leisure-time groups and in supporting the suppression of conflict. It has often been observed that particularly in residential contexts older adults avoid strong overt reactions to their neighbors and other group members. They tend to avoid emotional intensity; their antagonisms are muted and their confrontations indirect.

While supporting openness, one has to respect and accept this lower key of interaction. Student social workers need to appreciate that encouraging aggressive confrontation, as may be commonplace in groups serving younger people, or supporting expressions of divergent viewpoints, may not always be acceptable, even if there is an awareness of the endemic undercurrents that frequently exist among the residents and staff in homes for older people. For many residents who struggle to live private lives in public places, surviving in such close proximity to their neighbors requires bland or distanced relationships; open conflict would threaten precarious survival and security.

Herein lies a contradiction. For while it is better for a group to manage itself, a social work leader may question whether extreme tolerance for a group monopolist, for example, may communicate to the members the worker's low expectations and even a sort of disrespect for the group as a whole.

Confidentiality and Responsible Others

Aged participants are not likely to present material they would be unwilling to share, and the limits of confidentiality should be openly discussed (Appelbaum & Greer, 1993). When information must be passed on, it is helpful to discuss with the client how it should be presented. This solution has less meaning when the client is limited or forgetful, but he or she should nonetheless still be asked.

In sharing with the adult children of a person with dementia, the group worker may need to act as a surrogate ego, telling what the client would be willing to have told, as best as this can be understood. By not gossiping about older individuals, as adults sometimes do when discussing a small child, the social worker is modeling respect for the still-adult status of the disabled parent, an important consideration when the adult children may be struggling with concerns about their own aging and potential role reversals within the family.

In long-term care settings, students are sometimes reluctant to include members of the patient care staff when they are leading a group. Their rationale is that the presence of these persons may be inhibiting for the patients, whereas, in fact, it may be inhibiting for the novice group leader. Exclusion seems to show a lack of trust, both of the staff members themselves and of the group members' ability to deal with them. If there is a troubled relationship, generally it is better to have it where it can be openly observed.

One reason for including other staff members is to encourage their constructive interest in group activity. If time is taken to discuss the group with them before and after meetings, a major reason for their exclusion—the tendency of some to suppress the expression of negative feelings—can be checked.

The student's reminiscence group described earlier had its ups and downs. One morning the student telephoned that she would be arriving too late to start the group and asked the field instructor to take over. When the student arrived, she found the members, instead of reminiscing were eagerly rehearsing the names of the nursing aides who had accompanied them to the group. The student commented that the aides had never come when she led the group. Further inquiry showed that she had never asked them. In this group, the traditional material of reminiscence groups was abandoned in favor of information likely to secure the members better lives within the home.

Learning the names of the nursing assistants was a single example.

The reward came when the social worker arrived one afternoon and found one of the nursing aides surrounded by a circle of the more disabled patients, talking with them and encouraging them to address one another.

Empowerment and the Vulnerable Client

When dealing with dependent populations, there are three questions the practitioner must consider before embarking on advocacy.

First, will your intervention leave the client vulnerable to reprisals? This is no reason for not acting, but it does dictate a carefully thought-out strategy.

Second, what kind of changes does the client want? When one of the authors of this chapter administered the Philadelphia Geriatric Morale Scale to residents in two settings, one woman with a very low morale score nevertheless replied to the item that asked, "Where would you live if you could live where you wanted?" "Right here!" She saw the setting as the best arrangement available to her and would not have welcomed vigorous intervention. What she wanted was more respect from some of the nurses' assistants.

Third, what is the function of the complaint? Just as there are adult children who complain about the inconsiderate behavior of a parent but continue to reinforce it, there are older persons whose laments have a conversational quality. This does not mean that the complaints should not be taken seriously but only that they should be examined. Specificity is a clue, and so is willingness to act when fully supported. Either diffuseness or inaction indicates the need for deeper listening: You may not have heard what the client really said.

Levels of Directivity Within Groups of Older Adults

Groups with older adults should be framed within the context of older adult developmental issues and make use of lifelong wisdom of the group to problem solve, support, and promote well-being. In order to accomplish this, social workers need to feel comfortable altering their style, voice level, and physical presence when working with older adults. This is often challenging for students or inexperienced, self-conscious workers.

Certainly not all, but many older adults, particularly in residential settings, have mild to severe sensory and/or cognitive impairment. Thus, the social worker must adjust both their expectations of the client and group outcome as well as the way they structure and facilitate the group to the abilities of those clients. **Figure 29–1** provides a visual representation to help select how approaches to group leadership need to change depending upon the needs of the participants.

The horizontal axis of the diagram shows the levels or cognitive and/or sensory abilities of group members ranging from excellent to poor. The vertical axis of the diagram shows the level of directivity from low to high needed to lead the group effectively. This directivity needs to be fluid and may vary from person to person and change over the life of any one group. Numbers one, two, and three demonstrate the continuum of stages in which the leader needs to alter his or her communication and facilitation style.

At stage one the worker uses standard group techniques ranging from open discussion to formal therapy with explicit rules of confidentiality. Reminiscence and life review techniques as well as other approaches are easily understood and applied by the participants. If the social worker is seeking third-party reimbursement for such work, it is important to frame these approaches

Figure 29–1 LEVEL OF DIRECTIVITY IN GROUPS OF OLDER ADULTS

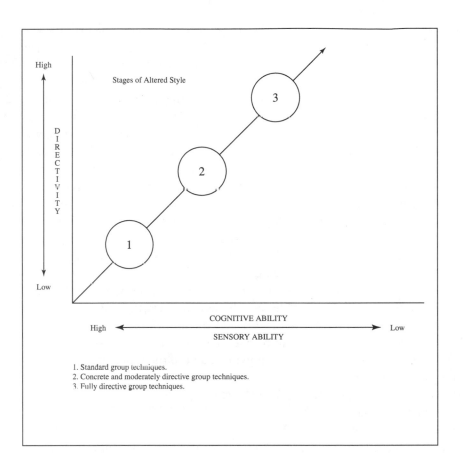

1. Standard group techniques.
2. Concrete and moderately directive group techniques.
3. Fully directive group techniques.

within established treatment modalities and the treatment plan. Reminiscence and life review approaches can be easily integrated within brief and cognitive behavioral models of therapy (Kunz, 2002a).

At stage two the worker should become more concrete and use more directive group techniques. Confidentiality may not be guaranteed on the part of the clients and the worker may need to respectfully redirect or otherwise shut down a participant in order to protect them from sharing what might be inappropriate in a group context. The worker must later follow-up on the issues the client had been dealing with by means of an individual approach or a referral.

The social worker will need to be more forceful in keeping the group on task and may need to be repetitive in communicating the purpose of the group and more frequently summarize the group progress. At this stage the worker must often "translate" between group members due to their sensory and/or cognitive impairment. It is helpful to include direct care staff to help some of the members communicate and focus on the group process. The worker must both slow down, but yet, maintain group momentum. Props are often needed to maintain group attention and appeal to members' more concrete level of cognitive development (Burnside, 1995; Kunz, 2002a).

This needed shift in facilitation style likely conflicts with expositions of group leadership found in many social work textbooks. The leader's success in resolving this conflict and facing the challenge of altering his or her physical and emotional presence will either make or break a group at this stage.

At stage three the worker must use fully directive group techniques. The level of "translation" between members now becomes even more repetitive. Often it requires the worker to move around the room physically to maintain group attention and connection between members, even to the point of connecting with residents who may not see, hear, or realize that someone else is there. Even more props are needed at this stage. The worker must connect the reactions and discussion that results to feelings and issues related to any of the stages of adult development. This is done for the group to better meet the emotional needs of each group member while at the same time tying these feelings and needs to the group as a whole. By structuring the group at the correct cognitive level the participants are able to make use of residual memories and skills resulting in rich and often surprising discussion and insight. Given the proper structure, the group process itself promotes a sense of well-being (and often more confident positive behavior) that often continues long past the period of time the client can remember what happened in the group (Feil, 1992; Kunz, 2002b).

Summary

From its early development in settlement houses and youth organizations, social group work gained its optimistic view of human nature, its commitment to fighting injustice, and its use of the group to help people learn new ways of coping with life's old and new challenges. Social group work was once a separate method within the profession, but today social workers are trained and prepared to intervene as needed with individuals, families, groups, or communities, a flexibility that fits them well for work with older people.

If they are to serve vulnerable older adults well, social workers leading groups in host settings must communicate with members of other professions. They must be sensitive to the situational factors that lead other professions to translate similar values somewhat differently.

The social worker in the group must deal with issues raised by the interface of social work values and the special characteristics and needs of very old people: respect for self-determination and the challenge of the reluctant participant; confidentiality and the need of family and caregivers to know; advocacy without damage to a dependent client's supporting systems; and the rights and varying needs of the individual and the group. Group leaders working with very frail or impaired older people need to learn that just as members' needs differ, so too must leaders adjust their leadership style to enable them to respond flexibly to each individual and to the group as a whole.

Exercises

EXERCISE 1

Interprofessional collaboration demands the ability to understand the feelings of the other. This exercise asks you to look at a situation in a nursing home from two points of view, that of the charge nurse and that of the social worker who comes once a week to lead a patient group.

For the first part, you are the nurse. Other members of the class will read aloud:

> *Physician:* Nurse, I have to examine Mrs. Smith right now. I don't have all day. Please get her ready.

> *Administrator:* Nurse, don't let that group stay in the room too long. We have to get it ready for the board meeting tonight.

> *Patient:* Help me, help me, help me, help me... (continues monotonously)

Beautician: Mrs. Brown's daughter wants her shampooed today so that she can take her out tomorrow. I can't do it unless you get her out of that group now.

Podiatrist: Nurse, surely you don't expect me to wait until Mrs. Green gets out of that group. You should have her feet soaking now so that she'll be ready when I get to her.

Daughter: After all, I drove down to see Mother. Surely she doesn't have to be in that group today.

Social worker: Nurse, Mrs. Jones seems to have had an accident. Could you get the aide to do something about it?

Explain to the group how the nurse feels.

In the second part, you are the social worker. You have arrived to find that only two group members are ready. Mrs. Ellis has gone off with her daughter. Mrs. Green is soaking her feet, waiting for the podiatrist, who has several other patients lined up and won't get to her for another half hour. The nurse has asked you to cut your group short today because someone else wants to use the room. Mrs. Smith is with the doctor, who chose this hour for his monthly visit. One of the two group members who appeared to be ready just had an "accident." You don't know why the aides couldn't have taken her to the bathroom first.

Explain to the group how the social worker feels.

EXERCISE 2

After attending one session, Mrs. Black announces that she does not belong in the group: "Those people are crazy." Mr. Ellis says he is too tired today; he'll let you know next time. Mrs. Rogers, who is always an active participant when she comes but is forgetful, has already begun a nap. Miss Marion, whom you persuaded to try it once, says she doesn't want to come again.

You respect the client's right to self-determination, but you feel that each of these persons needs the group activity, especially Mr. Ellis, who seems to be depressed and withdrawing.

How strongly would you act to persuade each of them to attend? What would be the determining factor in each case?

EXERCISE 3

Observe for at least an hour any small group of adults who customarily meet together that includes both younger and older members. This does not have to be a treatment group but can be an instrumental group, such as a committee or board. Tally the disagreements or confrontations that occur and note which members are involved and whether they disagree in a manner that is essentially direct, or indirect and friendly, pseudofriendly, or hostile. How do they use humor? Do disagreements occur more consistently between certain pairs? Afterwards, review your notes to see whether there was any difference in the way older and younger adults expressed disagreement.

Briefly summarize your findings and describe one exchange you observed that illustrates your conclusion. (Remember to protect the identity of the individuals involved unless they are public officials in an open meeting.)

EXERCISE 4

Mrs. Adams would like to attend the spring luncheon meeting of her church's women's group. In past years, members have made arrangements, well checked in advance, to pick her up at the nursing home. This year no one calls, possibly because her unsteadiness has been a source of concern. (She fell on the steps last year.) Mrs. Adams presents her problem in a moving manner to the student social worker, who agrees to help. Mrs. Adams is exultant. The student social worker is pleased at her pleasure. The charge nurse, only a little older than the student social worker, is outraged. She points out to Mrs. Adams that her physician has not okayed the trip and to the student social worker that she cannot transport Mrs.

Adams in her car. She points out that Mrs. Adams has medical problems that the student social worker does not understand. Then she calls the physician, reminding him of Mrs. Adams's fall last year, the brittleness of her diabetes, and her tendency to eat everything in sight on these occasions. Mrs. Adams tells everyone the nurse is treating her like a prisoner. The student social worker is crushed and resentful.

Describe the incident as each party might— Mrs. Adams, the student social worker, and the nurse. Which professional values might the nurse and the social worker have invoked and which might they have agreed on? How could each have handled it better?

References

Anderson, M. L., & Hill-Collins, P. (2001). *Race, class and gender: An anthology.* Belmont, CA: Wadsworth/Thomson Learning.

Appelbaum, P. S, & Greer, A. (1993). Confidentiality in group therapy. *Hospital Group Psychiatry, 44*(40), 311–312.

Association for the Advancement of Social Work with Groups. (2004). Retrieved July 1, 2004, from *www.aaswg.org*

Berlin, S. B. (2002). *Clinical social work practice.* Oxford, UK: Oxford University Press.

Berman-Rossi, T. (1994). *Social work: The collected writings of William Schwartz.* Itasca, IL: F. E. Peacock.

Burnside, I. (1995). Themes and props: Adjuncts for reminiscence therapy groups. In B. K. Haight & J. D. Webster (Eds.), *The art and science of reminiscing: Theory, research, methods, and applications.* Washington, DC: Taylor and Francis.

Chen, M., & Rybak, C. J. (2004). *Group leadership skills.* Pacific Grove, CA: Brooks/Cole.

Cohen, M. B., & Mullender, A. (1999). The personal in the political: Exploring the group work continuum from individual to social change goals. *Social Work with Groups, 22*(1), 21–39.

Corey, M. S., & Corey, G. (2002). *Group process and practice.* Pacific Grove, CA: Brooks/Cole.

Corey, G., Corey, M. S., Callanan, P., & Russell, J. M. (2004). *Group techniques.* Pacific Grove, CA: Brooks/Cole.

Council on Social Work Education (CSWE). (2004). Retrieved July, 2004, from *www.cswe.org*

Cox, E. O. (2002). Empowerment-oriented practice applied to long-term care. *Journal of Social Work in Long-term Care, 1*(2), 27–46.

Cox, E. O., & Parsons, R. (2000). Empowerment-practice: From practice value to practice model. In P. Allen-Meares & C. Garvin (Eds.), *Handbook of social work direct practice.* Thousand Oaks, CA: Sage.

Dobrof, R. (Ed.). (2002). *Advancing gerontological social work education.* Binghamton, NY: Haworth Press.

Doel, M., & Sawdon, C. *The essential group worker.* London, UK: Jessica Kingsley.

Ejaz, F. K., Knoelker, L. S., & Schurr, D. (2002). Family satisfaction with nursing home care for relatives with dementia. *Journal of Applied Gerontology, 21*(3), 368–384.

Fast, B., & Chapin, R. (2000). *Strengths-based care management for older adults.* Baltimore: Health Professions Press.

Feil, N. (1992). *V/F Validation: The Feil method, How to help disoriented old-old.* Cleveland, OH: Edward Feil.

Gitterman, A. (2002). Vulnerability, resilience, and social work with groups. In T. Kelly, T. Berman-Rossi, & S. Palombo (Eds.), *Group work strategies for strengthening resiliency* (pp. 19–33). Binghamton, NY: Haworth Press.

Gitterman, A., & Shulman, L. (2004). (Eds.). *Mutual aid groups, vulnerable populations and the life cycle* (Rev. ed.). New York: Columbia.

Gutierrez, L., Parsons, R., & Cox, E. (1998). *Empowerment in social work practice: A sourcebook.* Pacific Grove, CA: Brooks/Cole.

Health Insurance Portability and Accountability Act (HIPAA). (1996). Retrieved July 1, 2004, from *www.hhs.gov/ocr/hipaa*

Institute for Geriatric Social Work (IGSW). (2004.) Retrieved July 9, 2004, from *www.bu.edu/igs*

Kadushin, A., & Harkness, D. (2000). *Supervision in social work.* New York: Columbia University Press.

Kivnick, H., & Murray, S. (2001). Life strengths interview guide. *Journal of Gerontological Social Work, 34*(4), 7–32.

Kubie, S. H., & Landau, G. (1953). Group work with older people. New York: International Universities Press.

Kunz, J., & Larson-Utities, J. (1998). Comprehensive mental health treatment in long-term care. *Dimensions, 6*(4), 5–6.

Kunz, J. (2002a). Integrating reminiscence and life review techniques with brief cognitive behavioral therapy. In J. D. Webster & B. K. Haight (Ed.), *Critical advances in reminiscence work* (pp. 275–288). New York: Springer.

Kunz, J. (2002b). Targeted reminiscence interventions for older adults with dementia. *Journal of Geriatric Psychiatry, 35*(5), 25–44.

Lasch-Quinn, E. (1993). *Black neighbors: Race and the limits of reform in the American settlement movement, 1890–1945.* Chapel Hill, NC: University of North Carolina.

Lesser, J., Lazarus, L. W., Frankel, R., & Havasy, S. (1981). Reminiscence group therapy with psychotic geriatric patients. *The Gerontologist,* 21(3), 191–196.

Lund, M. (1998). The nurse ethicist. *Geriatric Nursing,* 19(6), 342–343.

McCormack, B. (2003). A conceptual framework for person-centred practice with older people. *International Journal of Nursing Practice, 9*, 202–209.

National Association of Social Workers (NASW). *Social group work with older people. Proceedings of seminar.* (1961). Lake Mohonk, New York: Arno Press.

National Association of Social Workers (NASW). 2004. Retrieved July 9, 2004, www.nasw.org

National Association of Social Workers (NASW). (1999). *The NASW code of ethics.* Washington, DC: Author.

Northern, H. (1998). Ethical dilemmas in social work with groups. *Social Work with Groups,* 21(1/2), 5–17.

Phillips, M. H., & Cohen, C. S. (2000). Strength and resiliency themes in social work practice with groups. In E. Norman (Ed.), *Resiliency enhancement* (pp. 128–142). New York: Columbia University Press.

Psychologists in Long-Term Care (PLTC). (2004). Retrieved July 9, 2004, www.wvu.edu/~pltc/PLTC

Rantz, M., & Connolly, R. (2004). Measuring nursing care quality and using large data sets in nonacute care settings: State of the science. *Nursing Outlook, 52*(1), 23–27.

Ronch, L., & Goldfield, J. (2003). *Mental wellness in aging.* Baltimore: Health Professions Press.

Rosow, I. (1974). *Socialization to old age.* Berkeley, CA: University of California Press.

Ryan, B. S., & Crawford, P. (2002). Creating loss support groups for the elderly. In S. Henry & J. F. East (Eds.), *Social work with groups* (pp. 151–162). Binghamton, NY: Haworth.

Schwartz, W. (1979). The social worker in the group. In B. R. Compton B. Galaway (Eds.), *Social work processes* (pp. 14–28). Homewood, IL: Dorsey.

Soltys, F. G., Reda, S., & Letson, M. (2002). Use of the group process for reminiscence. *Journal of Geriatric Psychiatry,* 35(1), 51–61.

Spencer, M., Lewis, E., & Gutierrez, L. (2000). Multicultural perspectives on direct social work. In P. Allen-Mears, & C. Garvin (Eds.), *Handbook of direct practice in social work: Future directions.* Thousand Oaks, CA: Sage.

Toseland, R. W. (1995). *Group work with the elderly and family caregivers.* New York: Springer.

U.S. Social Security Act, Amendments Section 1819 and 1919 (OBRA '87). Medicare and Medicaid: Requirements for long-term care facilities. *Federal Register,* Section 483:48826–48865 (September 26).

Williams, H. M. (2002). Social work skills in assisted living. *Journal of Social Work in Long Term Care,* 3(8), 5–8.

Wilson G. (1976). From practice to theory: A personalized history. In R. W. Roberts & H. Northern (Eds.), *Theories of social work with groups* (pp. 1–44). New York: Columbia University Press.

Zastrow, C. (1997). *Social work with groups.* Chicago: Nelson-Hall.

Resources

- Few papers on group work with older people are to be found in the journals dealing with groups, such as *Groupwork, International Journal of Group Psychotherapy, Journal of Specialists in Group Work*, and *Social Work with Groups*. On the other hand, practice-oriented journals dealing with gerontology do have papers on group work from time to time. Among these are *Clinical Gerontology, The Gerontologist*, and the *Journal of Gerontological Social Work*.

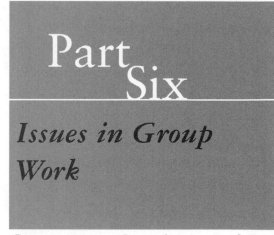

Part Six

Issues in Group Work

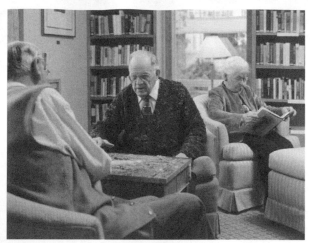

As with every therapeutic endeavor, issues arise that must be addressed by the practitioner. In Chapter 30, Gibson and Burnside present the importance of ongoing consultation and supervision for the practicing group leader. Neese highlights in Chapter 31 the ethical issues inherent in group work that must be addressed by the concerned practitioner.

Cross-cultural issues are also extremely important when working with older people from a variety of cultures and backgrounds. In Chapter 32, Anderson and Delgado point out the futility of group work with people from other cultures if the ethnic issues are not addressed. The section ends with two complementary chapters: Chapter 33, by Haight, highlights the importance of research in group work and the last chapter, Chapter 34, by Pierce, emphasizes the importance of evaluating the group work that we undertake.

Chapter 30

Consultation and Supervision

Faith Gibson
Irene Burnside

Key Words

- Directive
- Ego enhancement
- Feedback
- Mentor
- Responsibility for own learning
- Self-esteem
- Support
- Supervision
- Understanding

Learning Objectives

- Discuss six ways in which group work with older adults may differ from that with other age groups
- Discuss three pitfalls for new group leaders
- Explain the role of feedback given to students
- Discuss four ways to increase self-esteem in the learner
- Analyze one format for teaching group work

This chapter is about consultation in the specific area of group work with older adults and teaching and supervising students who are practicing group work (Proctor, 2000). Consultation is covered in the first part of the chapter, and the remainder is devoted to issues concerning the supervision and instruction of students. This latter section is intended for those who have never supervised students working with groups of older people. Supervision may be undertaken with an individual student, or in the case of coleadership, it is common for the supervisor to supervise both coleaders simultaneously.

Consultation

The literature of most helping professions abounds with content on consultation. However, there is little in the literature that is germane to consultation about group work with older adults. Therefore, basic general principles about consultation with application to working with older people will provide the framework for this discussion. A consultant is defined as one who gives professional advice or services (Merriam-Webster, 2004). In the helping professions consultation is the provision of expert advice, information or help by one professional person to another seeking guidance in the same field within a mutually supportive relationship.

The Growing Need

The rapid rate of technological change and its effects together with the awareness of underutilized, underdeveloped, and misused human resources has increased the demand for consultancy services in many fields. The growing and complex needs of many groups, including ethnic minorities and disabled and older people, often means that their requirements for services and assistance are growing faster than professionals are being prepared. One way of responding to this shortfall is to use consultants to support staff while they develop new knowledge and skills by means of on-the-job experience and work-based practice. A group work service for older people can provide practice experience to enable new or inexperienced staff and students in training to develop group work skills and knowledge. If supervision and support are not available from a member of staff, a visiting skilled consultant may be able to fulfill these roles and responsibilities (Gibson, 2004).

Characteristics of a Consultant

It is desirable that consultants should have conceptual sophistication, good interpersonal skills, and be confident in their work-related roles and skills. They need to be respected for their professional knowledge and practice wisdom and to be perceived as encouraging and supportive. The consultant should be knowledgeable about aging processes and the multidimensional needs of older people, group dynamics, and group work theory. Relevant theory is identified in Part 1. Consultants must be committed to advocating and using evidence-based practice. This means they must consistently seek to exercise conscientious and judicious use of evidence of current best group work practice in the advice and guidance they provide to others (Pollio, 2001).

Often consultants are asked to supply advice and information at short notice. Such instances could include a colleague requesting assistance regarding groups, or a director of nursing or an administrator asking for advice regarding establishing groups, or problems with existing group leadership in a facility. Consultants may also advise on teaching group work within an educational context. This may include advice on the content and structure of a group work curriculum, teaching group work in the classroom, securing and managing group work placements for students or staff, the assessment of group work training and practice, and the definition and establishment of acceptable standards of practice (Galinskey & Schopler, 1995). Another example would be for a consultant to be asked to observe a group in session to help the leaders improve their skills (Chen & Rybak, 2004). Two such examples are presented here.

EXAMPLE 1

A gerontologist with group work experience was conducting a seminar at a university. A young faculty member who was leading a group asked for some help in handling some of the behaviors in the group. She was especially frustrated by the monopolizing behavior of one of the men in the group. She requested that the consultant lead a portion of the group so she could sit back and observe. What she learned was that out of respect for the older adults, she hesitated to give feedback or intervene in behaviors such as monopolizing. When she compared her interventions to those of the consultant, she felt she had been too timid and too reluctant to intervene with the members and had not provided the leadership they needed.

EXAMPLE 2

An instructor was supervising a group of baccalaureate students in a day care center, all of whom were involved in leading groups. The director of the day care center called her aside to discuss a group-related problem. Two graduate students were coleading their first group of older people and were enthusiastic about it. The members, however, were less enthusiastic and wanted to quit the group, and she was not sure why. She asked the students if the instructor could sit in on their group to offer assistance and support them with suggestions that would help keep the group intact.

Some of the problems observed were: The coleaders sat next to one another so that the weaker members did not get support by having a leader close by them; the group met in a lounge with huge, soft sofas arranged in a large rectangle. This meant that they could not see or hear one another well. Several props were introduced together, which confused some members and encouraged simultaneous competing conversations. A man who had had a stroke, had difficulty speaking, and lacked confidence was directly asked a very specific question and was overcome with embarrassment. The leaders kept probing for feelings, which made some of the members anxious and fidgety. The lounge was noisy with people coming and going during the meeting and noises from outside intruded. It was clear that the needs of some of the members were not being met, and they were attending to please the director of the day care center.

The above are simple examples, readily identified and easily rectified. Issues of group process are usually more complex to master and group leaders need assistance to take responsibility for identifying their own strengths and weaknesses and relevant emotions rather than depending on the critique of an external authority figure.

Written reports of consultation sessions are important to provide a basis for continuing discussion. Either you are expected to solve all the problems (and then take the blame when they fail) or you are not taken very seriously and may be tolerated by some of the listeners only because someone above them in the hierarchy asked you to consult.

Because group work with older people is arduous, draining, and sometimes discouraging for the beginning group leader, considerable support is needed from an instructor or supervisor. This chapter gives students, instructors, health and social care workers, and volunteers an understanding of supervisory responsibilities vested in a clearly identified responsible person. Topics include the value of humor and feedback for students, pitfalls for new group leaders to avoid, anxiety and depression in new group leaders, how to increase self-esteem among new leaders, and some suggested formats for teaching group work.

Differences Between Older Adults and Other Age Groups

A leader who is new to working with older people in groups may, despite other group work experience, need some assistance in discovering the ways in which group work with older adults is both similar and different. Some of the differences are:

- Older people tend to be grateful and to express their appreciation to the leader in a variety of ways.
- The groups tend to be smaller—for example, four or six members if the group is composed of members with sensory disabilities and even smaller for people with dementia. Most leaders recommend groups sufficiently large to remain viable if some members become ill or die.
- The pace of the group may be slower.
- There are likely to be fewer struggles between members and leaders over power and control.
- Some goals may differ from other groups although many will be similar.
- Loss of all kinds is likely to be a recurring theme.
- The members will likely have multiple problems—physical, psychological, and socioeconomic.
- Sensory defects are frequent and sometimes severe.

- Physical ailments are many; a single member may have several.
- The physical environment of the meeting place is very important. It must be comfortable, accessible, and acceptable. Older group members generally poorly tolerate extreme temperatures, glare, and noise. (See **Table** 11–4 regarding the environment for cognitively impaired elders.)
- The leader may have to be very active, especially with groups of long-institutionalized people, and accept increased responsibility for convening meetings and helping members get to the group.

Older people may be initially reluctant to join a group and some may need considerable encouragement in the beginning phase, yet value the intimacy stage and dread termination.

- Socializing outside of group meetings can be very helpful and provide additional opportunities for enjoyment and satisfaction.
- Leaders are usually expected to share information about themselves.
- Older people tend to conserve energy; therefore, anxiety may be more difficult to assess in groups of aged persons.
- Physical dependence needs may be very high because of the frailty of group members or the extreme age of some participants.
- Transportation to and from the group (whether it is an in-house or an extramural group) can create many problems and requires meticulous planning.
- Daytime meetings are generally more acceptable than evening meetings.
- Groups should be planned around aged people's maximum-functioning portion of the day. If residents like to nap after lunch, that is not the best time for a group meeting.

- There may be a vast age difference between the leaders and the members.
- The subject of death and dying will come up frequently; death may occur within the group experience and will need to be openly addressed.
- Because of the poverty of many older people, those who could benefit from a group experience may not be able to afford it or have transportation available.
- Boredom and loneliness may be pervasive themes.
- Confrontation groups are usually not appropriate for older adults who need ego enhancement rather than confrontation.

In sum, group work with older people requires considerable involvement on the part of the leader who needs to be willing to take initiatives, offer reassurance and support, and patiently develop members' capacities for self-development and engaging in mutual aid (Corey & Corey, 2002). Other differences include the recurrence of specific themes, such as losses of many kinds and social isolation; some older people are more difficult to engage because of depression or sensory impairments; attention spans may be shorter because of physical or cognitive difficulties; group members may be on medications that affect mental alertness; they may forget to attend sessions; regular attendance may be difficult to maintain; group members need support and encouragement; and like younger people, they too have a great need to be listened to and to be accepted and understood (Corey, 2004).

Tasks of the Instructor or Supervisor

The instructor or supervisor of group work practice has several obligations to a student. The most important of which is to reduce a new leader's anxiety and to lend a vision of the possibilities inherent in group work with older people so that the leader can function reasonably confidently from the beginning. Here the terms *instructor* and *supervisor* are used interchangeably and without reference to whether they are employed by an educational institution or a service agency. Frequently a classroom teacher of group work may also follow the students into their practice agency to provide emotional support and additional teaching or instruction. Often too this person has responsibility for assessment of competence. In this case there should also be an identified agency-based staff member to whom the student relates concerning administrative matters. In some agencies, an identified staff member provides administrative support, educational guidance, and emotional support. This person is frequently known as a supervisor. Both types of learning experience may be offered on an individual basis. This is not essential, however, and group supervision, or a combination of individual and group supervision is very appropriate for either students or staff members practicing group work.

Advantages and disadvantages exist with either individual or group supervision and Kadushin and Harkness (2002) suggest that often a mixture of both proves fruitful. Group supervision is more economical of time. It is regarded as helpful for conveying information, exchanging views, and enlarging experience. It may trigger unhelpful competitiveness in students or be experienced as mutually supportive, providing the supervisor is sufficiently skilled in leading the group. Bernard and Goodyear (1998) and Bradley and Ladany (2001) reviewed the research literature on effectiveness of supervision, which is considered crucial for the delivery of high standards of practice.

Difficulties within the classroom may be mirrored by problems in the practice agency and vice versa. See Chapter 21 for a discussion about making links between students' experience of learning to function in a group work class and the experience of older members in groups that students are leading in practice agencies.

Humor and Understanding

The use of humor helps both students doing group work and student–instructor conferences. Often we become so grim and determined in our work with older people that we fail to see the joy and wit around us. Sometimes it takes an older person to teach the value of joy and humor. Irene Burnside cited an illuminating example from her first year of teaching. She described how she had a maverick student who was determined to change nurses, doctors, and agencies. The student bulldozed her way along and wondered why there was such chaos in her wake. One day when Burnside was trying to inject some realism and help her realign her ideals, she flared up: "Irene, you sound just like my mother!" Too weary for further explanation, Burnside asked her if she would change it to "grandmother" because at the moment her arthritis was bothering her. The student suddenly laughed, and thereafter their stormy relationship seemed to change for the better.

Students often hear their peers comment, "How dull," "How depressing," or "How do you stand it?" It becomes tiring after a while, continually defending one's interest in gerontology and working with older people. But students do need to find some rewards for themselves in this work, and instructors can give feedback to help the students find pleasure in group work.

As students begin to see traits they admire and respect in older people and discover the unique human qualities in each individual, they begin to appreciate their group work and their relationships with older adults. Not infrequently, students develop close relationships with aged clients and keep in touch long after student days have passed.

On one occasion, Burnside attended a student's wedding, which was held in a lovely park. The terrain was a bit rough, so during the reception she said to the 90-year-old grandmother of the bride, "Could I get you another glass of champagne?" The grandmother looked her squarely in the eye and said, "What's the matter, don't you think I can get it by myself?" (Burnside did not know the woman was leaving for vacation in Greece the next day.) When students begin to experience similar incidents and see the strengths, flair, courage, and uniqueness of so many older adults, they often become staunch advocates of the aged client.

Identifying Pitfalls for Beginning Group Leaders

Supervisors bear the responsibility for discouraging students without the appropriate background who may wish to take on the role of psychotherapist. The instructor should be alert for such a stance in a student and watch for excessive probing of group members, constant confrontations with members about behavior or statements made in meetings, and a desire to push in especially painful areas that are beyond their competence to explore. Although it seems to be true that older people reveal only what they wish, a new leader may confront them or aggressively challenge them, and the members may subsequently refuse to participate in the group. Holding a group to talking about taboo subjects is not the same as being aggressively confrontational. The balance, however, is a fine one, and acquiring the relevant skills needs practice and supportive encouragement (Shulman, 2002).

The supervisor also has to watch for occasions when new leaders' needs are usurping group needs. For example, a leader's need to help may end in infantilizing older people. Other leaders may give free rein to their curiosity and want the older person to reveal all while they sit back and share nothing. In the reverse situation, leaders use the group setting to vent their own problems and anxieties. It is not easy to teach the balance needed; students learn it as they make mistakes in practicing group work.

Feedback to Students

Feedback is crucial in teaching. One reason instructors or supervisors should give feedback to students is that they become a role model for students, who can then begin to give feedback to the older adults in their care. Many older persons suffer from lack of feedback, especially those who live alone. A second reason is that students do flourish with feedback. Students gain self-confidence with prompt, positive, and constructive feedback from a supervisor. There is no substitute for actual practice in leading a group.

Students should receive both positive and negative feedback on their performance with groups. How much of each should be given is up to the supervisor. Some students require a lot of encouragement; others need to be restrained because they come on too strongly. Skillful observation of each student is required to find out the mode of supervision that will maximize the student's potential. Every effort should be made to prevent failures, which foster discouragement and depression in a student leader. The instructor should bring out the best in each student. Some students have had so much negative feedback that they do not know what their best is, and imaginative ways may need to be found to develop their understanding and enhance their self-esteem (Duffy, 2001).

It is advisable to always present the positive comments first in the conferences or written evaluations. If you put the negative comments first, the student usually will not pay attention to the positive feedback that comes later (Kadushin & Harkness, 2002).

Recognizing Anxiety in New Group Leaders

The instructor must also be alert for anxiety in a new group leader, and the supervisor must help students understand the basis of their anxiety. Beginners often fear failure or are not sure what they can accomplish in a group. Therefore it is important to teach students how to tune in to the group and to their own feelings about the group in preparing for each session. Students also need to learn to manage endings, which like beginnings, are times of heightened emotion in groups (Birnbaum & Cicchetti, 2000; Shulman, 1999).

If a student has never been in an extended care facility before and the group meetings are to be held there, the student may have horrified initial reactions to everything from the smell to the behavior of the personnel. When students are indignant and their complaints seem unending, they can often be reminded that they are forgetting the aged persons; they are spending so much of their time and energy grumbling or coping with the staff that they have little energy left for creative work with the residents. This sort of behavior in a student may be one form of resistance. A student may hold back, as though stalling long enough will prevent having to go through the group experience. Procrastination is a common way for beginning group leaders to handle their anxiety. However, the instructor must also take responsibility when things are not going well. For example, if one gives vague, poor, incomplete instructions, the student can really get muddled trying to figure out what the assignment is or what the instructor expects.

Asking students what would help them most in their state of apprehension can bring a variety of requests—for example, just a desire to talk, to go for a cup of coffee, to go for a walk, to cry for a while. The instructor should try to respond to any such requests; launching a new leader well into group work is important just as successful beginnings are significant for group members and set patterns that carry on throughout the life of the group.

On the other hand, instructors must heed the concerns and criticisms of students about poor conditions and unacceptable standards of care and assist them to formulate and implement a response appropriate to the context and the issues causing concern.

Preventing Discouragement in New Leaders

Other reactions a group leader might experience include discouragement, concern over progress, and low self-esteem. Students beginning group work may become discouraged for a variety of reasons. Former students have identified some of these reasons as follows:

1. The student's lack of experience and knowledge may prevent them from recognizing and valuing their achievements in a new area of work.
2. The distressing living conditions of some older people where the student may be placed can be a factor.
3. The older people with whom the student is working may be depressed, because depression is endemic in late life, especially in nursing home residents.
4. The attitudes and behavior of some staff and doctors toward the patients may discourage a student.
5. Similarly, the attitude and behavior of the staff toward the student may cause distress.
6. As stated earlier, students may focus on aging relatives. A visit to parents and/or grandparents can suddenly make students aware of the aging process in their own families.
7. Deaths that occur in the agency (but outside the group) can cause grief and distress to group members and influence the mood and energy levels within the group.
8. Young students often get disheartened because of slow results or not meeting their goals (which often are set too high in the first place). Beginners have to be helped to get a more realistic view of

what they and the group can accomplish in the allotted time.

9. Ambitious students, when they do not get the grade they had hoped for in the group work experience, often get despondent.

10. Termination of the group experience and the relationship with the instructor can cause feelings of loss, especially if the student terminates both at the same time. Supervisors must be able to handle their terminations well and be able to guide students through the group termination experience. Role-modeling behavior is important here; students will tend to model their terminations with the group members in the way that classroom teachers of a group work course terminate their relationships with the students. Role modeling is still one of the most effective strategies used in group work teaching (Cohen & DeLois, 2001).

Increasing the Student's Confidence

Guiding new group leaders often requires pumping up deflated egos. Many students have low self-esteem and do not have a realistic idea of their assets and liabilities. If they have never led a group before, it takes time for them to view themselves in the role of group leader. Anxiety, lack of experience in group work, and fear of failure blend to exaggerate a new leader's trepidation. Positive rewards in the way of immediate feedback (either verbally or on written assignments) on student accomplishments seems to quickly help students.

Availability of the supervisor is also important, especially in the beginning of the group experience. The dependency needs of the new leader usually diminish rapidly if anxiety, depression, or low self-esteem are met with effective interventions by the supervisor and if sincere feedback, both constructive and corrective, is given very soon after each group meeting.

To provide effective interventions and feedback, the supervisor should attend student-led group meetings occasionally as an observer. Mastering the cast of characters, a formidable task in itself, is facilitated if the supervisor observes the group periodically or at least once. The student's written or verbal summary of the session often fails to capture the emotional flavor of the group, and ongoing audio or, preferably, videotapes are invaluable supervision aids.

Most supervisors find it helpful to observe the student leader within a group once or twice during a placement. The worth of such firsthand observation is illustrated by a student who was leading her first group and was having trouble with a man in his seventies who would interject statements with a sexual connotation that always brought the group and the leader to a sudden halt. The group was going smoothly; the residents were reminiscing; and the old man blurted out, "No matter how much you shake it, the last drop always ends up in your pants." Everything skidded to a stop, and two of the quiet, genteel women in the group stared at him incredulously, as though they were mentally playing the remark through again to make sure they had heard it right. During another meeting, an 80-year-old woman said during a lull, "You know, no man has a decent orgasm until he is 25 years old." While she startled the student leader and instructor, all the men in the group became noticeably more alert.

It seems that young students may be comfortable discussing sexuality with their peers and/or their instructor, but they can squirm noticeably when the subject of sexuality comes up in their group leadership. Sometimes they have to look at their own behavior. Are they overreacting? Are they unusually curious? Are they showing signs of disgust? Although the student wanted to change the man's behavior in the group, she failed to realize how much he kept everyone in that group on their toes. If she had convinced him to stop making such remarks, perhaps the listening and alertness of all the group members would have diminished. Students bent on changing behaviors need to understand and discuss thoroughly their rationale for wanting to achieve such changes. Moreover, the group belongs to its members, not the leader, and groups are usually well able to handle aberrant behaviors in ways acceptable to themselves.

Increasing a Leader's Knowledge Base

The preceptor must help the student to increase knowledge in two areas: the aging process and group process. Chapter 12 contains some of this necessary knowledge and gives practical suggestions regarding deficits in vision, hearing, taste, smell, and touch. Territoriality is also discussed. Chapter 11 offers detailed suggestions for creating the environment for group work with cognitively impaired older adults. There are many general group work texts concerned with group structure and process that will assist students understanding. Corey and Corey (2002), Northen and Kurland (2001), and Shulman (1999) are all recommended. Gitterman and Shulman (2004) writing on group work applications with a wide range of different people, ages, contexts and problems in living is also very relevant.

Emphasizing Individualization

Developing an appreciation of the unique characteristics of each person is as important in group work with older adults as it is with any other age group. Flexibility, consideration of individual interests, the demonstration of affection, and the reinforcement of control through the provision of a wide range of choices are all necessary aspects of group work with older people. It is important for the instructor to convey this understanding to students. Most of all, the instructor should indi-

vidualize the learning techniques with the student and provide a role model. Individualization begins at home (or in the classroom), because teachers often fail to practice with students the content they are endeavoring to teach. (See Chapter 2 for more on individual differences.)

Assisting Student Analysis

Supervisors play a critical role in assisting students to analyze and evaluate the group process in their practicum experiences. Because many refinements and changes may have to be made to the group in response to the age, abilities, disabilities, aspirations, and losses of older adults, the student needs to become sensitive to reading coded messages and metaphorical communications. This is generally true but has particular resonance when attending to the communications of people with dementia. They often communicate in two seemingly contradictory ways. They frequently speak more directly or more honestly because the thin veneer often used by younger people in which words are used to obscure meaning rather than convey meaning breaks down. People with dementia "tell it as it is." But they also often use metaphors and language more akin to poetry than the customary conventional rules of communication (Killick & Allan, 2001). It is by knowing and understanding the basics of communication and group process that the student can better understand what is the meaning of exchanges and what are the concerns of the group as a whole, and each member within it. Students also need to understand that the outcomes for groups of older persons might differ from those for groups of other ages. Students who expect unrealistic outcomes will be disappointed when they come to evaluate the outcomes of their groups.

Evaluation of the effectiveness of group work with the older adult is often concerned with global measures such as morale, life satisfaction, mental status, or ability to carry out activities of daily living. Other aspects of living are also important. These include communication skills, learning achievements, ability to relate to and assist others, resolution of past and present problems, and development of insight and the integration of troubled memories.

In order to promote positive outcomes, group leaders need to be aware of the way in which their actions affect the group. Outcomes should also be studied in relationship to the skill, expertise, attitudes, and education of the leader. Where the practice continues of allowing untrained personnel to lead groups of frail elderly people, it is essential that these leaders possess basic communication skills and some understanding of group dynamics and process. Their own attitudes about aging should also be examined as our attitudes ultimately shape our behaviors toward older individuals.

Suggested Formats for Teaching Group Work

Students provide information about group meetings to the instructor in the following ways:

- Process recordings—typed from audiotapes or by playing the audiotape to the instructor
- Logs or diaries written immediately after each meeting
- A video of the group meetings
- Critical incident analysis
- Discussion of meetings (the above methods are preferred to this)

Although there are many ways of learning to lead a group, it is useful to use structured formats when reporting group work (Kottler, 2001). The following checklist may be helpful for both supervisor and student.

1. Number of individuals in the group and availability of a sessional attendance list
2. Length of meetings
3. Number of meetings each week; duration in months
4. Days of the week meetings held
5. Number of men and women in the group (if group is not mixed, give rationale)
6. Age range
7. Disabilities that will be accepted
8. Whether confidentiality will be a ground rule stated by the leader or negotiated
9. Whether the group will have a single leader or coleaders
10. The theoretical framework(s) to be used to inform analysis, assist recording, and supervision
11. The special problems of the proposed group members, including:
    a. Attention span
    b. Communication or speech difficulties
    c. Diet regimens
    d. Ex-alcoholics
    e. Ex-drug addicts
    f. Hearing problems
    g. Impending death
    h. Incontinence
    i. Lack of social graces
    j. Loss of spouse
    k. Losses, such as economic or home
    l. Mental health problems, such as withdrawal, depression, or loneliness
    m. Physical health problems
    n. Vision problems
    o. Transportation problems
    p. Transportation issues
12. Whether support or supervision will be given and by whom
13. Arrangements for remuneration if relevant
14. Responsibilities for charting and reporting to the staff and doctor
15. Philosophy and rules of the agency that will influence the group leader and the group
16. Plans for terminating the group

17. Props, triggers, supplies, and materials that may be needed for the group
18. Payment for supplies
19. Requirements and arrangements for obtaining written consent for using recordings, photographs, and other materials obtained during the course of the group must be agreed on by students, their teachers, and agency administrators before a group commences. This must also include alternative arrangements for people who are unable to give consent because of impaired competence.

Supervisors or instructors bear the responsibility for double-checking the list to see that the items have been covered. In teaching, it is helpful if students give a rationale (and there may be several) for their choices. Giving reasons will help them think through the group experience more carefully.

If the supervisor or instructor prefers not to use tapes or process records, using the list format in Exercise 2 can expedite reporting for the student and reading by the supervisor. Agencies usually require students to write statements of goals and objectives, a task that students often find difficult. It is certainly one that makes them think very precisely about what they intend in terms of establishing and working with a group of older people. Most social work supervisory sessions are based upon written, audio, or, increasingly, video records, prepared by the student and scrutinized beforehand by the supervisor. Verbal accounts and critical reflection during supervisory sessions then augment discussion of these records.

Observation of direct practice has increased in recent years both as an educational/training tool and as a way of providing responsible accountability for professional practice. In a world of increasing bureaucratic controls, expanding private practice (over half of the members of the National Association of Social Workers, for example, are now in private employment), accountabil-

ity demands exerted by the managed care industry, and growing litigiousness, "eternal supervision" looms large. Kadushin and Harkness (2002) suggest that consultation rather than supervision offers qualified staff an effective means for safeguarding standards while preventing the erosion of professional autonomy.

Summary

This chapter deals briefly with consultation and in more detail with the tasks of supervision of group work practice. A supervisor should have a strong background in group work to be able to advise, instruct, and motivate the beginning group worker. Tasks of the supervisor include reducing students' initial anxiety, encouraging students to discuss their feelings that the group and its members arouse, and promoting their development of confidence and competence. Another responsibility is alerting them to the similarities and differences between group work with older people and group work with people of other ages. The supervisor also should advise students of the type of group they are qualified to handle and prevent them from assuming the posture of unqualified psychotherapists. In all these tasks, exercising humor and giving prompt feedback to the students are extremely important. This chapter also provides a detailed checklist to help both supervisors and new group leaders successfully prepare for and manage the group experience.

Exercises

EXERCISE 1

Draw up a chart with four columns headed Older adults, Adults in mid life, Young adults, and Adolescents. List the roles and responsibilities of a group leader working with groups comprising each age group. Identify common and specific features.

Exercise 2

Observe a group collecting accurate, meaningful data based on careful observation is important in analyzing the effectiveness of group work. Either group leaders or observers can use the following format. If you are an observer, you should keep in mind that your presence will alter the group process. You should also confer with the group leader to determine what the goals for that meeting were before you answer the questions on the list. If you are currently leading a group, thoughtfully analyze what happened. Ask your instructor or supervisor to read your answers and give you feedback. The last step is to analyze the feedback from your instructor or supervisor. Was it helpful? If so, why? If it was not helpful, consider why not.

Before the group meeting:

1. List attendance in the group.
2. Draw the seating arrangement of the group members. Describe any noticeable activity such as moving chairs, changing places, leaving the group, sitting on the periphery, and so on.
3. What was the group mood when you walked in? Were there any noticeable feelings evident in individuals? Were there any unusual events prior to the meeting, such as a death, an accident, a fire, an upset routine?

During the group meeting:

1. List the major themes and activities of the group meeting. If the mood of the group was related to the themes, explain.
2. Write one-paragraph descriptions of the mood and activities of the members and of the leader.
3. Describe one intervention that was goal directed. List the goal and the rationale for the intervention and evaluate its success.
4. Describe one verbal or nonverbal intervention that was unsatisfactory. Explain why you think it was unsatisfactory and why a correction is desirable. How could it have been handled differently?

After the meeting:

1. Did anything unusual occur immediately following the group meeting?
2. Did the participants continue their conversations as they left the meeting site.?
3. Did any participants or staff members subsequently mention any conversations or events connected with the meeting?

Future meetings:

1. List proposed future interventions and the rationale for each.
2. List questions or problems with which you think assistance is required.

Exercise 3

Get permission from a group you are leading or coleading to record a meeting on video. Then play it back to them. What are their reactions? Pretend you are a consultant, what will you recommend in future group meetings? What changes do you suggest the group leader(s) adopt and why?

Exercise 4

List the topics or themes that you regard as "taboo" in groups of older people. Why do you think this? What would assist you to feel better prepared for addressing these subjects as a group worker leading a group of older members?

References

Bernard, J. A., & Goodyear, R. K., (1998). *Fundamentals of clinical supervision* (2nd ed.). Needham Heights, MA: Allyn & Bacon.

Birnbaum, M., & Cicchetti, A. (2000). The power of purposeful sessional endings in each group encounter. *Social Work with Groups, 23*(3), 37–52.

Bradley, L., & Ladany, N. (Eds.). (2001). *Counselor supervision principles, process and practice* (3rd ed.). Philadelphia: Brunner-Routledge.

Chen, M., & Rybak, C. J. (2004). *Group leadership skills: Interpersonal process in group counseling and therapy.* Pacific Grove, CA: Brooks-Cole.

Cohen, M. B., & DeLois, K. (2001). Training in tandem: Co-facilitation and role modeling in a group work course. *Social Work with Groups,* 24(1), 21–36.

Corey, G. (2004). *Theory and practice of group counseling.* Belmont, CA: Brooks/Cole

Corey, G., & Corey, M. (2002). Groups for the elderly. In G. Corey, & M. Corey (Eds.), *Groups: Process and practice.* Pacific Grove, CA: Brooks-Cole.

Duffy, T. K. (2001). White gloves and cracked vases: How metaphors help group workers construct new perspectives and responses. *Social Work with Groups,* 24(3/4), 67–87.

Galinsky, M., & Schopler, J. (1995). Social group work competence: Our strengths and challenges. In R. Kurland, & R. Salmon (Eds.), *Group work practice in a troubled society: Problems and opportunities* (pp. 33–43). Binghamton, NY: Haworth Press.

Gibson, F. (2004). The past in the present: Using reminiscence in health and social care. Baltimore: Health Professions Press.

Gitterman, A., & Shulman, L. (Eds.). (2004). *Mutual aid groups, vulnerable populations, and the life cycle.* New York: Columbia University Press.

Kadushin, A., & Harkness, D. (2002). *Supervision in social work.* (4th ed.). New York: Columbia University Press.

Killick, J., & Allan, K. (2001). *Communication and people with dementia.* Philadelphia: Open University Press.

Kottler, J. A. (2001). *Learning group leadership: An experiential approach.* Needham Heights, MA: Allyn & Bacon.

Merriam-Webster. (2004). Merriam-Webster Online Dictionary, 11th edition, Merriam-Webster Inc. Company. Information retrieved 10/25/2004 *http://www.m-w.com/*

Northen, H., & Kurland, R. (2001). *Social work with groups.* New York: Columbia University Press.

Pollio, D. E. (2001). The evidence-based group worker. *Social Work with Groups,* 25(4), 21–35.

Proctor, D. (2000). *Group supervision: A guide to creative practice.* Thousand Oaks, CA: Sage.

Shulman, L. (1999). *The skills of helping individuals and groups.* Itasca, IL: Peacock.

Shulman, L. (2002). Learning to talk about taboo subjects: A lifelong professional challenge. In R. Kurland & A. Malekoff (Eds.), *Stories celebrating group work: It is not always easy to sit on your mouth* (pp. 139–150). Binghamton NY: Haworth Social Work Practice Press.

Chapter 31

Ethical Issues in Group Work

Jane B. Neese
Carole A. Winston

Key Words

- Ethics
- Values
- Bioethics
- Confidentiality
- HIPAA
- Informed consent
- Privacy

Learning Objectives

- List three ethical dilemmas commonly encountered in group work with older adults
- Define HIPAA and how HIPAA laws apply to group work
- Describe the relation of ethics to values and code of ethics
- Systematically analyze one ethical dilemma

This chapter focuses on ethical issues in group work and research with the aged. These issues exist in the overlap of several areas of concern, including gerontology, specialty professional practice (nursing, social work, counseling, and so on), theories governing group work, and research principles, but none of these areas alone provides sufficient guidance to the practitioner. The main focus of this chapter is on the ethical principles and the foundational values that support the principles in regard to both group treatment and implementation of research.

For both group work and research, informed consent and confidentiality are essential aspects, yet both can pose ethical dilemmas for the practitioner or researcher. According to Fehr (1999), one of the main elements in conducting an effective group is building trust based on confidentiality, which is discussed at the initial group meeting. Confidentiality and disclosure of group processes or issues are part of the initial group contract discussed prior to implementing any group. With older adults, discussion of confidentiality needs to continue not only in the first group session, but in subsequent group sessions. Likewise, informed consent in research with full disclosure of information, confidentiality, and possible anonymity requires repeated interactions to reach clarification with older adults (Levine, 2003).

Transfer this problem of confidentiality and informed consent to a geriatric setting, where some of the older adults who would benefit from participation would either be put off or unable to grasp the information being disclosed. Now, imagine that you wish to tape a group for teaching or research purposes. Some participants would be able to give consent, yet many would be unable to consent because they have conservators or guardians who would need to be contacted to provide consent. Of those older adults able to fully comprehend the informed consent, you may later contend with family members who object to their family member's participation in the group or the research study.

Values, Ethics, and Ethical Dilemmas

According to Volbrecht (2002), *ethics* is a dynamic and evolving process that involves reflection on our moral beliefs, values, and principles needed to make our society as civilized and productive as possible. Therefore, our ethical standards are grounded in our values as a society. *Values* are expressed by our beliefs and attitudes about what is important to us, whether it be a goal, an activity, a behavior, or an attribute (Volbrecht, 2002). A *principle* is a guideline from which more specific rules are derived (Haynes & Leners, 2004). *Ethical principles*, therefore, are based on "obvious moral truths" and are philosophical statements that guide behavior. An *ethical dilemma* occurs when there is a conflict between choices to uphold values, where each choice may be equally favorable or unfavorable. By definition and by the nature of ethical dilemmas, there is no one right solution (Haynes & Leners). For professional groups, ethical values and principles are developed through defining shared moral values and reaching a consensus of ethical principles within the professional organization. Both national organizations in social work and nursing have created codes of ethics, which are updated routinely by the members (Reamer, 2001).

Ethical codes are not only determined by practice area, but are also determined globally as an overview in approaching health care. In the late 1990s a multidisciplinary group composed of social workers, physicians, nurses, health care executives, academicians, ethicists, a jurist, an economist, and a philosopher met near Tavistock Square in London to discuss and ultimately prepare a statement of ethical principles (Berwick, Hiatt, Janeway, & Smith, 1997). Generally, these ethical principles were to offer guidance to all who are involved in health care and human services, including insurance agencies. The following are the seven overarching values and corresponding ethical principles (Berwick, Davidoff, Hiatt, & Smith, 2001):

- *Rights*—People have a right to health and health care.
- *Balance*—Care of individual patients is central, but the health of populations is also our concern.
- *Comprehensiveness*—In addition to treating illness, we have an obligation to ease suffering, minimize disability, prevent disease, and promote health.
- *Cooperation*—Health care succeeds only if we cooperate with those we serve, each other, and those in other sectors.
- *Improvement*—Improving health care is a serious and continuing responsibility.
- *Safety*—Do no harm.
- *Openness*—Being open, honest, and trustworthy is vital in health care.

These seven values and ethical principles are imbedded in the different professional practices.

Each professional group that engages in group work with older adults functions within their professional code of ethics developed and adopted by their respective profession. For social workers, the *Code of Ethics of the National Association of Social Workers* (National Association of Social Workers, 1999) provides the foundation of ethical principles of social work practice both at the baccalaureate and masters' level. In social work, for example, there are six shared values with corresponding ethical principles (see **Table 31–1**).

Similarly, nursing also has the *Code of Ethics for Nurses with Interpretive Statements* (American Nurses Association, 2001), which highlights cornerstone ethical principles guiding nursing practice in any nursing arena (see **Table 31–2**). Assimilating your professional code of ethics into your individual practice is paramount in any profession regardless of specialty area or population in which you practice. In many instances, an ethical dilemma arises from the conflict between the practitioner's professional code of ethics versus the decision made by an insurance company, a health care setting, or another health care or human service professional. Ethics committees are usually available for consultation in most hospital settings; however, for the individual practitioner in a private or group practice, an ethics committee is unlikely to be readily available. Therefore, networking with your professional group and reading current literature on ethical issues is important for those in solo practices.

In dealing with ethical dilemmas encountered in a hospital setting, private group practice, community setting, or in conducting research, the practitioner needs to understand that there are several ethical theories that guide how professionals view each conflict. The three most commonly used in health care and human service settings are: rule ethics, which are known more widely as the principles that guide bioethics; virtue ethics, which value moral considerations that arise in communities; and feminist ethics, which value equality and empowerment of communities (Volbrecht, 2002). Because rule ethics are the most frequently used ethical theory in health and human services, they and bioethics will be highlighted in this chapter. Bioethics comprises the following principles (Haynes & Leners, 2004):

- Beneficence—Helping others, promoting good
- Nonmaleficence—Do no harm
- Fidelity—Keeping promises, faithfulness
- Confidentiality—Respecting privacy
- Veracity—Truthfulness
- Accountability—Accepting responsibility for one's actions

In resolving an ethical dilemma, Volbrecht (2002) proposes the following framework to guide the practitioner. The first step is to identify the problem or issue and the people involved in the problem. The second step is to analyze the contextual factors which may involve political, economic, organizational, legal, or cultural aspects of the ethical dilemma. After identifying the problem and analyzing the context, the practitioner needs to explore the different possible options or solutions that are relevant to the dilemma. The fourth step is to apply your ethical

Table 31–1   Ethical Values and Principles in Social Work

1. Value: Service; Ethical principle: Social worker's primary goal is to help people in need and to address social problems.
2. Value: Social justice; Ethical principle: Social workers challenge social injustice.
3. Value: Dignity and worth of the person; Ethical principle: Social workers respect the inherent dignity and worth of the person.
4. Value: Importance of human relationships; Ethical principle: Social workers recognize the central importance of human relationships.
5. Value: Integrity; Ethical principle: Social workers behave in a trustworthy manner.
6. Value: Competence; Ethical principle: Social workers practice within their areas of competence and develop and enhance their professional expertise.

Source: National Association of Social Workers, 1999.

Table 31–2   CODE OF ETHICS FOR NURSES

1. The nurse, in all professional relationships, practices with compassion and respect for the inherent dignity, worth, and uniqueness of every individual, unrestricted by considerations, or social or economic status, personal attributes, or the nature of health problems.
2. The nurse's primary commitment is to the patient, whether an individual, family, group, or community.
3. The nurse promotes, advocates for, and strives to protect the health, safety, and rights of the patient.
4. The nurse is responsible and accountable for individual nursing practice and determines the appropriate delegation of tasks consistent with the nurse's obligation to provide optimum patient care.
5. The nurse owes the same duties to self as to others, including responsibility to preserve integrity and safety, to maintain competence, and to continue personal and professional growth.
6. The nurse participates in establishing, maintaining, and improving health care environments and conditions of employment conducive to the provision of quality health care and consistent with the values of the profession through individual and collective action.
7. The nurse participates in advancement of the profession through contributions to practice, education, administration, and knowledge development.
8. The nurse collaborates with other health professionals and the public in promoting community, national, and international efforts to meet health needs.
9. The profession of nursing, as represented by associations and their members, is responsible for articulating nursing values, for maintaining the integrity of the profession and its practice, and for shaping social policy.

Source: American Nurses Association, 2001.

decision process (i.e., bioethics, virtue ethics, feminist ethics, or your professional code of ethics). Finally, implement your plan and evaluate the outcomes (Volbrecht, 2002). Were you able to uphold your code of ethics? Did the plan support the desired results of promoting good and protecting the individual's privacy? Were you able to be truthful in discussing aspects of informed consent?

The Volbrecht framework provides a good model for analyzing ethical issues in group work, although the practitioner does need to recognize their code of ethics as well as the ethical theory that guides their practice. When applying this framework in a gerontologic context, the group leader should take into account not only the individual's ability to decide but also what he or she knows. There is a tendency to assume that everything that has been said has been heard, understood, and that all 80-year-old vocabularies have been updated. For example, when discussing the

group rules, the group leader may assume that the 80-year-old comprehends what the rules mean, when in actuality, the 80-year-old has heard but does not understand how the rules apply in the group setting. One of the benefits of Volbrecht's model is the ability to use the model with different sets of ethical theories and principles. If a practitioner espouses feminist ethics instead of bioethics, Volbrecht's model can still be used. In any ethical dilemma, outcomes and consequences of interventions should always be evaluated to find out whether or not individual's practices or a profession's principles need to be revised.

Each group develops its own rules and creates its own moral climate, but the leader plays a crucial role, and the group's norms must be ones he or she can live with. (This is not to say that the leader may not wince when a cantankerous member snarls at an intruder who seeks to join the group, "Get out! You don't belong here!") The good leader respects the strength of participants and refrains from rescuing needlessly, but the good leader also provides a floor of safety for all within the group.

Common kinds of ethical dilemmas that may arise for leaders are discussed in the following sections.

Leaders' duty to the group versus their duty to the individual. When the life of the group itself is at risk, the leader first preserves the group but then attends to the needs of the individual, with individual treatment if necessary. There are persons who are toxic to a group and, unrestrained, they may disrupt it beyond the members' power of restoration. This is especially possible when the disruptive individuals have paranoid ideation or when brain injury takes away their brakes, when their perseveration, agitation, or regression is simply more than the group can stand. Leaders will find these situations easier to deal with if they recall that any person with an unremitting need to break up a group is plainly unable to use that group in a healthy manner. The principle entailed is the good of the greatest number, but close behind it, is the worth of each individual.

Leaders' duty to provide democratic leadership versus their professional responsibility to intervene. Professional responsibility includes the duty to warn and to inform. No caring leader can be expected to stand by while the group runs off a cliff. Within reasonable bounds, groups, like individuals, have a right to learn from their own mistakes. Having sounded a few discreet caveats, the leader may wish to simply watch. Faith in the ability of all individuals to learn and to grow and trust that all persons have good motives as well as bad ones make this possible. Under extreme circumstances, however, the leader may elect to exercise her or his right to self-determination and not be a part of it. Metaphorically speaking, groups, even those whose members are in wheelchairs, can turn into lynch mobs. Such destructive behavior is ultimately destructive to the group that practices it. For example, members may turn on the confused, disoriented individuals least able to defend themselves and say, "You don't belong here!" This raises questions, of course, about the group's composition. Persons who are likely to be scapegoated within a group, should not be invited.

Leaders' obligations as employees and team members versus their duty to provide good professional services to the group. An example of this is when group leaders carefully selected members for a state hospital talking group, only to be asked by staff members if they could add an extra patient. They stepped into the room only to find eight pairs of indignant eyes fixed on the most disruptive patient on the unit. In this instance, the group leaders rose to the challenge—since the group members had to live in a dormitory with this patient—and helped members learn how they set off the very behavior they deplored. Keeping the disruptive one in the group was necessary to the treatment, but the initial byplay was between the group leaders and their staff teammates and had nothing whatever to do with the good of the group. Other situations might call for a quite different course of action. There are times to say no, but they should be carefully weighed. Sometimes the problem is not a value conflict but a poverty of solutions.

Leaders' obligation to ensure confidentiality versus their duty to protect patient welfare. This may be particularly difficult for nurses, because their code of ethics and job sanctions emphasize so strongly the duty to protect (Auton, 1999). In necessarily restrictive settings, such as prisons, conflict between confidentiality and welfare is handled by spelling out the limits of confidentiality at the very start. The leader points out that there are certain things, such as criminal activity and potential violence, which must be reported. Older adults in nursing facilities are unlikely to start a riot, but they have been known to take their own lives. A hierarchy of values does exist: an ultimate duty is to protect from grievous harm. Suicide risk must be reported. Other concerns also may properly belong in the resident's record, such as alterations in behavior or mood that may reflect untoward responses to medication or changing health status.

Most events can be charted in ways that present the participant more or less as he or she would like to be seen. You can test whether you have done so by envisioning that person reading his or her own record, as, indeed, he or she has every right to do. Nevertheless, there will be some things that belong in the chart that the person would rather you did not report. In these situations, there are two things you can do to preserve a remnant of trust: (1) report the facts but also record the client's own point of view, and (2) tell the participant that you must share your concern. The person's first intimation that you have mentioned her or his suicidal ideation should not be staff's removing scissors and razor.

More troublesome are those situations when the competence of a group member is being studied to determine whether a conservator is needed or when a decision has been made and evidence is being collected to make a case. Leaders, supplying information for these purposes, are haunted by the "don't squeal" norms of youth, and feel like betrayers. Here the course of action must be dictated by its consequences, assessed in terms of the member's ultimate need.

In conducting research with groups and with older adults, the researcher or group leader may experience several different ethical dilemmas.

Leaders' duty to the group versus their need to support research. Group leaders' duty to adhere to research protocols may be severely tested when the protocols are rigid and leaders feel locked into them. They often believe they are being forced to sacrifice some of the spontaneity, creativity, and fluidity of response they pride themselves on achieving. At the same time, if research is to move beyond anecdotal evidence, it is necessary to test theory under standardized conditions, which means, for example, that a 6-session group remains just that, no matter what crisis members are experiencing. Unfortunately, human behavior does not come in standard units, nor does distress wait outside the door. When a group member announces that she has just learned that her grandson has AIDS, she needs the group's support, not a prescheduled session on memories of life on the farm.

Researcher's duty to the older adult versus the need to protect research integrity. To maintain the integrity of the research procedures in ensuring consistency, the researcher may be confronted on whether or not to protect the consistency of the research versus to protect the safety or health of an older adult. For example, an older adult becomes seriously ill during the group session. To intervene and provide assistance to the ill older adult violates the research protocol and potentially excludes a participant from the study. On the other hand, the researcher is responsible for the safety, whether the safety issue is health or environmental, of the older adult participant.

Legal and Technical Considerations

Some decisions are taken out of the group leader's hand by overriding regulations. Laws and regulations can provide a protection, and to an impediment, or a cover. The Nursing Home Reform amendments and the Health Insurance Portability and Accountability Act (HIPAA) illustrate all three. The Nursing Home Reform amendments have benefited aged persons in residential care. They were needed because the rule of the market and the fear of litigation too often outweighed professional and personal ethics. The HIPAA law enables people to maintain health insurance coverage, but primarily has governed privacy and security of health care information.

When Congress was unable to convince the administration to protect the rights of nursing home residents, it forced the issue by outlining those rights within the law. The Nursing Home Reform amendments (OBRA '87) and the regulations derived from them deal quite directly with the rights to privacy, confidentiality, to be informed, to be free of abuse and exploitation, to receive treatment, and to refuse treatment (U.S. DHHS, 1991; Public Law 100–293, 1987). This was reinforced by the Patient Self-Determination Act (DHHS, 1992). All of this is clearly in the residents' interests.

Congress continued to struggle with privacy and security of patient-identified information as health and human services entered the computer age. Confidential patient information was being shared between health care agencies, insurance companies, and other agencies, not necessarily in the client's best interest. Not only does HIPAA address the security and privacy of health care information, but also HIPAA enables Americans to keep insurance as they change employment and limits the ability of insurance carriers to deny coverage for preexisting illnesses. HIPAA regulations, although passed in 1996, were not realized in practice until 2003. For practitioners working with older adults, HIPAA defines rules on standardizing electronic health care information and regulating the transmission of confidential information as well as guarding the security and privacy of the clients' record (Carter, Echols, & Stoll, 2004). Most Americans, whether young or old, find themselves signing privacy and confidentiality statements in any health or human service agency as well as when involved in research investigations. This is another example of how our laws regulate a professional ethical issue: confidentiality of the client.

Privacy is extraordinarily difficult to obtain even when the group is conducted in the setting for which these regulations are intended, the nursing facility or health care agency. Nursing facilities were designed less to promote privacy than to facilitate surveillance. Even settings designed for well older adults, such as senior centers and club houses in retirement communities, often lack meeting rooms with doors that shut. Nevertheless, the Nursing Home Reform amendments and HIPAA do recognize privacy as a goal.

For all the values the OBRA '87 and HIPAA regulations do support, there are times when a caring professional may experience them as an impediment. For example, when you are trying to persuade a depressed resident to join a group and she remains resolutely in her room. You cannot force her to join the group without her consent. Each time that health care information needs to be transmitted from one agency to a new agency, consent to share this information must be signed by the older adult or guardian. Any new treatment or procedure must be fully disclosed and understood by the older adult or guardian with a signed consent form.

OBRA '87 regulations also can become a cover. When the same reclusive resident firmly refuses to participate in any rehabilitative or recreational activities, staff need only to chart clearly and frequently that their persuasive attempts have failed to illicit consent to participate from the resident. Her refusal frees staff members of responsibility for her participation and deprives her of an opportunity to engage in an activity that might raise her spirits and diminish her depression. On the other hand, few group leaders would return to the 1970s when all residents were herded into treatment groups, willingly or not.

More important than any particular regulation is the shift in attitudes they compel. By giving even cognitively impaired residents the right to refuse, staff members recognize that residents are human beings with preferences and some capacity for sharing responsibility. This is liberating for all parties. In addition to laws governing privacy and security, there are laws mandating that health and human services professionals report reasonable suspicion of elder abuse. Failure to report can lead to fines, jail sentences, and loss of license for the professional. If group members in a nursing facility said that a staff member struck or otherwise verbally or physically abused a resident, the group leader would have to report this incident to the proper authorities. Reporting is a sobering process because of the penalties for the proven offender and is an expression of society's obligation to protect the frail and helpless. Nevertheless, the immediate response of colleagues and administration may be less than enthusiastic.

Considerations Relating to Age and Residential Factors

The Issue of Research

Two kinds of research are involved. First, there is the monitoring necessary to determine whether group and leader are meeting their goals. This presents no problems and, indeed, is obedient to the principles of accountability and good practice. The group leader may or may not share these findings with the group, but is under no obligation to do so. The purpose of this monitoring is to serve group members better.

The second is research intended to improve practice by examination of group outcomes. Closely related to this is using the group for teaching purposes to ensure future expertise in group leadership. Case material for the classroom and journal articles may be used freely as long as precautions are taken to protect the anonymity of participants. When audio- or videotaping is contemplated, informed consent and release of information must be secured, as required for any experimental research group. In conducting any type of research, whether it be a funded study or an innocuous survey conducted by a student, the researcher (faculty or student) must obtain permission from a human subjects committee. In large health care agencies, an internal review board (IRB) or human subjects committee is convened on a routine basis to examine all research

involving human or animal subjects. Smaller community agencies or private practices generally do not have an IRB committee available, but can request IRB committees in local hospitals or universities to review consent forms and research protocols prior to implementing a study or videotaping a group session.

If the participants are community residents in senior centers or similar settings, they usually can sign their own informed consents or release of information forms. If they are in day care or nursing facilities and impaired, the consent needed may be that of a conservator, guardian, or responsible family member. Courtesy would dictate an explanation to the resident of what the tape is for and who will see or hear it. Even when the resident has full capacity and signs on his or her own account, program directors or administrators may fear that family members will be upset. The safest course is to explain the project to those family members also and to note in the record that you have done so. The author has found that explanations to senior center administration, staff, as well as involved family members assist in generating more participation and provides opportunities for answering questions about confidentiality and privacy of identifiable information.

The Conditions of Aging

Although most aged people are healthy, active, and mentally alert, some are frail, unprotected, and functionally impaired. Persons dealing with them sometimes generalize one deficit from another, for example, assuming that those who do not hear very well do not think well either. Their very vulnerability imposes an increased responsibility on the group leader to see that all ethical standards are met.

Some very old persons who are otherwise quite alert process things more slowly. They also have bad days when things do not come as clearly: This is due to the frail body's inability to compensate for extra stress. The leader must take this into account, neither placing additional demands on them at these times nor rushing to conclusions about incapacity.

The group leader has both an opportunity and an obligation to help older persons achieve their full potential at each stage of life. Whenever possible, no one should be deprived of group services because of a lack of transportation; because of hearing or visual problems; or because of race, color, or ethnicity.

Some scapegoating in any human group seems inevitable, but no one should be scapegoated beyond bearing. The worker has an obligation to know who is brittle, to ease the entry of new members, to see that members are pleasantly challenged but not overwhelmed. Members also need to be protected against over-exposure of their own frailties, whether these are the emotional lability of the stroke patient, the aggression of the bully, or the endless whine of the chronically discontented.

Because the very old sometimes are reluctant to try new things they might enjoy, and because they fear demands on their waning energies, the group worker must gauge the difference between strong encouragement to participate and excessive pressure. This is true also of persons who are depressed. No one needs to remember this distinction between encouragement and coercion more than the group leader who is engaged in research.

Summary

Ethical violations in group work are less likely to occur because group leaders are unprincipled than because they take their own goodwill for granted and fail to examine the implications of their acts. All too often, grateful participants collude with them in what are really violations of their privacy, confidentiality, autonomy, and other values simply because group membership is so meaningful to them. The price of leadership is responsibility, and group leaders have a special obligation to be even more sensitive to participants' rights than the group members who trust them.

Exercises

EXERCISE 1

A member of your music group, Miss Brinkly, is 89 years old and hard of hearing, but you seat her right by the record player, and there is every evidence that she enjoys the group. The nursing assistants are eager to put the residents down for their naps and today, again, they have whisked Miss Brinkly off to bed. When you protest, they declare, "She can't hear anyway."

Miss Apley has little patience with people who talk when she is listening. Her command to you is curt, "If they can walk, tell them to get out. If they are in wheelchairs, push them out!" Mr. Seldon taps the time with his cane, and Miss Apley is glaring in his direction.

The following week, you arrive to find Miss Apley pacing in her wheelchair and several residents clustered outside the closed door of the meeting room. The group's meeting has been abruptly canceled: The administrator wants the room set up for the board meeting tonight. You'd like to continue this group because it's an activity the alert and the impaired can enjoy equally, but you feel your time is being wasted. You think you'll quit leading it.

Outline the ethical and value issues involved in each instance and tell what you would do.

EXERCISE 2

Mrs. Lambert comes to Wednesday group with bruises on both arms. Before group begins, you ask her what has happened. "I stumbled and bumped myself," she replies, but her roommate interposes, "Fran shook her because she was so slow." Mrs. Lambert shakes her head. "I fell," she says—although the location of the bruises makes this implausible. Fran is a nursing assistant. At this point, the group begins to gather. "Fran," begins Mrs. Pugh, hearing the name, "Fran's mean." "Yes," says Mr. Addison, "But she shouldn't argue with her." You know Fran will lose her job if you tell the director of nursing.

Describe the ethical, legal, and interpersonal issues entailed in reporting the bruises as possible evidence of resident abuse.

EXERCISE 3

Describe an ethical dilemma you have encountered in working with older persons. Analyze it using the Volbrecht's framework. First outline the ethical dilemma, the problem and the people involved in the problem. Identify the political, organizational, legal, and cultural issues surrounding the ethical dilemma. Explore all the different options or possible solutions to this ethical dilemma. Apply each solution or option to your identified ethical theoretical framework or professional code of ethics. Implement your plan and evaluate whether or not your outcomes were consistent with your ethical framework or professional code of ethics. In hindsight, how would you change the process?

References

American Nurses Association. (2001). *Code of ethics for Nurses with Interpretive Statements*. Washington, DC: Author.

Auton, L. M. (1999). Legal and regulatory issues in advanced practice nursing. In C. A. Shea, L. R. Pelletier, E. C. Poster, G. W. Stuart, & M. P. Verhey (Eds.), *Advanced practice nursing in psychiatric and mental health care* (pp. 159-184). St. Louis, MO: Mosby.

Berwick, D., Davidoff, F., Hiatt, H., & Smith, R. (2001). Refining and implementing the Tavistock principles for everybody in health care. *British Medical Journal, 323*, 616–620.

Berwick, D., Hiatt, H., Janeway, P., & Smith, R. (1997). An ethical code for everybody in health care. *British Medical Journal, 315*, 1633–634.

Carter, J., Echols, J., & Stoll, L. D. (2004). Economic aspects of health care. In L. Haynes, T. Boese, & H. Butcher (Eds.), *Nursing in contemporary society: Issues, trends, and transition to practice* (pp. 314–400). Upper Saddle River, NJ: Prentice Hall.

Fehr, S. S. (1999). *Introduction to group therapy: A practical guide*. New York: Haworth Press.

Haynes, L. C., & Leners, D. W. (2004). Professional values and ethical practice. In L. Haynes, T. Boese, & H. Butcher (Eds.), *Nursing in Contemporary Society* (pp. 106–126). Upper Saddle River, NJ: Prentice Hall.

Levine, R. J. (2003). Consent issues in human research. In E. J. Emanuel, R. A. Crouch, J. D. Arras, J. D. Moreno, & C. Grady (Eds.), *Ethical and regulatory aspects of clinical research* (pp. 321–330). Baltimore: The Johns Hopkins University Press.

National Association of Social Workers. (1999). *Code of ethics of the National Association of Social Workers*. Washington, DC: Author.

Public Health Service Amendments, U.S. Public Law 100–203. (1987).

Reamer, F. G. (2001). *Ethics in social work education*. Alexandria, VA: Council on Social Work Education.

U.S. Department of Health and Human Services (DHHS). (1991). *Federal Register, 56*(187), 48826–48879 (September 26).

U.S. Department of Health and Human Services (DHHS). *Health Care Financing Administration. 57 Fed. Reg.* 45,8194–82904 (March 6, 1992).

Volbrecht, R. M. (2002). *Nursing ethics: Communities in dialogue*. Upper Saddle River, NJ: Prentice Hall.

BIBLIOGRAPHY

Ahronheim, J. C., Moreno, J. D., & Zuckerman, C. (2000). *Ethics in clinical practice* (2nd ed.). Gaithersburg, MD: Aspen.

Davis, A. J., Aroskar, M. A., Liaschenko, J., & Drought, T. S. (1997). *Ethical dilemmas & nursing practice* (4th ed.). Stamford, CT: Appleton & Lange.

Emanuel, E. J., Crouch, R. A., Arras, J. D., Moreno, J. D., & Grady, C. (2003). *Ethical and regulatory aspects of clinical research: Reading and commentary*. Baltimore: The Johns Hopkins University Press.

Husted, G. L., & Husted, J. H. (2001). *Ethical decision making in nursing and healthcare* (3rd ed.). New York: Springer.

Resource

- The Web site found at *www.hhs.gov/ocr/hipaa/* is sponsored by the Office of Civil Rights through the Department of Health and Human Services. It offers a wide range of helpful guidance and technical assistance materials about the Privacy Rule. The OCR adds materials to this site, such as letters to health care providers highlighting educational materials and technical assistance information available at the Web site. The OCR also uses the Web site to respond to myths about the Privacy Rule to counteract the many rumors that circulate about how to implement HIPAA guidelines in practice, community, and educational settings.

Chapter 32

Cross-Cultural Issues in Group Work

E. Frederick
Anderson

Roger Delgado

Key Words

- Acculturation
- Coping
- Dignity/*dignidad*
- Familism
- Friendly conversation/*platica*
- Heterogeneity/homogeneity
- Hispanic/Latino older adults
- Institutional racism
- Jim Crow/de jure segregation
- Proverbs/sayings/methaphors/*dichos*
- Trusting in mutual trust/*confianza en confianza*
- Utilization of services

Learning Objectives

- Show how understanding the historical and contemporary experiences of older African-Americans and Hispanics can increase the effectiveness of group work with them
- Explain what respect means among African-American and Hispanic older persons, pointing out similarities and differences
- Discuss formal and informal modes of address, and explain the implications of respect and disrespect based on historical antecedents
- Describe three strategies for gaining initial rapport and recognition with Hispanic and African-American older adults
- Identify the stages of the group process in which cultural sensitivity is most crucial

The purpose of this chapter is to introduce group work strategies for direct practice with America's two largest minorities: African-Americans and Hispanics. Because both groups are complex, such an undertaking in one chapter must be succinct but informative.

The hopes, aspirations, and historical background of African-Americans and Latinos will be linked with effective approaches to working with them in groups. The authors hope that this exposure will encourage students and professionals alike to seek further information to enhance their abilities to gain rapport and work effectively with older individuals in both groups.

At the outset, it should be noted that African-Americans and Latinos are heterogeneous groupings that are often viewed monolithically in the professional literature. Failure to acknowledge intraethnic and interethnic differences seriously impairs a group worker's ability to relate to the many themes that might emerge in a diverse group of older Americans.

For the sake of clarity, each population will be discussed in turn, with attention to demographics, socioeconomic stresses, and life experiences that, together with coping styles, may affect members' responses to group work. Particular approaches will be suggested.

African-American Older Adults

Demographic Characteristics

From the statistics on infant mortality and morbidity to the statistics on longevity and old age, African-Americans are shown to be underserved and overrepresented among the impoverished and disenfranchised (National Urban League, 2004). The trends are so strong and compelling that they make it difficult for professionals who are socially distant from African-Americans to see anything in their heritage but social disorganization, chaos, and anomie. Nevertheless, blacks in the United States have exhibited remarkable resilience despite the barriers posed by unrelenting institutional racism. They have developed sources of informal support, turning first to family, church, and friends (National Urban League) and only secondarily to formal sources. Government and agencies sometimes have been quick to seize upon this intragroup self-reliance as an excuse for underservice (Estes, Biggs, & Phillipson, 2003). The extended African-American family is overstressed with multiple responsibilities and must live near elderly relatives in order to provide support (Gelfand, 2003).

African-American older adults represent a formidable population despite the pervasive and unrelenting institutional racism. Lack of access to well-paying employment has been a problem for a large number of black Americans throughout their lives and limits their income in retirement. Racial effects extend beyond income, however. Estes (2001) has reinforced an earlier observation in the previous edition of this text that poor blacks were less likely than low-income whites to have preventive medical care. It is hardly surprising that African-Americans suffer more strokes, cancer, and diabetes than whites and many of the poor outcomes are attributed to poverty and delayed care (Estes). Stanford, who deplores many black–white comparisons as suggesting that majority behavior is normative (Stanford & Yee, 1991), nevertheless concluded that the survival of so many to hardy old age was a tribute to their ability to cope (Stanford, 1992). African-Americans who reach 75 tend to outlive their white counterparts (Stoller & Gibson, 2000). This is referred to as the black–white crossover, because younger blacks are more at risk, while later their relative life expectancy increases.

The National Urban League's annual report entitled *The State of Black America: 2004* underscores the same early trends. However, the state of black America has worsened on several weighted index values in the National Urban League's annual reprise of this report. By all measures the status of Black Americans has declined in substantive areas, even though there has been begrudging progress in housing, health care, and education. The progress made is impacted by extreme retrenchment in the perception of basic and vital services as rights. In the Executive Summary of the report there is a table that is titled the "Equality Index." The Equality Index is operationalized in its preface: Assigning whites a weighted index value of 1, the Equality Index measures the disparities between blacks and whites in five key areas listed below. An index value of less than 1 means blacks are doing worse than whites in a particular category, while a value of 1 or above , means that they are doing equal or better. For example the index for total equality is .73 or 73% of their white counterparts. (See **Table 32–1**.)

Table 32–1 EQUALITY INDEX

Key area	Index value	Background and related statistics
Economics	.56	Fewer than 50% of black families own their own homes versus greater than 70% of whites
Homes	.45	Blacks are denied mortgages and home improvement loans at twice the rate of whites
Health	.25	On average, blacks are twice as likely to die from disease, accident, behavior, and homicide at every stage of life than whites; life expectancy for blacks is 72 years versus 78 years for whites
Education	.25	Teachers with less than three years experience teaching in minority schools at twice the rate that they teach in white schools
Social justice	.10	A black person's average jail sentence is six months longer than a white's for the same crime, e.g., 39 months versus 33 months
Civic engagement	1.45	Military volunteerism is 1.45, indicating that a substantially higher percentage of blacks volunteer in the military. This index score shows overrepresentation in the military by blacks relative to their percentage in the population and suggests the perception of the military as a way out of joblessness

Source: National Urban League, 2004a and 2004b.

The demographic context suggests insurmountable problems from birth to death. Yet there have been remarkable survival techniques rooted in the church, family and other social institutions that have mitigated the foreboding effects of the demographics (Day, 2002).

Historical Antecedents

John Hope Franklin's classic book entitled *From Slavery to Freedom* indicated how African-Americans were brought to the United States as chattels, and that circumstance left deep psychological and social wounds for the nation that are still in the process of healing (Franklin, 1974). Unrest in the cities suggests that those historical antecedents have resulted in institutional discrimination in jobs, education, family integrity, and myriad other areas that have only been simmering beneath the surface.

From their arrival in America, African-Americans have been tenacious in the defense of the family and their reliance on the church. Even under slavery, some black men bought their own freedom first with their extra labors and then that of their families. Those who could not buy their freedom struggled to stay together.

McAdoo (1999) said the black family has suffered three blows. With the hardships of Reconstruction, many freedmen left the South, separating themselves from the support of their extended families. A second exodus took place during the Great Depression of the 1930s, when younger adults migrated to the cities for work, sometimes leaving children and old people behind. The third blow to the black family was the social and economic disintegration that has spread through the cities since the mid-1970s. McAdoo says there was family stability on the plantation, where 75% of slave families had both parents present. She points out that in the 1940s, 82% of black families had two parents in the home. The single-parent family became a serious problem only in the late 1960s. Many black grandparents are shoring up the family by parenting their grandchildren (McAdoo).

The other pillar beside the family has been the church, which has served a multitude of functions. As slaves, African-Americans showed themselves to be ingenious in outwitting slave masters in order to achieve some solidarity. One strategy they employed was to adopt the Protestant church as a shield for religious meeting and discussion. There was little opportunity for group discussion among slaves outside the cover of the church according to the classic works by Mays and Frazier (Frazier, 1939; Mays, 1933). During Reconstruction, church membership provided many African-Americans with their first experience of property management and their first opportunities for leadership. Today, especially for the older generation, the church continues as a source of both instrumental and social support (McAdoo, 1999; Skinner, 2002).

Despite the resources of church and family, there are many continuing sources of stress. Skinner (2002) has pointed out that some areas of experience are unique to black Americans, especially history and the impact of racism, and that these must be taken into account in our explanations.

Stresses and Coping by Older Blacks

Every black American who is 60 years old today grew up during the years when segregation was enforced by both custom and law (de jure). Jim Crow regulations meant sitting at the back of the bus, separate washrooms, and living in ill-kept parts of town. Most—and all in the South—attended segregated schools. Because they were poor, they paid few taxes, which was then used as an excuse for inferior social provision. For exam-

ple, their teachers were paid less, because it was rationalized, "It costs them less to live." Under Jim Crow, there were many assaults on their dignity. Titles such as Mr. or Mrs. were never applied to blacks in the white press, and it was common for a white man, wanting service, to address a middle-aged African-American as "boy." The contrasts were very palpable and built into the very fabric of life.

The remarkable fact is that many African-Americans went to college and became physicians, lawyers, and teachers while others, less fortunate, nevertheless tilled their own land or wrested a living as tenant farmers, raised families, and formed islands of social support. Frazier's seminal work on the black family and Billingsley's follow up work in 1968 indicated that while the Caucasian family often did not welcome the aged and other kinspersons as permanent guests, the black family saw each additional member as an extra pair of hands (Billingsley, 1968; Frazier, 1939).

Today the stressors surrounding health, mental health, housing, work, transportation, and concern for younger generations continue and are mitigated to some extent by church and family networks (Gelfand, 2003). These voluntary sources cannot replace integral social services that should be universal entitlements for all elderly persons. The United States is the most reluctant welfare state among western nations. It continues to have an emergency or residual approach to social services as opposed to an institutional or primary prevention approach to social programs, including health care (Jansson, 2001).

When aged African-Americans in a mixed race group attempt to articulate their pain and the group leader, through ignorance or embarrassment, does not acknowledge it, the African-American member may simply tune out of the group or participate in a dysfunctional manner. Most black elders have developed inner radar that warns them when their interlocutors do not wish to listen to past racial slights. What these older African-Americans have to give the group is a lifetime of experience in coping, not only with racism but also with life.

During the assessment, the group leader needs to be aware of both the troubles and strengths of African-Americans to gain rapport. The leader should not bring up these issues precipitously, but if members raise them during the initial phase of the group, he or she should be prepared to acknowledge them.

Group Work Practice Techniques: Defining Goals and Establishing Rapport

Understanding the reason for the formation of a group is critical to the success of that group's endeavors. Groups in churches and senior centers may be formed for the purposes of reducing isolation, aiding the bereaved, discussing health care and other current issues, resolving problems arising from life transitions, or providing mutual support and education. A prospective leader should know that there are usually three phases associated with the formation, development, and tasks of a group that are of special importance when the participation of African-American older adults is sought.

PHASE ONE: GROUP FORMATION

It is important for the leader to be familiar with several key words as they affect African-Americans. Among these are *respect, pervasive institutional racism*, and *Jim Crow*.

Respect. In the remembered past, African-Americans were called by their first names instead of their surnames to reinforce a subordinate status. The X used by Malcolm X and many of Islamic faith is a reminder to all that the last names of African-Americans were taken from them and European names put in their place. Therefore, it is imperative that group members first address black individuals as Mr. or Mrs.

Jones instead of as Fred or Marie. Although using first names may appear friendly and informal, it may be perceived by African-Americans as disrespect. Older African-Americans do not refer to each other on a first name basis until they are given permission to do so or have known the other person for some time. It is better to start the group in a more formal manner.

Pervasive Institutional Racism. There are two forms of racism in this country: overt racism, which everyone can see, and covert racism, which is harder to identify unless you know the red flags. Group leaders who deal with the minority aged in general and with African-Americans in particular need to be aware of both kinds of racism and their implications for working with diverse groups. The process of gaining rapport entails understanding the impact of Jim Crow on the lives of older African-Americans.

Group leaders should use the beginning phase to allow themselves and the group to learn a bit more than usual about each participant. This will be an aid to planning with members the course the group is to take. Of particular importance during this phase is listening and letting the group *become* a group over several sessions.

PHASE TWO: TOPICAL DISCUSSION, INTERVENTION, OR TREATMENT

In phase two, it is important for the group leader to integrate what he or she has learned during the first phase into his or her leadership style. The key words *religion, coping behaviors, homogeneity*, and *heterogeneity* are crucial here.

Religion. Many black leaders are church trained or at least were raised in Protestant denominations. Even those who are more secular must deal with black churches (Mays, 1933). As any health care professional serving older black adults soon learns, churches can be a recruiting point and a source of infinite help. The outsider should be aware, however, that there are delicate politics and competition among them.

Many members of your small group may have strong spiritual beliefs that have helped them cope with life. Some of these beliefs may appear foreign to a generation that believes in moral relativism as opposed to moral absolutes of right and wrong. Moral relativism, a philosophy popularized by Jean Jacques Rousseau in the 18th century, posits that there are no right and wrong behaviors and that behavior is subject to the norms of a particular culture. Diametrically opposed to moral relativism is the philosophy of absolute morality or the religious notion that there is sinful behavior and nonsinful behavior. In this conservative religious frame there are no gray areas in moral conduct, only right and wrong. The leader must be prepared to accept views that may be at variance with conventional wisdom (Rousseau, 2004).

Homogeneity and Heterogeneity. While there are many general statements that may be made about older African-Americans, the most general statement that can be made is that they are not monolithic. They are quite heterogeneous in their outlook and experience. Each has overcome discrimination in his or her own manner. Therefore, the group leader should not be surprised to find that many of his or her African-American members, while appearing very liberal on certain topics, may be fiercely conservative on others. Intergroup and intragroup differences must be acknowledged in this phase to keep the group on track.

Warren in his classic work entitled *Black Neighborhoods* noted that African-American older adults who live in cities may be spatially compressed, but they are divided on the philosophy of life (Warren, 1975). The group leader should not take the opinions of one person as the gospel truth about what is transpiring in African-American communities. Keeping in mind the vantage point of the speaker and that person's social class often helps to clarify his or her statements.

Group leaders should not be surprised by African-American older adults who appear ethnocentric in their views. Ethnocentrism (group centeredness) appears in many organizations from the Sons of Norway to the Daughters of the American Revolution. Within one's own set, this "nationalism" is commonly considered group loyalty. It varies in degrees. What the group leader should do is listen carefully and observe where members of the group are on the task to be addressed and ensure that the unique needs of the group are addressed.

PHASE THREE: ENDING PHASE

Group leaders new to group dynamics often do an excellent job of initiating a group and facilitating it, but they have a hard time determining when it should be ended. When the group has achieved its goal, it should be either terminated or transformed into another entity that can provide its members new opportunities for further growth and development: it should not be continued when its purpose has been accomplished. When the group is to end, the leader must elicit from each member what it was about the group that made facilitated participation open the door to growth and change.

Hispanic Older Adults

This section focuses on the relevance of group process and group techniques for addressing the counseling needs of Hispanic older adults. Before more directly addressing the task at hand, it is useful to ascertain who the Hispanic aged are. In this chapter, the terms *Hispanic* and *Latino* are used as generic labels. It is important, however, for the reader to understand that there continues to be a lack of consensus regarding the preferability of each term. Sue and Sue (1990) use the term *Hispanic* to encompass individuals living in the United States who come or are of ancestry from Mexico, Puerto Rico, Cuba, El Salvador, the Dominican Republic, and other Latin American countries. Materials published on Hispanic older adults, to date, have primarily focused on Mexican-Americans and Puerto Ricans. The latter, as well as other specific ethnic group labels, will be used as appropriate to the group being discussed.

Demographic Characteristics

In Census 2000, 281.4 million residents were counted in the United States (excluding the Commonwealth of Puerto Rico and the U.S. island areas), of which 35.3 million (or 12.5%) were Hispanic. Mexicans represented 7.3%, Puerto Ricans 1.2%, Cubans 0.4%, and other Hispanics 3.6% of the total population (U.S. Census, 2000). Older Hispanics are the second-largest and most rapidly growing ethnic group in the United States. According to the 2000 census, there were 1,733,591 Hispanics 65 or older in the United States. Of these 58% were women and 42% were men. These older Latino adults constituted close to 5% of the Hispanic population in the United States (figures derived from the 2000 census). According to Villa and Torres-Gil (2001), while the population aged 65 and over in the United States is expected to increase 93% over the next three decades, the U.S. Latino elderly population will increase by 555%.

Sources of Stress

Older Hispanics face serious financial, health, and social problems. Hispanic older adults are substantially more likely than Americans in general to report serious financial problems. For health care practitioners, it is important to recognize that the well-being of aged Hispanics is tied closely to the underlying problems of poverty and poor health (Andrews, Lyons, & Rowland, 1992). Cubillos and Prieto (1987), in their demographic profile of Hispanic older adults, report that aged Hispanics are more likely than whites to suffer from chronic illness or disability, but are less likely to use formal long-term care services. They identify the need for the family, the government, community-based organizations, and the private

sector to work collectively to better serve the Hispanic aged.

In a telephone survey of 2,299 older Hispanics aged 65 and older (Andrews, 1989), it was found that although some Hispanic Americans have prospered, a great many still face a daily struggle, living on limited incomes and coping with poor health. In this survey, it was found that nearly three quarters of aged Hispanics have fewer than eight years of education; 4 in 10 do not speak English; and despite having worked throughout their lifetimes, their jobs offer low pay and no pension or health insurance benefits. It was further found that the most serious problems among aged Hispanics are not having enough money to live on (41%); being anxious or worried (41%); having too many medical bills (32%); and having to depend too much on others (30%).

There is a high prevalence of diabetes among Mexican-Americans 65 and over; approximately 23% report having been told by a doctor that they have diabetes compared with approximately 10% in the general population (Markides, Rudkin, Angel, & Espino, 1997). According to these authors, other diseases of high prevalence in Hispanics, including the elderly, include infectious and parasitic diseases, influenza, pneumonia, tuberculosis, and gallstone disease.

A national needs assessment study conducted by the National Association for Hispanic Elderly (Sanchez, 1992) found that older Hispanics reported mental health as their third most urgent need after general health and income. Some of the specific mental health problems cited included feelings of uselessness, dependency, and low self-worth; feelings of loneliness and isolation; problems in adjusting to U.S. culture; thoughts and fears of death; and problems in interpersonal relationships. In the same study it was recommended that programs designed to provide mental health services to ethnic minority elders consider the importance of cultural dynamics as a key to the provision of more effective services.

Vega and Alegria (2001) concluded that findings from recent studies suggested that Latinos such as Mexicans, Cubans, and Puerto Ricans generally immigrate or migrate with superior mental health status, compared to that of the total population of the United States. However, over time, Latinos experience an increased risk of mental health problems caused by the erosion of social support and traditional values. Aranda and Miranda (1997) suggested that using a social stress perspective helps to explain why older Hispanics may be at risk for developing psychological disorders as a result of migration and acculturation as well as minority group status. They add that migration is likely to disrupt attachments to supportive networks in the society of origin and to impose on the Hispanic immigrant the difficult task of incorporation into the primary groups of the host society. They go on to say that, depending on such factors as generational status and length of residency in the United States, the individual's life stresses may vary.

Utilization of Formal Human Services

One might expect that a group beset with a multitude of biopsychosocial stressors would utilize existing formal human services at a high rate. For a number of reasons, this has not been the case for older Hispanic adults. In a study that examined the use of formal helping networks (e.g., agency, counselor, psychologist, doctor, or priest) to meet the psychological needs of the Hispanic older adult (aged 55+ years), it was concluded that the Hispanic aged are in need of psychological services but underutilize them (Starrett, Todd, & Decker, 1989).

In a collection of articles about different aspects of aging in the Hispanic community, serious concern is expressed by Hispanic gerontologists because of the low-utilization rate of human and health care services by Hispanic aged (Sotomayor & Curiel, 1988). Miranda (1990)

posits that the underutilization of services by Hispanic older adults is caused by a wide range of structural barriers inherent in the service delivery system, such as the lack of cultural sensitivity in the design and delivery of services and the fragmented nature of continuing care services in the Hispanic community.

The Hispanic Family as Informal Support

While some writers believe that the extended family has been and continues to be the most important institution for Hispanics (Sotomayor & Applewhite, 1988), others posit that the weakness in the explanation that older Hispanics underutilize social services because they continue to have access to extended family support is that it does not consider the influence of urbanization on the extended family; romanticizes the reality of the barrio where families are, in actuality, poor, thereby limiting the feasibility of mutual economic support; does not acknowledge the differential responses from service providers in the dominant Anglo-American society to minority communities; and, lets service providers off the hook for providing needed services to Mexican-American elders (Krajewski-Jaime, 1990).

Although there are, in fact, many positive aspects to the expressive and instrumental support received by Hispanic elders from the family as a social support system when it is available, Arevalo (1989) points out that in many instances, Latino families have become acculturated and nuclear and do not feel that they should support their oldest members. Markides and Krause (1986), in a study of intergenerational support for older Mexican-Americans in a three-generation sample of 1,125 respondents, found that while older Mexican-Americans were often engaged in strong helping networks with their children, not all intergenerational support exchanges were beneficial, as dependency often resulted in psychological distress.

Cox and Monk (1990), in their examination of experiences and support networks of black and Hispanic caregivers of family members with dementia, found that both formal and informal support networks were used interchangeably. However, they also found an increased use of formal supports when available, followed by a decreased use of informal supports such as family. Aranda and Miranda (1997) posit that the social supports of the Hispanic elderly as we see them today are the result of a combination of sociodemographic, sociohistorical, and ethnic change and health status variables that are complexly related to one another. The notion that acculturation may have a direct influence on mental health, as well as an indirect effect through social support, is in need of further examination.

Group Work with Older Hispanics

Burnside (1994) has stated that group work is one form of treatment that is effective with older adults and that it should be considered in prevention and maintenance aspects of the health care of older persons. However, as with other counseling services that only recently have been made available to Hispanic elders, the use of group work is a novel experience. A review of the literature on the use of group work, group therapy, and self-help groups with Hispanic elders reveals modest but encouraging efforts. Acosta and Yamamoto (1984), in their examination of the utility of group work practice for Hispanic Americans, particularly those who are primarily unacculturated and monolingual Spanish-speaking, found that the consideration of cultural factors in conducting group work is crucial for maximizing effectiveness along with the use of behavioral and experiential approaches. Miranda (1991), in an exploration of mental health status among Hispanic older adults and avenues for improving mental health services to this population, advocates the use of natural support networks or self-help groups.

Mayers and Souflee (1990–1991), in their discussion of two approaches that can be used by social service providers to link and strengthen the social support system of aging Mexican-Americans, recommended the use of mutual aid, self-help, and informal network strategies. The model proposed delineates the various roles that human service professionals can play in Mexican-American support groups. Sanchez (1992), in a review of mental health issues affecting the aged Hispanic population, also recommended the use of lay groups and informal support networks within the community.

In summary, there is a dearth of written documentation regarding the use of group work and group therapy with Hispanic elders. Thus, the practitioner with an interest and need to provide such services may be quite unclear about how to develop and provide effective services to Hispanic older adults within the context of a group. The following section attempts to provide the reader with a selective review of issues that may be considered in efforts to provide group work or group therapy to older Hispanics. It is assumed that the worker is already familiar with basic principles, processes, and techniques of group work or group therapy.

Culturally Relevant Issues

In recent years, there has been increased attention to cultural factors in the delivery of mental health services to ethnically diverse populations. What is still lacking, however, is material that addresses strategies for counseling specific ethnic groups. In the case of Hispanic older adults, such a need is especially acute. One of the ongoing challenges to the development of practice-related materials for working with Hispanics is the latter group's intergroup/intragroup heterogeneity and cultural diversity; thus, recommendations made here must be considered within such a cultural milieu.

Given the ethnic diversity of Latino elders, it is difficult to present a how-to approach for providing social group work to older adults of Mexican-American, Puerto Rican, Cuban, and other Latino ethnic backgrounds. The effort here is, therefore, to provide the reader with a selective list of potentially relevant issues for consideration and possible exploration when providing group work services to Latino elders.

Historical Experiences

In addressing the aging process in general and the effects of minority experiences on aging, Moore (1971) postulated that each minority group has a special history; the special history has been accompanied by discrimination; a subculture has developed; coping structures have developed; and rapid change is occurring. Woodruff and Birren (1983) pointed out that the historical memory of each group has been unique. Conquest, prolonged conflict, and annexation are antecedents linking the history of the Native Americans and Mexicans; dehumanizing enslavement and its special institutional forms in America are unique to blacks; varied immigration and migration patterns of the Asian and Hispanic peoples have resulted in a cycle of recruitment, exploitation, and exclusion. Suffice it to say, it is important for human services professionals to explore with Hispanic aged clients any long-term significance of cumulative historical experiences as it relates to their ability and willingness to use services, especially when rendered by nonminority service providers.

Level of Acculturation

Acculturation is a complex interactional process involving both members of the cultural group undergoing change and members of the host culture. In a model proposed by Mendoza and Martinez (1981), it was suggested that efforts to understand sociocultural adjustment consider four propositions:

1. There are different patterns of acculturation:
   a. cultural resistance, defined as an active or passive resistance to alternate cultural norms, while maintaining native customs
   b. cultural shift, defined as a substitution of native customs with alternate cultural norms
   c. cultural incorporation, defined as an adaptation of customs from both native and alternative cultures
   d. cultural transmutation, defined as an alteration of native and alternate cultural practices to create a unique subcultural entity.
2. Acculturation is multidimensional and therefore not a construct that can be analyzed by a single measurement or necessarily generalized from a cluster of correlated variables.
3. Many acculturating individuals are multifaceted.
4. As a dynamic process, acculturation reflects not only changes that occur as a function of time and exposure to an alternate culture but also reflects changes that are dictated by contextual factors.

Valle (1980), in a discussion of guidelines for cross-cultural curriculum design, presents an acculturation continuum that posits traditional (reflecting values, norms, language, customs of the culture of origin), bicultural (reflecting incorporation of both ranges), and assimilated (reflecting values, norms, and so forth, of the host society) levels of acculturation. Cuellar, Harris, and Jasso (1980), in efforts to conceptualize and operationalize level of acculturation, have developed an Acculturation Rating Scale for Mexican-Americans (ARSMA). The scale is able to differentiate five distinct types of Mexican-Americans based on level of acculturation: very Mexican, Mexican-oriented bicultural, true bicultural, Anglo-oriented bicultural, and very anglicized. The measurement of acculturation on ARSMA is based on the dimensions of language familiarity and usage, ethnic interaction, ethnic pride and identity, cultural heritage, and generational proximity.

When assessing the consequences of acculturation for older adults, it is important to look at both the positives and negatives. For example, Markides et al. (1997) point out that acculturation has been shown to be associated with risk factors for chronic disease such as hypertension, but as a positive influence for both diabetes and obesity.

Applewhite and Daley (1988) assert that human service professionals need to be aware of the rich diversity of peoples within the Hispanic aged population. They further add that professionals need to locate or position individuals and groups they seek to serve within this broad Hispanic elderly population. Specific individuals and groups may to a large degree share many characteristics, life experiences, needs, and aspirations with other Hispanic elderly. At the same time, each individual and group will have unique "common sense knowledge" and distinct perspectives that must be considered if the professional is to fully understand the manner in which Hispanic elderly define, constitute, and order reality.

Some Suggestions for Working with Latino Older Adults

Counselors and other mental health professionals who work with Latino clients are strongly urged to recognize that many psychological and social factors within their culture influence the efficacy of the counseling experience. Level of acculturation determines the use of bilingual-bicultural or monolingual-monocultural group work interventions with Latinos. However, with Latino older adults, especially those who have not yet become highly acculturated, there are several cultural areas that need to be considered and addressed throughout the various stages of the helping process (i.e., establishing the relationship, problem identification and assessment, facilitating therapeutic change, evaluation, and termination). Because most clients who terminate counseling prematurely do so within the initial sessions, the primary focus of the present discussion is on suggestions for establishing the relationship.

PRELIMINARY TASKS

Because most older Latinos have not been through the experience of individual or group counseling, it is important for the worker to:

1. Give a brief description of the purpose and objectives of the group
2. Explore the client's expectations and the reason for participation in the group
3. Clarify and resolve any existing conflict in purpose and expectations to enhance therapeutic goodness of fit
4. Discuss the principle of confidentiality as related to group process and content
5. Assess the existence of both intrapsychic and extrapsychic factors in the client's biopsychosocial problem situation
6. Determine the need for the possible utilization of other support systems, both formal and informal
7. Discuss with the client the need for the use of specific interventions and projected duration of the intended social group work experience

RESPETO (RESPECT)

Due to cultural socialization experiences, older Latinos expect to be treated with respect by all, but especially by younger human service professionals. This gives rise to one of the reasons why special care must be exercised in how the older client is addressed (i.e., with respect, as in Señor Garcia/Mr. Garcia; Señora Lopez/Mrs. Lopez). Correct pronunciation of the client's name is also important; needless to say, the ongoing mispronunciation of a client's name by the worker can be counterproductive to the establishment of client—worker rapport.

DIGNIDAD (DIGNITY)

Associated with *respeto* is the older individual Latino's belief that what makes a person good and respected is an inner dignity (*dignidad*). Thus, the worker who is able to acknowledge and show respect for the client's *dignidad* through both verbal and nonverbal actions is able to help reduce initial client resistance while also establishing trust and personal and professional credibility. Such rapport is especially essential since for some Latino older adults, the seeking of psychological–emotional support outside the family may seem tantamount to being disloyal and dishonoring the family's pride and dignity.

VERGUENZA (SHAME)

Latino elders may be especially vulnerable to experiencing *verguenza* or shame when they are compelled, even by extenuating circumstances, to resort to the use of professional counseling services for personal problems and/or when the family support system is unable, unwilling, or unavailable to serve as the helping resource. The discussion of personal problems within a therapeutic group context may, initially, give rise to the experiencing of *verguenza* by the older Latino at both the individual and the family level.

CONFIANZA EN CONFIANZA (TRUSTING IN MUTUAL TRUST)

Velez (1980) posits that *confianza en confianza* (trusting in mutual trust), a term that denotes mutualistic generosity, intimacy, and personal investment in self and others, may be used by the helping professional as a resource for reducing resistance and building the client–worker relationship.

PLATICA (FRIENDLY CONVERSATION)

One of the strategies recommended for facilitating communication with Hispanic Americans is the use of *platica* (social conversation), especially during the initial phase of an interview (Valle, 1980). Such helper-initiated conversation can be used to enhance the expressive, and eventually the instrumental, aspects of the helping relationship. It may be particularly useful for *platica* to be personalized so that it relates to recent or current events and activities that might be of interest or relevant to both the client and the worker. In addition to serving as a warm-up for a group session, the use of platica can also communicate to the client that he or she is still a person. *Platica* can be useful even though the worker will not be able to engage every member of the group during any given group session. Engaging group members in *platica* also presents the group leader as a socially gracious host, something that has special meaning in Latino culture.

USE OF *DICHOS/REFRANES* (PROVERBS/SAYINGS)

Zuniga (1992) and Falcov (1998) suggested that the appropriate and timely use of *dichos* (culturally relevant folk sayings) can be a very useful way of facilitating communication in counseling. Zuniga suggested that the use of *dichos* that exist in Mexican-American and other Latino cultures offers the clinician culturally viable tools for mitigating resistance, enhancing motivation, reframing problems, and for providing a therapeutic ambience that contributes to culturally sensitive treatment. Aviera (1996), who has conducted numerous *dichos* groups at Metropolitan State Hospital with Spanish-speaking men and women, ages 18 to 65, with diverse psychiatric conditions, stated that the use of culturally relevant *dichos* effectively facilitates building rapport, decreases defensiveness, enhances motivation and participation in therapy, improves self-esteem, helps to focus attention, stimulates emotional exploration and articulation of feelings, helps develop insight, and assists in the exploration of cultural values and identity. Examples of *dichos* utilized by Aviera include: "*Caras vemos, corazones no sabemos*" (Faces we see, but [what is in] hearts we don't know), and "*Mas vale tarde que nuca*" (Better late than never). Aviera recommended that the selection of dichos be related to the client's level of acculturation. One of several mottos used by Aviera for the *dichos* groups was "*Dichos son el juicio de su gente*" (Dichos are the wisdom of your people).

Familism Within the Group

One of the major themes associated with Latinos is the importance of the family, both nuclear and extended (when available), as a valuable source of emotional support. One of the desirable outcomes of a group is that it functions as a system for mutual aid. Schwartz (1961) defined a *social work group* as "An enterprise in mutual aid, an alliance of individuals who need each other, in varying degrees, to work on certain common problems. The important fact is that this is a helping system in which the clients need each other as well as the worker" (p. 19). It is conceivable that for Latino older adults, a well-functioning group, such as the one in **Figure 32–1**, may come to represent something akin to a surrogate family. Thus, in this sense, prior positive cultural socialization experiences with the family group as a valuable resource may enhance the older Latino client's ability to benefit from participation in a social work group. Among the curative factors in groups that Yalom (1985) identifies, one, altruism, would seem to have special relevance to the Latino elderly.

Summary

The use of social group work with minority elders can be a method for quality service delivery. Admittedly, there are many different types of groups and settings for practice. However, regardless of the type of group, setting, or background of the service provider, it is imperative that the history of aged minority clients be acknowledged and explored as appropriate. It is also recommended that group facilitators make a sensitive and concerted effort to explore, understand, and utilize the cultural strengths of minority older adults.

Although it often is tempting to place people into categories, it is critical for human service providers to understand that there is a great deal of cultural diversity within and among groups of minority elders. Thus, while generalizations are helpful, the group worker still must determine the individual preferences of each member. Therapeutic strategies recommended in this chapter may be applicable to some African-American and some Hispanic older adults but not to others and certainly not to all minorities, although certain concerns, such as the desire for respect, are common to all (see Figure 32–1). Because there continues to be a dearth of empirical data and literature on how to serve older minority adults, the group leader's own cultural

Figure 32–1

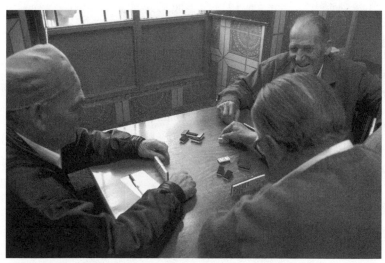

©Gary Conner/PhotoEdit

Like African-American and Hispanic elders, and many other older adults, these older adults may consider group informality, like using first names, as disrespectful.

sensitivity and willingness to learn are important. As a final point, the importance of enhancing the multilevel empowerment of older minority clients at the individual, family, group, and broader levels cannot be overemphasized.

Exercises

EXERCISE 1

In a small group of four to seven participants, discuss the statement, "We are all human, and we all have some uniquenesses and differences. But being human, we have a lot in common." What are some of the differences and similarities among the people in your small group as reflected by ethnicity or race?

EXERCISE 2

In a small group, discuss what you think you know about African-American and Hispanic elders; conversely, discuss with members of your small group any gaps in your knowledge and how you might be able to acquire knowledge and skills for enhancing the provision of group work services to African-American and Hispanic older adults.

EXERCISE 3

Conduct an interview with a minority elder and explore areas of life satisfaction as well as past and current sources of psychosocial stress. How does the interviewee cope with stress (i.e., personal, informal, and formal resources used)? What types of services are needed to resolve the major stressors being experienced by your interviewee?

EXERCISE 4

In a small group of five to eight people, discuss the meaning of a variety of generic and culturally specific *dichos*/proverbs. The purpose for this exercise is to facilitate discussion, compare and contrast the meanings of *dichos*/proverbs, and enhance cultural understanding and sensitivity. It is recommended that the facilitator have a source book of *dichos*/proverbs to use as an initial baseline of information.

References

Acosta, F. X., & Yamamoto, J. (1984). The utility of group work practice for Hispanic Americans: Ethnicity in social group work practice [Special issue]. *Social Work with Groups, 7*(3), 63–73.

Andrews, J. W. (1989). *Poverty and poor health among elderly Hispanic Americans*. Baltimore: Commonwealth Fund Commission on Elderly People Living Alone.

Andrews, J. W., Lyons, B., & Rowland, D. (1992). Life satisfaction and peace of mind: A comparative analysis of elderly Hispanic and other elderly Americans. *Clinical Gerontology, 11*(3/4), 21–42.

Applewhite, S. R., & Daley, J. M. (1988). Cross-cultural understanding for social work practice with the Hispanic elderly. In S. R Applewhite (Ed.), *Hispanic elderly in transition: Theory, research, policy, and practice* (pp. 3–16). New York: Greenwood.

Aranda, M. P., & Miranda, M. R. (1997). Hispanic aging, social support, and mental health. In K. S. Markides, & M. R. Miranda (Eds.), *Minorities, aging and health* (pp. 271–294). Thousand Oaks, CA: Sage.

Arevalo, R. (1989). The Latino elderly: Visions of the future. In R. Arevalo & R. Delgado (Eds.) [Special issue].*California Sociologist: Journal of Sociology and Social Work, 12*(1),1–7.

Aviera, A. (1996). "Dichos" therapy: A therapeutic use of Spanish language proverbs with hospitalized Spanish-speaking psychiatric patients. *Cultural Diversity and Mental Health, 2*(2), 73–87.

Billingsley, A. (1968). *Black families in white America*. Englewood Cliffs, NJ: Prentice-Hall.

Burnside, I. (1994). Education and preparation for group work (pp. 65–74). In I. Burnside & M. C. Schmidt (Eds.), *Working with older adults: Group process and techniques* (3rd ed.). Boston: Jones & Bartlett.

Cox, C., & Monk A. (1990). Minority caregivers of dementia victims: A comparison of black and Hispanic families. *Journal of Applied Gerontology, 9*(3), 340–354.

Cubillos, H. L., & Prieto, M. M. (1987). *Hispanic elderly: A demographic profile*. Washington, DC: National Council of La Raza, Policy Analysis Center.

Cuellar, J. B., Harris, L. C., & Jasso, R. (1980). An acculturation scale for Mexican-American normal and clinical populations. *Hispanic Journal of Behavioral Science, 2*(3),199–218.

Day, K. (2002). *Prelude to struggle: African-American clergy and community organizing for economic development in the 1990's*. Lanham, MD: University Press of America.

Estes, C. L. (2001). *Social policy and aging: A critical perspective*. Thousand Oaks, CA: Sage.

Estes, C. L., Biggs, S., & Phillipson, C. (2003). *Social theory, social policy and ageing*. Philadelphia: Open University Press.

Falicov, C. J. (1998). *Latino families in therapy: A guide to multicultural practice*. New York: Guilford Press.

Franklin, J. H. (1974). *From slavery to freedom: A history of the Negro*. New York: Knopf.

Frazier, E. F. (1939). *The Negro family in the United States*. Chicago: University of Chicago Press.

Gelfand, D. E. (2003). *Aging and ethnicity: Knowledge and services*. New York: Springer.

Jansson, B. S. (2003). *The reluctant welfare state: American welfare policies—past, present, and future*. Belmont, CA: Brooks/Cole/Thompson Learning

Krajewski-Jaime, E. R. (Ed.). (1990). *Empowering Mexican-American elderly. An ecological model to plan culturally sensitive services* [Special issue]. Monograph Series (2). East Lansing: Geriatric Education Center of Michigan, Eastern Michigan University.

Markides, K. S., & Krause, N. (1986). Older Mexican Americans. *Generations, 10*(4), 31–34.

Markides, K. S., Rudkin, L., Angel, R. J., & Espino, D. V. (1997). Health status of Hispanic elderly. In L. G. Martin & B. J. Soldo (Eds.), *Racial and ethnic differences in the health of older Americans* (pp. 285–300). Washington, DC: National Academy of Sciences.

Mayers, R. S., & Souflee, F. (1990–91). Utilizing social support systems in the delivery of social services to Mexican-American elderly. (Applications of social support and social network interventions in direct practice) [Special issue]. *Journal of Applied Social Science, 15*(1), 31–50.

Mays, B. E. (1933). *The Negro's church*. New York: Russells.

McAdoo, H. P. et al. (Eds.). (1987). Blacks. In A. Minahan, *Encyclopedia of social work* (18th ed., pp. 194–206). Silver Spring, MD: National Association of Social Workers.

McAdoo, H. P. (Ed.). (1999). *Family ethnicity: Strength in diversity*. Thousand Oaks, CA: Sage.

Mendoza, R. H., & Martinez, J. L. (1981). The measurement of acculturation. In A. Baron, Jr. (Ed.), *Explorations in Chicano psychology* (pp. 71–82). New York: Holt.

Miranda, M. (1990). Hispanic aging: An overview of issues and policy implications. (In U.S. DHHS Publication. HRS-P-DV 90-4). *Minority aging: Essential curricula content for selected health and allied health professions* (pp. 609–622). Washington, DC.

Miranda, M. (1991). Mental health services and the Hispanic elderly. In M. Sotomayor (Ed.), *Empowering Hispanic families* (pp. 141–154). Milwaukee, WI: Family Service of America.

Moore, J.W. (1971). Situational factors affecting minority aging. *The Gerontologist, 11*(1), 88–93.

National Urban League (2004). The state of black America. [Executive summary]. Washington, DC: National Urban League. *http://www.nul.org/pdf/sobaexec.pdf*

National Urban League. (2004). The state of black America. [Abstract]. Washington, DC: National Urban League. *http://www.nul.org/pdf/sobaastract.pdf*

Rousseau, Jean-Jacques. (2004). Retrieved from *http://www.en.wikipedia.org/wiki/Moral_relativism*

Sanchez, C. D. (1992). Mental health issues: The elderly Hispanic. *Journal of Geriatric Psychiatry, 25*(1), 69–84.

Schwartz, W. (1961). *The social worker in the group. New perspectives on services to groups: Theory, organization, and practice* (pp. 7–34). New York: National Association of Social Workers.

Skinner, J. (2002). *Multicultural measurement in older populations.* New York: Springer

Sotomayor, M., & Applewhite, S. R. (1988). The Hispanic family and the extended multi-generational family. In S. R. Applewhite (Ed.), *Hispanic elderly in transition: Theory, research, policy, and practice* (pp. 121–133). New York: Greenwood.

Stoller, E. P., & Gibson, R. C. (2000). *Worlds of difference: Inequality in the aging experience* (3rd ed). Thousand Oaks, CA: Pine Forge Press (Sage).

Sotomayor, M., & Curiel, H. (Eds.). (1988). *Hispanic elderly: A cultural signature*. Edinburg, TX: Pan American University Press.

Stanford, E. P. (1992). *Beyond the graying of America: Who cares?* San Diego, CA: San Diego State University Press.

Stanford, E. P, & Yee, D.L. (1991). Gerontology and the relevance of diversity. *Generations 15*(4), 11–14.

Starrett, R. A., Todd, A. M., & Decker, J. T. (1989). The use of formal helping networks to meet the psychological needs of the Hispanic elderly. *Hispanic Journal of Behavioral Science, 11*(3), 259–273.

Sue, D. W., & Sue, D. (1990). *Counseling the culturally different: Theory and practice*. New York: Wiley.

U.S. Bureau of the Census. (2000). *The Hispanic population: Census 2000 brief*. Washington, DC: U.S. Government Printing Office.

U.S. Department of Human Health Services. (1990). *Minority aging: Essential curricula content for selected health and allied health professions* (pp. 433–452). (DHHS No. HRS-P-DV 90-4). Washington, DC.

Valle, R. (1980). Social mapping techniques. A preliminary guide for locating and linking to natural networks. In R. Valle & W. Vega (Eds.), *Hispanic natural support systems* (pp. 113–121). Sacramento, CA: State of California Department of Mental Health.

Vega, W. A., & Alegria, M. (2001). Latino mental health and treatment in the United States. In M. Aguirre-Molina, C. W. Molina & R. E. Zambrano (Eds.), *Health issues in the Latino Community* (pp. 179–208). San Francisco, CA: John Wiley & Sons.

Velez, C. G. (1980). Mexicano/Hispanic support systems and confianza: Theoretical issues of cultural adaptation. In R. Valle & W. Vega (Eds.), *Hispanic natural support systems* (pp. 45–54). Sacramento, CA: State of California Department of Mental Health.

Villa, V. M., & Torres-Gil, F. M. (2001). The later years: The health of elderly Latinos. In M. Aguirre-Molina, C. W. Molina & R. E. Zambrano (Eds.), *Health issues in the Latino community* (157–178). San Francisco: John Wiley and Sons.

Warren, D. (1975). *Black neighborhoods: An assessment of community power.* Ann Arbor, MI: University of Michigan Press.

Woodruff, D. S., & Birren, J. E. (1983). *Aging: Scientific perspective and social issues.* Pacific Grove, CA: Brooks/Cole.

Yalom, I. D. (1985). *The theory and practice of group psychotherapy* (3rd ed.). New York: Basic Books.

Zuniga, M. E. (1992). Using metaphors in therapy: Dichos and Latino clients. *Social Work, 37*(1), 55–61.

BIBLIOGRAPHY

Applewhite, S. R (Ed.). (1988). *Hispanic elderly in transition: Theory, research, policy, and practice.* New York: Greenwood.

Barresi, C. M., & Stull, D. (Eds.). (1993). *Ethnic elderly and long-term care.* New York: Springer.

Falicov, J. C. (1998). *Latino families in therapy: A guide to multicultural practice.* New York: Guilford Press.

Markides, K. S., & Mindel, C. H. (1987). *Aging and ethnicity.* Newbury Park, CA: Sage.

Markides, K. S., Rudkin, L., Angel, R. J., & Espino, D. V. (1997). Health status of Hispanic elderly. In L. G. Martin, & B. J. Soldo (Eds.), *Racial and ethnic differences in the health of older Americans.* Washington, DC: National Academy of Sciences.

Chapter 33

Research Issues in Group Work

Barbara Haight

Key Words

- Data collection
- Informed consent
- Team model
- Practitioner-researcher model
- Process recording
- Record of service
- Sample
- Standardized research scales
- Summary recording

Learning Objectives

- Identify two reasons for research into group services
- List and describe two common recording or data collection methods
- Develop two hypotheses (questions) relevant to your work with a group
- Evaluate the process of a group session based on the records of service and summaries of recordings

The Issue of Research

Some authors believe that research is not the domain of people practicing group work while others believe research is necessary (Burnside & Schmidt, 1994). If one is treating patients, then knowing the outcome effect of the treatment is not only necessary, it is mandatory. We would not take or prescribe medicine without knowing that the medicine was effective for the identified illness. So why would we do less for psychosocial interventions such as groups? Why would we continue with group interventions if we don't even know that they work? We are not only wasting our time, we are wasting the time of the participants who come to a group. The idea of not evaluating group process and outcomes through research is unethical. Without research, we don't know what we're doing or why we are doing it.

Thus, we come to this chapter with the notion that research informs practice and practice informs research. The whole job of practice and research may be too burdensome for one person but it is an ideal project for a team composed of a researcher and a practitioner. In a national Delphi study, Burnette, Morrow-Howell, and Chen (2003) ranked priorities for gerontological research in social work. Intervention research received the highest priority rating. Specifically, 83% of the social workers voted for developing and testing psychosocial interventions across specific populations and conditions. Nurses concur that nursing research is interdependent with nursing practice, like the strands of a double helix (Grady, 2002).

A wealth of knowledge exists naturally within the rich, dynamic world of practice. The creation of knowledge need not rest within the exclusive domain of professional researchers, but can become part of the daily routine of practice. To create knowledge, practitioners should continually assess their own practice and become active researchers, not merely consumers of research. With practice experience and a careful monitoring of practice approaches, group services can improve and become more effective. However, randomized clinical trials remain the accepted standard for testing health care interventions (Dunbar-Jacob & Schron, 2002) and such trials should be used more frequently.

In addition to accepting groups as therapeutic, practitioners should pay attention to the systematic evaluation of group outcomes. Evaluation is the process of obtaining information about the end product of a program or process (Miller, 1991). Program evaluation is a specific domain of research that is goal or outcome oriented and designed to ascertain whether one achieved service objectives. (See chapter 34.) The following practitioner–researcher model guided the thinking of many group workers in the past. Thus, this chapter presents the practitioner–researcher model, along with the concept of a team approach.

Practitioner–Researcher Model

Practitioners generally consider research and practice as two separate endeavors without sharing a common base or framework. However practice and research do share a similar intellectual orientation, which has been identified as either the problem-solving process or the nursing process (Stanley & Beare, 1999). When practitioners approach a problem, they engage in an assessment/intervention process that includes the following steps:

1. Identifying the problem
2. Collecting relevant information
3. Interpreting the information
4. Understanding the problem
5. Formulating the problem's cause
6. Selecting, implementing, and evaluating an appropriate intervention

The problem-solving process used by researchers is analogous to the one used by practitioners and involves:

1. Identifying the problem
2. Reviewing the literature
3. Developing a hypothesis
4. Selecting a research design
5. Collecting data
6. Analyzing data
7. Making conclusions
8. Disseminating results
9. Applying to practice (Burns & Grove, 2001)

In general, the above listing takes a broad view of research and proposes that knowledge for practice can be generated through a systematic review of the practitioner's usual activities. Such knowledge-building activities need not be costly, need not rely on complex research methodologies, and should not deprive clients of needed services.

Group Practice

Group work practitioners need to become familiar with the practitioner–researcher model in order to contribute to the growth of group work practice. Group practice evaluation can contribute to knowledge of process and outcome. Evaluation also can be used to obtain information needed to plan groups, monitor group membership, develop new groups, and test for service effectiveness (Miller, 1991). Practitioners wish to understand, for example, why members do or do not attend group meetings, under what conditions interventions succeed or fail, and whether service goals and objectives are achieved. Evaluation of practice can illuminate the usefulness of specific group modalities, improve skills, and enable group workers to share their knowledge with others doing similar work.

Before starting to collect data, practitioners should decide the specific focus of the evaluation and decide what information is needed to answer the questions identified by the practitioner. Theoretical concepts need to be clearly defined and stated in terms that can be measured. For example, the practitioner should clearly define outcomes and establish criteria to measure effective service. In other words, what is a successful or unsuccessful intervention? What standard will be used to ascertain whether clients' mood or behavior has been affected by the group intervention? Specifically, if a practitioner wishes to evaluate whether group members' expressions and feelings of depression were changed by the intervention, then the depression criteria must be defined so that depression can be clearly evaluated before and after the intervention.

Group Members (Sample)

The research sample generally consists of the members of a group who have been informed in advance about the research protocol. The sample participants are group members who have indicated their willingness to participate in the study by signing a consent form. The sample participants should be assured of confidentiality and protection from physical and mental harm. These points are part of a professional code of ethics that guides practice research, as it guides clinical practice itself.

Record Keeping

Group practitioners keep written records of their group meetings. For most group workers, the written record is the key instrument for systematically collecting pertinent information. Records document information about clients and hold practitioners accountable for services performed. Generally, records include the reasons for service, the service process, and future service recommendations. Records also include professional observations, client information, and a description of group interactions. For some time, practitioners have been urged to look to the record to generate data from the records they keep because such records provide an empirical approach. Records are a valuable though underused tool for gathering data.

Practitioners can monitor their own practice directly if they write or dictate information about group members, process, and services rendered directly into the record. There is a trend toward standardizing records to facilitate computerization of data. Computerization of data may have a major impact on practice evaluation research as it will make data collection less cumbersome and hence the research process more accessible to practitioners. Nevertheless, practitioners often find that record keeping is troublesome, time consuming, and a burdensome complicated task. Some complain that record keeping is a burdensome and complicated task.

Also, practitioners often lack time to record completely and don't know what should be included in records. Despite frustrations with record keeping, good records are a standard and convenient vehicle for monitoring practice. A variety of record-keeping instruments are useful for group workers. These instruments include:

1. *Process recordings*—Detailed step-by-step narratives of a group's development. Although time consuming, these provide rich detail and help the leader analyze interactions that occur during group sessions.
2. *Summary recordings*—A more focused and selective form of recording. These focus

on critical incidents that occur in a group and are used after each session to monitor a group's progress. Generally, workers prefer using summary recordings rather than process recordings to indicate what has transpired in group sessions, because summary recordings are less time consuming and are more focused. However, whether using process or summary recordings to monitor practice, it is preferable for the group leader to record information about the group soon after each session while recalling events and dynamic processes.

3. *Record of service*—Asks the group worker to identify the main problem or theme that emerges from the group sessions and records the responses of the group leaders to the problem.

4. *Group prospectus*—A special tool to evaluate and explore difficulties in the formation of new groups. Practitioners often work with groups that terminate prematurely, experience poor attendance, or do not seem to meet members' needs. Such group problems are often the result of inadequate planning. The group prospectus evaluates the process in the formation of new groups. It consists of seven parts: agency context, purpose, structure, pregroup contact, need, composition, and content.

5. *Observer/recorder*—An observer may be used to record information about the group process. Automated monitoring devices such as audio- and videotape recorders can also be an effective although unedited method of collecting information about groups.

6. *Client report*—Composed by one or more members, they can also participate in evaluating service effectiveness by directly reporting changes in behavior or affect

to the practitioner or by completing questionnaires. However, client self-reporting may not be accurate or consistent.

7. *Standardized scales*—Evaluating the service through objective, standardized scales that measure specific affect or behavior such as depression, memory, social interaction, or activities of daily living (Miller, 1991). Standardized instruments are considered the most valid and reliable means to gather data about service effectiveness and about changes in client affect or behavior. Yet, practitioners are disinclined to use such measures because they have had inadequate training in their correct administration.

Team Approach to Research

A team approach to research can provide both the practitioner and the researcher with the best of both worlds. The practitioner has ready access to a population, is a known and trusted professional, and is familiar with the population. The researcher knows the research process, knows how to write a proposal, knows how to gain funding if necessary, and knows about data analysis and data application. Both practitioner and researcher need each other to conduct a successful research project that evaluates a group intervention.

Occasionally, collaborative research projects do not work. Larson (2003) wrote of disincentives in collaborative research and listed four problem areas: increased time needed for communication, the lack of clarity regarding leadership (and authorship), the need for sharing resources and revenues, and the possible incidence of partners who do not fulfill their commitment. She states that two major characteristics of successful collaboration are effective leadership and taking time to problem solve before the collaboration begins.

Before the team can begin the process, there are many points to consider. For example, what are the purpose and goals of the project? What are the expected outcomes? How will the team measure the outcomes? What is the best way to get the answers to these questions? Following is the workplan for an actual team project, best illustrated in an abbreviated form by **Tables 33–1 and 33–2**, showing the separate tasks of the researcher and the practitioner.

Duties of the Team

REVIEWING THE LITERATURE

The researcher and the practitioner refine the purpose through an in-depth literature review. They should ascertain that the question is important and remains unanswered. A thorough review of existing scientific literature is essential for designing research (Yin, Zhou, & Bashford, 2002). Conn et al. (2003) suggested that researchers extend their searches beyond mere computer-based searches to achieve a systematic and comprehensive search. O'Mathuna (2000) agreed that an accurate presentation and review of original research articles is necessary to make evidence-based decisions. Upon completion of the search, the researcher writes a summary of the literature review that serves as the basis for examining the question and choosing a theory. The researcher shares the literature review with the practice partner so that the practice partner can talk intelligently about the topic while communicating with agencies and participants. Both the researcher and the practitioner continue to work diligently in their own areas of expertise but they meet often to share ideas and to keep each other informed.

FINDING A MODEL OR THEORY

Why is theory important? Theory explains the links between variables, integrates knowledge, leads to prediction, and provides process and understanding in accounting for empirical findings. In gerontological/sociological publications, there is a limited use of theory (McMullin, 2000).

McMullin states that old theories must be reworked to be useful. Bengston, Rice, and Johnston (1999) suggest that the decline of general theory results from the quest for a grand theory and the drive for solutions without theory. Fortunately, there are scholars who continue to buck this trend and provide appropriate theories for gerontology (Hooker & McAdams, 2003). And, if an appropriate theory is not available, there are models that can diagram the expected change. Also, current federal support for translational research emphasizes a closer link among theory, intervention studies, and evidence-based practice (Pillemer, Suitor, & Wethington, 2003).

DESIGN AND METHODOLOGY

While the researcher is looking for a theory, the researcher must also consider the design. Before the team chooses the variables, states the hypothesis, and finds appropriate measures, the researcher must consider the design. The design guides the investigation and is like a musical score informing a symphony performance. The design indicates the way the project will play out. If the team expects change in group members as a result of participating in the group process, then the group members will need to be tested at the start and finish of the process. That part of the design is pretest and posttest. Next the study must be controlled to show that the expected change was the result of the intervention. Control exists when there is a comparison group of like participants and the outcomes of one group are compared to the other. Thus, the design of choice is pretest, posttest with experimental and control groups. Those who do not participate in the intervention are in the control group. The researcher compares the mean scores of each group to one another to see which group has decreased or increased, depending on how the instruments are constructed to measure the changes desired as a result of the intervention.

The researcher must then state a hypothesis. The hypothesis is a statement that predicts the

Table 33–1   THE TEAM RESEARCH PROCESS FOR THE RESEARCHER

Formulate a problem

Review the literature

Select a theory or model

Formulate research objectives or hypothesis

Define major variables

Identify limitations and assumptions

Select a research design and method

Define the population and sampling size

Formulate a recruitment plan

Develop a plan for data collection and analysis

Gain protection of human subjects

Implement the plan

Supervise the project

Tabulate and analyze the results

Write a report

Communicate findings

Aublish

Table 33–2   THE TEAM RESEARCH PROCESS FOR THE PRACTITIONER

Agree to the identified problem

Review a summary of the literature

Search for an appropriate practice setting

Present the proposal to the practice setting, families, and other concerned individuals

Collaborate with researcher on issues

Gain approval and entrée

Select a practice team

Participate in ethics and research training with the team

Implement the plan

Supervise the practice of the intervention

Contribute to formulating conclusions and practice recommendations

Publish

Apply findings to evidence-based practice

---

direction of change and states the cause of the change. An example of one hypothesis is:

> Older adults who participate in a group intervention will decrease depression more than older adults who do not participate in a group intervention.

In group work, there are three functions to consider when designing a project: the process of the group conversation and activities, the outcomes of the process, and the functioning of the group. More than likely, the researcher will want to measure each of these functions that operate within one intervention. To do this, the researcher must use a combination of methods: a survey method to measure group functioning, a qualitative method to measure the process, and a quantitative method to measure the outcomes. Three different methods will answer the questions. Another name for mixed-method research is triangulation. *Triangulation* refers to a combination of methods and combines data from

more than one source. Triangulation is a legitimate research strategy in that it yields completeness and confirms the quantitative data, providing details that would be unavailable from one method alone (Risjord, Dunbar, & Moloney, 2002). Following is an explanation of the three methods used in this project: survey, qualitative, and quantitive.

SURVEY METHOD

Surveys directly question individuals. The hardest part of the survey method is asking the precise questions that will give the required data. The easiest part of doing a survey with a group is that the survey can be administered while the group is still meeting, therefore yielding a possible 100% response rate. Someone other than the people running the group should conduct the survey. This person should, however, be someone who knows about older people. The researcher should make sure, for example, that there is enough light to read the questions, there is no glare from the paper, there is dark, large print that is easy to see, and that the questionnaire is below the eighth-grade reading level. If one is working in a geographic area with a low literacy rate, it is helpful to read the questions to the participants and to mark the answers for them.

There are many criteria to consider when creating the survey questions. The questionnaire should be appealing and user-friendly (Sleutel, 2001). The questions should be simple and clear, eliciting the needed information. Questions such as the following will collect informative responses: Did the participants enjoy attending the group? Did they like the way the group was led? Did they think the leader was open, and a good listener? Did they think the leader used leadership skills to run the group? What would they like to change? Asking the questions of a variety of people and then correcting the questions as the survey is developed should help craft valid questions. When creating the questionnaire, the researcher must think about how the data will be analyzed and entered into a computer so that data entry is a clear and simple process.

Qualitative Method. The second method is the qualitative method uses the words of the group participants as data, hence the qualitative researcher studies the conversation of the group members. There are many ways to do qualitative research (Gubrium & Holstein, 2002). Content analysis is a useful way to analyze qualitative data and to look for common meanings within the words of the participants. Pure qualitative research demands much rigor and is difficult to apply to the group process. An important point for the researcher to remember when transcribing group work tapes is that the researcher must consider the pattern within the conversation of each member and within the whole group. The leader is also an important factor in the dynamics of the group and can't be disallowed (Carey, 1994).

Although it is difficult to do pure qualitative research in a group, recordings of the process will yield much additional data and understanding.

For example, if a group member becomes more depressed after the intervention, the data from the survey and the qualitative recordings will help the team to understand the negative change: Did the group member enjoy the group? Did the group accept the member? Each of those questions and answers will help the group leader to understand group failure as well as success and add to the evidence base of group practice.

If the team has audio-recorded the sessions, it will be necessary to hire a transcriber to transcribe the tapes. Subsequently, the team must decide how to analyze the data. A content analysis will provide an objective and systematic description of the salient points of the group process. A content analysis may be done by hand or with software designed for qualitative analysis. Looking at the process and outcomes together provides richer information. Thurmond (2001) reminds us that triangulation will not strengthen a flawed study but researchers should use more than one method if it contributes to a better understanding of the study. Sandelowski and Barroso (2002) stress the importance of presenting the results so that both researchers and practitioners easily understand them.

Quantitative method. The third method used is the quantitative method. The quantitative method uses numbers and statistics to look for change between and within groups and individuals for comparative purposes. Basically, the quantitative method looks at the effects of the intervention on selected research variables. Thus the team must decide what change to expect as a result of the group process. For example, does the team expect to decrease depression, improve communication, modify behavior, or increase activity?

Reliable and valid instruments exist to measure outcomes. Another review of the literature and a look at the actual instruments can help determine the choice. A careful review of the literature and consideration of the actual instruments that are constantly being updated can help determine the most appropriate selection

(O'Rourke & Tuokko, 2003). The measures chosen must be valid, meaning they test the true outcome, and reliable, shown to be effective over time in other studies.

DATA ANALYSIS AND SAMPLE SIZE

A statistician is an important member of any research team. Early on, the statistician should check the proposal and review the questionnaires for ease of data entry. The statistician should advise regarding the number of participants needed for a reasonable effect size (Cohen, 1988). The effect size tells how many subjects are needed to demonstrate significant differences between groups. The statistician also looks at the design and suggests the appropriate statistical analysis for the design. (For example, to measure group improvement over time from pretest to posttest, the numbers comprising the scores are entered into the computer, and the computer calculates averages [mean scores]). Look at the mean scores for each group, looking for change within the group, thus providing a gain score for the group. Then, compare the gain scores between the control and the experimental group. Use a test or analysis of covariance (ANCOVA) to look for significant differences between the groups. The quantitative method provides one way of knowing if the intervention is effective. Triangulation, using more than one method or mixed methods, provides other ways of knowing and renders a clear picture of the individual's experience in the group.

PROJECT PLAN

The project plan sets out the details for conducting the project and is also known as the procedure. The project plan serves as a blueprint for conducting the project, starting with agency contact, group recruitment, and random assignment of participants to each condition. The plan delineates the manner of testing, identifies the people who will do the testing, and tells how the questionnaires (instruments) used for the testing will be handled. Then, the plan specifies the intervention for the experimental group—describing the leader, the number of participants, the process, the themes to be discussed in group, and so on. The plan describes the procedure for the control group in the same detail. If there is training required for the people who run the groups, the training becomes a part of the procedure as well. The plan provides instruction for posttesting, handling of instruments, and separation (actual departure) of the leader from the group. If previously uninformed people are working with the team to run the group, then the team needs to make a separate booklet of the project plan so that each group leader will have a precise plan for doing the work.

RECRUITMENT

How one intends to recruit is part of the proposal plan (Davis, Broome, & Cox, 2002). If fliers or advertising in the newspaper is used for recruiting, the Institutional Review Board (IRB) must approve the advertisements.

It is often difficult to recruit and retain underrepresented minorities (Findlow, Prohask, & Freedman, 2003). To enhance recruiting, Areans, Alvidrez, Nery, Estes, and Linkins (2003) suggest an easy-to-reach site, some choice in group participation, and a consumer approach of meeting the needs of the community. Signing the informed consent is a barrier to recruitment, as some older people just don't like to sign papers. DiMattio (2001) suggested that research reports should include strategies for recruitment because women as well as minorities are underrepresented in research studies.

PROTECTING HUMAN SUBJECTS

Although the research plan is ready to implement, the project cannot start until a human subject review board has reviewed the plan and approved it. There are often stringent guidelines applied to the research process, which is an advantage to research because the guidelines really do protect subjects. The guidelines emphasize protecting the participants in a research project, guarding their privacy, and completely disclosing all parameters of the project to the participants.

All research workers in the project must have training in human subject research. More than likely, the practice partner will not have that background, so the research partner is responsible for providing a tutorial and making sure all other workers in the project are knowledgeable. In most universities today, researchers must take an ethics tutorial before being allowed to begin a research project. These tutorials can be found on the Web, and anyone with access to the Web can get them (Belmont Report, 1998).

While preparing the project for review by the Institutional Review Board, the researcher must also create an informed consent form for the participants to sign, indicating their approval to participate in the project and allowing the research team to use the data obtained. The informed consent document should fully inform the prospective participants of the way they will be involved. If the project uses audio-recordings, the consent should state that the participant's conversation in the group will be recorded. Further, the consent should be written at or below the eighth-grade reading level.

IMPLEMENTING THE PROJECT

Implementing the project will require the services of both team members. While the researcher has been writing and gaining IRB approval for the study, the practitioner has been busy contacting agencies, meeting people, and generally recruiting people to participate in the project. The team will administer the instruments that measure outcomes. During the project, the researcher will supervise the project and the practitioner will provide supervision to the group leaders. The researcher and the statistician will enter the data into the computer. When the project is complete and the data entered and analyzed, using a statistical package such as SPSS, the team will meet again to discuss presenting and publishing the material. Both team members will present and publish the data.

Summary

Group work is a valued practice modality that serves the needs of a diverse, aged, population. Professionals from many disciplines use a variety of group interventions in community and institutional settings. These professional practitioners have access to a wealth of information about the effectiveness of various group approaches with older people in the group records that they are obliged to keep as responsible practitioners. They also have an important role in the development of knowledge about group practice with the aged. As practitioners become acquainted and comfortable with the practitioner–researcher model, or the team model, the potential for contributing to the knowledge base of practice increases substantially. The team model outlined stages in planning and implementing a program of qualitative and quantitative evaluation of a group intervention and stressed the need for obtaining ethical approval by IRB and written informed consent by participants. Practitioners and researchers will undoubtedly agree that effective practice is predicated on knowledge, and that helping aged people through groups means knowing why, how, and when groups are effective.

Exercises

EXERCISE 1

Write a summary record of a group meeting. Analyze the major themes that emerge from discussion. How does this meeting reflect other concerns? What else do you need to know, and how would you go about finding this data?

EXERCISE 2

Apply program evaluation techniques: The director of a local senior citizens' center notices that the seniors come and eat their hot meal at midday but they do not relate well to one another on a personal or social level. The seniors seem socially isolated and leave the center quickly after they eat. You were hired as a group facilitator. For two months, you direct socialization groups. Your practice instincts tell you that group intervention is working. However, you want to find a more scientific way to determine if your practice is effective in increasing the socialization of your elderly clients. What do you do?

References

Areans, P., Alvidrez, J., Nery, R., Estes, C., & Linkins, K. (2003). Recruitment and retention of older minorities in mental health services research. *The Gerontologist, 43*(1), 36–44.

Belmont Report. (1998). FDA. Retrieved May 1, 2002, from *http://ohrp.osophs.dhhs.gov/humansubjects/guidance/belmont.htm*

Bengston, V., Rice, C., & Johnson, M. (1999). Are theories of aging important? Models and explanations in gerontology at the turn of the century. In V. Bengston & K. Schaie (Eds.), *Handbook of theories of aging* (pp. 3–20). New York: Springer.

Bliss, D. (2001). Mixed or mixed up methods? *Nursing Research, 50*(6), 331.

Burnette, D., Morrow-Howell, N., & Chen, L. (2003). Setting priorities for gerontological social work research: A national Delphi study. *The Gerontologist, 43*(6), 828–838.

Burns, N., & Grove, S. (2001). *The practice of nursing research.* Philadelphia: W. B. Saunders & Co.

Burnside, I., & Schmidt, M. (1994). *Working with older adults: Group process and techniques* (3rd ed.), Boston: Jones & Bartlett.

Campbell, D., & Stanley, J. (1966). *Experimental and quasi-experimental designs for research.* Boston: Houghton-Mifflin.

Carey, M. (1994). The group effect in focus groups: Planning, implementing, and interpreting focus group research. In J. E. Morse (Ed.), *Critical issues in qualitative research methods.* Thousand Oaks, CA: Sage.

Cohen, J. (1988). *Statistical power analysis for the behavioral sciences.* Hillsdale, NJ: Lawrence Erlbaum Associates.

Conn, V., Isaramalai, S., Rath, S., Jantarakupt, P., Wadhawan, R., & Dash, Y. (2003). Beyond MEDLINE for literature searches. *Journal of Nursing Scholarship, 35*(2), 177–183.

Davis, L., Broome, M., & Cox, R. (2002). Maximizing retention in community-based clinical trials. *Journal of Nursing Scholarship, 34*(1), 47–54.

DiMattio, M. (2001). Recruitment and retention of community-dwelling aging women in nursing studies. *Nursing Research, 50*(6), 369–373.

Dunbar-Jacob, J., & Schron, E. (2002). Ancillary studies in clinical trials. *Nursing Research, 51*(5), 336–338.

Grady, P. (2002). Making a difference: Connecting research to practice. *Nursing Outlook, 50*(6), 224.

Gubrium, J., & Holstein, J. (Eds.). (2002). *Handbook of Interview Research.* Thousand Oaks, CA: Sage.

Hooker, K., & McAdams, D. (2003). Personality reconsidered: A new agenda for aging research. *The Gerontologist, 58*(B6), 296–304.

Larson, E. (2003). Minimizing disincentives for collaborative research. *Nursing Outlook, 51*(6) 267–271.

McMullin, J. (2000). Diversity and the state of sociological aging theory. *The Gerontologist, 40*(5), 517–531.

O'Mathuna, D. (2000). Evidence-based practice and reviews of therapeutic touch. *Journal of Nursing Scholarship, 32*(3), 279–286.

O'Rourke, N., & Tuokko, H. (2003). Psychometric properties of an abridged version of the Zarit Burden Interview within a representative Canadian caregiver sample. *The Gerontologist, 43*(1), 121–127.

Pillemer, K., Suitor, J., & Wethington, E. (2003). Integrating theory, basic research and intervention: Two case studies from caregiving research [Special issue]. *The Gerontologist, 43*(1), 19–27.

Risjord, M., Dunbar, S., & Maloney, F. (2002). A new foundation for methodological triangulation. *Journal of Nursing Scholarship, 34*(3), 269–275.

Sandelowski, M., & Barroso, J. (2002). Finding the findings in qualitative studies. *Journal of Nursing Scholarship, 34*(3), 213–219.

Sleutel, M. (2001). Conducting survey research at nursing conferences. *Nursing Research, 50*(6), 379–383.

Stanley, M., & Beare, P. (1999). *Gerontological Nursing* (2nd ed.). Philadelphia: F. A. Davis.

Thurmond, V. (2001). The point of triangulation. *Journal of Nursing Scholarship, 33*(3), 253–258.

Warren-Findlow, J., Prohaska, T., & Freedman, D. (2003). Challenges and opportunities in recruiting and retaining underrepresented populations into health promotion research [Special issue 1]. *The Gerontologist, 43*, 37–46

Yin, T., Zhou, Q., & Bashford, C., (2002). Burden on family members: A meta-analysis of interventions. *Nursing Research, 51*(3), 199–208.

Chapter 34

Evaluation Issues in Group Work

Thomas W. Pierce

Key Words

- Process evaluation
- Outcomes evaluation
- Stakeholder
- Goals of evaluation
- Group goals and objectives
- Measurement
- Research design
- Quantitative analysis
- Qualitative analysis
- Recommendations

Learning Objectives

- To identify the major steps involved in planning and conducting a program evaluation
- To anticipate decisions in planning an evaluation
- To identify the stakeholders in an evaluation
- To use the results of an evaluation to improve a group service for older adults

Introduction

Organizations sponsoring groups for older adults increasingly have come to rely on formal evalua-tions of these programs in order to provide the best services possible within the limits of available resources. Program evaluation is used to provide information about the specific goals of a group, the methods used to achieve these goals, and the degree to which group members experience outcomes consistent with these goals. This information can then be used to inform decisions about the initiation, continuation, and improvement of these programs.

Unfortunately, the people in the best position to acquire information about the activities and accomplishments of a group—its leaders and organizers—may not be familiar with the accepted standards, practices, and limitations of program evaluation. To address this issue of unfamiliarity, this chapter will provide an intro-duction to the various steps involved in conduct-ing an effective evaluation. Specifically, it will describe: (a) the goals one might reasonably set for an evaluation, (b) the types of decisions involved in planning that evaluation, (c) methods com-monly used to determine whether a group is achieving its stated goals, and (d) factors that evaluators should take into account when making recommendations. While acknowledging that a single chapter cannot provide a comprehensive overview of program evaluation, my goals are to help readers anticipate the dozens of decisions they will face when planning an evaluation and to recommend additional sources of information concerning the evaluation process.

Settings for Evaluation

This chapter will address two situations in which groups for older adults are evaluated. First, as part of an internal review, a group might be evaluated by the parent organization that administers the service (for example, a local chapter of the Alzheimer's Association that evaluates the effectiveness of its caregiver support groups). Second, a group may be evaluated to fulfill a requirement for funding provided by an external source. Evaluation in these two situations can vary significantly in terms of method and emphasis, but is motivated by the common goal of making the activities of the group accountable to the persons and organizations that support and depend on it.

Internal Review of a Program

It is reasonable to expect that periodically an organization that dedicates resources to maintaining a service will want to determine whether that service is achieving its stated goals. Internal evaluation of a group will likely be concerned both with the outcomes of group participation and with the process through which the group achieves these outcomes. The process component of an evaluation is concerned with describing how a group functions and describing the people it serves, whereas the outcomes component focuses on determining whether a group has produced significant positive changes in the members of that group. The emphasis in outcomes assessment is on quantitative analysis of characteristics such as skills, abilities, mood, knowledge, or quality of life. By using both process and outcome measures to determine what a group does and how well it is doing, the evaluator is in a position to recom-

mend changes that may help the group function more effectively.

Strengthening Funding Proposals

Group leaders seeking funding from an external source will almost certainly find that their applications are more competitive when they include a clear description of how they plan to measure the effects of their program. It is the applicant's responsibility to convince the potential funding source of three things. First, there is an unmet need for the group in the community. Second, the group will be conducted in a manner that meets this need. Third, it will be possible to assess the degree to which the group meets these needs. Program evaluation in this context is focused on the very reasonable question of whether the people funding the program are receiving what they paid for. The more confident a funding agency is that it will be able to obtain an answer to this question, the more comfortable it will be in providing financial support for the group.

Risks and Benefits of Evaluation

Before proceeding with an evaluation, group leaders should first address the question of whether to conduct a formal evaluation at all. Although evaluation can result in significant benefits to groups for older adults, there are significant costs and risks that need to be taken into account. For example, even the most well executed of evaluations will demand a significant commitment of time and money. Unless there is a clear commitment on the part of group leaders to use the results to make changes in the way a group is conducted, or unless evaluation is a requirement for new or continued funding, the costs of evaluation may outweigh the benefits. Moreover, an evaluation that is poorly planned or poorly executed can result in destructive outcomes that can include: (a) incorrect recommendations regarding the continuation of a program, (b) declines in leadership/staff morale, (c) missed opportunities to identify ways of better serving group members, and (d) a waste of time and financial resources. Given the significant costs and risks associated with evaluation, one should only be conducted when adequate resources are available.

Planning an Evaluation

Planning is the most important step in evaluation because it is here that the bulk of the decisions have to be made. Unfortunately, there is no way to prepare the reader for every issue that might arise in planning an evaluation. However, one way of grounding the process is to remember that the evaluator's job is to anticipate the questions that the people reading the final report will want answered. Evaluation planning consists of identifying these questions and then providing a detailed description of how the evaluator will collect the data to answer them.

Identifying the Stakeholders in the Evaluation

When planning an evaluation it is important to consider whom the evaluation is for and whom it will be about. At a minimum, these "stakeholders" will include the older adults who participate in the group, the person(s) responsible for organizing and leading the group, and the persons and organizations who provide financial support. If one defines *stakeholder* more broadly, one could also include persons and organizations in a position to refer an older adult to the group (for example, a local chapter of the Alzheimer's Association refers a caregiver to a support group), as well as older adults in the community who may be in a position to benefit from the group at some point in the future. It also may be useful to collect data from people who: (a) declined to participate in the group, or (b) began participation in the group, but dropped out. Even though it may be difficult to

locate these individuals, they may have important suggestions for how to make the group useful to a wider range of people.

Determining the stakeholders in an evaluation is important for several reasons. First, it helps the evaluator identify those persons who are in the best position to provide information regarding the manner in which the group operates, as well as its impact on group members and the community as a whole. Second, inclusiveness in obtaining input from stakeholders is important because people who are not included in the planning phase of an evaluation may be less invested in providing high quality information or in taking the recommendations of the evaluation seriously (Patton, 1997). Third, the methods used to collect and analyze data, as well as the style of presentation of the final report, will depend on the backgrounds of the people who will ultimately read and make decisions on the basis of the report.

Define the Overall Goal of the Evaluation

Evaluation is a goals-driven process that is useful only to the extent that it leads to better delivery of services to older adults. These goals can vary widely from one setting to another. For example, the sponsors of a group might wish to compile information about the number and types of people being served in order to demonstrate that the community is utilizing the group. Alternatively, a parent organization might choose to evaluate a group because of questions regarding its continued viability. In the first example, the primary question is whether people are using the program. In the second example, the primary questions are whether the program produces positive outcomes and at what cost. Different questions will demand different measures and different methods for data collection. Consequently, the first thing to make clear in planning an evaluation is its purpose. Once this overall goal has been established, its achievement should drive every planning decision from that point on.

What Information Should Be Collected?

A number of authorities on program evaluation draw a distinction between collecting descriptive information regarding the manner in which a group functions (evaluation of process) and determining whether participation in the group is associated with positive or negative outcomes (evaluation of outcomes) (e.g., Posavac & Carey, 2003; Weiss, 1998). This distinction largely boils down to one between what the group does versus what the group has accomplished. The next two sections address, in turn, the collection of process and outcome data.

PROCESS INFORMATION

An evaluator's task in collecting process information is to determine who is using the group and how the group functions. There are several potential sources of information from which to draw. First, program records may provide information regarding: (a) the number of members who attended the group in each of the years covered by the evaluation, (b) the length of time members attended the group, (c) reasons why members stopped attending the group, and (d) descriptive information about each group member, including gender, race, age, and years of education.

If the group has not maintained records at this level of detail, alternative means for obtaining this information can be explored. Surveys distributed to current and past group members may be used, although a low return rate will raise questions about the degree to which the results accurately describe attendees as a whole. Alternatively, phone or in-person interviews may yield higher participation rates than surveys, although this method can be time consuming and expensive for the evaluator.

Qualitative methods can also provide valuable information for evaluators. Qualitative approaches, with their emphasis on narrative data, lend themselves best to understanding the process of how a group functions, although they can also provide important information regarding outcome performance. An evaluator who includes a qualitative component as part of data collection might ask group members, group leaders, and others a set of open-ended questions and obtain their verbal or written responses. These questions might probe: (a) participants' understanding of the purpose of the group, (b) their description of what happens in group meetings, (c) their views regarding strengths and weaknesses of the group, and (d) participants' assessment of how the group has impacted their lives. These open-ended questions allow the evaluator to learn about aspects of the group that are not assessed in surveys or standardized questionnaires and about positive or negative outcomes that were not anticipated by the persons who organized the group.

Qualitative methods used to analyze such narrative data demand a great deal of time and skill. Evaluators not familiar with such approaches are strongly encouraged to consult one or more sources devoted specifically to applying these methods. References to several excellent resources are provided at the end of this chapter.

OUTCOME INFORMATION

Outcome measures are used to determine whether members of a group experienced positive or negative changes as a result of participation. The natural starting point in deciding which outcomes to assess is to identify the goals for the group. In other words, the evaluator has to be able to list the specific ways in which group members are expected to change. For example, let's say that the organizers of a support group for Alzheimer's caregivers have identified three areas in which they hope attendees will show improvement: perceived social support, mood, and general knowledge of the disease. These three intended outcomes comprise the core of the topics or constructs that need to be evaluated. Thus, the evaluator will need to find a way to measure each of these constructs.

In many cases, a clear statement of intended outcomes will already be available—perhaps from a grant proposal used to obtain initial funding for the group or from a proposal to the board of directors of the organization sponsoring the group. If no such mission statement exists, the evaluator will have to work with the people most familiar with the group to create the equivalent of a mission statement. This, in itself, may be a worthwhile by-product of an evaluation. If it becomes evident that a clear set of program objectives cannot be identified, it may not be possible to evaluate a program in terms of outcomes (Grembowski, 2001).

One additional point to consider in deciding which program objectives and outcomes to assess is that it may be necessary to collect information from persons who are not currently involved with the group. For example, a group receiving nutrition education may only meet for a limited number of sessions (for example, McClelland, Bearon, Fraser, Mustian, & Velazquez, 2001). If a specific objective of the program is to help older adults make better long-term nutrition decisions, an evaluator may decide to assess nutrition habits and knowledge at least six months after participants have completed the program. Moreover, they might compare these results to those obtained from persons who never attended the group. Alternatively, if community awareness of the group is an important objective, evaluators will likely need to assess whether: (a) members of the target population and (b) professionals in a position to refer an older adult to this group are familiar with the program.

At this initial stage in the planning process, the evaluator should strongly consider getting input from the various stakeholders (for example, group leaders and members, members of a board of directors) regarding the choice of outcomes to be assessed. Not only will this provide a sense of ownership in the evaluation process, but may contribute valuable information regarding additional outcomes that should be assessed.

Provide Operational Definitions for Constructs

After selecting the set of constructs to be assessed, the evaluator will need to provide an operational definition for each of these constructs. An operational definition is the researcher's statement about how they will measure a particular construct. For example, an operational definition might be a score from a standardized test (for example, a person's score on the Beck Depression Inventory as an operational definition of depression) or it might take the form of a behavioral benchmark such as the amount of weight that an older person in a fitness group is able to lift.

There are a number of advantages to using quantitative data to describe constructs. First, questionnaires, surveys, and performance measures are available to assess a wide variety of outcomes (for example, depression, social support, and cognitive function). Second, collecting data from a quantitative measure often does not require a large investment in time either for the persons providing the information or for the evaluator. Third, standardized protocols for administering and scoring these measures increase the level of objectivity associated with data collection. Fourth, using a standardized instrument enables evaluators to compare the scores of people in their group to those obtained: (a) from other groups of people participating in the same type of program, (b) from people in the general population, or (c) from the members of the same group at different points in time.

There are a number of test characteristics that the evaluator should consider when selecting a measurement instrument. First, the instrument should be reliable. The term *reliability*, in the context of research, refers to the consistency of the measurement tool (Rust & Golombok, 1999). There are two senses in which a measure is expected to be reliable. First, a measure is said to have test-retest reliability if there is a strong positive correlation between scores obtained from the same set of people at two different times of testing. In other words, a measure has test-retest reliability when participants provide roughly the same scores when given the same measure twice.

Another criterion for evaluating the reliability of a measurement instrument is internal consistency. Internal consistency refers to the degree to which the items that make up a test or questionnaire are measuring the same thing. Coefficient alpha, a commonly reported measure of internal consistency, represents an average correlation among the items that comprise a test or subtest. A benchmark for evaluating the internal consistency of a measure is that the value for coefficient alpha should be greater than .70 (Kerlinger & Lee, 2000).

A second consideration for an evaluator when selecting an assessment instrument is that the measure should be valid. The validity of a measurement tool refers to whether the instrument is measuring what it is supposed to measure (Rust & Golombok, 1999). A good place to start in determining if a measure is valid is to examine the publication where the measure was first introduced to the field. This might be a journal article or a testing manual that is sold with the instrument. One of the many ways to establish the validity of a new measure is for its authors to report correlation coefficients between the new measure and previously established measures. For the new measure to be valid it should be strongly correlated with other measures of the same construct and should not be correlated with measures of clearly different constructs (Campbell & Fiske, 1959). For example, a measure of depression has evidence of validity when it is strongly correlated with other measures of depression, but not with measures of other constructs, such as introversion/extroversion or intelligence.

A third factor to consider when selecting a measurement instrument is the amount of time required for administration. A useful rule of thumb is that an evaluator should attempt to limit the time for data collection to no more than an hour. Anything more than this presents risks to the quality of the data due to fatigue and boredom on the part of the participant. In addition, the more time required for participants to complete a battery of measures, the less likely they will be to finish it. This places the evaluator in the uncomfortable position of having to leave out potentially useful measures that could add significantly to their information base. It also makes it difficult for the evaluator to include more than one measure of the same construct. Unfortunately, these are the kinds of choices that evaluators are forced to make.

Design of the Evaluation

The design for data collection refers to the evaluator's plan for when to collect data and from whom to collect it. There are many possible designs for use in program evaluation and excellent comprehensive descriptions of these are provided in Grembowski (2001) and Weiss (1998). In general, the choice of design dictates the types of questions the evaluation will be able to address. This section presents four designs that are commonly used for program evaluation.

POSTTEST ONLY WITH NO COMPARISON GROUP

In this design, the evaluator obtains scores from group members after they have completed the group or have attended it for a specified amount of time. This design is relatively easy to implement and can provide useful information regarding the process through which the group functions (for example, did the group leader encourage focused or wide-ranging discussions?). However, this design is of limited value for assessing outcomes because the evaluator is unable to compare the scores of group members to those of people who have not attended the group.

Figure 34-1 provides a pictorial representation of this design. In **Figures 34–1** through **34–4**, circles represent points where data are collected from group members and squares represent points where data are collected from the members of a comparison group.

POSTTEST ONLY WITH A COMPARISON GROUP

In this design, the mean scores for group members are compared to the mean scores for a comparison sample of persons who have not participated in the group. The comparison sample, commonly referred to as a control group, should be matched as closely as possible to the members of the group on such variables as age, gender, level of education, socioeconomic status, and the reasons why that person was initially referred to the group (for example, number of years in a caregiving role). This design allows the evaluator to draw conclusions about differences between persons who have and have not attended the group. However, because data are collected from each person only once, they do not provide information about whether attending the group is associated with positive changes in scores.

PRETEST–POSTATTENDANCE WITH NO COMPARISON GROUP

In this design, outcome measures are administered to group members both before and after they have attended the group. This design, commonly referred to as a longitudinal design, allows the evaluator to assess the degree to which group members display significant changes in outcome measures from one point in time to another. Although there is no comparison group, per se, members serve as their own matched source of comparison. The primary limitation of this design is that it is difficult to know whether or not it was participation in the group that caused the changes in the scores or whether the changes were due to some other factor (Kerlinger & Lee, 2000). For example, in a group for older bereaved adults, it is possible that depression scores improve merely because of the passage of time, not due to any benefit produced by the group.

PRE-TEST–POST-TEST WITH A COMPARISON GROUP

Of the four designs discussed in this chapter, the one with the fewest limitations has pre- and posttesting for members of the group, as well as for members of a comparison group. The amount of time between pre- and post-testing is the same for both sets of people. Inclusion of a comparison

Figure 34-1

Posttest only with no comparison group.

	Pre-Test	Post-Test
Group Members	No data	◯

Figure 34-2

Posttest only with a comparison group.

	Pre-Test	Post-Test
Group Members	No data	◯
Comparison Group	No data	☐

Figure 34-3

Pretest—Postattendance with no comparison group.

	Pre-Test	Post-Test
Group Members	◯ → ◯	
Comparison Group	No data	No data

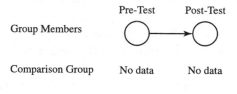

Figure 34-4

Pretest—Posttest with a comparison group.

	Pre-Test	Post-Test
Group Members	◯ → ◯	
Comparison Group	☐ → ☐	

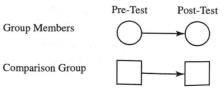

group allows the evaluator to eliminate competing explanations for why scores on outcome measures change over time (for example, natural remission of depression). The pattern of results that best supports the effectiveness of the group is one in which group members demonstrate improvements on outcome measures that are significantly greater than those displayed by members of the comparison group.

Data Collection and Analysis in Evaluation

Administration of Measurement Instruments

ADHERENCE TO ETHICAL STANDARDS

As in all research settings involving human participants, the evaluator has a number of ethical responsibilities. First, all persons providing data should give their informed consent to participate. Participants should know who is collecting the information and for what general purpose, although the evaluator does not necessarily need to reveal the expected results of the study. The evaluator should make participants aware of the risks and benefits associated with their participation and with the fact that they may end their participation at any time without penalty. An informed consent document should also make it clear that any information the participant provides will remain confidential (Kerlinger & Lee, 2000).

A second general category of ethical responsibility concerns the issues of bias and dishonesty during the course of evaluation. It is the evaluator's ethical responsibility to collect, analyze, and interpret data without regard to: (a) previously held beliefs about the effectiveness of the program, or (b) pressure from a particular constituency to reach a positive or negative conclusion about the group.

FOLLOW THE ESTABLISHED PROTOCOL

Before data collection begins, evaluators should generate a detailed plan for how they will collect their data. This plan includes: (a) a list of the people from whom data will be collected, (b) the measures that will be administered to each person, and (c) the time frame for collecting the data. Every member of the evaluation team should receive training in the administration of standardized measures and they should make every effort to follow the established protocol.

Data Analysis

There are many approaches to data analysis and selection of the appropriate statistical tools will vary depending on the questions asked. However, there are several guidelines that evaluators can use to organize their efforts. First, they should start with the list of questions the evaluation was intended to answer and work their way through the list one question at a time. Second, the evaluator should keep it simple. There is no need to use a statistical approach that is more complicated than the question demands. One very good reason to keep things simple is that there is a limit to the mental effort that a reader of an evaluation report will be able to expend. Using simple methods to answer simple questions will allow readers to more carefully consider the implications of the data, rather than spend their time trying to understand a needlessly complex method for presenting or analyzing data.

Procedurally, it is recommended that the evaluator begins their quantitative analysis by obtaining descriptive information regarding the people being served by the group. For example, how many people participated in each of the last three years? What are the demographics of group members in terms of gender, race, socioeconomic status, level of education, and distance traveled to attend group meetings? How do the demographics of the people attending the group differ from those of the general population? How many people started the group, but then dropped out? For these people, is information available about why they stopped attending the group? Is the number of participants being served consistent with projected usage estimates made when the group started? What is the average length of time that people spend on a waiting list before joining the group? Frequency counts and percentages should be adequate for categorical variables such as gender and race. However, descriptive statistics (mean, median, and standard deviation) need to be used to describe results for continuous variables, such as age.

After describing the people in the group, the next set of questions concerns the degree to which attendees experience positive or negative changes as a result of group membership. The selection of statistical tools to answer this question depends on: (a) the design of the evaluation study, and (b) the level of statistical sophistication of the people who will produce and read the report. Obviously, to assess change one has to have data from at least two points in time. An example of this scenario might be one in which outcome measures were administered to group members when they first started to attend the group and then a second time after they had been attending for a specific length of time (for example, six months). One simple way to present these data would be to first determine the degree of change for each individual member and then to calculate a mean change score for the entire group. This would enable the evaluator to report a finding such as "scores on the Beck Depression Inventory decreased by an average of 3.3 points." A more sophisticated approach to reporting these results would be to perform a test of whether the average amount of change in the scores was statistically significant (that is, not just due to chance). Readers unfamiliar with the various options for performing tests of statistical significance, such as a t-test or analysis of variance (ANOVA), should consult one of the references on data analysis provided at the end of this chapter.

Another scenario might be one in which the evaluator has collected outcome data from two groups: persons who attended the group and persons who did not. In this situation each group of people provided data on only one occasion. Separate independent-sample t-tests can be used to determine whether there is a significant difference between the mean scores for the two groups on each outcome measure. As indicated earlier, this test can only speak to differences between group members and nonmembers. It cannot be used to infer that participation in the group caused a change in the scores.

One thing to bear in mind when using tests of statistical inference, such as a t-test or ANOVA, is that they may require a relatively large sample size in order to detect a significant effect. This means that if an evaluator is working with data from a small sample (that is, 15 or fewer people) the results from a statistical test may fail to be significant, even though the average degree of change in the scores is well within the range of what group organizers were hoping for. In such cases, it is quite likely that conducting the same analysis with a larger sample size would result in a statistically significant finding, perhaps at some point in the future after more people have participated in the group. At this point, however, the evaluator will have to base his or her assessment on a descriptive presentation of the data.

If no one from the evaluation team is in a position to conduct the appropriate statistical analyses it may be possible to recruit a volunteer with these skills from the business community or from the faculty at a local college or university. The evaluation team should anticipate this need in its funding proposal by providing the name and qualifications of the individual who will conduct the required analyses.

Conclusions and Recommendations from Evaluations

Perform an Analysis of the Goals-to-Reality Fit Regarding Program Outcomes

After data analysis has been completed, the evaluator is finally in a position to draw conclusions about the status and performance of the group. A logical starting point is to consider each of the previously stated goals and objectives. An evaluator might begin by listing the evidence both supporting and failing to support each separate goal. For example, one goal of a caregiver support group might be to increase participants' degree of perceived social support. If results show that scores for a measure of social support increase significantly from pretest to posttest, the evaluator has evidence that this particular objective has been met. Unfortunately, there are no set rules for stating when a goal has or has not been met. This decision will depend on the amount of weight the evaluator places on each source of information, as well as on the confidence the evaluator has in the accuracy of each piece of evidence.

Next, the evaluator must make an overall judgment regarding the "fit" between the goals for a group and the reality of what the group actually accomplished. Again, there is no formula for making this decision. Even a legalistic criterion, such as "preponderance of evidence," is one where two people could look at the same evidence and reach different conclusions. Ultimately, the evaluator will have to weigh the available information and make a subjective decision. Evaluation can and should be informed by objective data, but, in the end, it retains the human element of people forming opinions based on the evidence available.

Analysis of Process Information

Although the primary emphasis at this stage of the evaluation is on outcome data, the importance of process data should not be overlooked. For example, if the data from outcome measures do not support the effectiveness of the group with respect to one or more goals, the evaluator must make a judgment regarding the reason for this negative finding. One possibility is that the underlying theoretical basis for using the group to produce the desired change was flawed. If this is the case, no group using that particular method, no matter how dedicated or well trained its leaders, could have successfully met the stated goals. A second possibility is that the underlying strategy behind the group was sound, but the method was not executed effectively by the persons conducting the group. Careful comparisons of the methods used by the group and the methods proscribed by its originators can reveal whether the group actually functioned the way it was supposed to. Distinguishing between these two possibilities is critical for deciding whether: (a) to discontinue the group because there is no sound theoretical basis for expecting it be effective, or (b) to maintain the group, but to make modifications in the way it is implemented.

Recommending Change

If the evaluation team has identified an aspect of the group that needs to be improved, it is reasonable to expect it to make a set of recommendations for how to remedy the situation. This does not preclude group leaders and members from proposing alternative solutions, but it does indicate that evaluation is intended to help address problems, not merely to identify them. Additionally, one productive result of evaluation is that group leaders can often use recommendations from past evaluations as the basis for requests for additional funding or additional resources from internal or external sources.

On the practical side, recommendations should be specific enough to enable group organizers to generate a plan to address areas that need improvement. For example, the recommendation that "The group leader needs to be better organized" is not as helpful as more specific suggestions, such as "Group leader should: (a) provide an outline/agenda for each session, (b) have a plan for what will be accomplished in each group meeting, (c) be on time for all sessions." It is also helpful for evaluators to present a list of acceptable alternatives for how to address concerns and to direct group organizers to resources of which they might not be aware. For example, an evaluator might recommend that group organizers take advantage of consulting services that might be available through a national organization (for example, Gerontological Society of America).

Follow-Up and Follow-Through

There are a number of things that group leaders can do to prepare for the next evaluation. After the report is written, it is useful to think about ways to make the next evaluation more productive and efficient. For example, group leaders might solicit information from other stakeholders about their reactions to the evaluation both in terms of how it was conducted and its findings. Essentially, the stakeholders are asked to evaluate the evaluation. This exercise can address questions such as whether the evaluation: (a) presented an accurate description of the accomplishments of the group, (b) was fair and unbiased, (c) allotted adequate time to complete the review, and (d) provided criticisms or recommendations that have the potential to produce positive changes in how the group functions. This information can be used to anticipate the need for additional measurement tools or to collect information from a source that was overlooked in the just-completed evaluation.

For example, a postevaluation review might indicate that inadequate record keeping had made it difficult to determine the number and characteristics of group members over the period of time covered in the evaluation. Finally, the group should respond to all recommendations made by the evaluation team. The response to a specific recommendation may be to: (a) implement it, (b) modify it, or (c) provide a compelling justification for not implementing it. The group's willingness and ability to improve performance on the basis of constructive criticism will likely be assessed during the next evaluation.

Summary

Evaluation has become an accepted and expected part of justifying the resources needed to initiate and maintain group services for older adults. Through careful planning, attention to detail in collecting data, and sound judgment in drawing conclusions, evaluators can play an important role in improving the quality of these programs.

Exercises

EXERCISE 1

Select a group for working with older adults. What arguments would you make in favor of conducting an evaluation of that group? What points would you make in arguing against evaluating the group?

EXERCISE 2

Identify the major outcome goals of the group. Provide operational definitions for each of these outcome goals.

EXERCISE 3

Develop a time line for conducting an evaluation of the group. Outline each step in the process, list the resources you think you would need to complete each step, and state the amount of time you think you would need to complete each step.

References

Campbell, D. T., & Fiske, D. W. (1959). Convergent and discriminant validation by the multitrait-multi-method matrix. *Psychological Bulletin, 54*, 81–105.

Grembowski, D. (2001). *The practice of health program evaluation*. Thousand Oaks, CA: Sage.

Kerlinger, F. N., & Lee, H. B. (2000). *Foundations of behavioral research* (3rd ed.). Fort Worth, TX: Harcourt College.

McClelland, J. W., Bearon, L. B., Fraser, A. M., Mustian, R. D., & Velazquez, S. (2001). Reaching older adults with nutrition education: Lessons learned during the Partners in Wellness pilot project. *Journal of Nutrition for the Elderly, 21*, 59–72.

Patton, M. Q. (1997). *Utilization-focused evaluation: The new century text* (3rd ed.). Thousand Oaks, CA: Sage Publications.

Posavac, E. J., & Carey, R. G. (2003). *Program evaluation: Methods and case studies* (6th ed.). Englewood Cliffs, NJ: Prentice-Hall.

Rust, J., & Golombok, S. (1999). *Modern psychometrics: The science of psychological assessment* (2nd ed.). New York: Routledge.

Weiss, C. H. (1998). *Evaluation: Methods for studying programs and policies* (2nd ed.). Upper Saddle River, NJ: Prentice-Hall.

BIBLIOGRAPHY

Program Evaluation

Grembowski, D. (2001). *The practice of health program evaluation*. Thousand Oaks, CA: Sage.

Patton, M. Q. (1997). *Utilization-focused evaluation: The new century text* (3rd ed.). Thousand Oaks, CA: Sage.

Posavac, E. J., & Carey, R. G. (2003). *Program evaluation: Methods and case studies* (6th ed.). Englewood Cliffs, NJ: Prentice-Hall.

Royse D., Thyer, B. A., Padgett, D. K., & Logan, T. K. (2001). *Program evaluation: An Introduction* (3rd ed.). Belmont, CA: Brooks/Cole.

Weiss, C. H. (1998). *Evaluation: Methods for studying programs and policies* (2nd ed.). Upper Saddle River, NJ: Prentice-Hall.

Analysis of Quantitative Data

Abrami, P. C., Cholmsky, P., & Gordon, R. (2001). *Statistical analysis for the behavioral sciences: An integrative approach*. Boston: Allyn & Bacon.

Howell, D. C. (2002). *Statistical methods for psychology* (5th ed.). Pacific Grove, CA: Wadsworth Group.

Welkowitz, J., Ewen, R. B., & Cohen, J. (2000). *Introductory statistics for the behavioral sciences* (5th ed.). Fort Worth, TX: Harcourt Brace College.

Analysis of Qualitative Data

Creswell, J. W. (2003). *Research design: Qualitative, qualitative, and mixed-methods approaches* (2nd ed.). Thousand Oaks, CA: Sage Publications, Inc.

Denzin, N. K., & Lincoln, Y. S. (2000). *The handbook of qualitative research* (2nd ed.). Thousand Oaks, CA: Sage Publications, Inc.

Murray, M., & Chamberlain, K. (1999). *Qualitative health psychology: Theories and methods* (3rd ed.). Thousand Oaks, CA: Sage.

Patton, M. Q. (2002). *Qualitative research and evaluation methods* (3rd ed.). Thousand Oaks, CA: Sage.

Web Sites

Basic Guide to Program Evaluation
   http://www.mapnp.org/library/prog_mng/prog_mng.htm #anchor1680928/

The Program Manager's Guide to Evaluation
   http://www.acf.hhs.gov/programs/core/pubs_reports/ prog_mgr.html

Resources

- **Action National Volunteer Agency** 806 Connecticut Avenue, NW, Washington, DC 20525. Telephone: 800-424-8867 or 202-634-9424. This is the federal umbrella agency that administers the Retired Senior Volunteer Program (RSVP) as well as Foster Grandparents and Senior Companions. RSVP is its largest program and it recruits volunteers for community agencies.
- **Administration on Aging (AOA)** *www.aoa.dhhs.gov* The U. S. Administration on Aging, located in the Department of Health and Human Services is the federal focal point and advocate agency for older persons and their concerns. Responsible for national policy, program development and program implementation serving older adults.
- **Age Exchange** *www.age-exchange.org.uk* Reminiscence Centre, 11 Blackheath Village London SE3 UK. Reminiscence theatre, publications, exhibitions and training. Contact address for UK Reminiscence Network and European Reminiscence Network

- **Alzheimer's Association**, 919 North Michigan Ave, Suite 1100, Chicago, IL. 60611 (800) 272 3900 *www.alz.org*
- **Alzheimer's Disease Education and Referral Center (ADEAR)** *www.alzheimers.org*
- A clearinghouse sponsored by the National Institute on Aging with a quarterly newsletter, *Connections* and other publications.
- **Alzheimer's Disease International** *www.alz.co.uk* or *info@alz.co.uk* 45/46 Lower Marsh Street, London SE1 7RG UK
- **Alzheimer's Outreach** *http://www.zarcrom.com/users/alzheimers*
- **American Art Therapy Association** *www.arttherapy.org* A national association dedicated to the belief that the creative process involved in making of art is healing and life enhancing. The AATA has established standards for art therapy education and practice, and seeks to enhance the practice of art therapy.

- **American Association for Retired Persons (AARP)** *www.aarp.org* 1909 K Street, NW, Washington, DC 20049. A non-profit membership organization dedicated to addressing the needs and interests of persons 50 and older. Seeks to enhance the quality of life for all by promoting independence, dignity and purpose. Provides a Talent Bank, 1909 K Street, NW, Washington, DC 20049. It sponsors a number of programs for volunteers. Its Talent Bank identifies volunteers and refers them to agencies nation-wide.
- **American Dance Therapy Association (ADTA)** *www.adta.org* Telephone: (410) 997 4040 Maintains a registry of qualified therapists, monitors standards of education and experience, publish the American Journal of Dance Therapy.
- **American Music Therapy Association (AMTA)** *www.musictherapy.org* Promotes the development of the therapeutic use of music in rehabilitation, special education and community settings and is committed to the advancement of education, training, professional standards, credentials and research in support of the music therapy profession.
- **American Psychological Association**
- **American Public Health Association (AHPA)** *www.apha.org* The oldest and largest organization of public health professionals in the world. Brings together a variety of professionals in a multidisciplinary environment to promote professional exchange, study and action.
- **American Self-Help Group Clearinghouse** *http://mentalhelp.net/selfhelp/* Offers a guide that has been developed to act as a starting point for exploring real-life support groups and networks that are available throughout the world and in local communities.

- **American Society on Aging (ASA)** *www.asaging.org* Suite 511, 833 Market Street, Room 511, San Francisco, CA 94103-1824. Telephone: (415) 974 9600. A non-profit organization committed to enhancing the knowledge and skills of those working with older adults and their families. Publishes Generations.
- **American Society of Group Psychotherapy and Psychodrama** *www.asgpp.org* or *asgpp@ASGPP.org* Telephone: (609) 452 1339
- **American Therapeutic Recreation Society** *www.atra-tr.org* 1414 Prince Street, Suite 204, Alexandria, VA 22314 (703) 683 9420
- **Association for the Advancement of Social Work with Groups, Inc. (AASWG)** *www.aaswg.org* A not-for-profit international organization of group workers and friends concerned with advocacy and action in support of practice, education, research and writing about social work with groups.
- **Association for Gerontology in Higher Education (AGHE)** *www.aghe.org* Dedicated to increasing commitment of and fostering the development of higher education in the field of aging through education, research and public service.
- **Association of Personal Historians** *www.PersonalHistorians.org*
- **Caregivers** *www.caregivers.com*
- **Children of Aging Parents (CAPS)** *http://www.CAPS4caregivers.org* Telephone: 1-800-227-7294
- **Council on Social Work Education (CSWE)** *www.cswe.org* Non-profit national association representing individual members and graduate and undergraduate programs of professional social work education. A special project within CSWE, SAGE-SW —Strengthening Aging and Gerontological

Education for Social Work is focused on preparing social work education for the aging of American society.

- **ElderCare Online** *http://www.ec-online.net*
- **Elders Share the Arts and National Center for Creative Aging** *www.eldersshare the arts,org* or *http://www.creative aging.org/index.cfm* 138 South Oxford, Brooklyn NY 11217 Telephone: (718) 398 3870. Undertakes inter-generational arts and oral history-based programs with community groups, performances, exhibitions, publications and training programs.
- **European Reminiscence network** (see Age Exchange).
- **Family Caregiver Alliance** *http://www.caregiver.org* Telephone: 1-800-445-8106
- **Friends and Relatives of the Institutionalized Aged** *http://www.fria.org/contact_us.html*
- *http://www.fria.org/consumers_family.html* Focuses on New York State but provides information of wider interest and is a long-standing advocacy group. Telephone: 212-732-5667
- **Gerontological Society of America (GSA)** *www.geron.org* 1275 K Street NW, Suite 350, Washington, DC 20005-4006. A non-profit professional organization providing researchers, educators, practitioners and policy makers with opportunities to understand, advance and use basic and applied research in aging to improve the quality of life as one ages.
- **Grandparents Information Center** *www.aarp.org/grandparents/searchsupport/.*
- **Health Insurance Portability and Accountability Act** of 1996, *www.hhs.gov/ocr/hipaa/*
- **Institute for Human Values in Aging** *www.HRMoody.com* Publishes Human values in aging newsletter.

- **International Federation for Retirement Education** *www.infre.org*
- **International Institute of Reminiscence and Life Review** *jkunz@staff.uwsuper.edu* c/o John Kunz, 102 Main, Center for Continuing Education/Extension, Belknap & Catlin, PO Box 2000 University of Wisconsin - Superior. Telephone: 715-394-8529
- **International Longevity Center** *www.HRMoody.com* or *www.ilcusa.org/pub/news.htm* Publisher and distributor of Human Values in Aging Newsletter.
- **International Psychogeriatric Congress Secretary**, 3127 Greenleaf Avenue, Wilmette, IL 60091
- **Legacy Center** *thelegacycenter@yahoo.com* Dedicated to preserving stories, values and meaning for individuals, communities and organizations. 612-333-2833
- **Memories in the Making®** *www.alz.org/chapter/orangecounty* c/o Alzheimer's Association, Orange County, CA. 2540 N. Santiago Blvd., Orange, CA 92867. Information: Sam Heinly (714) 283 1984
- **National Adult Day Services Association (ADSA)** *www.nadsa.org*
- **National Association for Dramatherapy** *www.nadt.org* or *nadt@dmg-dc.com* 733 15th Street NW 330, Washington, DC 20005. Telephone: (202) 966 7409
- **National Association for Poetry Therapy** 12950 NM 5th Street, Pembroke Pines, FL 33028-3102 (954) 499 4333 *www.poetrytherapy.org* or *NAPTstarr@aol.com* Toll Free: (866) 844.NAPT
- **National Center for Creative Aging** (see Elders Share the Arts) *http://www. creativeaging.org/index.cfm*

- **National Coalition of Creative Arts Therapies Associations**
  http:www.nccata.org/ 93 Edwards St. New Haven, CT 06515 An alliance of professional associations dedicated to the advancement of the arts as therapeutic modalities. Its website also provides contact information for six associations: American Art Therapy Association, American Dance Therapy Association, American Music Therapy Association, American Society of Group Psychotherapy and Psychodrama, National Association for Drama Therapy, and National Association for Poetry Therapy.
- **National Council on Aging (NCOA)**
  www.ncoa.org 409 Third Street, SW, Washington, DC 20024. Dedicated to promoting the dignity, self-determination, well being and contributions of older persons.
- **National Council on Social Work Education** *www.ncswe.org*
- **National Endowment for the Arts**
  http://www.arts.gov/resources/Accessibility/OlderResources.html 1100 Pennsylvania Avenue, NW Washington, DC 20506 Telephone: (202) 682-5532 TTY: (202) 682-5496 Link to information about seniors and the arts including the arts and aging resource list.
- **National Family Caregivers Association**
  http://www.nfcacares.org Telephone: 1-800-896-3650
- **National Institute on Adult Daycare**
  Promotes standards for adult day care. Washington, DC:
- **National Institute on Aging (NIA)**
  www.nia.nih.gov One of the 25 institutes and centers of the National Institutes of Health, and leads a broad scientific effort to understand the nature of aging, and to extend the healthy active years of life.
- **National Institute of Mental Health**
  5600 Fisher's Lane, Room 15C-05 Rockville MD. 20857. Telephone: (301) 443 4513
- **National Long-term Care Ombudsman Resource Centre** *http://www.ltcombudsman.org/static_pages/ombudsmen.cfm* This site provides a listing of all state ombudsman programs.
- **National Mental Health Association**
  1021 Prince Street, Alexandria VA 22314-2971. Telephone: (800) 969 6642. Provides information, support and referrals on many mental health issues, publications and educational programs to educate the public about mental health issues in later life.
- **National Preretirement Education Association** *www.npea.com*
- **National Remotivation Therapy Organization Inc. (NRTO)**
  www.remotivation.com
- **National Retirement Education Foundation** *www.nrea.com*
- **National Urban League**
  http://www.nul.org/pdf/sobaexec.pdf
- **SeniorNet** *www.seniornet.org* A non-profit organization founded to provide older adults education for and access to computer technologies to enhance their lives and to enable them to share their knowledge and wisdom.
- **Senior Spectrum** *www.seniorspectrum.com*
- **Timeslips Creative Storytelling Project, Center on Age and Community**
  www.timeslips.org University of Wisconsin-Milwaukee. Regional training, training manual, videos, performances and exhibitions. Telephone: (414) 229 2732
- **U. S. Bureau of the Census**
  http://www.census.gov/population

- **U.S. Department of Health and Human Services Center for Disease Control and Prevention and National Center for Health Statistics** Atlanta GA.
- **The United Way** Contact the local United Way office for referrals of would-be volunteers *www.unitedway.org*
- **Validation Training Institute Inc.** *www.vfvalidation.org*
- **Well Spouse Foundation** *http://www.wellspouse.org* 1-800-838-0879
- **White House New Freedom Commission** *www.whitehouse.gov* Information on policy statements, issues and news information. Makes recommendations to enhance the delivery of mental health services to all individuals and focuses on people with disabling conditions receiving equitable and appropriate services.
- **World Confederation of Physical Therapy** *www.wcpt.org*

Index

A

Acculturation, 452–453
Acculturation Rating Scale for
Mexican Americans (ARSMA),
452
Action-oriented groups, 5
Active listening, 51
Activities
for adult day care participants,
293
in board-and-care homes, 304
cooking, 322–323
creative, 314
life-skills, 322–323
for people with dementia,
145–146
Activities of daily living (ADLs),
10, 21
Activity groups, 5
Activity theory, 8
Acute care settings
educational groups in, 343
group development procedures
for, 347–350
overview of, 341–343
patient population groups in,
344–346
psychoeducational groups in, 343

self-help groups in, 343
social workers and, 406
support groups in, 343–344
telehealth support groups in, 344
Addams, Jane, 371
Administrative support, 98–99,
105
Adult day care services
caregiver support groups and,
296–297
community resources for, 297
as continuum of care, 290
explanation of, 289–290
group process in, 291–296
historical background of,
288–289
models of, 289
overview of, 287
participant needs in, 293
settings for, 291
Advocacy, 404–405
Advocacy groups, 88
Aesculapius, 370
Affection, 65, 66
African Americans
demographic characteristics of,
444–445
families and, 445–446

as group, 443–444
group work practice techniques
for, 447–448
historical antecedents of,
445–446
life expectancy for, 9
stressors on, 446–447
Age-specific groups, 34
Ageism, 21
Aging
accouterments of, 156
adaptive strategies for, 195
considerations regarding,
440–441
normal changes due to, 14–16
present state of, 3
process of, 67
psychological and social growth
and, 332
Aging theories
activity, 8
continuity, 8
developmental, 8–9
disengagement, 8
explanation of, 7–8, 302
Agitation, 89–91
Alcoholic beverages, 324–325
Alcoholics Anonymous, 333, 334

487

Photo Credits